The Physician's Guide to

DEPRESSION &
BIPOLAR DISORDERS

The Physician's Guide to

DEPRESSION & BIPOLAR DISORDERS

DWIGHT L. EVANS, MD

Ruth Meltzer Professor and Chairman
Department of Psychiatry
Professor of Psychiatry, Medicine and Neuroscience
University of Pennsylvania Health System
Philadelphia, Pennsylvania

DENNIS S. CHARNEY, MD

Dean of Research
Anne and Joel Ehrenkranz Professor
Departments of Psychiatry, Neuroscience, and
Pharmacology and Biological Chemistry
Mount Sinai School of Medicine
New York, New York

LYDIA LEWIS

President
Depression and Bipolar Support Alliance
Chicago, Illinois

McGraw-Hill
MEDICAL PUBLISHING DIVISION

New York   Chicago   San Francisco   Lisbon   London   Madrid   Mexico City
Milan   New Delhi   San Juan   Seoul   Singapore   Sydney   Toronto

The Physician's Guide to Depression & Bipolar Disorders

1 2 3 4 5 6 7 8 9 0   DOC/DOC   0 9 8 7 6 5

ISBN 0-07-144175-1

This book was set in Garamond by International Typesetting and Composition.
The editors were Janet Foltin and Christie Naglieri.
The production supervisor was Catherine H. Saggese.
Project management was provided by International Typesetting and Composition.
The text designer was Marsha Cohen.
The cover designer was Pehrsson.
The index was prepared by Pat Perrier.
RR Donnelley was printer and binder.

This book is printed on acid-free paper.

Library of Congress Cataloging-in-Publication Data

The physician's guide to depression and bipolar disorders / editors, Dwight L. Evans,
    Dennis S. Charney, Lydia Lewis.—1st ed.
        p. ; cm.
    Includes bibliographical references and index.
    ISBN 0-07-144175-1
    1. Depression, Mental. 2. Manic depressive illness. 3. Depression,
Mental—Complications. 4. Manic depressive illness—Complications. I. Evans, Dwight L.
II. Charney, Dennis S. III. Lewis, Lydia.
    [DNLM: 1. Depressive Disorder—diagnosis. 2. Bipolar Disorder—diagnosis. 3. Bipolar
Disorder—therapy. 4. Depressive Disorder—therapy. WM 171 P5778 2005]
RC537.P52 2005
616.89′5—dc22   2005049148

Dedicated to all patients with mood disorders and to the Depression and Bipolar Support Alliance

Contents

SECTION V

Immunologic and Infectious Diseases / 375

SECTION VI

Special Topics / 437

Contributors

BRAD A. ALFORD, PhD
Professor of Psychology
Department of Psychology
University of Scranton
Scranton, Pennsylvania
Chapter 3

KELLY C. ALLISON, PhD
Research Assistant Professor
Weight and Eating Disorders Program
Department of Psychiatry
University of Pennsylvania School
  of Medicine
Philadelphia, Pennsylvania
Chapter 7

AARON T. BECK, MD
University Professor
Department of Psychiatry
University of Pennsylvania School
  of Medicine
Philadelphia, Pennsylvania
Chapter 3

SUSAN R. BERGESON
Vice President
Depression and Bipolar Support Alliance
Chicago, Illinois
Chapter 20

MARC R. BLACKMAN, MD
Chief
Endocrine Section
Laboratory of Clinical Investigation
Intramural Research Program
National Center for Complementary and
  Alternative Medicine
National Institutes of Health
Bethesda, Maryland
Chapter 18

GIOVANNI CIZZA, MD, PhD, MHSc
Principal Investigator
Clinical Endocrinology Branch
National Institute of Diabetes and Digestive and
  Kidney Disease
Bethesda, Maryland
Chapter 8

DEAN G. CRUESS, PhD
Associate Professor
Department of Psychology
University of Connecticut
Storrs, Connecticut
Chapter 16

FRANK deGRUY, III, MD, MSFM
Chair
Department of Family Medicine
University of Colorado School of Medicine
Aurora, Colorado
Chapter 1

MAHLON R. DeLONG, MD
W.P. Timmie Professor
Department of Neurology
Emory University School of Medicine
Atlanta, Georgia
Chapter 13

DANIEL P. DICKSTEIN, MD
Clinical Research Fellow
Pediatrics and Developmental
  Neuropsychiatry Branch
Mood and Anxiety Disorders Program
National Institute of Mental Health
Bethesda, Maryland
Chapter 4

DWIGHT L. EVANS, MD
Ruth Meltzer Professor and Chairman
Department of Psychiatry
Professor of Psychiatry, Medicine
  and Neuroscience
University of Pennsylvania Health System
Philadelphia, Pennsylvania
Chapter 6

MYLES S. FAITH, PhD
Assistant Professor
Weight and Eating Disorders Program
Department of Psychiatry
University of Pennsylvania School
  of Medicine
Philadelphia, Pennsylvania
Chapter 7

JANINE GIESE-DAVIS, PHD

Senior Research Scholar
Department of Psychiatry and
    Behavioral Sciences
Stanford University School of Medicine
Stanford, California
    Chapter 15

ROBERT N. GOLDEN, MD

Stuart Bondurant Professor and Vice Dean
School of Medicine
Chair, Department of Psychiatry
University of North Carolina at Chapel Hill
Chapel Hill, North Carolina
    Chapter 17

PAUL E. HOLTZHEIMER, III, MD

Assistant Professor
Department of Psychiatry and Behavioral Sciences
Emory University School of Medicine
Atlanta, Georgia
    Chapter 13

LAURA HOOFNAGLE

Publications Manager
Depression and Bipolar Support Alliance
Chicago, Illinois
    Chapter 5

KAREN E. JOYNT, MD

Resident in Internal Medicine
Department of Medicine
Duke University Medical Center
Durham, North Carolina
    Chapter 10

ANDRES M. KANNER, MD

Professor of Neurological Sciences
Rush Medical College
Director, Laboratory of Electroencephalography and
    Video-EEG-Telemetry
Associate Director, Section of Epilepsy
    and Clinical Neurophysiology and Rush
    Epilepsy Center
Rush University Medical Center
Chicago, Illinois
    Chapter 14

SUZAN KHOROMI, MD, MHS

Laboratory of Clinical Investigation
Intramural Research Program
National Center for Complementary and
    Alternative Medicine
National Institutes of Health
Bethesda, Maryland
    Chapter 18

K. R. R. KRISHNAN, MD, CHB

Professor
Department of Psychiatry and Behavioral Sciences
Chair, Department of Psychiatry and
    Behavioral Sciences
Duke University Medical Center
Durham, North Carolina
    Chapter 10

OLADIPO A. KUKOYI, MD

Assistant Professor
Departments of Family Medicine and Psychiatry
University of Iowa School of Medicine
Iowa City, Iowa
    Chapter 11

ELLEN LEIBENLUFT, MD

Chief
Unit on Affective Disorders
Pediatrics and Developmental
    Neuropsychiatry Branch
Mood and Anxiety Disorders Program
National Institute of Mental Health
Bethesda, Maryland
    Chapter 4

JANE LESERMAN, PHD

Professor
Department of Psychiatry
University of North Carolina at Chapel Hill
Chapel Hill, North Carolina
    Chapter 16

LYDIA LEWIS

President
Depression and Bipolar Support Alliance
Chicago, Illinois
    Chapter 5

CONSTANTINE G. LYKETSOS, MD, MHS

Professor of Psychiatry and Behavioral Sciences
Codirector, Division of Geriatric Psychiatry
    and Neuropsychiatry
Department of Psychiatry and
    Behavioral Sciences
School of Medicine
Johns Hopkins University
Baltimore, Maryland
    Chapter 12

WILLIAM M. McDONALD, MD

JB Fuqua Chair for Late-Life Depression
Associate Professor, Department of Psychiatry and
    Behavioral Sciences
Emory University School of Medicine
Atlanta, Georgia
    Chapter 13

JENNIFER M. MEEGAN, BA
Post-Baccalaureate Intramural Research Student
Intramural Research Program
National Institute of Dental and Craniofacial Research
National Institutes of Health
Bethesda, Maryland
Chapter 18

SAMANTHA MELTZER-BRODY, MD, MPH
Assistant Professor
Department of Psychiatry
University of North Carolina at Chapel Hill
Chapel Hill, North Carolina
Chapter 17

ANDREW H. MILLER, MD
Professor
Department of Psychiatry and Behavioral Sciences
Director, Psychiatric Oncology
Winship Cancer Center
Emory University School of Medicine
Atlanta, Georgia
Chapter 15

BARBARA E. MOQUIN, MSN, APRN, BC-P
Senior Research Nurse Specialist
Laboratory of Clinical Investigation
Intramural Research Program
National Center for Complementary and Alternative Medicine
National Institutes of Health
Bethesda, Maryland
Chapter 18

DOMINIQUE L. MUSSELMAN, MD, MS
Associate Professor
Department of Psychiatry and Behavioral Sciences
Emory Univesity School of Medicine
Atlanta, Georgia
Chapter 6

CHARLES P. O'BRIEN, MD, PhD
Vice Chair
Department of Psychiatry
University of Pennsylvania Health System
Research Director, VA Mental Illness Research
Education and Clinical Center
Philadelphia Veterans Affairs Medical Center
Philadelphia, Pennsylvania
Chapter 19

CHRISTOPHER M. O'CONNOR, MD, FACC
Professor, Department of Medicine
Associate Professor, Department of Psychiatry and Behavioral Sciences
Chief, Division of Clinical Pharamcology
Department of Medicine
Duke University Medical Center
Durham, North Carolina
Chapter 10

JOHN M. PETITTO, MD
Professor
Department of Psychiatry, Neuroscience and Pharmacology & Therapeutics
McKnight Brain Institute
University of Florida
Gainesville, Florida
Chapter 16

DANIEL S. PINE, MD
Chief
Section on Developmental Affective Neuroscience
Mood and Anxiety Disorders Program
National Institute of Mental Health
Bethesda, Maryland
Chapter 4

CHARLES L. RAISON, MD
Assistant Professor
Departent of Psychiatry and Behavioral Sciences
Emory University School of Medicine
Atlanta, Georgia
Chapter 15

ROBERT G. ROBINSON, MD
Paul W. Penningroth Professor and Head
Department of Psychiatry
University of Iowa
Roy J. and Lucille A. Carver College of Medicine
Iowa City, Iowa
Chapter 11

PAUL B. ROSENBERG, MD
Assistant Professor
Division of Geriatric Psychiatry and Neuropsychiatry
Department of Psychiatry and Behavioral Sciences
School of Medicine
Johns Hopkins University
Baltimore, Maryland
Chapter 12

DAVID R. RUBINOW, MD
Chief
Behavioral Endocrinology Branch
National Institute of Mental Health
Bethesda, Maryland
Chapter 9

A. JOHN RUSH, MD
Professor & Vice Chair for Research
Betty Jo Hay Distinguished Chair in Mental Health
Rosewood Corporation Chair in Biomedical Science
Department of Psychiatry
University of Texas Southwestern Medical School
Dallas, Texas
Chapter 2

PETER J. SCHMIDT, MD

Chief
Unit on Reproductive Endocrine Studies
Behavioral Endocrinology Branch
National Institute of Mental Health
Bethesda, Maryland
Chapter 9

THOMAS L. SCHWENK, MD

Professor and Chair
Department of Family Medicine
University of Michigan Health System
Ann Arbor, Michigan
Chapter 1

DAVID SPIEGEL, MD

Jack, Lulu and Sam Willson Professor in the School
    of Medicine
Associate Chair, Department of Psychiatry and
    Behavioral Sciences
Stanford University School of Medicine
Stanford, California
Chapter 15

JEFFREY P. STAAB, MD, MS

Assistant Professor of Psychiatry
Departments of Psychiatry and Otorhinolaryngology—Head
    and Neck Surgery
University of Pennsylvania School of Medicine
Philadelphia, Pennsylvania
Chapter 6

ALBERT STUNKARD, MD

Professor of Psychiatry
Department of Psychiatry
University of Pennsylvania School of Medicine
Philadelphia, Pennsylvania
Chapter 7

MADHUKAR H. TRIVEDI, MD

Professor and Director
Mood Disorders Research Program and Clinic
Department of Psychiatry
University of Texas Southwestern Medical School
Dallas, Texas
Chapter 2

Preface

The Physician's Guide to Depression & Bipolar Disorders is the first edited volume addressing the relationship between depression and chronic medical illness. Only recently have medical professionals and public authorities acknowledged depression as a growing international public health problem, yet depression in the clinical setting remains under-recognized and under-treated. Even less attention has been paid to the relationship between comorbid depression and disease, despite growing evidence that their connection has significant medical and societal consequences. This volume addresses this gap in our knowledge by bringing together in a single location the most up-to-date information on this complex subject.

What is generally known about the relationship between depression and chronic illness can be briefly summarized. Depression is very common in chronic medical illness, hindering recovery, increasing functional impairment, contributing to the costs of treating disease, and worsening prognosis. Depression may even figure as a causal factor in the onset and course of certain medical conditions and, conversely, certain chronic diseases may be a risk factor for depression because of psychosocial stressors, functional impairment, and other biologic mechanisms. Depression and medical illness coexist with a decidedly bidirectional nature.

The genesis of this volume is found in two recent events. In November 2002, the Depression and Bipolar Support Alliance, the world's largest patient advocacy organization, convened a 2-day multidisciplinary consensus conference in Washington, DC, including nearly 50 medical and public policy experts to present and discuss the expanding body of information on comorbid depression and medical illness. The following year, *Biological Psychiatry* devoted its August 1, 2003

issue to this burgeoning issue in the psychiatric and medical fields.

This book extends the work of these two important efforts. It summarizes under one cover the available knowledge about the intertwinings of depression, bipolar disorder, and disorders related to the endocrine and metabolic, cardiovascular and cerebrovascular, neurologic, and immunologic systems. Emphasis is on describing the epidemiology, etiology, diagnosis, and treatment of comorbid depression with specific disorders. As the chapters clearly indicate, the relationship between comorbid depression and medical illness is better understood for some diseases than others. The intent of this volume is to clearly describe the state of current knowledge for each disorder discussed, and stimulate future inquiries where gaps in our understanding exist.

The Physician's Guide to Depression & Bipolar Disorders is written for a broad audience. Readers who could benefit from the contents include psychiatrists, psychologists, and other health care professionals who treat patients with mental and behavioral health disorders, as well as physicians in virtually all medical and surgical specialties, whose patients might be affected by depression, bipolar disorder, and a range of mood disorders. The fact that symptoms of depression are often indistinguishable from those of co-occurring illnesses makes it imperative that clinicians acquire a more precise understanding of how depression and other chronic medical conditions impact each other, as well as how the treatments for each may influence the other. An overarching theme is that there should never again be a valid reason for not aggressively seeking out and treating depression in medically ill patients.

This book is also written for investigators working in the full range of biomedical sciences, including basic, patient-oriented, epidemiologic, health services, and public policy research. Given the relatively nascent status of the field, enterprising investigators may use this book as a blueprint for future action in those areas where our knowledge is yet limited and where additional research may bear fruit. Much more research is needed to better understand the bidirectional relationship between depression and chronic medical illness and identify possible common pathogenic, mechanistic pathways that link these two medical conditions. There is still much work to be done, and much opportunity for those who wish to dive in.

The organization of the book is straightforward.

- Section I presents basic information on the prevalence, diagnosis, and psychopharmacologic and psychotherapeutic treatment of depression and bipolar disorder in adults, adolescents, and children, including a chapter illuminating the importance of patient empowerment in recovery. This Section is oriented primarily to physicians and other health care professionals not specifically trained in the care of patients with mental illness, but it is also useful for specialists in depression and bipolar disorder as a concise summary of what is currently known in the field.
- Sections II–V cover the epidemiology, underlying biologic and physiologic mechanisms, diagnosis, and treatment of comorbid depression and specific disorders:

- Section II—Disorders of endocrinology and metabolism, with particular attention to diabetes, obesity, osteoporosis, and reproductive endocrinology.
- Section III—Cardiovascular and cerebrovascular disorders, with particular attention to cardiovascular disease and stroke.
- Section IV—Neurologic disorders, with specific attention to Alzheimer's disease, Parkinson's disease, and epilepsy.
- Section V—Immunologic and infectious diseases, with particular attention to cancer and HIV/AIDS.
- Section VI covers several special topics, including comorbid depression and chronic pain and substance abuse, the use of complementary and alternative medical therapies in treating mood disorders, and principles clinicians can adopt to facilitate recovery from mental illness.

We hope that the clinician and the researcher find this volume both timely and informative, and useful as a guide to a better understanding of the relationship between depression and bipolar disorder and chronic medical illness.

Dwight L. Evans, MD
Dennis S. Charney, MD
Lydia Lewis

The Physician's Guide to

DEPRESSION &
BIPOLAR DISORDERS

SECTION I

General Principles:
Prevalence Diagnosis
and Treatment

CHAPTER 1

Diagnosis and Treatment of Depression and Bipolar Disorder in a Primary Care Setting

FRANK DEGRUY, III AND THOMAS L. SCHWENK

The primary care physician has substantial responsibility for the effective diagnosis and treatment of patients with unipolar and bipolar depressive disorder. Why this is and whether it is desirable are the subjects of considerable controversy. Some health policy experts consider this reality to be less than ideal, and the result of an inadequate mental health care system with poor access to an overtaxed psychiatric workforce. However, most observers believe the care of patients with mental illness by primary care physicians is not only inevitable but desirable, because of the desire of patients to seek comprehensive care for both medical and psychiatric problems from a single source, and the benefits of integrating comprehensive care for all primary care problems by a single clinician.[1] Perhaps most fundamentally, patients seeking care for mental illness in primary care settings differ in several critical ways from those in mental health care settings.[2,3]

As has been documented repeatedly in large, community-based and practice-based surveys,[2,4] there is a concentrating phenomenon between the prevalence of clinical depression in the community (2–4%) and its prevalence in community-based primary care medical practices (6–8%). This concentrating effect continues from the primary care to the mental health office. However, in addition to this quantitative difference, there is also a qualitative difference between patients seen by the primary care physician and those seen in a mental health care setting. Depressed patients seen in primary care settings have different clinical and socioeconomic features than those seen in psychiatric settings.[5] For this reason, while many of the recommendations and guidance in this book apply to all patients with unipolar and bipolar depression and will not be duplicated here, there are some special features of their care in primary care settings that will be addressed specifically in this chapter.

The following questions regarding the diagnosis of depression patients in primary care, as well as attention to case management and collaborative approaches to management, will be addressed in this chapter, with a focus on bipolar disorder since issues related to the care of patients with unipolar depression have been addressed in detail recently.[6]

1. What is the epidemiology of unipolar and bipolar depression in primary care?
2. What are the clinical consequences, especially of delayed diagnosis or inadequate treatment, of depression in primary care?
3. What are common presentations of and barriers to diagnosis of depression in primary care?
4. What is the relationship between medical comorbidity and depression in the care of depressed patients in primary care?
5. How can depression be accurately and efficiently diagnosed, including clinical and psychosocial clues to its diagnosis and the role of screening and case finding?
6. What are the general issues in the management of depressed patients in primary care, including structured approaches to collaborative care and management models that lead to improved quality of care?

1. What is the epidemiology of unipolar and bipolar depression in primary care?

The epidemiology of depression in primary care can be best described as a series of nested populations. In the National Comorbidity Study,[4] 30–40% of the general population was found to have a lifetime criterion-based depressive disorder, of which most had major depressive disorder and most were women. Approximately 10–20% of the general population will consult a primary care physician for mental health problems in the course of a year.[7] About 10–40% of all primary care patients will have a criterion-based psychiatric disorder, of which most (90%) are mood and anxiety disorders and substance abuse.[8] There are some special groups, such as primary care patients who are high utilizers of medical services, who have rates of psychiatric illness in the range of 40–50%, often undiagnosed. This high utilization could be physician-initiated and occur because of medical comorbidity, but is more often patient-initiated

based on a highly somatizing approach to distress, with little recognition by the patient (and frequently by the physician) of the underlying psychiatric illness. In practice-based studies, approximately a third of patients who screen positive for depression on symptom-based questionnaires, or 12–14%, have criterion-based depressive diagnoses, mostly major depressive disorder and minor depression. However, of these over 40% are only mildly and/or transiently depressed.[9]

Bipolar disorder was thought until recently to be relatively rare in the general population, and therefore in the primary care population as well, with the prevalence of bipolar disorder with overt mania perhaps 0.5–1% in the general population and 2–3% in primary care. A psychiatric epidemiologic study from the Netherlands using a criteria-based diagnostic interview (the Composite International Diagnostic Interview or CIDI) found a community-based lifetime prevalence of bipolar disorder (mostly bipolar I) of 1.9%, of which a quarter had sought no care for their mental illness, formal or informal.[10] However, concurrent U.S. data suggest that bipolar disorder is present in 3–4% of the general population[11] and, when defined more broadly and mostly with hypomania (bipolar II), may be present in 5–7% of primary care patients.[12,13] This prevalence would represent 25–40% of all patients with clinical depression and anxiety.[14–16] At the very least, of those patients in primary care thought to have unipolar major depressive disorder, 10–20% may have bipolar illness,[2] again mostly bipolar II illness with hypomania rather than the more classic bipolar I disease seen in psychiatric settings with obvious mania.[14–17] A French multicenter study found that 45% of depressed outpatients had bipolar disorder when followed longitudinally and with particular attention to bipolar symptoms and criteria.[18] Some studies suggest that, of primary care patients with depression who are followed longitudinally, up to 30% may eventually be diagnosed with bipolar illness,[14,17,19] in most of whom the diagnosis is significantly delayed.

From a primary care perspective, the definition of bipolar disorder should be functionally broadened, at least for the purpose of identifying patients requiring more careful assessment, to include a category of patients who appear to have unipolar depression but are treatment-resistant, who present to the physician for medical care only when depressed as opposed to when they are experiencing mania or hypomania, and who suffer from agitation, irritability, and impulsivity, and may be more suicidal as a result. They often do not respond to typical antidepressant regimens, although the classic warnings about unmasking mania in undiagnosed bipolar patients do not apply. Instead, patients become anxious, agitated, and restless and appear to be "activated," although in fact they are simply hypomanic. These patients may represent up to 25–30% of all depressed primary care patients who are identified and treated by primary care physicians, and may be disproportionately represented in treatment-resistant and otherwise under-treated subpopulations.[19]

2. What are the clinical consequences, especially of delayed diagnosis or inadequate treatment, of depression in primary care?

The under-diagnosis and delayed diagnosis of unipolar depression are well-known and well-described phenomena.[20,21] In general, primary care physicians make a structured and documented diagnosis of depression in only about 50% of patients who meet DSM criteria in a structured interview. However, many of these patients have relatively mild and transient distress and symptoms that do not make a significant incremental contribution to their overall morbidity and disability.[2,3,5] Overall, patients with significant major depression who are undiagnosed in primary care have increased rates and expense of unnecessary health care utilization, poorer outcomes for a wide range of chronic diseases (i.e., diabetes mellitus, coronary artery disease, arthritis, stroke, and cancer, see later for a more complete discussion of depression and

medical comorbidity), significant functional impact on work and home roles, and an increased risk of recurrence and chronicity.[22] A recent study of a large population of patients with chronic and recurrent depression who received care from only primary care physicians found that about a quarter were not treated aggressively to wellness, although most were satisfied with their care and most physicians stated a commitment to treating to full wellness.[23] This study suggests that both patients and physicians are not as committed to treating to full function and wellness in depression as they might be in other chronic diseases, and that there may be different systemic barriers to such treatment than for other chronic medical care. Regarding bipolar disorder more specifically, a patient-based self-report survey of bipolar patients found that over two-thirds were initially misdiagnosed. Misdiagnosed patients saw a mean of 4 physicians before an accurate diagnosis was made.[11] Half of these patients had a delay in diagnosis of at least several months, and many up to 2 or 3 years.

Overall societal costs for depression are in the range of $40–50 billion/year, most of which is attributable to work absence, increased medical care utilization and functional impact.[24] Other studies suggest that the cost of bipolar disorder alone is in the range of $24–45 billion/year, with the latter figure including indirect costs such as lost income, decreased productivity in home and work roles, and the opportunity costs of suicide.[16,25,26] It is not clear if this is incremental to or overlaps with the cost quoted earlier for depression as a whole of $40–50 billion. The medical cost for a single patient with a nonresponsive or chronic form of bipolar disorder was estimated to be over $600,000.[26] These patients experience a high level of unemployment because of difficulty in making and maintaining work commitments, disrupted personal and social relationships, and significant legal problems, often related to alcohol abuse which is common in these patients as a form of self-treatment for agitation and anxiety. Substance abuse is present in 40–50% of bipolar patients.[27] The World Health Organization lists bipolar disorder as one of the top 10 disorders (sixth) reducing quality-adjusted life years.[28] A self-report survey (convenience sample) conducted by a patient advocacy organization[29] found that 57% of bipolar patients were unemployed, with a median household income of less than $15,000 ($2000). One-third were divorced or separated. A similar survey of respondents responding positively to the Mood Disorders Questionnaire (MDQ) found that over half had lost their job involuntarily (compared to a quarter of MDQ-negative respondents), and 26% had legal problems (compared to 5% of MDQ-negative respondents).[30,31]

Clinically, a delay in diagnosis of either unipolar or bipolar depression, and the resultant prolonged neurotransmitter dysfunction, may lead to an increased level of mood dysregulation and an increased risk of recurrence and chronicity. This kindling phenomenon, with increased sensitivity to future external stressors, leads to depressive events of increased severity, increased chronicity with decreased responsiveness to antidepressants (or, in the case of bipolar disorder, decreased responsiveness to lithium,[32] an increased risk of suicide, and decreased functional status, including a negative synergism with concomitant medical comorbidity such as cardiac, endocrinologic, or rheumatologic disease. There is some suggestion that long delays in diagnosis may lead to increased functional impairment even when the patient is treated to euthymia,[33] as well as the somewhat counterintuitive concept that bipolar II patients have higher levels of dysfunction and disability than do bipolar I patients,[34] perhaps because of longer delays in diagnosis and a lower likelihood of full treatment to remission.

3. What are common presentations of and barriers to diagnosis of depression in primary care?

Despite recent improvements in the diagnosis and treatment of depression by primary care physicians, depressed patients continue to suffer from substantial barriers to their accurate diagnosis, including the following:[21]

1. Stigmatization by friends, family members, coworkers, and employers as having a "psychiatric" (interpreted by many to mean less well-defined, less worthy, less able to be confirmed objectively, and/or more related to individual character or motivation) rather than a "medical" diagnosis (correspondingly interpreted by many to be more worthy of sympathy, less likely to be self-induced, and more able to be diagnosed and measured objectively).
2. The greater time required by physicians to make an accurate diagnosis.
3. The relatively lower reimbursement for mental health care provided by some health insurance plans to primary care physicians.
4. The lack of effective and efficient referral resources for primary care physicians.
5. Competing priorities in primary medical care in which other medical diagnoses compete more effectively for the time and attention of both patient and physician (because they are more *worthy*).[35]
6. A sense by many patients that mental illness is not something requiring medical attention or will/should resolve on its own.

The diagnosis of bipolar disorder is further complicated by its perception as being infrequent or even rare by many primary care physicians, and a sense that it is even less the responsibility of the primary care physician than is unipolar depression. Until recent studies described earlier expanded the concept of bipolar epidemiology to include a larger number of patients with hypomania and other forms of agitated depression not responsive to usual depression treatment regimens, primary care physicians diagnosed patients with bipolar I disease infrequently and referred most of them, if possible, to psychiatrists because of the primary care physician's perception that these patients required more complex medication regimens, experienced high rates of suicidal ideation and completed suicides, and were less responsive to usual treatment regimens.

Depression typically presents in primary care with a wide range of somatic and psychosocial complaints, including some or all of the following:[36]

1. Fatigue
2. Pain such as headache or low back pain
3. Various organ systems and somatic complaints such as dizziness or weakness
4. Sleep disturbance
5. Vague organ dysfunction such as nausea or constipation
6. Coexistent but related diagnoses such as irritable bowel syndrome, chronic fatigue, or fibromyalgia
7. Poor recovery from serious medical comorbidity (such as an inability to return to work following myocardial infarction)
8. Memory and cognitive dysfunction
9. Learning and attentional problems
10. Relationship disruption

Depressed patients rarely complain at an initial visit of mood disturbance or the possibility of a depressive diagnosis. Practice-based studies of depression in primary care can screen literally hundreds of consecutive patients before finding a patient who will give his/her primary reason for visiting the physician as depression, despite the fact that 30–40% of those patients will screen positive for significant depressive symptoms (see above). Primary care patients are often unaware of, or actively oppose, the possibility of a mental illness diagnosis, and frequently feel stigmatized by such a diagnosis because they are being evaluated by a "medical" professional. They frequently deny (often appropriately so) the existence of sadness since depression in the primary care setting is more about functional loss than mood disturbance. They interpret their distress more in terms of physical symptoms, particularly chronic pain, weakness, fatigue, and cognitive dysfunction.

Bipolar patients rarely present when they are in a manic or hypomanic phase, because they often enjoy the associated energy and grandiose feelings, and do not perceive such sensations or feelings to be a medical problem. Instead, they present during a depressed phase with some of the symptoms noted earlier. If diagnosed, they are often labeled as having unipolar depression. The diagnosis of bipolar disorder may be uncovered later as the patient is followed longitudinally or is treatment-resistant to the monotherapy usually used for unipolar depression.[17] The most common situation in primary care in which the physician should consider the possibility of undiagnosed bipolar disorder is the patient thought to have unipolar disorder who does not respond to typical antidepressant regimens used in primary care, has substantial side effects to several medication regimens, has been diagnosed previously and/or raises the issue of attention deficit hyperactivity disorder, or complains of distractability, insomnia, flights of ideas, bursts of goal-directed activities or speech, irritability, or social anxiety. Careful questioning for hypomanic symptoms is essential, as is triangulation of the patient's reports with data from family members and friends when possible.[16] Certain features are particularly helpful in distinguishing unipolar from bipolar depression, including a sudden onset of symptoms, an earlier age of onset (i.e., adolescence as opposed to the third decade of life which is the modal decade for the onset of unipolar depression), and a family history of bipolar disorder or more than one family member with suicidality or substance abuse.

4. What is the relationship between medical comorbidity and depression in the care of depressed patients in primary care?

There are extensive relationships between chronic medical disease and depression, with biologic, epidemiologic, clinical, preventive, and/or therapeutic connections between depression and cardiovascular disease, HIV infection, diabetes, obesity, dementia, cerebrovascular disease, cancer, and chronic pain.[22]

These relationships have been reviewed in detail.[37] The relevance of these relationships to primary care physicians derives from four generic and consistent relationships which apply to all or most of the chronic medical illnesses listed earlier:

1. Depression and chronic medical illness are commonly comorbid.
2. Depression adversely affects recovery, rehabilitation, and prognosis for many chronic medical illnesses.
3. Chronic medical illness is a strong risk factor for the development of depression.
4. Depression is a strong risk factor for the development of several chronic medical illnesses.

These relationships are of particular importance to primary care physicians in the care of patients with coronary artery disease, diabetes, cerebrovascular disease, HIV disease, and cancer. A selective review of these relationships relative to the four principles listed earlier follows.

The relationship between depression and cardiac disease, particularly coronary artery disease, is perhaps the most studied. Several connections between depression and coronary artery disease in the pathophysiology of both conditions, their bidirectional associative or possibly even causal relationships, and the influence of one on the other's treatment and rehabilitation suggest that primary care physicians should frequently think about coexistent depression when caring for patients with the new onset of angina, unstable coronary syndromes, and rehabilitation from myocardial infarction. Depression is associated with an increased risk of developing coronary artery disease, an increase in both short-term and long-term mortality following myocardial infarction, and a decrease in successful rehabilitation following myocardial infarction.[38] Patients with depression and coronary artery disease have a two- to threefold greater risk for developing future cardiac events than do those without depression. In those patients with depression, the risk of developing newly diagnosed coronary artery disease is roughly twice as likely compared to patients without depression. These studies control for a wide range of known cardiac risk factors.[39] Similarly, across a wide range of research designs and populations studied, depression, particularly clinical depression as opposed to subclinical syndromes, is as strong a predictor or a stronger predictor than other traditional cardiac risk factors for short-term and long-term prognosis following myocardial infarction. At least seven potential mechanisms have been proposed to explain this relationship:[40]

1. Noncompliance by depressed patients with known preventive, therapeutic, and rehabilitative interventions in cardiac disease.
2. The clustering of behavioral and clinical risk factors known to be common in both depressed and heart disease patients, such as smoking and sedentary lifestyle.
3. Dysregulation of the hypothalamic-pituitary-adrenal (HPA) axis, including non-suppression and dysregulation of cortisol synthesis and release.
4. Decreased heart rate variability.
5. Altered immunologic and inflammatory regulation, with an increase in proinflammatory cytokines.
6. Platelet activation leading to hypercoagulable states.
7. Psychologic stress, presumably working through some of the earlier mechanisms as intermediate steps.

All of these mechanisms come under the purview and responsibility, at least to some extent, of primary care physicians. What is not known is whether structured depression treatment programs can reduce this risk, improve recovery and rehabilitation, or favorably alter prognosis. Selective serotonin and mixed receptor agents, as well as psychotherapeutic regimens are safe in patients with cardiac disease, but there are no studies yet of sufficient power to demonstrate an improved outcome of heart disease in patients whose depression is treated.

Depression is strongly associated with the development of diabetes mellitus, type 2, and may be associated with a poorer prognosis and an increased risk of developing diabetic complications. While the prevalence of depression in diabetic patients appears to be increased, there is some confusion regarding the degree of increase, and whether it applies to patients with both type 1 and type 2 diabetes mellitus.[41] The prevalence of criterion-based, clinical depression in diabetic patients is roughly 8–20%, with most studies showing a range of 9–14%, which is increased over the 4–6% rate in nondiabetic patients in most practice-based primary care studies. Patients with antecedent depression have a roughly 2–2.5 times increased risk, after controlling for a wide range of risk factors common to both depression and diabetes, of developing type 2 diabetes over the subsequent 10–12 years.[42,43] Subsequent to the diagnosis of diabetes in patients with depression, the adequacy of diabetic control is of lesser quality, presumably due to some or all of the same health behavior and biological mechanisms as suggested for the relationship between depression and coronary artery disease earlier. Dysregulation in the synthesis and release of cortisol, catecholamines, growth hormone and glucagon, increased production of proinflammatory cytokines, and altered glucose transport all have a negative impact on control and complications. There are no controlled studies of the effective treatment of depression leading to improved outcomes in diabetic patients, although both psychopharmacologic and psychotherapeutic approaches are generally safe.

Poststroke depression has long been known to be a common association, the treatment of which has been associated with improved functional status and rehabilitation success.[44] The prevalence of depression in poststroke patients is approximately 20%, which is substantially higher than that of the general population, roughly similar to that in diabetes and coronary artery disease (as discussed earlier), and less than that in HIV(+) patients (see further). The diagnosis of depression in patients recovering from stroke is controversial because many of the symptoms and signs which could be assigned to the criterion-based diagnosis of depression are common in stroke patients without depression, such as fatigue, weight change, appetite change, anhedonia, and sleep disturbance (similar to the situation in diagnosing depression in patients with cancer). The general recommendation in the primary care setting is to assign all appropriate symptoms to the possible diagnosis of depression so as to increase the level of suspicion and higher likelihood of accurate diagnosis, albeit at the risk of occasional overdiagnosis, i.e., improving sensitivity even at the slight expense of specificity. Studies have varied over time regarding whether the commonly believed increased risk of depression in patients with left hemisphere stroke is actually true, but recent meta-analyses have confirmed this association. Recent studies have also suggested that clinical depression increases the subsequent risk of suffering a stroke, with relative risks in the 2.5–3.5 range.

The presence of depression in stroke patients is associated with significant impairment in activities of daily living and cognitive function, as well as with an increased risk of subsequent mortality by three to four times. Several controlled trials of antidepressants have shown expected benefits on depression in poststroke patients, as well as improvements in cognitive function, and other trials have shown the effectiveness of typical antidepressants in preventing depression in poststroke patients who were treated shortly after stroke onset. Similar to the situation with coronary artery disease, there are no rigorous trials showing a reduction in the risk of subsequent stroke from the premorbid treatment of clinical depression.[44]

The relationship between depression and human immunodeficiency infection (HIV) or AIDS is somewhat more ordinary, in a sense, than in other chronic diseases, although no less important. There is an increased risk for major depression, or other clinical depressive syndromes, in HIV(+) patients, particularly women, with prevalence rates for clinical depression in

HIV(+) women ranging as high as 40–60%, and most studies clustering in the 20–30% range. Rates in HIV(+) men are significantly lower, 6–10% in most studies, which is somewhat parallel to similar gender differences in prevalence rates in HIV(-) populations. All of these studies suffer from sample size and methodologic issues, including varying definitions of depression, depressive symptoms, and time frames, as well as differences in disease stage.[45] Most studies suggest that depression and stress can exacerbate HIV infection, including a more rapid progression of disease. While it is possible that this is reflective of a simple association between progression of a disease with an ominous prognosis and the resultant psychosocial dysfunction and emotional impact, it appears that depression predates the progression, including preceding a decrease in CD4 cell counts. The presence of coexistent depression appears to be associated with an increased risk of mortality, similar to the relationship with coronary artery disease. Similar to the potential mediating mechanisms for other chronic diseases, as described earlier, most research in HIV infection focuses on the mediating effect of depression on immunologic parameters, and dysregulation of the HPA axis, cortisol, and catecholamines. Substance P, a potent neurokinin for which antagonists have been shown to have antidepressant effects, has also been implicated in HIV progression and serum levels have been shown to be increased in HIV(+) patients. Some or all of these mechanisms may be related to viral replication, apoptosis, and/or cytokine release. As with other chronic diseases, all usual psychopharmacologic and psychotherapeutic approaches to depression are safe and as effective as in other populations.

5. How can depression be accurately and efficiently diagnosed, including the role of screening and case finding?

Primary care physicians often base their approach to and understanding of depression on experiences from medical school and residency training which are usually based in psychiatric and specialty mental health settings. Unfortunately, these lessons are often lost in the primary care setting where patients present differently and have different medical, socioeconomic, and demographic features.[2,3,5] Depressed patients in psychiatric settings compared to those in primary care settings have more psychologic insight, are more inclined to seek and receive mental health care, are younger and more likely male, have a higher socioeconomic status, and have more psychosocial and marital support. The absence of these clinical and demographic factors in primary care patients all contribute to the persistent problem of under-diagnosis and under-treatment in primary care. Primary care patients are unlikely to raise the possibility of mental illness when seeking care from a primary care physician, and are more likely to focus on somatic symptoms as a "ticket for admission." Some patients may be overtly hostile to the possibility of mental illness as an explanation for their symptoms. Conversely, a study of British general practitioners showed that patients who raise the possibility of a psychiatric diagnosis early in the office visit are more likely to be accurately diagnosed with depression.[46]

The diagnosis of depression, either unipolar or bipolar, can be facilitated if the primary care physician targets case-finding efforts to patients with new major medical diagnoses, patients with chronic or recurrent pain complaints for which the pathophysiology is unclear, patients with fatigue and similar complaints such as dizziness, weakness, or sleep disturbance, patients who are labeled as a "problem" or "difficult" because of recurrent vague complaints without apparent diagnosis or resolution, patients who have frequent patient-initiated visits for vague indications, patients whose lack of energy and interpersonal behavior act as an "energy sump" that pulls energy and enthusiasm out of the physician and office personnel and leaves them depleted and discouraged, patients with a significant past or family history of major depression, and patients who respond positively to any question about lack of interest or energy, mood changes, sleep disturbance, cognitive dysfunction, or a concern about depression.[6,21]

A two-question approach to case-finding in patients with the above features, or in other patients in whom depression is suspected, has been explored and its value confirmed in several studies.[47] The two questions address the mood and anhedonia criteria in the DSM IV-TR case definition for major depressive disorder:

1. During the past month have you often been bothered by feeling down, depressed, or hopeless?
2. During the past month have you often been bothered by little interest or pleasure in doing things?

A New Zealand study of general practice patients found a likelihood ratio for a positive test of 2.9 and for a negative test 0.05, with a sensitivity of 97% and specificity of 67%.[48] The use of a two-question case-finding instrument like this is essentially equivalent to the physician simply remembering to frequently include DSM IV-based questions in his/her exploration of vague somatic symptoms for which the differential diagnosis is large and complex.

The role of broad, unselective screening, as opposed to targeted case-finding, is controversial because of the relatively high sensitivity but low specificity of most screening instruments used for unipolar depression.[49] The United States Preventive Services Task Force (USPSTF), which previously had found insufficient evidence to recommend screening adults for depression in primary care,[50] now recommends screening but only if appropriate systems are in place to support subsequent accurate diagnosis and effective treatment and follow-up.[51] Their review of a wide range of screening instruments found little to recommend one instrument over another, with all questionnaires measuring various aspects of mood, symptoms and stresses.

In support of the critical importance of adequate treatment and follow-up, a systematic review of several commonly used screening questionnaires in primary care settings found no evidence for an improvement in psychosocial outcomes from routine screening. There was no evidence of an increased accuracy in diagnosis in patients who screen positive, and no evidence that increased recognition led to an increased likelihood of treatment or more effective treatment.[52] Perhaps for these reasons, a review of 434 managed care organizations in 60 U.S. markets found that only 14.9% required any sort of screening for mental illness, including depression.[53] Conversely, a cost-utility analysis of depression screening in primary care, in which a self-administered questionnaire was followed by an unstructured provider assessment, showed that, while annual or periodic screening was extremely expensive and cost nearly $200,000 per quality-adjusted life-year for annual screening and over $50,000 for screening every 5 years, the cost for one-time assessment was only $32,000 per quality-adjusted life-year.[54] Based on this analysis, the study recommended one-time assessment, which fits well with the targeted case-finding recommendations described earlier, based on certain triggers or clues in the clinical presentation that are associated with an increased likelihood of depression as the cause.

The USPSTF noted that the two-question screen described earlier may be as reasonable as longer questionnaires with 20 or more items which require several minutes to complete.[51] A meta-analysis of the operating characteristics of 11 standard and well-known screening questionnaires found an average administration time of 1–5 min, with a median likelihood ratio for positive results of 3.3 and for negative results of 0.19.[55] These performance characteristics suggest that any of the several instruments available would have reasonable clinical value in sorting through the large volume of primary care patients presenting with a wide range of possible depressive symptoms or markers. Other recent reviews[56,57] have focused on the operating characteristics of specific questionnaires in specific populations, including the PHQ-9 which is commonly used in primary care settings. The USPSTF could make no recommendation about screening for depression in children or adolescents, because of insufficient study of the issue in primary care settings.

Bipolar disorder may be more accurately diagnosed in patients with past episodes of mania or hypomania (especially in patients whose relatives and friends can provide additional perspectives on the patient's behavior and history), in patients with a positive family history for bipolar disorder, substance abuse and suicide, and in patients who are treatment-resistant to monotherapy for unipolar depression and have a high level of agitation, restlessness, and insomnia. Little is known about screening for bipolar disorder in primary care. As noted earlier, the epidemiology of bipolar disorder in primary care appears to be changing, because of changes in disease patterns and/or in classification nomenclature.

The apparent marked increase in prevalence of bipolar II in primary care, characterized by hypomania and treatment-resistant agitated depression rather than manic cycling, suggests that questionnaires designed to detect hidden bipolar I features in patients seen in psychiatric settings may have little value in primary care. For example, a commonly used bipolar screening questionnaire, the Mood Disorder questionnaire (MDQ), was studied in the outpatient psychiatric setting by screening 198 patients (mostly bipolar I) who were subsequently assessed with a structured, DSM criterion-based telephone interview.[31] A cutoff of 7 (out of 13) items scoring positively resulted in a fairly high specificity of 0.90 but a sensitivity of only 0.73. Given the markedly lower prevalence of bipolar disorder in primary care compared to psychiatric settings, even a relatively high specificity results in a positive predictive value for the use of the MDQ in primary care settings that is almost certainly too low to be of use. The relatively low sensitivity will similarly result in a negative predictive value of low clinical value in a low prevalence population such as that found in primary care. It is discouraging to primary care physicians to know that a "positive" score on a screening questionnaire has a low (less than 50%) likelihood of being confirmed on follow-up interviewing or referral, both of which are cumbersome, time-consuming, and expensive. The development of a brief bipolar screening instrument that performs relatively well in primary care settings of low prevalence is critical to improving upon the current underdiagnosis of bipolar disorder by primary care physicians.

In summary, an intermediate strategy for screening for unipolar depression, consisting of targeted case-finding for those patients whose clinical presentation and the presence of risk factors suggest the possibility of depression, may be the most optimal combination of efficiency and effectiveness. It is logistically difficult and discouraging to physicians to implement a broad-based screening program in all or most primary care patients, because, despite the favorable operating characteristics of many instruments, the false positive rate is still high. Even under the best of circumstances, the positive predictive value of most questionnaires and brief screens is barely over 50%, and the high rate of false positive responses generates expensive and labor-intensive follow-up.[49] A targeted case-finding approach, however, does put a greater burden on primary care physicians to have a low threshold for raising the possibility of depression, and either asking a few targeted questions or administering a structured questionnaire. The high prevalence of depressive symptoms, although not necessarily a clinically significant diagnosis, in most primary care practices suggests that the physician should be doing this for as many as a quarter to a third of all adult patients. Similarly, a targeted strategy for assessing patients with markers for bipolar disease, particularly treatment-resistant depressed patients who have significant agitation and anxiety, with a focus on past and family history and gathering additional clinical information from family members and friends, may be aided by the MDQ, recognizing that both positive and negative predictive value may not be optimal in a primary care setting.

6. What are the general issues in the management of depressed patients in primary care, including structured approaches to collaborative care and management models that lead to improved quality of care?

In the usual daily practice of caring for depressed patients, primary care physicians infrequently practice guideline-concordant care. For example, patients with a first episode of depression tend to receive treatment for an inadequate duration and patients who meet criteria for maintenance therapy are often inadequately treated.[58] These examples of nonadherence to guidelines are neither unique to depression nor to primary care.[59–61] Nevertheless, the structure of primary care and of the larger health care system in which it is embedded make structured, guideline-concordant, high-quality care for certain chronic diseases almost impossible to achieve. The primary care setting has been designed principally to care for acute problems, where the patient presents with acute symptoms that can be effectively treated with a brief course of therapy, e.g., acute cystitis, appendicitis, or a scalp laceration. If the acute problem is sufficiently severe or complex to require the expertise of a consultant or the mobilization of additional resources and technologies, access is usually relatively efficient, integration is usually smooth, effective communication is usually available, and high-quality care can often be achieved.

The care of depression, as a complex chronic disease, does not work like this. For over two decades primary care physicians have been exhorted to follow fairly simplistic recommendations, derived from controlled clinical trials conducted in psychiatric settings, and the results have been disappointing.[62] Simply referring all depressed patients to a mental health professional for care has likewise been shown to result in inadequate care, principally because so many patients do not complete the referral process,[63]

and because many patients prefer to integrate all chronic disease care in the primary care setting.

The reasons for these failures can be understood by comparing the features of this approach to depression care to the principles of the chronic disease management model.[64] This model acknowledges that chronic diseases are difficult to manage in the primary care setting as it is currently structured, even if efficacious pharmacotherapy is available, and that additional resources are necessary to overcome this difficulty. With an acute problem, the diagnosis is relatively straightforward, criterion-based, and grounded in an accepted pathophysiologic model; treatment is based on clinical trials conducted with patients and in settings similar to those in practice; and resolution is readily measured and achievable in a short period of time (even in a single visit). In contrast, chronic diseases tend to persist for months or years; are not cured so much as managed while they wax and wane in intensity; require adherence to a regimen even when symptoms have improved or resolved; and may require repeated assessments over time to optimize the therapeutic regimen.

In order for primary care physicians to effectively and efficiently manage chronic problems such as depression, six requirements must be met:

1. There must be a means of identifying patients whose disease process can be altered in a way that improves outcome on a long-term basis.
2. The patient must be activated and educated, or those characteristics can be taught or imbued to the patient.
3. The clinician must be similarly activated, educated, and motivated, particularly to value the care of chronic disease which is less dramatic in its response, less likely to be cured, and often less remunerative in its rewards.
4. A care manager is required to monitor progress, address adverse events, and ensure follow-up.
5. The care manager requires a database that tracks patients, treatment programs, required assessments, and special issues.

6. There must be available consultation with mental health specialists that is convenient and includes effective bi-directional communication as well as an educational function by which the primary care physician's repertoire of skills can grow and improve.

The benefits and consequences of these six principles are relatively self-evident, but a brief expansion may be helpful. Targeted case finding is important because patients do not present complaining of depression, as discussed earlier. However, even targeted case finding is time-consuming and labor-intensive, and structured systems and funding for such a practice function would markedly enhance its long-term viability. Patient activation has been extensively incorporated into chronic disease management protocols, and is thought to be effective, although, again, not without cost. In chronic disease care, patients are the ultimate authorities on their disease, and their active engagement in all treatment and monitoring decisions is critical. A knowledgeable clinician is obviously critical, with a particular focus on management protocols and their rationale, the kinds of problems to anticipate and effective responses, and a selection of strategies for managing less common questions and problems which occasionally arise after usual approaches have been tried.

The care manager is the central element of any chronic disease management program, and is appearing more frequently in modern primary care practice. The care manager can be an office nurse, a specially trained receptionist, or a health professional with more focused training (i.e., social worker, health educator). She will usually function across many chronic diseases, because of the breadth of care in most primary care offices. Her principal function is to engage the patient in the management plan, to maintain contact with the patient periodically to assess progress and symptom status, and to answer questions and deal with problems as they arise. The care manager's primary tool and support technology is a sophisticated electronic medical record and associated health care database, although even a simple box of index cards—a tickler file—can be developed and is far superior to the physician's mental recall. The essential function of any database is to remind the care manager when it is time for a follow-up call or visit to assess progress and answer questions. Access to a speciality consultant is necessary for those times that the evaluation or management goes beyond the expertise of the primary care clinician, or when standard management protocols do not address unusual responses or treatment-resistant situations. Shared or collaborative models of care, in which both the primary care clinician and the mental health specialist have scheduled appointments with the patient on an alternating basis have been shown to be effective.[65]

So what might the care of a patient with unipolar or bipolar depression in primary care look like? First, one might expect to find incorporated into the routine intake and check-in process a case-finding protocol for those patients at high risk for depression, specified according to known medical, psychosocial, and demographic risk factors. Each practice would have to design the most efficient and effective approach to this critical first function, so as to deploy limited resources with the least disruption and cost. Positive findings would result in a more detailed, structured interview by the physician, or possibly an intermediate assessment by the care manager. Once a diagnosis had been made, the primary care clinician would use the care manager as well as electronic and audiovisual resources to explain the diagnosis and its consequences, with a subsequent exploration of the patient's reactions, beliefs, and preferences for treatment. This conversation would inform a subsequent discussion of management options and agreement on a plan of management. Such an approach would require one or more longer visits, which would be reimbursed at a higher and special rate that accounts for the fact that the effective care of depression benefits the larger health care system financially through reduced costs in other medical care and to the patient's employer.

The care plan would likely involve one or more pharmacotherapeutic agents, psychotherapy, or both, and perhaps a set of adjunctive activities such as physical exercise. The care manager and the depression consultant might be brought into this case in a number of ways. The care manager may be present during this initial visit—indeed, may conduct it herself—or may be introduced to the patient after the treatment plan is established. The mental health consultant may routinely meet all patients enrolled for depression care, but more likely would be called in if a complication or difficulty arose. Within a few days of initiating treatment, the care manager, armed with the care plan and knowledge of the patient's symptom profile, is now responsible for making contact with the patient, confirming her understanding and commitment to the care plan, and probing for any difficulties associated with medication or other aspects of treatment. One of the most common times for a depressed patient to prematurely discontinue therapy is within a few days of beginning a medication, when the patient is experiencing side effects but no benefits. The care manager can provide protocol-guided advice according to the clinical situation, as well as psychosocial and educational support. Another common time for primary care patients to discontinue therapy prematurely is after a few weeks if there is no evidence of improvement. This might be the time when the depression database reminds the care manager to again contact the patient and remind her that improvement comes slowly.

There are a number of ways the mental health consultant can contribute to the care of depressed primary care patients. The specific form the primary clinician/consultant collaboration actually takes depends on financial and organizational features of the specific health plan, volume and logistics issues, and interpersonal working relationships and clinical compatibility. The following represent a sampling of potential roles for the mental health consultant.

1. Consult in the case of diagnostic dilemmas.
2. Confirm the initial choice of therapy.
3. Consult in the case of treatment failure or other therapeutic difficulties.
4. Meet with the depression care team (or the practice clinicians) regularly to review protocols and address requested clinical topics.
5. Meet for case conferences, chart reviews, and scheduled clinical consultations.
6. Schedule routine brief meetings with all patients enrolled in depression care, and make recommendations for changes in treatment approach as indicated.

Most primary care patients prefer to receive care for depression and other mental problems in their primary care setting, as part of their comprehensive care for a broad range of acute and chronic medical problems. Primary care physicians and mental health professionals whose goal is to provide the most effective, efficient, guideline-concordant care for depression possible will find that designing practice protocols and collaborative approaches as described earlier will make this care productive, satisfying and a model for how other common and complex chronic diseases should be managed.

REFERENCES

1. Knesper D, Riba M, Schwenk TL. *Primary Care Psychiatry*. Philadelphia, PA: W.B. Saunders, 1997.
2. Coyne JC, Fechner-Bates S, Schwenk TL. Prevalence, nature and comorbidity of depressive disorders in primary care. *Gen Hosp Psych* 1994;16: 267–276.
3. Schwenk TL, Klinkman MS, Coyne JC. Depression in the family physician's office: What the psychiatrist needs to know. The Michigan depression project. *J Clin Psych* 1998;59S:1–7.
4. Kessler RC, McGonagle KA, Zhao S, et al. Lifetime and 12-month prevalence of DSM-III-R psychiatric disorders in the United States: Results from the National Comorbidity Survey. *Arch Gen Psychiatry* 1994;51:8–18.
5. Schwenk TL, Coyne JC, Fechner-Bates S. Differences between detected and undetected patients

in primary care and depressed psychiatric patients. *Gen Hosp Psych* 1996;18:407–415.

6. Schwenk TL, Terrell LB, Harrison RV, et al. Depression, University of Michigan Health System Clinical Practice Guideline, *http://www.med.umich.edu/i/oca/practiceguides/depress/depress04.pdf*, accessed July 1, 2004.

7. deGruy F. Mental health care in the primary setting. In: Donaldson MS, Yordy KD, Lohr K N, et al. (eds.), *Primary Care: America's Health in a New Era*. Washington, DC: National Academy Press, 1996.

8. Spitzer RL, Williams JB, Kroenke K, et al. Utility of a new procedure for diagnosing mental disorders in primary care. The PRIME-MD 1000 study. *JAMA* 1994;272:1749–1756.

9. Klinkman MS, Coyne JC, Gallo SM, et al. False positives, false negatives, and the validity of the diagnosis of major depression in primary care. *Arch Fam Med* 1998;7:451–461.

10. ten Have M, Vollebergh W, Bijl R, et al. Bipolar disorder in the general population in The Netherlands: Results from The Netherlands Mental Health Survey and Incidence Study (NEMESIS). *J Affect Disord* 2002;68:203–213.

11. Hirschfeld RM, Calabrese JR, Weissman MM, et al. Screening for bipolar disorder in the community. *J Clin Psych* 2003;64:53–59.

12. Akiskal HS. The prevalent clinical spectrum of bipolar disorders: Beyond DSM-IV. *J Clin Psychopharmacol* 1996;16(2 Suppl 1):4S–14S.

13. Akiskal HS, Bourgeois ML, Angst J, et al. Re-evaluating the prevalence of and diagnostic composition within the broad clinical spectrum of bipolar disorders. *J Affect Disord* 2000;59 (Suppl 1): S5–S30.

14. Manning JS, Haykal RF, Connor PD, et al. On the nature of depressive and anxious states in a family practice setting. *Compr Psychiatry* 1997;38: 102–108.

15. Ghaemi SN, Sachs GS, Chiou AM, et al. Is bipolar disorder still underdiagnosed? Are antidepressants overutilized? *J Affect Disord* 1999;52: 135–144.

16. Glick ID. Undiagnosed bipolar disorder: New syndromes and new treatments. *Prim Care Companion J Clin Psychiatry*. 2004;6:27–33.

17. Manning JS, Connoro PD, Anjali S. The bipolar spectrum: A review of current concepts and implications for the management of depression in primary care. *Arch Fam Med* 1998;7:63–71.

18. Allilaire JF, Hantouche EG, Sechter D, et al. Frequency and clinical aspects of bipolar II disorder in a French multicenter study: EPIDEP. *Encephale* 2001;27:149–158.

19. Manning JS, Haykal RF, Akiskal HS. The role of bipolarity in depression in the family practice setting. *Psychiatr Clin North Am* 1999;22: 689–703.

20. Hirschfeld RM, Keller MB, Panico S, et al. The National Depressive and Manic-Depressive Association consensus statement on the undertreatment of depression. *JAMA* 1997;277:333–340.

21. Schwenk TL. Diagnosis of late life depression: The view from primary care. *Biol Psychiatry* 2002;52:157–163.

22. Evans DL, Charney DS. Mood disorders and medical illness: A major public health problem. *Biol Psychiatry* 2003;54:77–180.

23. Schwenk TL, Evans DL, Laden SK, et al. Treatment outcome and physician-patient communication in primary care patients with chronic, recurrent depression. *Am J Psych*. 2004 Oct;161(10): 1892–901.

24. Simon GE. Social and economic burden of mood disorders. *Biol Psychiatry* 2003;54:208–2154.

25. Wyatt RJ, Henter I. An economic evaluation of manic-depressive illness: 1991. *Soc Psychiatry Psychiatr Epidemiol* 1995;30:213–219.

26. Begley CE, Annegers JF, Swann AC, et al. The lifetime cost of bipolar disorder in the U.S.: An estimate for new cases in 1998. *Pharmacoeconomics* 2001;19:483–495.

27. Regier DA, Farmer ME, Rae DS, et al. Comorbidity of mental disorders with alcohol and other drug abuse: Results from the Epidemiologic Catchment Area (ECA) Study. *JAMA* 1990;264: 2511–2518.

28. Murray CJ, Lopez AD. Global mortality, disability, and the contribution of risk factors: Global Burden of Disease Study. *Lancet* 1997;349:1436–1442.

29. Hirschfeld FM, Lewis L, Vornik LA. Perceptions and impact of bipolar disorder: How far have we really come? *J Clin Psychiatry* 2003;64:161–174.

30. Calabrese JR, Hirschfeld RM, Reed M, et al. Impact of bipolar disorder on a U.S. community sample. *J Clin Psychiatry* 2003;64:425–432.

31. Hirschfeld RM, Williams JB, Spitzer RL, et al. Development and validation of a screening instrument for bipolar spectrum disorder: The Mood Disorder Questionnaire. *Am J Psychiatry* 2000; 157:1873–1875.

32. Swann AC, Bowden CL, Calabrese JR, et al. Differential effect of number of previous episodes of affective disorder on response to lithium or divalproex in acute mania. *Am J Psychiatry* 1999; 156:1264–1266.

33. MacQueen GM, Young LT, Robb JC, et al. Effect of number of episodes on wellbeing and functioning of patients with bipolar disorder. *Acta Psychiatr Scand* 2000;101:374–381.

34. Robb JC, Cooke RG, Devins GM, et al. Quality of life and lifestyle disruption in euthymic bipolar disorder. *J Psychiatr Res* 1997;31:509–517.

35. Klinkman MS. Competing demands in psychosocial care. A model for the identification and treatment of depressive disorders in primary care. *Gen Hosp Psychiatry* 1997;19:98–111.

36. Kroenke K, Spitzer RL, Williams JB, et al. Physical symptoms in primary care: Predictors of psychiatric disorders and functional impairment. *Arch Fam Med* 1994;3:774–779.

37. Lewis L. Recognizing and meeting the needs of patients with mood disorders and comorbid medical illness: A consensus conference of the Depression and Bipolar Support Alliance. *Biol Psych* 2003;54:181–183.

38. Kaufman PG. Depression in cardiovascular disease: Can the risk be reduced? *Biol Psych* 2003; 54:187–190.

39. Carney RM, Freedland KE. Depression, mortality, and medical morbidity in patients with coronary heart disease. *Biol Psych* 2003;54:241–247.

40. Joynt KE, Whellan DJ, O'Connor CM. Depression and cardiovascular disease: Mechanisms of interaction. *Biol Psych* 2003;54:248–261.

41. Musselman DL, Betan E, Larsen, et al. Relationship of depression to diabetes types 1 and 21: Epidemiology, biology, and treatment. *Biol Psych* 2003;54:317–329.

42. Eaton WW, Armenian H, Gallo J, et al. Depression and risk for onset of type 2 diabetes: A prospective population-based study. *Diabetes Care* 2002;25:464–470.

43. Kawakami N, Tkatsuka N, Shimuza H, et al. Depressive symptoms and occurrence of type 2 diabetes among Japanese men. *Diabetes Care.* 1999;22:1071–1076.

44. Robinson RG. Postroke depression: Prevalence, diagnosis, treatment, and disease progression. *Biol Psych* 2003;54:376–387.

45. Cruess DG, Evans DL, Repetto MJ, et al. Prevalence, diagnosis and pharmacological treatment of mood disorders in HIV disease. *Biol Psych* 2003;54:307–316.

46. Wright AF. A study of presentation of somatic symptoms in general practice by patients with psychiatric disturbance. *Br J Gen Pract* 1990;40: 459–463.

47. Whooley MA, Avins AL, Miranda J, et al. Case-finding instruments for depression: Two questions are as good as many. *J Gen Intern Med* 1997;12:439–445.

48. Arroll B, Khin N, Kerse N. Screening for depression in primary care with two verbally asked questions: Cross sectional study. *Br Med J* 2003;327:1144–1146.

49. Schwenk TL. Screening for depression in primary care: A disease in search of a test. *J Gen Intern Med* 1996;11:437–439.

50. U.S. Preventive Services Task Force. *Guide to Clinical Preventive Services*, 2nd ed. Baltimore, MD: Williams & Wilkins, 1996.

51. U.S. Preventive Services Task Force Now Finds Sufficient Evidence to Recommend Screening Adults for Depression. Press Release, May 20, 2002. Rockville, MD: Agency for Healthcare Research and Quality. *http://www.ahrq.gov/news/press/ pr2002/deprespr.htm* (accessed July 6, 2004).

52. Gilbody SM, House AO, Sheldon TA. Routinely administered questionnaires for depression and anxiety: A systematic review. *Br Med J* 2001;322: 406–409.

53. Garnick DW, Horgan CM, Merrick EL, et al. Managed care plans' requirements for screening for alcohol, drug, and mental health problems in primary care. *Am J Managed Care* 2002;8: 879–888.

54. Valenstein M, Vigtan S, Zeber JE, et al. The cost-utility of screening for depression in primary care. *Ann Intern Med* 2001;134:345–360.

55. Williams JW, Polly Noel PH, Cordes JA, et al. Is this patient clinically depressed? *JAMA* 2002;287: 1160–1170.

56. Sharp LK, Lipsky MS. Screening for depression across the lifespan: A review of measures for use in primary care settings. *Am Fam Phys* 2002;66: 1001–1008.

57. Nease DE, Malouin JM. Depression screening: A practical strategy. *J Fam Pract* 2003;52: 118–124.

58. Katz SJ, Kessler RC, Lin E, et al. Medication management of depression in the United States and Ontario. *J Gen Intern Med* 1998;13:77–85.

59. Meyers DG, Steinle BT. Lipid screening and treatment by cardiologists have not improved. *Kans Med* 1997;97:14–17.
60. Cabana MD, Rand CS, Powe NR, et al. Why don't physicians follow clinical practice guidelines? A framework for improvement. *JAMA* 1999;282:1458–1465.
61. Lehman AF, Steinwachs DM, Dixon LB, et al. Patterns of usual care for schizophrenia: Initial results from the Schizophrenia Patient Outcomes Research Team (PORT) Client Survey. *Schizophrenia Bull* 1998;24:11–20.
62. Kessler RC, Berglund P, Demler O, et al. National Comorbidity Survey Replication. The epidemiology of major depressive disorder: Results from the National Comorbidity Survey Replication (NCS-R). *JAMA* 2003;289:3095–3105.
63. Olfson M. Primary care patients who refuse specialized mental health services. *Arch Intern Med* 1991;151:129–132.
64. Bodenheimer T, Wagner EH, Grumbach K. Improving primary care for patients with chronic illness: The chronic care model, Part 2. *JAMA* 2002;288:1909–1914.
65. Katon W, Russo J, Von Korff M, et al. Long-term effects of a collaborative care intervention in persistently depressed primary care patients. *J Gen Intern Med* 2002;17:741–748.

CHAPTER 2

Strategies and Tactics in the Treatment of Depression

A. John Rush and Madhukar H. Trivedi

▶ INTRODUCTION

Randomized-controlled trials (RCTs) have established the efficacy of many medications and several depression-targeted, time-limited psychotherapies.[1-3] This scientific evidence is derived from studies of groups of depressed patients. Clinicians, however, must apply this group-based knowledge to individual patients. In so doing, several strategic and tactical decisions must be made, which constitute the focus of this chapter. Strategic treatment choices refer to which treatment to choose initially, and for those who do not respond, which treatment to choose next. Tactics refer to how these treatment choices are to be implemented. Tactics include: (1) procedures to enhance patient adherence, (2) measurement of outcomes, (3) timely dose adjustments, and (4) timely declaration of treatment failure should it occur. This chapter provides strategic and tactical recommendations for the treatment of clinical depression based on available clinical research.

The optimal management of depression often entails more than one treatment attempt, since no single treatment is a panacea, and since there is clear evidence of heterogeneity in terms of response to a particular treatment. Some patients respond best to one treatment, while

for others an entirely different treatment is necessary. Therefore, a multistep treatment plan is often needed to identify the best treatment for a specific patient. Specifically, the initial treatment will not be sufficient to achieve complete symptom remission in many patients. In fact, efficacy trials reveal that only about 50% of outpatients with nontreatment resistant, nonpsychotic major depressive disorder (MDD) initially treated with either a single antidepressant medication or a time-limited, depression-targeted psychotherapy[4,5] will have a clinically significant benefit or a response typically defined as at least a 50% reduction in baseline symptom severity[6-9] in trials lasting 8–10 weeks. Unfortunately, symptom remission or the virtual absence of depressive symptoms (the goal of treatment) occurs in only 30–35% of patients with the initial treatment. A multistep treatment plan facilitates the timely implementation of appropriate revisions in treatments (e.g., switching from one treatment to another or adding a second treatment to the first), which can be expected for many depressed patients.

The use of a multistep, strategic treatment plan also helps to make treatment more consistent, efficient, and effective by providing specific objectives for each treatment step and a measure to assess how well each objective is being met.[10] Furthermore, such a plan helps both clinicians and patients to focus on essential steps to achieve and sustain symptom remission. This focus is especially important because depressed patients can overwhelm practitioners with the number and magnitude of psychosocial difficulties, as well as their depressive symptoms.

Several decisions must be made before selecting a specific initial treatment. Figure 2-1 provides an overview of these decisions.

Determining that Treatment is Indicated

Establishing the diagnosis and assessing symptom severity is essential prior to initiating treatment. Milder, nonchronic forms of MDD may respond, or even remit in the short term, with

supportive clinical management *without* the use of antidepressant medication or formal psychotherapeutic interventions. For example, modestly symptomatic depressed outpatients with MDD achieved a similar degree of reduction in depressive symptoms when treated with pill-placebo plus clinical management as with imipramine, though remission rates may be lower than with medication.[11] It should be noted, however, that those who responded to placebo plus clinical management fared poorly over the subsequent 18-month naturalistic follow-up study.[12]

Depressed patients who respond best to nonspecific treatment typically have been depressed for a short time (e.g., 1–2 months),[13] have few or no prior episodes, have few concurrent psychiatric and general medical conditions (GMCs) (uncomplicated depressions), and have mild symptoms that minimally impair daily function.[6] For these mild, uncomplicated, brief,

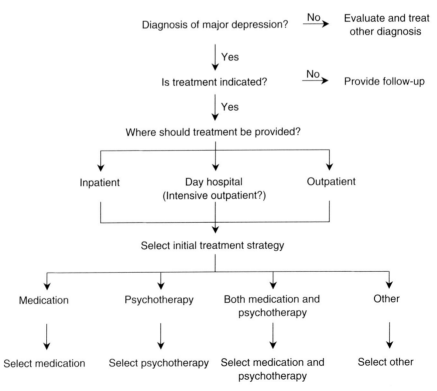

Figure 2-1. Strategic treatment decisions.

nondisabling depressions, an extended evaluation may be clinically useful. Some of these patients will develop a worsening of their depression, in which case treatment is clearly indicated. A small proportion may have symptomatic improvement and even remission. However, careful follow-up for these patients is very important, since some will subsequently develop a more severe depression that does require treatment.

Choosing the Treatment Setting

The first decision in initiating treatment entails choosing the treatment setting (e.g., outpatient, day hospital, or inpatient setting). The preferred setting depends on (1) the imminent risk of suicide, (2) the patient's capacity to recognize and follow instructions or recommendations as an outpatient (e.g., psychotic features such as hallucinations or delusions may recommend inpatient or intensive outpatient care), (3) the availability of psychosocial resources, (4) the level of psychosocial stressors, (5) the degree of functional impairment, and (6) the presence of other conditions (e.g., substance dependence,

cardiac disease) that may be better managed in inpatient settings in some cases.

Who should provide the treatment depends on the capacity of the provider and care system to provide what is needed, as well as on patient preference. Most depressed patients can be successfully treated as outpatients in a primary care setting. Typically, depressed patients requiring psychiatric care present diagnostic problems, have severe depressive or psychotic symptoms, have not responded adequately (i.e., remitted) to one or two prior treatment trials by nonpsychiatrists, or have initially remitted but subsequently relapsed while continuing treatment. Psychiatric care is also usually called for with patients who require special treatments, such as electroconvulsive therapy (ECT), light therapy, monoamine oxidase inhibitors (MAOIs), or complex medication regimens.[6]

Phases and Objectives of Treatment

Treatment is divided into acute, continuation, and maintenance phases (Fig. 2-2). Acute treatment aims at symptom remission and restoration

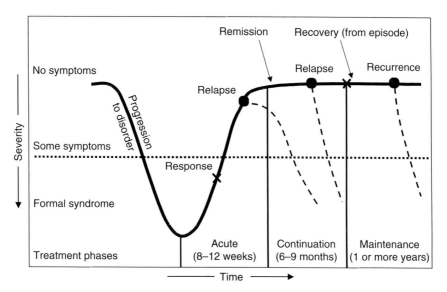

Figure 2-2. Phases of treatment. (Source: Adapted from Depression Guideline Panel, 1993.)

of psychosocial functioning (also an objective of the continuation phase). Sustained symptomatic remission is the goal of acute treatment for depression, and sustained remission is the goal of longer-term treatment for two major reasons.[1,14–24] Patients whose depressions remit fully will function better on a day-to-day basis,[25–27] and they have a better prognosis (lower likelihood of and longer time to relapse or recurrence),[1,28–31] as compared to those patients whose depressions improve but for whom some depressive symptoms remain (i.e., residual symptoms). While the major objective of acute treatment is symptom remission, psychosocial function typically also improves and returns to a normal level if remission is achieved,[27] though this recovery may not occur completely until after several weeks or even 1–2 months of symptom remission have been achieved.[32] On the other hand, it is also widely recognized that sustained symptomatic remission may be difficult to achieve.[33]

Continuation phase treatment aims at preventing relapse (a return of the index episode). For medication, continuation phase treatment is always recommended. Continuation phase psychotherapy may also be needed (see below).

Maintenance phase treatment aims at preventing new episodes (recurrences). A history of recurrent (three or more episodes) major depression or bipolar disorder places the patient at a higher risk for recurrent depression in the future. Patients with recurrent or chronic depressions are typically candidates for maintenance treatment.

▶ SELECTING AMONG MEDICATION, PSYCHOTHERAPY, OR THE COMBINATION

Strategic choices involve the selection of a treatment, whereas tactical choices are made to implement optimally the treatments. The three most common major acute phase treatment strategic approaches include medication, psychotherapy, or the combination of medication and psychotherapy. For some patients, light therapy may also be an option.[34] For the severely ill, those with psychotic symptoms (hallucinations or delusions), or those with an insufficient benefit from several treatment trials, ECT may be needed.[6]

Once an overall treatment strategy (e.g., medication, psychotherapy, the combination) is chosen, a specific treatment (e.g., a specific medication or psychotherapy) is selected. This initial treatment selection is implemented and, depending on response, subsequent revisions in the treatment plan are made. For example, doses are changed, medications are switched or added, or psychotherapy is added to medication. When the patient responds adequately to the medication in the acute phase, whether used alone or with psychotherapy, the same medication at the same dose is used in the continuation phase to prevent a return of the index episode (a relapse). If psychotherapy alone proves to be effective, continuation phase psychotherapy may or may not be needed (see below).[35,36]

Whatever acute phase treatment strategy is selected, it is very useful to define the treatment objective(s) (i.e., target symptoms and psychosocial function) with patients. The strategy chosen should be implemented for a sufficient time (see below) and at a sufficient dose (usually maximally tolerated dose) to achieve symptom remission. If patients understand what to expect, they can better collaborate in determining whether or not the objectives are met. With defined objectives, clinicians can more clearly decide if the initial treatment choice(s) were appropriate (i.e., Were the objectives met?). As a result, subsequent strategic revisions in the treatment plan, such as switching or augmenting treatments, or extending the treatment period, can be implemented in a timely fashion.

Factors to Consider in Selecting Among Acute Strategies

Several factors affect the probability of reaching remission (or response), the time needed to achieve remission (or response), or the durability of the remission (or response) once it is achieved. For medication, psychotherapy, or the combination of both, the presence of concurrent Axis I (psychiatric syndromes), II (personality disorders), or III (GMCs) disorders, the prior course of illness (e.g., chronic illness vs. brief illness), the level of psychosocial support, the degree of treatment resistance, pretreatment symptom severity, and patient preference may all play a role in achieving a remitted state.

When more concurrent psychiatric,[37] personality,[38,39] or general medical[40–42] conditions are present at the beginning of treatment, remission seems to be less likely or it may take longer to achieve, with any of the three treatment strategies. Personality disorders (Axis II) often accompany depression, though the diagnosis of a personality disorder in the depressed patient may be unreliable. The presence of a personality disorder does not contraindicate treatment for the depression. The personality disorder may prolong the time to response or remission, interfere with adherence, or reduce the likelihood of obtaining a response or remission, with either medication or psychotherapy. In general, the presence of personality disorders suggests a more guarded prognosis than in their absence. Furthermore, personality disorders may represent a higher risk for subsequent depressive relapse or recurrence even if the depression initially responds to treatment.

Course of Illness

The initial choice of psychotherapy, medication, or the combination (psychotherapy and medication) depends in part on the prior course of the depressive illness, since a prominent history of chronic or frequently recurrent depressive episodes recommend maintenance treatment, which itself should have established long-term efficacy. Presently, most antidepressant medications have established efficacy in longer-term treatment based on placebo-controlled, randomized trials. Thus, medication is the preferred

maintenance treatment of chronic or recurrent depressions.[6] For dysthymic disorder, that is often complicated by recurrent major depressive episodes, evidence also supports the efficacy of maintenance medication to prevent recurrences.[43–45] Maintenance medication treatment will also more likely be needed for patients who have a history of incomplete remission (residual symptoms between major depressive episodes).[26,28,29,46,47] If maintenance medication treatment is expected, medications with fewer long-term side effects (e.g., sedation, weight gain) are preferred.

In addition, some evidence suggests that long-standing, more chronic depressions will take longer to remit or may be less likely to remit with various treatments.[37,43,48]

While the need for longer-term maintenance treatment typically recommends that medication (alone or combined with psychotherapy) be the initial treatment, maintenance psychotherapy (especially interpersonal and cognitive therapy) also appears to be effective in those who respond or remit initially.[49,50] Importantly, there is growing evidence that psychotherapy, at least for some patients, will improve prognosis, even after the therapy is discontinued.[50]

Life Events

The presence or absence of current stressful life events should not influence whether medications or psychotherapy or which medications are selected. Once symptom reduction is achieved, depressed patients are typically better able to manage these complex life circumstances. On the other hand, the presence of such chronic, disturbing life circumstances (e.g., chronic marital discord, spousal abuse) logically argues for stronger consideration of combined treatment initially, to obtain both complete symptom remission or full psychosocial restoration.[51,52] In addition, Nemeroff et al.[53] found that chronically depressed patients who reported parental loss or abuse in childhood had a better response to psychotherapy than to medication. Thus, such a history may recommend psychotherapy (alone or combined with medication).

Personality Disorders

When a personality disorder is present, the initial use of both psychotherapy and medication is recommended, or alternatively, the addition of psychotherapy if maximal symptom reduction with medication is not obtained with medication alone or if psychosocial impairment remains. For example, once depressive symptoms have largely subsided with medication alone, psychotherapy may be added to address directly the personality disorder. This recommendation rests on inferences from studies[47,51,52] that indicate that cognitive-behavioral therapy (CBT) to address *residual depressive symptoms* following a response leads to a far better longer-term prognosis (see Rush and Thase[49] for a review of the indications for psychotherapy).

Psychosocial Support

Greater levels of current psychosocial support generally increase the likelihood of response or remission, perhaps because the depressive illness has not yet become so severe or chronic that it has resulted in loss of friends, spouse, or employment.

Symptom Severity

For severely ill depressed patients, medication alone has established efficacy, whereas psychotherapy alone has not been well studied. Thus, for severe depressions psychotherapy alone is not as predictably effective as medication.[6] In the context of depressed outpatients seen in primary care settings, however, recent evidence suggests that symptom severity was

not related to the likelihood of response to cognitive therapy.[54]

For less severe, less complex depressions, there is little evidence that the combination of medication and formal psychotherapy produces symptomatic relief greater than that obtained with either treatment alone.[6] In general, the less severe, less chronic, and less complex the depression, the greater the role for patient preference, because evidence upon which to base the selection between psychotherapy (time-limited, targeted type) and medication is largely absent.

Treatment Resistance

The degree of treatment resistance (usually gauged by the number of previously well-delivered but ineffective treatment trials) seems to affect both the likelihood of and time to achieve remission independent of initial depressive symptom severity.[55] The level of treatment resistance may also affect the stability of the remitted state (e.g., see Nierenberg et al.[56]). Consequently, when implementing each treatment step in the treatment plan, clinicians should consider a history of treatment resistance as an indicator that recommends longer treatment trials or perhaps the use of medications at higher doses, to ensure that those patients who might benefit from each treatment are provided the treatment in a fully adequate fashion. In addition, treatment resistance recommends a combination of medication and psychotherapy.

Patient Preference

In spite of patients being better informed about the treatment of depression, some are still adamantly opposed to medication, whereas others are equally opposed to psychotherapy. Some patients even insist on a particular medication or a specific form of therapy. When empirical evidence does not strongly point toward psychotherapy or medication alone, it is entirely reasonable to respect these preferences, given the apparent equivalency among these approaches for many depressed outpatients. While patients may exercise their first preference initially, a contingency plan should be developed should the first treatment be ineffective.

▶ SELECTING A SPECIFIC ANTIDEPRESSANT MEDICATION

Overview

Once the decision is made to choose antidepressant medication (alone or combined with psychotherapy) as the initial strategy, several factors should be considered in selecting a specific medication. Factors that help to inform the selection of the antidepressant medication include comparative efficacy, previous treatment responses in the patient or family members, presenting symptoms, safety and side effects, potential for drug interactions, dosing convenience (to enhance adherence), concurrent psychiatric disorders, personality disorders, concurrent GMCs, and patient preference.

Efficacy

Overall, the efficacy of the antidepressant medications appears to be equivalent. Some,[57–59] but not other reports[6,43] suggest that for some patients, agents that block both norepinephrine and serotonin reuptake (so-called dual action agents or serotonin-norepinephrine reuptake inhibitors or SNRIs) may be slightly more likely to produce remission than more selective single action agents in 8-week, acute phase trials. Some inpatient studies[60–65] have found that such dual action agents are more effective than more selective agents (the selective serotonin reuptake inhibitors [SSRIs]). These data would argue for selecting a dual action agent in the more severely depressed outpatients, though the greater efficacy of dual action agents has not been established prospectively in outpatients in primary care. In fact, a recent small primary care study did not reveal venlafaxine (a dual action agent) to be more effective than escitalopram (a selective SSRI).[66] The small sample size and the less than appropriately aggressive dosing of both agents may have precluded finding a between-treatment difference. In a second, randomized-controlled trial with larger fixed doses,[67] the two drugs again were not different, though the sample size of roughly 100/group may have precluded detecting small differences in remission rates.

Previous Treatment Responses

A patient's prior treatment history is important because a prior good response to a specific medication typically predicts that the same medication, at the same dose, will be well tolerated and will result in a good response in the future. If a first-degree relative has responded well to a tricyclic antidepressant (TCA) or an MAOI, a better response to the same class of agents can be expected in the patient.[68] However, for the newer antidepressants, whether a family history of response to a particular drug or drug class predicts response to the same drug/drug class for the patient has not been evaluated, though clinicians often use such a history in first-degree relatives to select the same agent for the patient.

Presenting Symptoms

Some presenting symptoms inform the decision as to medication choices. For example, when depression is associated with psychotic symptoms, both an antidepressant medication and an antipsychotic agent are recommended because this combination is more effective than an antidepressant alone.[6] Amoxapine alone is also effective in psychotic depression. ECT is also highly effective for psychotic depression, but it is not usually a first-line treatment though it is useful for patients for whom medications are not effective.[3,6]

For depressions with atypical symptom features (such as overeating, oversleeping, weight gain in the context of a mood that is still reactive to daily events), the SSRIs[69,70] or bupropion[71] seem to have efficacy. The MAOIs, however, have the most robustly defined efficacy, and they are known to be more effective than the TCAs based on randomized-controlled trials.[6] The MAOIs though, pose significant management issues given the needed dietary proscriptions and cardiovascular side effects.

Safety and Side Effects

Safety in overdose is an important issue, especially early in treatment. Thus, agents with better safety in overdose are preferred.[21] In addition, medications with lower acute and longer-term side effects are preferred, because side effects account for 50–65% of patient attrition in both the short and longer term.[72] If maintenance medication is anticipated, long-term side effects such as weight gain or sexual side effects, are especially important when selecting an initial antidepressant medication since these side effects may lead to attrition from longer-term treatment. Patients should be advised as to which side effects to anticipate, and be encouraged to report side effects as early as possible. Management of side effects may include lowering the dose, switching medications, or treating the side effects with an additional medication.

Short-term side effects are sometimes used to select among the antidepressants. For example, a more sedating antidepressant may be preferred for more anxious depressed patients, while a more activating antidepressant may be thought to be better for more psychomotor-retarded patients. The available evidence, however, does not support this practice.[33,73–76] That is, the attempt to match side effects to presenting symptoms does not result in better efficacy.

Alternatively, some clinicians aim to match the initial side-effect profile with presenting symptoms to increase adherence early on. That is, patients with marked insomnia or anxiety are thought to gain some immediate relief of these symptoms before the full antidepressant effect is realized, and are, therefore, more likely to adhere to a sedating treatment.[77] This belief is also not supported by empirical data. Furthermore, even if short-term side effects seem to be beneficial, longer-term side-effect burden must be considered. For example, initially sedating antidepressants often continue to be sedating in the longer run, which could increase treatment discontinuation during continuation or maintenance therapy.

Potential for Drug Interactions

When choosing among antidepressant medications, the potential for drug interactions should be considered. For example, depressions often accompany GMCs that require specific nonpsychotropic medications. Some antidepressants inhibit the P450 isoenzyme system(s) and, therefore, affect (typically reducing) the metabolism of other medications.

To illustrate, fluoxetine, paroxetine, and bupropion block the cytochrome P450 2D6 isoenzyme system. They will, therefore, increase the blood levels of medications (e.g., selected TCAs, neuroleptics and so on) that depend highly on the 2D6 system for their metabolism. Other antidepressants (e.g., nefazodone) inhibit other P450 systems (e.g., the 3A/4 system). Information on the effects of different antidepressants on the P450 systems is available in the Physicians' Desk Reference (PDR).[78]

Dosing Convenience

Most antidepressants can be administered once a day, which is associated with better adherence than more frequent dosing. Adherence can be enhanced by having the patient link the time to take the medication to predictable daily routines (such as breakfast or dinnertime).

Concurrent Psychiatric Disorders

When the depression is accompanied by another concurrent psychiatric disorder, the initial target of treatment may be either the depression or the concurrent nonmood disorder. That is, the nonmood disorder may dictate the treatment plan and medication choice. For example, if the depression is accompanied by obsessive-compulsive disorder (OCD), treatments for the OCD are selected. If effective, treatment for the OCD usually results in remission of the depression. Specifically, clomipramine or an SSRI may be preferred when both OCD and MDD are present. Similarly, when MDD co-occurs with generalized anxiety disorder, panic disorder, posttraumatic stress disorder, or an eating disorder, medications that have established efficacy in each of these conditions are preferred initially over the antidepressants for which efficacy with the concurrent psychiatric disorder has not been established.[6]

When the depression is accompanied by substance abuse, the possibility of a substance-induced mood disorder must be considered. In such cases, a careful prior history may reveal that for some patients, the depression has never occurred without the presence of active substance abuse. In such cases, a several week period of abstinence is likely to lead to remission of the depressive symptoms (if they are substance induced) without the use of an antidepressant medication. Some of these patients, however, will continue to have persistent depressive symptoms even after several weeks of abstinence. In this case, an independent mood disorder should be diagnosed and treated with antidepressants, psychotherapy, or the combination targeted at the depression.

Concurrent General Medical Conditions

Since GMCs often accompany depression, GMCs are risk factors for developing depression. In the presence of depression, the outcome of these GMCs is often worsened,[79] including an increase in both the morbidity and mortality of the associated GMC.[7] Therefore, treatment of the depression is indicated, though management may be more complex and time-consuming than for uncomplicated depressions (i.e., those without concomitant GMCs). The principles that guide treatment for depressions without GMCs generally apply when GMCs are present. Choosing among the medications for depressed patients with GMCs is influenced by factors such as prior response to antidepressant treatments, the relative medical safety and tolerability of the medications, and the potential for drug-drug interactions.

Patient Preference

Since the evidence does not strongly differentiate among the antidepressant medications based on efficacy, and since poor adherence is a common obstacle to achieving remission, patient preference can play a key role in selecting among the antidepressants (as long as there is no medical contraindication to the agent). Patients are more likely to adhere to a treatment when they have participated in its selection.

▶ TACTICAL ISSUES IN MEDICATION TREATMENT

Tactics refer to treatment procedures that are implemented to ensure that an adequate treatment trial at an adequate dose is conducted for an adequate time period with optimal adherence. It is extremely useful to anticipate common problems that are likely to be encountered during treatment and to apply specific tactics to overcome these problems. These problems include adherence, side effects, use of adjunctive medication, inadequate dosing, inadequate duration of treatment, and the inaccurate evaluation of outcomes (failure to measure symptom changes).

Enhancing Adherence

Difficulties with adherence are common in routine care. Poor adherence is probably responsible for more unsuccessful treatment attempts than is the selection among different medications.[80] Adherence can be affected by (1) the nature and severity of side effects, (2) the conscious or unconscious meanings patients attach to taking medication(s), or (3) the desire to leave treatment (medication or psychotherapy) once improvement is achieved—perhaps because of the shame and stigma that still surround depression.[72] The best predictor of adherence is prior history of adherence.

Adherence is not related to gender, educational level, or socioeconomic status.[80] Whether the presence of concomitant psychiatric or general medical illnesses affects adherence is unclear, though personality disorders (longstanding history of difficulties developing or maintaining supportive interpersonal relationships) likely reduce adherence.

Obstacles to adherence should be anticipated and planned for, even prior to prescribing medication (or initiating psychotherapy). Adherence to treatment for depression is increased if patients are educated at the outset about the aims of treatment and the treatment plan (e.g., the objectives of treatment and the anticipated treatment period). Adherence checks should be a routine part of each visit. More frequent visits or brief telephone calls (e.g., weekly vs. biweekly), especially in the first weeks of treatment, improve adherence by providing support and encouragement, and if needed, by providing timely interventions to reduce untoward side effects (e.g., adjunctive medications or dose reduction). These contacts also serve to counter demoralization and pessimism that may impair adherence, and to provide information to overcome short-term concentration and recall problems that are part of the depressive episode. Adherence obstacles should be revisited routinely when beginning both the continuation and maintenance phases of treatment and when changing treatments.

Side Effects

Side effects, in general, are most often encountered within the first weeks of treatment initiation, or when medication doses are increased. Idiosyncratic or serious adverse side effects (e.g., seizures, allergic reactions), although uncommon, are also most likely encountered within the first several weeks of treatment. Some side effects (e.g., sedation) are dose-dependent and can usually be reduced by decreasing the dose or slowing the rate of dose escalation. Moderate side effects, when encountered, argue for holding the dose and allowing time for physiologic adaptation, which often results in fewer and less severe side effects. Some side effects (e.g., orthostatic hypotension) are less dose-dependent, and tolerance to them is unlikely. In these cases, gradual dose escalation is less useful, and a change in treatment may be indicated. Finally, the use of adjunctive medication may be needed so that an increase in the antidepressant dose can be achieved, when at least some symptomatic benefit has occurred.

Adjunctive Medication

Adjunctive medications are often combined with antidepressant medications to (a) provide rapid relief of associated symptoms (e.g., anxiolytics to reduce anxiety; sedative hypnotic to improve sleep) or to (b) treat side effects of the antidepressant medication. While some clinicians prescribe adjunctive medications when the antidepressant medication is initiated in the hope of providing immediate symptom relief, most patients will not require adjunctive medication. Therefore, it is preferable to determine prospectively whether there is a need for it. For example, many SSRIs, bupropion, and other agents may increase insomnia or cause sedation. One cannot predict which of these side effects will occur in a specific patient.

Another disadvantage is associated with routinely prescribing adjunctive medications at the initiation of antidepressant treatment. If adverse side effects occur when both medications are begun together (e.g., an allergic rash), it will be unclear as to whether these side effects were caused by the antidepressant or the adjunctive medication. Thus, both medications have to be stopped, and clinicians are naturally reluctant to restart the antidepressant alone because it could, in fact, have caused the adverse event.

In addition, some adjunctive medication will impact some of the criterion depressive symptoms by which the effect of acute treatment is measured, thereby, reducing the certainty of whether a full antidepressant response has been obtained (at least until the adjunctive medication is discontinued). When the adjunctive medication is discontinued, some return of symptoms or side effects may occur. In addition, adjunctive medications may cover side effects that, if observed, would lead to either dose adjustments or switching treatments. For example, the initial use of both a sedative-hypnotic and fluoxetine to prevent insomnia may confound the decision to either decrease the dose or switch to an alternative agent. In short, adjunctive medications may obscure information needed to make strategic decisions. It is more logical to wait to determine whether the adjunctive medication is needed, rather than automatically prescribe it from the outset.

Dosing Issues

Medication must be provided at an adequate dose for a sufficient duration that the maximal benefit is realized. Underdosing of medication is common. Most medications are started at lower doses, and doses are raised to find the maximally tolerated dose. Gradual dose escalations are important to enhance adherence by reducing unacceptable initial side effects. While the TCAs were associated with a roughly once-a-week visit frequency for outpatients as doses were adjusted, for most of the newer agents (e.g., the SSRIs, bupropion, mirtazapine) dosing is less complicated, dose increments are fewer,

and the proper dose is more easily attained earlier due to better side-effect profiles.[77] In fact, for some antidepressants (e.g., escitalopram, fluoxetine), the starting dose may be the therapeutic dose for many patients.

Timely and appropriate dose adjustments are essential to maximize the chances of achieving remission. When and whether to make dose adjustments are affected by drug metabolism, pharmacokinetics, drug interactions, and side effects. Some patients metabolize certain drugs more rapidly or more slowly than do others. Slow metabolizers encounter more side effects earlier, and at lower doses. Fast metabolizers may experience virtually no side effects, even with rather large doses. Overly aggressive dosing with associated elevated blood levels may cause arrhythmias, seizures, delirium, or other symptoms. Therapeutic blood levels in general are not of routine clinical value in most patients, though they may be informative in patients without an adequate response to selected agents or with substantial intolerability to multiple agents.[6]

In general, studies have failed to show a statistically significant difference with higher doses of most of the newer antidepressants (e.g., SSRIs or bupropion).[81] Venlafaxine, however, has a clear dose response curve since higher dose groups (i.e., 150–225 mg/day; 300–395 mg/day) demonstrated greater improvement than lower dose groups (75 mg/day).[82] Even with the SSRIs, however, some studies have found that a proportion of patients unresponsive to a standard dose of fluoxetine responded when a higher dose was used.[83,84] Thus, even for agents such as fluoxetine or escitalopram that do not have an established dose response curve, dose increases in some patients will help to achieve maximal effect.[83] There is no evidence that higher doses beyond the range recommended by package labeling, are associated with higher response or remission rates. Thus, in the context of good tolerability, doses should be raised to the maximum allowed by the label if lower doses do not result in remission.

Duration of Treatment

Once a medication trial is begun, it should last at least 4–6 weeks to determine whether the medication will produce a benefit. On the other hand, a 10–12 week trial may be needed to define the full extent of symptom reduction that is possible. About 2/3 of patients who ultimately respond will show at least some benefit (>25% reduction in symptoms) by 4–6 weeks if dosage is adequate. If the patient has not had at least a 20% reduction in symptom severity by 4 weeks, the likelihood of a response in 8 weeks is about 20% (assuming that adequate dosages were used).[85,86] Dose elevation is indicated in the context of an inadequate therapeutic effect at therapeutic doses with modest side effects after 4–6 weeks, or if there is a prior history consistent with rapid drug metabolism and minimal side effects are noted along with minimal benefit after 4 weeks.

What if minimal benefit is noted after 6 weeks of treatment? Extending the initial trial further may be indicated in some patients (i.e., those with >30% reduction in baseline symptoms by 6 weeks, or those with prior unsuccessful medication trials that have been shorter than 6 weeks).

Measuring Outcome

Because the aim of treatment is full symptom remission (not just an improvement or a response), careful interviewing and the use of a symptom rating scale can be extremely useful to determine whether symptom remission has been reached. Recall that symptom remission results in better functional[27] and a better prognosis[26,46,87] than simple improvement. Since less than half of depressed outpatients will achieve remission with the initial treatment, a second treatment trial (either an augmentation or a switch) will be common place.[6]

A specific assessment of core depressive symptoms is preferred over a clinical global judgment because such an assessment increases recognition of residual symptoms by both the patient and clinician.[88] The measurement of depressive symptoms, when combined with an assessment of side effects, helps to inform the clinical decision as to whether to continue, raise the dose, or change to a second treatment approach.[6]

A range of self-reports or clinician ratings is useful in this regard.[89] Easy to use self-report depression ratings include the Beck Depression Inventory-II,[90] the Quick Inventory of Depressive Symptomatology-Self-Report (QIDS-SR$_{16}$),[91–93] and the Patient Health Questionnaire (PHQ) (Appendix 2-1).[94]

These scales are recommended over older self-reports (e.g., Zung Depression scale) because the older scales do not measure all nine criteria symptom domains (sad mood, concentration, energy, and so on) used to diagnose a major depressive episode. The QIDS-SR$_{16}$ and the PHQ each have a range of 0–27 with easily recalled categories of severity (0–5 none; 6–10 mild; 11–15 moderate; 16–20 severe; ≥21 very severe). The QIDS-SR$_{16}$ has been shown to have a high correspondence with a clinician-rated matching version—the QIDS-C$_{16}$.[93,95] Both the QIDS-SR$_{16}$ and the QIDS-C$_{16}$ are in the public domain and are available in multiple languages (www.ids-qids.org). While a self-report can often substitute for a clinician rating, a self-report is *not* recommended with psychotic patients or those with neurocognitive impairments due to degenerative neurologic conditions, delirium, or toxic states.

▶ SECOND TREATMENTS

Recognizing an Unsatisfactory Response to the Initial Acute Phase Medication

The initial acute medication treatment may fail because of misdiagnosis, poor patient adherence, inadequate dosing, insufficient duration of the treatment trial, unacceptable side effects, idiosyncratic adverse events, or simple lack of efficacy given adequate dose, duration, and tolerability.

If the initial treatment is ineffective after appropriate dose adjustment and at least a 6-week trial, a diagnostic reevaluation is recommended. In some cases an occult general medical or substance abuse condition may be found with reinterviewing before proceeding to a second antidepressant treatment. Having confirmed the diagnosis, one next ascertains that adherence has been acceptable (and specifically that substances of abuse have not interfered with the effect of the antidepressant treatment). Having established adequate adherence, the next step is to ascertain that the dose and duration of the initial treatment trial have been adequate. If the diagnosis was correct, the proper dose and treatment duration was achieved, adherence was adequate, and yet the treatment was ineffective, one can conclude that the depression was "treatment resistant" (at least to one treatment).

Treatment resistance, a common problem for patients with MDD, may range from mild to severe.[96] Mild resistance includes an unsatisfactory response (i.e., lack of symptom remission) with a single antidepressant trial. More severe resistance entails inadequate responses to two or more monotherapy trials and even several augmentation trials. Methods to rate the degree of resistance based on the number and types of adequately delivered treatment trials are available.[3,97,98] Some investigators have recommended that treatment resistance not be declared until inadequate responses to two adequately delivered trials of two different classes of antidepressants have been established.[99,100]

To ensure that the treatment was actually given at an adequate dose for an adequate duration, before moving to the second treatment, one can refer to proposed criteria for both adequate doses and adequate treatment durations. Adequate durations range from 4 to 12 weeks.[97,101] Nearly all agree that adequate doses must be at least at minimal dosage found in RCTs to distinguish the medication from placebo in major depression.[102] Most investigators[103,104] recommend that one to two dose escalations be

tried before declaring treatment resistance, though a failure to achieve a >25% reduction in symptoms by 6 weeks is fairly strong evidence of resistance (i.e., few of these patients will achieve full remission).

The third element in the declaration of treatment resistance (and, therefore, the need for a second treatment) entails the definition of an acceptable treatment outcome. While a clinically significant improvement (a response) may recommend continuing the initial treatment, the goal of treatment is remission.[102] Recall that response without remission is associated with significant residual symptoms that interfere with work, family and social activities[25,26–28,105] and higher and earlier relapse or recurrence rates.[29,30] Lack of a significant reduction in symptoms (at least 20% by 6 weeks, or 30% by 8 weeks) is an indication that remission is unlikely. A lack of response by 12 weeks is a signal to change treatments (i.e., to consider the patient resistant to the first treatment).

If the depression does not respond adequately to the first treatment, properly provided, then strategic treatment options include switching to an alternative treatment (different medication or psychotherapy), or continuing the initial medication and adding to it (either psychotherapy or another medication). Obviously augmentation is an option only if the initial treatment is well tolerated (Fig. 2-3).

Stage I	Inadequate response to one monotherapy
Stage II	Inadequate response to two adequate monotherapy trials (different classes)
Stage III	Stage II resistance plus inadequate response to one augmentation trial
Stage IV	Stage III resistance plus inadequate response to a second augmentation trial
Stage V	Stage IV resistance plus inadequate response to bilateral ECT

Figure 2-3. Staging treatment resistance. (Source: Adapted from Thase ME, Rush AJ. *J Clin Psychiatry* 1997;58(Suppl 13):24; Souery D, et al. *Eur Neuropsychopharmacol* 1999;9:83.)

The Pros and Cons of Switching versus Augmenting

Whether to switch from the initial treatment to a new treatment or to augment the first treatment with a second rests on the need for simplicity, the response and tolerability associated with the initial treatment, prior treatment history, and patient preference. Augmentation treatments may be inexpensive, easily implemented, and response often occurs within 2–4 weeks. On the other hand, augmentation likely will increase side effect burden; evidence for the efficacy of augmentation is sparse, and if augmentation is effective, it is not clear how long it should be continued. Augmentation is likely better accepted if the initial treatment has achieved some meaningful benefit without substantial side effects. Whether the degree of benefit with the initial treatment affects the efficacy of different augmentation treatments is not clear. From a practical perspective, patients who have benefited significantly (but not remitted) with the initial treatment may prefer augmentation over switching, as they value the benefit already achieved.

Switching to a new treatment may entail a period of several weeks to attain a full effect, and, in rare cases, a washout period for safety reasons (e.g., switching from fluoxetine to an MAOI). In general, a minimal benefit from the initial treatment combined with substantial side effects would recommend a switch.

Whether switching or augmenting is more effective is not known.[3,6] For example, a switch within the SSRI class[106–109] seems likely to achieve a 50% response rate, but a switch to another class also seems to be effective based largely on uncontrolled, open trial evidence (see below).

▶ SWITCHING MEDICATIONS

If intolerable side effects were encountered with the first antidepressant medication, switching to another antidepressant is obviously required. In these cases, a switch to a different class makes logical sense. When considering a switch in the context of nonresponse (but acceptable side effects) with the first treatment, switching to an antidepressant of the same class or another class is a consideration. Some believe that switching from one agent that affects a specific neurotransmitter system to one that affects another neurotransmitter system (e.g., a switch from a serotonin reuptake blocker to a selective norepinephrine reuptake blocker) will be more effective than switching to another agent affecting the same neurotransmitter system, though there are no double-blind, controlled clinical trials to evaluate this choice.[110] Secondly, as noted earlier, whether a switch to a dual action agent (e.g., one that inhibits both serotonin and norepinephrine reuptake) will be more effective than a switch to another selective agent (e.g., a selective serotonin or norepinephrine reuptake inhibitor) has not been well studied (see below). The third option is to switch to an agent with a different therapeutic mechanism of action than the initial failed agent. Whether this is more effective than switching to an agent with a similar mechanism of action as the initial agent is not clear except for TCAs and MAOIs. Several studies of TCAs and MAOIs have shown that a switch from a TCA to an MAOI is more effective than a switch from one TCA to another.[111–113] Whether this principle applies to the newer agents is not known.[114]

Based largely on studies of TCAs or MAOIs or on nonmasked, open trials, a switch from one medication class to another for those not responding to the first treatment is associated with response rates of 50% (and perhaps 20–30% remission rates).[3,98,115] If a subsequent switch (a third monotherapy treatment step) is needed, some estimate that about 25–35% will respond;[116] this estimate is based entirely on clinical impression.

Switching from One SSRI to Another

There are few controlled trials of patients switched from an initial SSRI to a second SSRI.

Several uncontrolled studies[107–109,117,118] have found participants not responding to the initial SSRI had a 42–61% response rate to the second SSRI. However, it has been suggested that markedly lower response rates to a switch within SSRIs would be observed when the failure to respond is documented prospectively, when medication doses were adjusted upward for the initial SSRI, and when only those who did not respond to (as opposed to those who were intolerant to) the first SSRI were included in the studies. A double-blind study[116] of MDD patients with a history of resistance to two previous antidepressant treatments (mostly SSRIs) found a last observation carried forward (LOCF) response rate for venlafaxine of 45% and a 36% response rate for paroxetine—LOCF. Remission rates were 37% for the venlafaxine-treated patients and 18% for the paroxetine-treated patients.

In the only well-controlled, multisite trial,[119] chronically depressed outpatients were administered either imipramine or sertraline for 12 weeks. In the face of nonresponse to the initial agent, in the context of tolerating the agent for 12 weeks, patients were switched to the alternate medication for an additional 12 weeks (double-blind). Significant improvement rates were found for both second step treatment groups; 44% responded to the sertraline-to-imipramine switch, while 60% responded to the imipramine-to-sertraline switch. Remission rates were 23% for imipramine following sertraline, and 32% for sertraline following imipramine. A higher rate of attrition due to side effects was found with imipramine (9%) than sertraline (0%) when they were used as second step treatments.

Switching from SSRIs to Other Newer Agents

A survey of 400 U.S. psychiatrists found that the most common next step in the management of nonresponders to an SSRI was the switch to a non-SSRI antidepressant.[120] While switching from an SSRI to bupropion is a popular strategy among psychiatrists,[120] little literature forms the basis for this practice. A small, naturalistic, open study compared a switch from an SSRI (citalopram) to bupropion SR, bupropion SR to citalopram, and the combination of both medications. The combination was associated with a 28% remission rate as compared to a 7% rate for either bupropion SR or citalopram alone.[121] Another open trial (29 subjects) of a switch to bupropion SR following incomplete response to 8–12 weeks of fluoxetine found a remission rate of 23%.[122]

Venlafaxine was evaluated in an open study of 84 consecutive treatment-resistant depressed patients with a history of at least three previous unsuccessful medication trials.[56] A 30–33% response rate was found. Another open study of depressed patients with a documented history of unsatisfactory improvement after at least 8 weeks of an adequately dosed antidepressant, venlafaxine resulted in a 58% response rate.[123]

Switching from an SSRI to mirtazapine was evaluated in an open multicenter study[124] to find a 48% response rate with the mirtazapine switch (15–45 mg/day) in 103 patients who had either not tolerated or not responded to SSRI treatment. The efficacy of mirtazapine was comparable among the SSRI nonresponders ($n = 76$) and the SSRI-intolerant patients ($n = 18$).

Switching from SSRIs to Older Agents

As noted earlier, a switch from sertraline to imipramine was effective among sertraline nonresponders in a blinded controlled study (response rate: 44%), though a placebo control was not used to compare against the response rate for imipramine.[119]

Switching Among Older Agents

Several studies have examined the efficacy of MAOIs in the treatment of patients who had not responded to TCAs.[115] In a crossover study of patients with mood-reactive, nonmelancholic, depression, of 46 patients previously unresponsive to imipramine who completed phenelzine treatment, 31 (67%) responded to phenelzine, while of 22 patients previously unresponsive to phenelzine who completed imipramine treatment, nine (41%) responded to imipramine.[111]

In sum, the idea of switching from one failed medication to another (or therapy) is supported largely by open trial data. However, the RCTs available (largely with the older agents) support a switch either within a class (e.g., one SSRI to another) or between classes of medications. Whether there is a preferred next best step following inadequate benefit to or another first step medication is not known.

▶ AUGMENTATION OPTIONS

Augmentation broadly refers to adding a second treatment (medication, psychotherapy, or somatic treatment) to the initial agent to enhance its antidepressant effect. The augmenting agent may or may not be an effective antidepressant when it is used alone. Sometimes the term "combination" treatment has been used to designate the use of two different agents, each of which is an effective antidepressant when used alone. Augmenting agents include lithium, thyroid supplements, stimulants, bupropion, buspirone, pindolol, folic acid, alpha$_2$-antagonists, estrogens, and atypical antipsychotics, among others.

Lithium

Lithium is an effective augmenting agent as documented in prospective, randomized, placebo-controlled, blinded trials, since its first use by De Montigny and colleagues as an augmenting agent to TCAs in 1981.[125] Lithium (0.1 meq/L) may work by enhancing serotonin turnover and induce a short-term effect.[126]

Meta-analyses of placebo-controlled trials and systematic reviews[127] reveal that approximately 50% of patients will respond to lithium augmentation within 2–6 weeks when dosed at 800 mg/day of lithium carbonate or a dose sufficient to produce a level of >0.5 meq/L. The odds ratio of responding to lithium augmentation as compared to placebo) is 3.3.[128]

Lithium, generally used at 600–900 mg/day, to achieve a level of ≥0.4, seems to be sufficient for response,[126] which is typically seen within 2–3 weeks. Further improvement may be seen over the ensuing 4 weeks.[129] It is not clear how long lithium augmentation should be continued, though at least 12 months, based on a double-blind, placebo-controlled study, has been recommended.[130]

Lithium augmentation has been studied in controlled trials with TCAs and MAOIs, though lithium augmentation with SSRIs also seems to be effective.[131–133] Practical issues limit the use of lithium augmentation in practice, given its narrow therapeutic window and the need to monitor lithium levels, as well as thyroid and renal function. Common side effects with lithium include excessive thirst, polyuria, memory problems, drowsiness, fatigue, tremors, weight gain, and gastrointestinal disturbances, especially at higher doses (>0.8 meq/L).

Some recommend that lithium augmentation be considered first-line when the depression does not respond to one or more standard antidepressant monotherapies.[127] A small ($n = 35$) randomized, placebo-controlled trial[134] did not find lithium augmentation to be effective in patients who had not responded to multiple antidepressants and who had also not responded to a 6-week prospective trial of nortriptyline. This finding suggests that lithium augmentation may be most useful in modestly treatment-resistant depressions.

Thyroid Hormones

Thyroid hormone augmentation is also an effective augmenting agent based on a positive meta-analysis[135] of eight controlled studies (4 double-blind placebo-controlled) of triiodothyronine (T3) augmentation in TCA treatment-resistant major depression. Patients treated with T3 were twice as likely to respond compared to controls. Similarly, Joffe reviewed 11 studies where T3 was used to augment response in TCA nonresponders, and reported that overall T3 augmentation was effective in 55–60% of patients.[136] However, not all studies have been positive.[137,138] Triiodothyronine (T3) seems to be more effective than thyroxine (T4).[139,140] The average daily dose of T3 is 37.5 μg, with a range of 25–50 μg/day. In a randomized-controlled trial, T3 augmentation was as effective as lithium augmentation in patients who had not responded to a TCA; more than 50% of patients responded.[141] Reports of T3 augmentation of SSRIs are limited.[142] As with lithium, there is less information available regarding combination with the newer antidepressants.

Pindolol

Pindolol, a beta-blocker with serotonin-1A (5-HT1A) receptor antagonistic properties, has been combined with SSRIs to block the initial auto-inhibitory process involving the 5-HT1A receptors, thereby causing an earlier or enhanced antidepressant effect. Initial open-label studies suggested that pindolol might be an effective augmenting agent,[143,144] but most controlled studies[145–148] have not been positive. Artigas and colleagues suggested that pindolol might shorten the latency of onset of SSRIs in the treatment of depression.[149]

While pindolol has typically been used at 7.5 mg/day (2.5 mg tid), PET imaging studies suggest that this dose is likely suboptimal.[150,151] Adverse effects such as insomnia, irritability, and anxiety have been reported at doses of 7.5 mg/day, though generally this dose is well tolerated. Higher doses, however (e.g., 15–25 mg), are associated with an increased risk of adverse cardiac effects. Pindolol augmentation should be discontinued if there is no response after 2 weeks, as further response is unlikely,[152] and the dose of pindolol should be tapered off over 2–4 weeks.

Buspirone

Buspirone, an azaspirone, is approved as an anxiolytic for generalized anxiety disorder. The anxiolytic effect is thought to be due to its activity as a partial agonist at the postsynaptic 5-HT1A receptor. It may also exert mild antidepressant effects through potentiation of serotonin transmission. When used alone, buspirone has modest antidepressant efficacy.[153–156]

Case reports and open-label case series suggest a positive antidepressant effect when buspirone is used to augment SSRIs.[157–162] The typical dose is 30 mg/day, but up to 60 mg can safely be used. However, neither of two 6-week randomized, placebo-controlled trials found buspirone augmentation to be effective.[163,164] On the other hand, neither study was conclusive. One study[155] had a high placebo response rate, and efficacy for buspirone was suggested in the second study for the more severely depressed patients.[163,165]

Stimulants

Stimulants, such as dextroamphetamine, methylphenidate, or pemoline, have been used to augment antidepressant treatment in patients with only a partial response to antidepressants, despite the lack of controlled data for standard stimulants. Open trials and case reports suggest that methylphenidate and amphetamine may usefully augment the SSRIs, TCAs, or even the MAOIs.[166–172] The use of stimulants has been limited by the risk of abuse associated with these drugs and their schedule II classification.

More recently, modafinil, a novel psychostimulant with a lower abuse potential and schedule IV status, is available for excessive daytime sleepiness associated with narcolepsy. The mechanism of action of modafinil is unknown. Unlike other stimulants, modafinil is highly selective for the CNS targets with little effect on dopaminergic activity in the striatum. A small retrospective case series[173] and an open-label study[174] suggested that 100–200 mg/day of modafinil may be an effective augmenting agent for depression. A preliminary double-blind, placebo-controlled study found modafinil to be a useful adjunct therapy for the short-term management of residual fatigue and sleepiness in patients who were partial responders to antidepressant therapy.[175]

Atypical Antipsychotic Medications

Both risperidone and olanzapine have 5-HT2A antagonist properties, which may enhance the action of serotonin, and, therefore, augment the antidepressant effects of the SSRIs.[176–178] The combination of SSRIs and atypical antipsychotics seems to have synergistic effects on the release of dopamine and norepinephrine.[179]

Small, open-label studies suggest that risperidone may augment the SSRIs in nonresponding depressed patients.[180,181] A small 8-week double-blind prospective trial of depressed patients who had not responded to three prior treatments found that augmenting fluoxetine with olanzapine produced significantly greater reduction in depression with either olanzapine or fluoxetine alone in these treatment-resistant patients.[178] A meta-analysis of two controlled studies found olanzapine augmentation of fluoxetine to be effective over 8 weeks.[182] Open-label trials suggested the efficacy of ziprasidone in patients with treatment-resistant depression (TRD).[183] One open-label pilot study has also suggested efficacy for quetiapine augmentation in patients with severe depression who had not responded to 4 weeks treatment with citalopram.

Atypical antipsychotic agents have significant side effects. This fact, combined with the modest evidence for efficacy of these agents to augment the antidepressants, recommends caution, and perhaps a second opinion, before proceeding with their use.

Bupropion

Bupropion, a dopamine and norepinephrine modulator,[184] is widely used clinically to augment the efficacy of SSRIs or venlafaxine. Case reports, retrospective analyses, and open-label studies suggest efficacy for this strategy.[121,122,185–188] In a small, nonrandomized, open-label trial, combining bupropion-SR with citalopram, was more effective than switching to other medications.[121] In a prospective, open study, about 60% of outpatients resistant to fluoxetine had a full or partial response to bupropion-SR augmentation.[122] In spite of the lack of definitive, prospective evidence, bupropion is the preferred augmentation strategy by psychiatrists in partial responders to SSRIs.[189] Bupropion is also effective in reducing serotonin-mediated sexual side effects found with SSRIs.[190,191]

Estrogen

It has been suggested that estrogen may be an effective augmenting agent to treat depressed women, possibly due to its effects on the serotonergic system[192] as reported in animal studies and studies in postmenopausal women without hormone replacement therapy (HRT). However, the evidence is sparse and inconsistent.[192] Two early studies[193,194] failed to find a benefit of estrogen augmentation of TCAs. Four nonrandomized studies of HRT to treat SSRI nonresponse[195–198] suggested that estrogen may augment the antidepressant effect of SSRIs.

Folic Acid

Major depression is commonly associated with low plasma and red cell folate levels, and patients with low folate levels respond less well to antidepressant treatment.[199–202] A recent review of all randomized trials that compared treatment with folic acid or 5′-methyltetrahydrofolate acid to an alternative for patients with MDD[203] found two studies ($n = 151$) that revealed efficacy for adding folate.[204] While folate alone is not an effective antidepressant, folate may be a useful augmentation option.

Mirtazapine

Mirtazapine enhances central noradrenergic and 5-HT1 serotonergic neurotransmission via blockade of α_2-adrenergic auto- and heteroreceptors, without directly affecting serotonin reuptake. Longer-term use of mirtazapine may increase serotonergic neurotransmission by desensitizing inhibitory α_2-heteroreceptors located on serotonergic nerve terminals.[205]

A double-blind, placebo-controlled study of mirtazapine augmentation in 26 outpatients with treatment-resistant depression[206] found remission rates were 45.4 and 13.3% for active drug and placebo groups, respectively (statistically significant). This study is limited by small sample size, diagnostic heterogeneity, and the variety and dose ranges of the primary antidepressants.

Tricyclic Antidepressants

Nelson et al. suggested that treatment with both fluoxetine and desipramine is a rapid and effective strategy for the treatment of major depression based on a small, open-label study.[207] Another small ($n = 41$), double-blind, controlled study compared a dose increase of fluoxetine with lithium or desipramine augmentation in patients with partial or nonresponse to 8 weeks of fluoxetine (20 mg/day).[84] Dose elevation was significantly better than either augmentation strategy. In a larger follow-up study with three similar treatment groups, there was no difference in response rates across the three treatments, though dose escalation with fluoxetine was numerically superior.[208]

Dopamine Agonists

Preclinical and clinical evidence suggests that dopamine may play a role in the development and treatment of depression.[209] Pramipexole, a dopamine D_2/D_3 receptor agonist, has traditionally been used in Parkinson's disease in conjunction with L-dopa. There is some evidence that pramipexole used alone has antidepressant activity. In a double-blind placebo-controlled study,[210] pramipexole was an effective and safe treatment for depression. By the end of the 8-week trial subjects receiving pramipexole had significantly greater improvement in their depressive symptoms from those receiving a placebo. Similarly, pramipexole also has demonstrated antidepressant effects in patients with Parkinson's disease and depression.[211] In terms of augmentation, a few studies suggesting efficacy of pramipexole are available.

A retrospective chart review of pramipexole as an adjunctive medication in bipolar and unipolar depression found that approximately 44% of patients benefited over a 6-month period,[212] which was similar to the 68% response rate in another 16-week naturalistic prospective study with adjunctive pramipexole.[213] More recently, a small, double-blind, placebo-controlled study of pramipexole added to mood stabilizers in treatment-resistant bipolar depression,[214] resulted in a 67% (8/12) response rate for pramipexole as compared to a 20% (2/10) response rate for a placebo. The mean percent reduction in depressive symptoms was more than twice as great for pramipexole (48%) as compared to the placebo (21%). Thus, pramipexole may be an effective augmenting agent for SSRIs. In addition, pramipexole may also be helpful for the SSRI-associated sexual dysfunction side effects.

Pergolide

Pergolide is a mixed dopamine-1/dopamine-2 (D_1/D_2) receptor agonist that is used to treat Parkinson's disease. The addition of pergolide to an antidepressant was associated with response in 11 out of 20 patients in an open trial.[215]

Lamotrigine

Lamotrigine, a novel anticonvulsant, has been shown to be an effective antidepressant in a double-blind, placebo-controlled study of for patients in the depressed phase of bipolar I disorder.[216] Two small, placebo-controlled trials of lamotrigine versus placebo as an adjunctive treatment to paroxetine[217] or fluoxetine[218] in TRD were suggestive of efficacy, but neither study was definitive.

Nonpharmacologic Treatments

Psychotherapy as an Augmentation

Cognitive-behavioral therapy is depression-targeted and focuses on current problems and issues rather than the past. Studies have shown that CBT appears to reduce residual symptoms in depression and ultimately reduces the risk of relapse.[47,51,52,219,220] In a study by Ward et al., the authors found that brief psychotherapy (such as nondirective counseling or cognitive-behavior therapy) was a more effective treatment for depression than usual care in the short term, but after 1 year there was no difference in the outcome (see later).[221]

Exercise

The positive effect of exercise as a monotherapy or as an augmentation for depression has been investigated. Population studies have revealed a correlation between physical activity level and mental health in both younger and older adults.[222,223] In addition, individuals who exercise at moderate amounts and intensities have increased longevity,[224,225] and reduced risk of coronary disease,[226] stroke,[227] diabetes,[228] and various cancers.[229,230]

Each of three separate meta-analyses have documented the positive effect of exercise on depression.[231,232] These meta-analyses included data from both randomized and nonrandomized studies that compared exercise to no treatment or to other available treatments. A more critical recent systematic review and metaregression analysis[233] of RCTs using exercise as an intervention in the management of depression, concluded that data were insufficient to

determine whether exercise was effective in reducing symptoms of depression due to the lack of high quality research in this area.[233]

On the other hand, one randomized-controlled trial has found 16 weeks of an aerobic exercise program used alone was as effective as antidepressant medication in older patients with MDD.[234] A 6-month follow-up of these patients revealed that subjects in the exercise group had significantly lower relapse rates ($P = 0.01$) than those in the medication group following completion of acute treatment.[235] The recent Depression Outcomes Study of Exercise randomized-controlled trial found that a public health dose of individually conducted aerobic exercise given three to five times a week for 12 weeks when used alone was an effective treatment for MDD in adults between 20 and 45 years.[236] Another 10-week randomized-controlled trial reported that exercise was an effective augmentation to antidepressant medication in reducing depressive symptoms in older people who were partial responders to treatment.[237] Significantly more patients in the exercise group (55%) had at least a 30% decline in symptoms as compared to 33% in the control group.

In sum, there are a large number of potentially useful augmenting agents. No one augmenting agent is known to be more effective than another. Augmenting agents that have been most rigorously evaluated (lithium, thyroid hormone) have been used largely with older agents (TCAs, MAOIs). Augmenting agents most widely used with the newer agents include bupropion and buspirone. Psychotherapy should also be considered as an augmentation given controlled trials indicating efficacy and the potential for longer-term benefit.[50] If the augmentation is effective, subsequent removal of the agent may provide an empirical test of whether it should be continued.

▶ PSYCHOTHERAPY

Formal psychotherapy aims at specific treatment objectives, and is to be distinguished from general clinical management that is part of any medication treatment. General clinical management includes explaining the diagnosis, the treatment objectives, the treatment plan, and the anticipated treatment period to the patient, as well as general counseling and management to enhance adherence and manage side effects, and a regular assessment (preferably a symptom measure) to determine whether the treatment objectives are being met. Clinical management may involve consulting both the patient and significant other(s) to obtain a history, to assess the clinical outcome, and to provide for patient support.

Indications

Formal psychotherapy, when used alone to treat depression, addresses a range of aims including: symptom remission, psychosocial restoration, and the prevention of relapse/recurrence in the continuation/maintenance phases (similar to medications). Psychotherapy trials aimed at depressive symptom remission typically enter somewhat less severely ill patients than do medication trials. Therefore, efficacy data (see further) would recommend psychotherapy alone for mild to moderate depressions, though a study in primary care[54] did not find differential benefit from cognitive therapy depending on pretreatment depressive symptom severity.

When used in combination with medication, psychotherapies may target the above objectives or other objectives, such as medication adherence, psychosocial concomitants or sequelae of the disorder (e.g., marital discord, occupational difficulties), or residual depressive symptoms. Formal psychotherapy to increase adherence may be indicated for those with significant prior or current adherence difficulties and those with relatively fixed negative attitudes toward medication treatment. Formal psychotherapies to ameliorate psychosocial difficulties often found with depression may include individual, family, couples, or occupational therapies. Evidence suggests that such treatments, when used in combination with medication to control symptoms, result in improvement of the targeted area (e.g., marital counseling improves marriages).[49]

Efficacy

Acute treatment with cognitive (CT), interpersonal (IPT), or behavioral (BT) psychotherapy alone is an effective treatment to reduce the symptoms of MDD. These therapies usually result in response rates comparable to those found with antidepressant medication alone in acute RCTs.[6,7,238] These depression-targeted, time-limited psychotherapies produce better symptom response than waiting-list controls.[6,49,239]

Choosing Among the Psychotherapies

There are no clinically useful predictors by which to choose from among the available, time-limited psychotherapies,[49] though time-limited therapies are preferred over time-unlimited therapies given their established efficacy, and because medication is an effective alternative if time-limited psychotherapy fails. A meta-analysis of RCTs of short-term, psychodynamic therapy suggested a lower response rate for this modality than for the more reeducative therapies, but firm conclusions from these studies cannot be drawn given their inherent methodological difficulties.[6] There is no firm evidence that psychotherapy alone is preferred over medication when the depression is accompanied by a concurrent Axis II disorder, though such a recommendation makes clinical sense.

Declaring an Unsatisfactory Response to Acute Phase Psychotherapy

When psychotherapy is used alone, it should be tried for a predefined time period and symptomatic outcomes should be assessed (as with medication treatment) to provide for a timely revision in the treatment plan if symptom remission is not achieved. Just as with medication, psychotherapy alone should result in a symptom remission. A symptomatic response (without full remission) should not be viewed as a satisfactory outcome since medications may add to the efficacy of the therapy.[6,48]

When to decide that the psychotherapy used alone will not result in remission is somewhat unclear. Some patients respond early, whereas others appear to take 8 to 10 weeks to respond to therapy. In general, about 8 weeks of weekly therapy should be provided. If less than a 25% reduction in symptoms has occurred, it is unlikely that remission will be achieved without additional treatment in most patients.[54] However, partial response (25–49% reduction in baseline symptoms) by week 8 argues for further extending the trial period (perhaps up to 16 weeks). As with medication, if a patient inappropriately discontinues psychotherapy while symptomatic, it is advisable to try to reengage him or her, because the depression has not remitted and, consequently, the prognosis is poor.

Second Treatment Following Psychotherapy Alone

What treatment should follow if psychotherapy alone is ineffective? Medication, given its established efficacy, is the next best logical step. A recent report[240] found that roughly 50% of chronically depressed patients who tolerated but did not respond to nefazodone responded to 12 weeks of a form of cognitive therapy used as a second step treatment. The psychotherapy may be continued (if at least partially effective) or discontinued once medication is begun. Whether a different kind of psychotherapy would be effective if the initial form of psychotherapy was not effective has not been evaluated.

▶ MEDICATION COMBINED WITH PSYCHOTHERAPY

Indications

Logically, three different pathways may lead to the use of combined treatment: (1) use of the combination at the outset of treatment; (2) the addition of psychotherapy when there is only a partial benefit to medication alone (i.e., psychotherapy to augment medication); or (3) the addition of medication in the context of partial response to psychotherapy alone (i.e., medication augmentation of psychotherapy).

Medication and formal psychotherapy may be combined at the outset, though the efficacy of this practice is not substantiated by RCTs for patients with nonchronic, uncomplicated forms of MDD. That is, this combination treatment seems not to produce greater acute symptomatic benefits than that achieved with either treatment used alone (for metaanalytic findings, see Depression Guideline Panel,[6] Thase et at.[241]). On the other hand, even for these less complex forms of depression, the combination may be a consideration if a broader spectrum of action is the aim of using the combination (e.g., both symptom reduction and psychosocial restoration). Therefore, initiating both medication and psychotherapy at the outset of acute treatment would be called for if the targets of each treatment were defined as distinct, and both targets were to be addressed (e.g., medication to control symptoms and psychotherapy and marital therapy to address marital problems, or adherence therapy to enhance adherence).

Clinical impression and recent "megaanalyses"[241] also suggest certain indications for the combined treatment approach. Specifically, more severely or chronically depressed patients[48] may especially benefit from the combination. In addition, combination treatment may be preferable to either treatment alone (1) when there is a coexisting Axis II disorder, (2) when there is a chronic or recurrent pattern with incomplete interepisode recovery,[48] or (3) when the patient is discouraged and demoralized, as well as clinically depressed.[6,49,241] Combined treatment may also be indicated for patients with a greater treatment resistance.[242]

Indications for adding psychotherapy when there is a partial response to medication might include persistent cognitive, self-esteem, or interpersonal difficulties if the remediation has been effective for other core depressive symptoms. In general, especially for patients with little prior treatment, both diagnosis and medication management require time for the patient to collaborate in the optimal use of the medication. Thus, it is often simpler initially to begin with medication and clinical management and then, subsequently, add formal psychotherapy if symptom remission is incomplete or psychosocial problems remain after an adequate medication trial.

Psychotherapy may be added to medication even some months following symptom response to further reduce symptomatology and improve functioning, but when to add it is a clinical judgment depending, in part, on the duration and severity of the psychosocial and functional difficulties, the presence of Axis II disorders, and patient preference. Psychosocial and functional improvements occur weeks to months following symptom responses, whether by either medication alone or psychotherapy alone,[32] though substantial functional improvement does occur within 4–8 weeks of symptomatic improvement associated with medication alone.[27] Since psychosocial improvements follow symptom response to medication, a 4–8-week observation period to evaluate the full effects of medication alone on psychosocial function seems logical, before deciding to add psychotherapy, in most cases. Obviously, the need for psychotherapy to redress psychosocial difficulties becomes clearer if symptom control has been achieved for a period of time, yet psychosocial problems continue.

Efficacy

Combined treatment with antidepressant medication and psychotherapy is more effective than either medication or time-limited, targeted psychotherapy alone for chronically depressed patients.[48] A large multisite outpatient trial randomized patients to nefazodone, Cognitive Behavioral Analysis System of Psychotherapy (CBASP),[243] or the combination. CBASP is a time-limited approach specifically designed for the treatment of chronic depression. Response rates were 48% for nefazodone, 48% for CBASP, and 73% for the combination (intent-to-treat sample), while remission rates were 30, 33, and 48%, respectively. Thus, the combination of nefazodone and CBASP increased both response and remission rates. Another 6-month randomized clinical trial[244] compared antidepressant medication ($n = 84$) with the combination of antidepressant medication plus psychotherapy ($n = 83$) in ambulatory patients with MDD.[244] At 24 weeks, the success rate was 40.7% in the pharmacotherapy group and 59.2% in the combination group. In another large 20-week randomized-controlled trial, Paykel et al. compared antidepressant treatment alone to antidepressant treatment plus cognitive therapy in a group of depressed patients ($n = 158$) who were partial responders to antidepressant medication alone.[47] The addition of the therapy (cognitive therapy) significantly reduced the relapse rate over 17 months from 47 to 29%.

Second Treatment Following Medication Plus Psychotherapy

When the combination of both medication and psychotherapy does not produce remission, given evidence that either switching or augmenting one medication with another may be effective, either a medication switch or the addition of a second medication while continuing psychotherapy would be logical next steps.

► CONTINUATION PHASE TREATMENT

Indications

Continuation phase medication is always recommended, whether medication is used alone or combined with psychotherapy in acute treatment, because early medication discontinuation is associated with a higher relapse rate compared with later medication discontinuation.[6] Continuation phase medication is recommended at the same dose found to be effective in acute phase treatment.[21,245]

Continuation treatment typically lasts 4–9 months. The length of the continuation period, in theory, depends on the length of the prior episode. Continuation treatment aims at preventing the return of the index episode until its natural course, as determined by its physiology and biology, would have ended spontaneously. Therefore, patients with longer prior episodes (e.g., 15 months) whose current depressive episode has lasted only 2 months, for example, would be candidates for at least 11 months of continuation phase treatment, assuming that successful acute phase treatment required 2 months. For patients with psychotic depressions, continuation phase treatment may need to be extended or maintenance treatment should be considered (especially if there has been a prior episode of psychotic depression).

Efficacy

Few studies address the question of whether to continue psychotherapy following response to acute phase combined treatment. Continuation phase psychotherapy is recommended following successful response to acute phase psychotherapy when used alone for those with longer-standing depressions to reduce relapse rates.[36] In addition, as noted earlier, psychotherapy may be added to continuation medication if psychosocial or depressive symptom residua are present and not ameliorated by medication alone.[47,51,52]

Discontinuing Treatment

If continuation phase medication is to be discontinued, a gradual medication taper of 2–4 weeks is recommended for those serotonin reuptake blocking agents with shorter half-lives (e.g., paroxetine, venlafaxine) in order to reduce discontinuation symptoms.[246]

► MAINTENANCE PHASE TREATMENT

Indications

Maintenance treatment aims at preventing new episodes (recurrences) and thus is appropriate for recurrent or chronic depressions, but not for single-episode, MDD. The decision to provide maintenance treatment depends on the prior course of illness and other risk factors for recurrence.

Those with recurrent MDD will, on average, suffer one major depressive episode (MDE) every 5 years.[7,247] A substantial number of patients with MDD (20–35%) will have a chronic, unremitting course.[7,247] Chronic depressions often begin with early-onset dysthymic disorder (onset prior to age 18). Patients with early onset dysthymic disorder then subsequently develop recurrent depressive episodes, from which full remission (with treatment) is unlikely. Patients with antecedent dysthymia and those with incomplete recovery between depressive episodes (i.e., persons with residual interepisode symptoms) are very likely to have recurrent episodes in the future. Chronic depressions may be more difficult to treat initially, or they may have more symptom breakthrough in maintenance treatment.[26,46,248]

Whether to recommend maintenance treatment for those with only two major depressive episodes is less clear. Potential factors that recommend maintenance treatment in such situations are previous incomplete interepisode recovery between the prior two depressive episodes, since that course is associated with higher relapse rates.[6,26,46,87] If two episodes have occurred within the last 3 years, or if there is a positive family history for recurrent depression or bipolar disorder, a higher likelihood of an earlier new episode (recurrence) seems to be present than for patients without such histories. Thus, maintenance treatment may be more strongly considered in such cases. Certainly, these factors need to be weighed by clinicians and patients together to decide on the advisability of maintenance treatment. If maintenance treatment is not implemented, careful monitoring of symptoms is recommended to detect early the development of a new depressive episode. Early detection of a new episode will shorten the length of the episode if treatment is implemented.

Efficacy

Maintenance treatment with medication is more effective than placebo in virtually all studies to date.[249,250] Strong evidence suggests that those patients with three or more major depressive episodes are candidates for maintenance phase treatment.[45,251] Indeed, even at 5 years in highly recurrent MDD, maintenance medication has prophylactic efficacy.

Psychotherapy alone as a maintenance treatment has efficacy.[251] Frank and coworkers[251] (in adults) and Reynolds and colleagues[45] (in the elderly) found that maintenance phase interpersonal psychotherapy (IPT),[253] even in patients with highly recurrent forms of MDD, can delay recurrences, such that psychotherapy alone may usefully provide a medication-free interlude in a medication maintenance regimen for selected patients (e.g., those planning to become pregnant, those needing surgery, and so on). Medications, however, appear to be most effective at prolonging the well interval. When maintenance treatment is called for based on prior history of chronicity or recurrence, medication treatment (alone or in combination with psychotherapy) should be considered an essential part of acute phase treatment.

Management Issues in Maintenance Treatment

Several problems may be encountered in maintenance (and continuation) phase treatment of depression: (1) symptom breakthrough, (2) intercurrent general medical illnesses requiring medication, or (3) pregnancy.

When symptom breakthrough is mild and time-limited, only support, reassurance, and perhaps a dose adjustment is needed.[245] If symptom breakthrough is profound, prolonged, disabling, or unresponsive to dose adjustments and reassurance, practitioners must decide how it should be treated in the absence of randomized-controlled trial evidence. Perhaps the simplest approach is to augment the current medication with an additional medication, though which medication (or therapy) is called for is not known. Some believe that an SSRI may be augmented with bupropion or buspirone for symptom breakthrough (see above). However, any of the above-noted augmenting agents are a consideration. If medication augmentation proves to be effective, then the augmenting medication may be discontinued after a time to empirically evaluate whether it is necessary over the longer term. If the augmenting medication fails, then switching to a different treatment may be needed for profound symptom breakthrough. Symptom breakthrough may also be addressed with psychotherapy, but this option has not been formally studied. Perhaps psychotherapy would be indicated if the symptoms were caused by disturbed interpersonal relationships or life events (e.g., divorce or unemployment).

Pregnancy may be managed with continuing medication, or preferably with a drug-free period. In this case, given the evidence for the efficacy of IPT alone in maintenance treatment,[45,251] IPT without medication may provide a clinically useful drug-free period. The development of other general medical illnesses and the need for nonpsychotropic medications during continuation and maintenance phase treatment are common occurrences.

These circumstances need to be managed, taking into account pharmacokinetics and drug interactions with continuation/maintenance medication.

Discontinuing Medication

When to discontinue maintenance medication treatment is unclear. Some patients may require years of maintenance mediation. As noted earlier, if agents with a short half-life that block serotonin reuptake are used, a gradual taper of the dose over 2–4 weeks is helpful in avoiding discontinuation symptoms. Once medication has been discontinued (after either continuation or maintenance treatment), monthly symptom monitoring for the first 6 months after discontinuation is useful as this time period is of particular risk for recurrences.

▶ GUIDELINES AND ALGORITHMS

Wide variations in clinical practice procedures have been recognized in the treatment of depressed patients,[254,255] as well as in general medicine. Clinical practice guidelines for the treatment of depression have been developed for primary care[6,7] and psychiatric practitioners[1,6,7,14–24] with the aim of improving the quality of care and clinical outcomes, by reducing undesirable practice variations and enhancing preferred practice procedures.

Defining Guidelines

The Institute of Medicine[256] defines *practice guidelines* as "systematically developed statements to assist practitioners and patient decisions about appropriate health care for specific clinical circumstances" (p. 8). Examples of practice guidelines for depression include those by the American Psychiatric Association,[1,257] the Agency for Health Care Policy and Research (AHCPR) for depression in primary care,[6,7] and

the World Federation of Societies of Biological Psychiatry.[18,19]

Algorithms, clinical pathways, or *disease management protocols* are more specific than guidelines; they often recommend specific treatments to be delivered in particular sequences. Algorithms are cognitive tools that aim to assist, but not limit, clinical decision-making.[24,258,259] Algorithms not only specify the *strategies* (i.e., which treatments to use and in what order or sequence) but also recommend *tactics* (i.e., how to implement each treatment strategy) of treatment. A treatment algorithm often provides a flow chart to that specifies the recommended treatment steps (and treatment choices at each step). The steps are taken based on a patient's clinical status and prior treatment response.

Both scientific evidence and clinical judgment form the basis for algorithm recommendations, because the scientific evidence is insufficient as a sole source for recommending treatments. As with guidelines, however, algorithms can only provide group-based guidance. Clinicians must be knowledgeable enough, however, to adapt, modify, or ignore the algorithm or guideline recommendations for a specific patient in order to optimize clinical outcomes and to provide safe care. Since algorithms provide even more specific recommendations than guidelines (e.g., they may specify the starting dose and rate of dose adjustment), there is an even greater need for sophisticated basic and clinical knowledge and for substantial clinical experience by the algorithm user, to ensure the safe and proper adaptation of recommendations to individual patients.

While patients who do not remit with the first treatment present a major public health challenge,[260] very few RCTs that compare different treatments for depressions not remitting after even one initial antidepressant treatment are rare, as noted earlier.[103,261] As a result, clinical practice guidelines or algorithms that suggest different second or third treatment steps rest largely on clinical consensus or on open uncontrolled trials,[2,3,21,262] and most practice guidelines do not recommend only one specific "next-step" treatment or even a highly specific treatment sequence.[1,6,7] Additional scientific evidence is strongly needed by which to define the most specific, effective next-step treatment options for treatment-resistant MDD. Such evidence should improve clinical outcomes and may reduce the cost of care.[263–265]

Implementing Guidelines

The efficient and diligent implementation of algorithms or guidelines may require substantial revisions in practice procedures. For many depressions, a chronic (rather than acute) disease management approach is needed. Such programs are often used for patients with other chronic general medical disorders such as diabetes or asthma. Chronic disease management programs include four essential elements: (1) practice design features, (2) patient education, (3) expert care (i.e., guideline-based care), and (4) information systems.[263–267] *Practice design features* include appropriate appointment setting, reminders to patients to keep appointments, follow-up procedures for missed appointments, and the specification of specific roles for different members of a multidisciplinary care team. *Patient education* involves providing information about the disorder and the treatment options. This information is designed to establish realistic expectations about the possible treatment outcomes, to develop skills in self-management and behavioral change, to maximize the use of social supports, and, most importantly, to develop a clinician-patient partnership in the long-term management of the disorder. *Expert care* requires education and decision support for clinicians along with easy access to consultation should problems/obstacles arise. *Information systems* are needed to provide reminders and feedback to both clinicians and patients. For example, the use of a simple outcome measure to inform providers and patients of the effect of the treatment will facilitate timely revisions in the treatment plan. Easy and rapid access to new research that could

affect treatment decisions, as well as better systems to reduce the paperwork burden also improves the efficiency and potentially the effectiveness of the treatments. Deficits in one or more of these critical parameters will likely affect clinical outcomes.

Effectiveness of Guidelines

In the last decade, researchers have begun to evaluate prospectively the clinical effects and costs entailed in implementing practice guidelines for depression in primary care[266,268–271] and psychiatric settings.[10,104,264,265,272] Furthermore, a few controlled trials have been conducted to evaluate which treatment choices are preferred for patients who do not respond or remit with one or more prior treatments (e.g., Shelton et al.[178]). A large ongoing multisite trial, Sequenced Treatment Alternatives to Relieve Depression (STAR*D)[103,261] (www.star-d.org), will compare a range of treatment options in depressed patients who do not respond adequately to one or more previous treatments.

Primary Care Studies

Katon and colleagues[268] were the first to compare guideline-based care for depression with treatment as usual (TAU) in a primary care (PC) setting. These studies used the treatment guidelines for nonpsychotic MDD developed by the Agency for Health Care Policy and Research.[6] To conduct the study, they also provided resources typically not available in PC settings to implement the guidelines. This so-called "collaborative care" model included the provision of staff to assess patient symptomatic outcomes, ready access to psychiatric consultation, and sufficient staff to guide/assist the primary care providers to implement the guidelines.[270,273] This initial study revealed positive benefits for this guideline-based collaborative care approach.

In a more recent report, enhanced care also entailed more patient education and greater visit frequency with a psychiatrist. This study revealed that more patients stayed in collaborative, guideline-based treatment than in TAU, and that patients in collaborative care had larger reductions in depressive symptoms and were more likely to have recovered at 3 and 6 months, than were patients in TAU.[273] Continued improvement in depression was noted up to 28 months for the moderate severity group. For the high severity group, benefits were noted at 6 and 12 months. No increase in the cost of care was noted for the collaborative group.[273]

These positive findings were corroborated by a recent multisite study (Improving Mood-Promoting Access to Collaborative Treatment [IMPACT][271]) that compared a collaborative care management program ($n = 906$) with a multi-step treatment medication algorithm in PC settings for elderly outpatients with MDD versus TAU ($n = 895$). This study provided a depression care specialist (DCS) who screened patients, assisted in the clinical diagnosis and in the regular measurement of symptoms with the PHQ[274] at each clinic visit, followed patients to ensure adherence, and who provided patient education, and for selected patients, Problem Solving Therapy (PST).[275] Medications were delivered based on a prespecified three-step medication algorithm, consistent with depression guidelines[1] and algorithms (e.g., Crismon et al.[21]).

Over a 12-month period following entry into treatment, 45% of the intervention patients responded as compared to 19% in the TAU group. The intervention group had greater rates of treatment for depression, greater satisfaction with care, lower depression severity, less functional impairment, and greater quality of life. The net cost increase was $550/patient/year. The collaborative care studies and the IMPACT study have demonstrated the effectiveness of guideline-based care for depression, and the benefit of modifying practice procedures to ensure the delivery of guideline-based care in primary care settings.

Psychiatric Setting Studies

Further evidence of the clinical benefit of algorithms as compared to TAU comes from the Texas Medication Algorithm Project (TMAP).[10,104] TMAP was the first study to evaluate a chronic disease management program, which included guided medication treatment algorithms in psychiatric outpatients with schizophrenia, bipolar, or MDD treated in the public mental health sector. The intervention included specific medication treatment algorithms,[10,21,104,276–278] the regular systematic assessment of symptoms and side effects at each medication visit, the provision of a patient/family educational program,[279] and the provision of additional staff (a Clinical Coordinator) to provide a more frequent visits, closer follow-up of patients, patient/family education, and to guide physicians in the implementation of the medication algorithms. For depressed patients, clinicians used a clinician-rated and self-report scale [91,93,280] to measure depression at each treatment visit to gauge the benefit achieved with each treatment step in the algorithm. Results[10] revealed a substantial clinically and statistically greater benefit in terms of depressive symptoms, function, and side effect burden for the algorithm group ($n = 175$) as compared to TAU ($n = 175$).

Taken together, results from primary and specialty care studies to date on guideline-based care of depressed patients recommend (1) the adoption of a chronic disease management approach to these patients, (2) the diligent assessment of clinical outcomes (e.g., depressive symptoms), and (3) the development of a specific treatment plan should the initial or subsequent treatments not produce the desired outcome (symptom remission). On the other hand, available evidence is indeed sparse for deciding what the next best step is for a specific patient. Determining the best treatment remains a trial and error approach, attempting to find the best tolerated, safest, and most effective treatment for the individual patient. When to combine medications, which medications to combine, and when to switch medications—as opposed to augmenting one with another is under active study (www.star-d.org).

▶ SOMATIC TREATMENTS (ECT)

While the vast majority of depressed patients will not need to consider somatic treatments such as ECT, though ECT still plays a key role for depressed patients in those with substantial levels of treatment resistance. The safety and efficacy of ECT has been well established.[6] However, ECT does have cognitive side effects that can be reduced by the use of ultra brief pulse, unilateral stimulation.[281,282] ECT is typically used for acute phase treatment. Medications—perhaps preferably nortriptyline and lithium combined—must be used following the achievement of remission with ECT.[99] Additional somatic treatments are under development. They include repetitive transcranial magnetic stimulation (rTMS)—a nonconvulsive means of stimulating selected areas of the central nervous system that does not require anesthesia,[283,284] magnetic seizure therapy—a method to reduce facial seizures that may not have significant cognitive side effects,[285] and vagus nerve stimulation (VNS).[286–290]

▶ CONCLUSIONS

Major depressive disorder is a heterogeneous syndrome—heterogeneous in terms of etiology, response to treatment, and underlying neurobiology and pathophysiology. Luckily, a wide range of potentially effective treatments are available. However, no treatment is a panacea. The evidence suggests that only 30–40% of depressed outpatients who begin a medication or psychotherapy will remit. Even the combination of both only 50% will remit with the first treatment trial. Remission rates may be even lower for those patients with more chronic (prolonged) major depressive episodes or for those with concurrent general medical, psychiatric disorders, or personality disorders.

Since no treatment is universally effective, it is wise to plan initially for at least two acute phase treatment trials at the outset so that patients may avoid becoming inappropriately discouraged when the first treatment is not fully effective. Such inappropriate discouragement may lead to attrition. In addition to the treatment plan, substantial evidence suggests that specific treatment tactics be used to obtain an optimal outcome and appropriate attention to patient adherence. These tactics include patient (and often family) education, a careful titration of the medication used to maximize benefit while minimizing side effects, regular evaluation of depressive symptoms to enhance the chances of remission, and the appropriate use of adjunctive medication. Establishing explicit goals and following a stepwise treatment plan or algorithm may help both practitioners and patients to obtain the best outcomes, especially since treatment algorithms (or more specific guidelines) for MDD appear to have efficacy.[10,273]

The treatment of depressed patients can be very satisfying for both the patient and the clinician. The approach is analogous to the treatment of other chronic GMCs. The majority of patients, with several treatment attempts, can achieve remission. For more complex, treatment-resistant patients, a second opinion, the combination of medication and psychotherapy, and more complex pharmacologic approaches may be required.

▶ APPENDIX 2-1

The 16-item quick inventory of depressive symptomatology-self-report (QIDS-SR$_{16}$).

STAR ✶ D CLINIC VISIT

QIDS-SR16
Self-Assessment

☐ update

Patient ID ⊔_⊔_⊔_⊔_⊔_⊔_⊔_⊔_⊔_⊔_⊔ Date ⊔_⊔ / ⊔_⊔ / ⊔_⊔_⊔_⊔
MM   DD   YYYY

Level ⊔_⊔
Week in level ⊔_⊔

CHECK THE ONE RESPONSE TO EACH ITEM THAT BEST DESCRIBES YOU FOR THE PAST SEVEN DAYS.

During the past seven days...

1. Falling Asleep:

☐ 0   I never take longer than 30 minutes to fall asleep.

☐ 1   I take at least 30 minutes to fall asleep, less than half the time.

☐ 2   I take at least 30 minutes to fall asleep, more than half the time.

☐ 3   I take more than 60 minutes to fall asleep, more than half the time.

2. Sleep During the Night

☐ 0   I do not wake up at night.

☐ 1   I have a restless, light sleep with a few brief awakenings each night.

☐ 2   I wake up at least once a night, but I go back to sleep easily.

☐ 3   I awaken more than once a night and stay awake for 20 minutes or more, more than half the time.

3. Waking Up Too Early:

☐ 0   Most of the time, I awaken no more than 30 minutes before I need to get up.

☐ 1   More than half the time, I awaken more than 30 minutes before I need to get up.

☐ 2   I almost always awaken at least one hour or so before I need to, but I go back to sleep eventually.

☐ 3   I awaken at least one hour before I need to, and can't go back to sleep.

4. Sleeping Too Much:

☐ 0   I sleep no longer than 7–8 hours/night, without napping during the day.

☐ 1   I sleep no longer than 10 hours in a 24-hour period including naps.

☐ 2   I sleep no longer than 12 hours in a 24-hour period including naps.

☐ 3   I sleep longer than 12 hours in a 24-hour period including naps.

During the past seven days...

5. Feeling Sad:

☐ 0   I do not feel sad.

☐ 1   I feel sad less than half the time.

☐ 2   I feel sad more than half the time.

☐ 3   I feel sad nearly all of the time.

Please complete either 6 or 7 (not both)

6. Decreased Appetite:

☐ 0   There is no change in my usual appetite.

☐ 1   I eat somewhat less often or lesser amounts of food than usual.

☐ 2   I eat much less than usual and only with personal effort.

☐ 3   I rarely eat within a 24-hour period, and only with extreme personal effort or when others persuade me to eat.

7. Increased Appetite:

☐ 0   There is no change from my usual appetite.

☐ 1   More frequently I feel a need to eat than usual.

☐ 2   I regularly eat more often and/or greater amounts of food than usual.

☐ 3   I feel driven to overeat both at mealtime and between meals.

Please complete either 8 or 9 (not both)

8. Decreased Weight (Within the Last Two Weeks):

☐ 0   I have not had a change in my weight.

☐ 1   I feel as if I have had a slight weight loss.

☐ 2   I have lost 2 pounds or more.

☐ 3   I have lost 5 pounds or more.

9. Increased Weight (Within the Last Two Weeks):

☐ 0   I have not had a change in my weight.

☐ 1   I feel as if I have had a slight weight gain.

☐ 2   I have gained 2 pounds or more.

☐ 3   I have gained 5 pounds or more.

STAR ★ D CLINIC VISIT

QIDS-SR16
Self-Assessment

☐ update

Patient ID ⊔⎵⎵⎵⎵⎵⎵⎵⎵⎵⎵⊔   Date ⊔⎵⎵⊔ / ⊔⎵⎵⊔ / ⊔⎵⎵⎵⊔
MM   DD   YYYY

Level ⊔⎵⊔
Week in ⊔⎵⊔
level

During the past seven days...

10. Concentration/Decision Making:

☐ 0   There is no change in my usual capacity to concentrate or make decisions.

☐ 1   I occasionally feel indecisive or find that my attention wanders.

☐ 2   Most of the time, I struggle to focus my attention or to make decisions.

☐ 3   I cannot concentrate well enough to read or cannot make even minor decisions.

11. View of Myself:

☐ 0   I see myself as equally worthwhile and deserving as other people.

☐ 1   I am more self-blaming than usual.

☐ 2   I largely believe that I cause problems for others.

☐ 3   I think almost constantly about major and minor defects in myself.

12. Thoughts of Death or Suicide:

☐ 0   I do not think of suicide or death.

☐ 1   I feel that life is empty or wonder if it's worth living.

☐ 2   I think of suicide or death several times a week for several minutes.

☐ 3   I think of suicide or death several times a day in some detail, or I have made specific plans for suicide or have actually tried to take my life.

13. General Interest

☐ 0   There is no change from usual in how interested I am in other people or activities.

☐ 1   I notice that I am less interested in people or activities.

☐ 2   I find I have interest in only one or two of my formerly pursued activities.

☐ 3   I have virtually no interest in formerly pursued activities.

During the past seven days...

14. Energy Level:

☐ 0   There is no change in my usual level of energy.

☐ 1   I get tired more easily than usual.

☐ 2   I have to make a big effort to start or finish my usual daily activities (for example, shopping, homework, cooking, or going to work).

☐ 3   I really cannot carry out most of my usual daily activities because I just don't have the energy.

15. Feeling Slowed Down:

☐ 0   I think, speak, and move at my usual rate of speed.

☐ 1   I find that my thinking is slowed down or my voice sounds dull or flat.

☐ 2   It takes me several seconds to respond to most questions and I'm sure my thinking is slowed.

☐ 3   I am often unable to respond to questions without extreme effort.

16. Feeling Restless:

☐ 0   I do not feel restless.

☐ 1   I'm often fidgety, wringing my hands, or need to shift how I am sitting.

☐ 2   I have impulses to move about and am quite restless.

☐ 3   At times, I am unable to stay seated and need to pace around.

MAQ

If your doctor has prescribed medicine(s) for your depression, how often in the past week have you missed taking the medicine(s)? (Include all times whether you forgot, misplaced the pills, or decided not to take the medicine) Please check one.

☐ Never

☐ Rarely

☐ Sometimes

☐ Less than Half the Time

☐ About Half the Time

☐ Somewhat More than Half the Time

☐ Very Often

☐ Nearly All the Time

☐ All the Time

STAR ✶ D CLINIC VISIT

QIDS-SR16
Self-Assessment

☐ update

Patient ID └┴┴┴┴┴┴┴┴┴┴┘   Date └┴┴┘ / └┴┴┘ / └┴┴┴┘

MM   DD   YYYY

Level └┴┘

Week in └┴┘
level

QIDS-SR16 SCORING SHEET

To Score the QIDS-SR16:

└┴┘   1. Enter the highest score on any 1 of the 4 sleep items (1–4 above)

└┴┘   2. Item 5

└┴┘   3. Enter the highest score on any 1 appetite/weight item (6–9)

└┴┘   4. Item 10

└┴┘   5. Item 11

└┴┘   6. Item 12

└┴┘   7. Item 13

└┴┘   8. Item 14

└┴┘   9. Enter the highest score on either of the 2 psychomotor items (15 and 16)

└┴┴┘   **Total Score (Range: 0–27)**

REFERENCES

1. American Psychiatric Association. Practice guideline for the treatment of patients with major depressive disorder (revision). *Am J Psychiatry* 2000;157(Suppl 4):1–45.
2. Rosenbaum JF, Fava M, Nierenberg AA, et al. Treatment-resistant mood disorders. In: Gabbard GO (eds.), *Treatments of Psychiatric Disorders*, 3rd ed. Washington, DC: American Psychiatric Press, 2001, pp. 1307–1384.
3. Thase ME, Rush AJ. Treatment-resistant depression. In: Bloom FE, Kupfer DJ (eds.), *Psychopharma-cology: Fourth Generation of Progress*. New York: Raven Press, 1995, pp. 1081–1097.
4. Riso LP, Thase ME, Howland RH, et al. A prospective test of criteria for response, remission, relapse, recovery and recurrence in depressed patients treated with cognitive behavior therapy. *J Affect Disord* 1997;43:131–142.
5. Rush AJ, Thase ME. *Psychotherapies for Depressive Disorders: A Review. WPA Series in Evidence and Practice in Psychiatry*, 2nd ed., Vol. 1: *Depressive Disorders*. Chichester, UK: Wiley 2002.
6. Depression Guideline Panel: *Clinical Practice Guideline*, No. 5: *Depression in Primary Care,*

Vol. 2: *Treatment of Major Depression.* Rockville, MD: U.S. Department of Health and Human Services, Public Health Service, Agency for Health Care Policy and Research, AHCPR Publication No. 93-0551, 1993.

7. Depression Guideline Panel: *Clinical Practice Guideline*, No 5: *Depression in Primary Care*, Vol. 1: *Detection and Diagnosis* U.S. Department of Health and Human Services, Public Health Service, Agency for Health Care Policy and Research, AHCPR Publication No. 93-0550, 1993.

8. Jarrett RB, Rush AJ. Short-term psychotherapy of depressive disorders: Current status and future directions. *Psychiatry* 1994;57(2):115–132.

9. Fava M, Davidson KG. Definition and epidemiology of treatment-resistant depression. *Psychiatr Clin North Am* 1996;19:179–200.

10. Trivedi MH, Rush AJ, Crismon ML, et al. Clinical results for patients with major depressive disorder in the Texas Medication Algorithm Project. *Arch Gen Psychiatry* 2004;61(7):669–680.

11. Elkin I, Shea MT, Watkins JT, et al. National Institute of Mental Health Treatment of Depression Collaborative Research Program. General effectiveness of treatments. *Arch Gen Psychiatry* 1989;46:971–982.

12. Shea MT, Elkin I, Imber SD, et al. Course of depressive symptoms over follow-up. Findings from the National Institute of Mental Health Treatment of Depression Collaborative Research Program. *Arch Gen Psychiatry* 1992;49:782–787.

13. Khan A, Leventhal RM, Khan SR, et al. Severity of depression and response to antidepressants and placebo: An analysis of the Food and Drug Administration database. *J Clin Psychopharmacol* 2002;22(1):40–45.

14. Altshuler LL, Cohen LS, Moline ML, et al. The Expert Consensus Guideline Series. Treatment of depression in women. *Postgrad Med* 2001; (Spec No):1–107.

15. American Academy of Child and Adolescent Psychiatry. Practice parameters for the assessment and treatment of children and adolescents with depressive disorders. *J Am Acad Child Adolesc Psychiatry* 1998;37(Suppl 10):63S–83S.

16. Anderson IM, Nutt DJ, Deakin JFW. Evidence-based guidelines for treating depressive disorders with antidepressants: A revision of the 1993 British Association for Psychopharmacology guidelines. *J Psychopharmacol* 2000;14:3–20.

17. Ballenger JC. Clinical guidelines for establishing remission in patients with depression and anxiety *J Clin Psychiatry* 1999;60(Suppl22):29–34.

18. Bauer MS, Whybrow PC, Angst F, et al. World Federation of Societies of Biological Psychiatry (WFSBP) guidelines for biological treatment of unipolar depressive disorders, Part 1: Acute and continuation treatment of major depressive disorder. *World J Biol Psychiatry* 2002;3:5–43.

19. Bauer MS, Whybrow PC, Angst F, et al. World Federation of Societies of Biological Psychiatry (WFSBP) guidelines for biological treatment of unipolar depressive disorders, Part 2: Maintenance treatment of major depressive disorder and treatment of chronic depressive disorders and subthreshold depressions. *World J Biol Psychiatry* 2002;3:69–86.

20. Canadian Psychiatric Association Network for Mood and Anxiety Treatments. Clinical guidelines for the treatment of depressive disorders. *Can J Psychiatry* 2001;46(Suppl 1):5S–90S.

21. Crismon ML, Trivedi M, Pigott TA, et al. The Texas Medication Algorithm Project: Report of the Texas Consensus Conference Panel on Medication Treatment of Major Depressive Disorder. *J Clin Psychiatry* 1999;60(3):142–156.

22. Hirschfeld RM, Keller MB, Panico S, et al. The National Depressive and Manic-Depressive Association consensus statement on the undertreatment of depression. *JAMA* 1997;277(4): 333–340.

23. Reesal RT, Lam RW, CANMAT Depression Work Group: Clinical guidelines for the treatment of depressive disorders. II. Principles of management. *Can J Psychiatry* 2001;46(Suppl 1): 21S–28S.

24. Trivedi MH, DeBattista C, Fawcett J, et al. Developing treatment algorithms for unipolar depression in cyberspace: International Psychopharmacology Algorithm Project (IPAP). *Psychopharmacol Bull* 1998;34:355–359.

25. Judd LL, Paulus MP, Wells KB, et al. Socioeconomic burden of subsyndromal depressive symptoms and major depression in a sample of the general population. *Am J Psychiatry* 1996; 153:1411–1417.

26. Judd LL, Akiskal HS, Maser JD, et al. A prospective 12-year study of subsyndromal and syndromal depressive symptoms in unipolar major depressive disorders. *Arch Gen Psychiatry* 1998; 55:694–700.

27. Miller IW, Keitner GI, Schatzberg AF, et al. The treatment of chronic depression, part 3: Psychosocial functioning before and after treatment with sertraline or imipramine. *J Clin Psychiatry* 1998;59(11):608–619

28. Judd LL. The clinical course of unipolar major depressive disorders. *Arch Gen Psychiatry* 1997;54(11):989–991.

29. Paykel ES, Ramana R, Cooper Z, et al. Residual symptoms after partial remission: An important outcome in depression. *Psychol Med* 1995;25: 1171–1180.

30. Rush AJ, Trivedi MH. Treating depression to remission. *Psychiatr Ann* 1995;25:704–705, 709.

31. Van Londen L, Molenaar RP, Goekoop JG, et al. Three- to 5-year prospective follow-up of outcome in major depression. *Psychol Med* 1998; 28(3):731–735.

32. Mintz J, Mintz LI, Arruda MJ, et al. Treatments of depression and the functional capacity to work [published erratum appears in *Arch Gen Psychiatry* 1993 Mar;50(3):241]. *Arch Gen Psychiatry* 1992;49:761–768.

33. Rush AJ, Batey SR, Donahue RM, et al. Does pretreatment anxiety predict response to either bupropion SR or sertraline? *J Affect Disord* 2001;64(1):81–87.

34. Lam RW, Kennedy SH. Evidence-based strategies for achieving and sustaining full remission in depression: Focus on meta-analyses. *Can J Psychiatry* 2004;49(3 Suppl 1):17S–26S.

35. Blackburn IM, Moore RG. Controlled acute and follow-up trial of cognitive therapy and pharmacotherapy in out-patients with recurrent depression. *Br J Psychiatry* 1997;171:328–334.

36. Jarrett RB, Basco MR, Risser R, et al. Is there a role for continuation phase cognitive therapy for depressed outpatients? *J Consult Clin Psychol* 1998;66(6):1036–1040.

37. Fava M, Uebelacker LA, Alpert JE, et al. Major depressive subtypes and treatment response. *Biol Psychiatry* 1997;42(7):568–576.

38. Ezquiaga E, Garcia A, Pallares T, et al. Psychosocial predictors of outcome in major depression: A prospective 12-month study. *J Affect Disord* 1999;52(1–3):209–216.

39. Viinamaki H, Hintikka J, Tanskanen A, et al. Partial remission in major depression: A two-phase, 12-month prospective study. *Nord J Psychiatry* 2002;56(1):33–37.

40. Iosifescu DV, Nierenberg AA, Alpert JE, et al. The impact of medical comorbidity on acute treatment in major depressive disorder *Am J Psychiatry* 2003;160(12):2122–2127.

41. Keitner GI, Ryan CE, Miller IW, et al. 12-month outcome of patients with major depression and comorbid psychiatric or medical illness (compound depression). *Am J Psychiatry* 1991;148: 345–350.

42. Keitner GI, Ryan CE, Miller IW, et al. Recovery and major depression: Factors associated with twelve-month outcome [see comments]. *Am J Psychiatry* 1992;149:93–99.

43. Keller MB, Gelenberg AJ, Hirschfeld RM, et al. The treatment of chronic depression, part 2: A double-blind, randomized trial of sertraline and imipramine. *J Clin Psychiatry* 1998;59(11): 598–607.

44. Kocsis JH, Friedman RA, Markowitz JC, et al. Maintenance therapy for chronic depression. A controlled clinical trial of desipramine. *Arch Gen Psychiatry* 1996;53:769–774.

45. Reynolds CF III, Frank E, Perel M, et al. Nortriptyline and interpersonal psychotherapy as maintenance therapies for recurrent major depression. A randomized controlled trial in patients older than 59 years. *JAMA* 1999;281:39–45.

46. Judd LL, Akiskal HS, Maser JD, et al. Major depressive disorder: A prospective study of residual subthreshold depressive symptoms as predictor of rapid relapse. *J Affect Disord* 1998; 50:97–108.

47. Paykel ES, Scott J, Teasdale JD, et al. Prevention of relapse in residual depression by cognitive therapy: A controlled trial. *Arch Gen Psychiatry* 1999;56(9):829–835.

48. Keller MB, McCullough JP, Klein DN, et al. A comparison of nefazodone, the cognitive behavioral-analysis system of psychotherapy, and their combination for the treatment of chronic depression. *N Engl J Med* 2000;342(20):1462–1470.

49. Rush AJ, Thase ME. Psychotherapies for depressive disorders: A review. In: Maj M, Sartorius N (eds.), *WPA Series. Evidence and Experience in Psychiatry, Vol. 1. Depressive Disorders.* Chichester, UK: Wiley, 1999, pp. 161–206.

50. Hollon SD, Jarrett RB, Nierenberg AA, et al. Psychotherapy and medication in the treatment of adult and geriatric depression: Which monotherapy or combined treatment? *J Clin Psychiatry* 2005;66(4):455–468.

51. Fava GA, Rafanelli C, Grandi S, et al. Prevention of recurrent depression with cognitive behavioral therapy: Preliminary findings. *Arch Gen Psychiatry* 1998;55:816–820.

52. Fava GA, Rafanelli C, Grandi S, et al. Six-year outcome for cognitive behavioral treatment of residual symptoms in major depression. *Am J Psychiatry* 1998;155(10):1443–1445.

53. Nemeroff CB, Heim CM, Thase ME, et al. Differential responses to psychotherapy versus pharmacotherapy in patients with chronic forms of major depression and childhood trauma. *Proc Natl Acad Sci U S A* 2003;100(24):14293–14296

54. Schulberg HC, Raue PJ, Rollman BL. The effectiveness of psychotherapy in treating depressive disorders in primary care practice: Clinical and cost perspectives. *Gen Hosp Psychiatry* 2002;24(4):203–212,

55. Sackeim HA, Keilp JG, Rush AJ, et al. The effects of vagus nerve stimulation on cognitive performance in patients with treatment-resistant depression *Neuropsychiatry Neuropsychol Behav Neurol* 2001;14(1):53–62.

56. Nierenberg AA, Feighner JP, Rudolph R, et al. Venlafaxine for treatment-resistant unipolar depression. *J Clin Psychopharmacol* 1994;14: 419–423.

57. Detke MJ, Lu Y, Goldstein DJ, et al. Duloxetine 60 mg once daily dosing versus placebo in the acute treatment of major depression. *J Psychiatr Res* 2002;36(6):383–390.

58. Detke MJ, Lu Y, Goldstein DJ, et al. Duloxetine, 60 mg once daily, for major depressive disorder: A randomized double-blind placebo-controlled trial. *J Clin Psychiatry* 2002;63(4):308–315.

59. Fava M, Mallinckrodt CH, Detke MJ, et al. The effect of duloxetine on painful physical symptoms in depressed patients: Do improvements in these symptoms result in higher remission rates? *J Clin Psychiatry* 2004;65(4):521–530.

60. Danish University Antidepressant Group. Citalopram: Clinical effect profile in comparison with clomipramine. A controlled multicenter study. *Psychopharmacology* (Berl) 1986;90(1):131–138.

61. Danish University Antidepressant Group. Paroxetine: A selective serotonin reuptake inhibitor showing better tolerance, but weaker antidepressant effect than clomipramine in a controlled multicenter study. *J Affect Disord* 1990;18:289–299.

62. Danish University Antidepressant Group. Moclobamide: A reversible MAO-A-inhibitor showing weaker antidepressant effect than clomipramine in a controlled multicenter study. *J Affect Disord* 1993;28:105–116.

63. Vestergaard P, Gram LF, Kragh-Sorensen P, et al. Therapeutic potentials of recently introduced antidepressants. Danish University Antidepressant Group. *Psychopharmacol Ser* 1993;10: 190–198.

64. Fuglum E, Rosenberg C, Damsbo N, et al. Screening and treating depressed patients. A comparison of two controlled citalopram trials across treatment settings: Hospitalized patients vs. patients treated by their family doctors. Danish University Antidepressant Group. *Acta Psychiatr Scand* 1996;94(1):18–25.

65. Danish University Antidepressant Group (DUAG). Clomipramine dose-effect study in patients with depression: Clinical end points and pharmacokinetics. *Clin Pharmacol Ther* 1999; 66(2):152–165.

66. Montgomery SA, Huusom AK, Bothmer J. A randomised study comparing escitalopram with venlafaxine XR in primary care patients with major depressive disorder. *Neuropsychobiology* 2004;50(1):57–64.

67. Bielski RJ, Ventura D, Chang CC. A double-blind comparison of escitalopram and venlafaxine extended release in the treatment of major depressive disorder. *J Clin Psychiatry* 2004; 65(9): 1190–1196.

68. Rush AJ, Kupfer DJ. Strategies and tactics in the treatment of depression. In: Gabbard GO, Atkinson SD (eds.), *Treatments of Psychiatric Disorders*, 2nd ed. Washington, DC: American Psychiatric Press, Vol. 1, 1995, pp. 1349–1368.

69. Jarrett RB, Schaffer M, McIntire D, et al. Treatment of atypical depression with cognitive therapy or phenelzine: A double-blind, placebo-controlled trial. *Arch Gen Psychiatry* 1999;56: 431–437.

70. Pande AC, Birkett M, Fechner-Bates S, et al. Fluoxetine versus phenelzine in atypical depression. *Biol Psychiatry* 1996;40:1017–1020.

71. Nierenberg AA, Alpert JE, Pava J, et al. Course and treatment of atypical depression. *J Clin Psychiatry* 1998;59(Suppl 18):5–9.

72. Lin EHB, Von Korff M, Katon W, et al. The role of the primary care physician in patients' adherence to antidepressant therapy. *Med Care* 1995;33:67–74.

73. Rush AJ, Trivedi MH, Carmody TJ, et al. Response in relation to baseline anxiety levels in major depressive disorder treated with bupropion

sustained release or sertraline. *Neuropsychopharmacology* 2001;25(1):131–138.

74. Rush AJ, Carmody TJ, Haight BR, et al. Does pretreatment insomnia or anxiety predit acute response to bupropion SR? *Ann Clin Psychiatry* 2005;17:1–9.

75. Trivedi MH, Rush AJ, Carmody TJ, et al. Do bupropion SR and sertraline differ in their effects on anxiety in depressed patients? *J Clin Psychiatry* 2001;62(10):776–781.

76. Simon GE, Heiligenstein JH, Grothaus L, et al. Should anxiety and insomnia influence antidepressant selection: A randomized comparison of fluoxetine and imipramine. *J Clin Psychiatry* 1998;59:49–55.

77. Mulrow CD, Williams JW Jr., Trivedi M, et al. Treatment of Depression: Newer Pharmacotherapies. Evidence Report/Technology Assessment No. 7. (Prepared by the San Antonio Evidence-based Practice Center based at the University of Texas Health Science Center at San Antonio under Contract 290-97-0012). AHCPR Publication No. 99-E014. Rockville, MD: Agency for Health Care Policy and Research, 1999.

78. Medical Economics Company. *Physicians' Desk Reference.* Montvale, NJ: Medical Economics Company, 2004.

79. Evans DL, Charney DS. Mood disorders and medical illness: A major public health problem. *Biol Psychiatry* 2003;54(3):177–180.

80. Basco MR, Rush AJ. Compliance with pharmacotherapy in mood disorders. *Psychiatr Ann* 1995;25:269–270, 276, 278.

81. Preskorn SH, Lane RM. Sertraline 50 mg daily: The optimal dose in the treatment of depression. *Int Clin Psychopharmacol* 1995;10: 129–141.

82. Kelsey JE. Dose-response relationship with venlafaxine. *J Clin Psychopharmacol* 1996;16(3 Suppl 2):21S–26S.

83. Fava M, Rosenbaum JF, Cohen L, et al. High-dose fluoxetine in the treatment of depressed patients not responsive to a standard dose of fluoxetine. *J Affect Disord* 1992;25:229–234.

84. Fava M, Rosenbaum JF, McGrath PJ, et al. Lithium and tricyclic augmentation of fluoxetine treatment for resistant major depression: A double-blind, controlled study. *Am J Psychiatry* 1994; 151(9):1372–1374.

85. Nierenberg AA, McLean NE, Alpert JE, et al. Early nonresponse to fluoxetine as a predictor of poor 8-week outcome. *Am J Psychiatry* 1995;152: 1500–1503.

86. Quitkin FM, Petkova E, McGrath PJ, et al. When should a trial of fluoxetine for major depression be declared failed? *Am J Psychiatry* 2003; 160(4):734–740.

87. Judd LL, Akiskal HS, Paulus MP. The role and clinical significance of subsyndromal depressive symptoms (SSD) in unipolar major depressive disorder. *J Affect Disord* 1997;45:5–17.

88. Biggs MM, Shores-Wilson K, Rush AJ, et al. A comparison of alternative assessments of depressive symptom severity: A pilot study. *Psychiatry Res* 2000;96(3):269–279.

89. Rush AJ, Pincus HA, First MB, et al. *Task Force for the Handbook of Psychiatric Measures.* Washington, DC: American Psychiatric Association, 2000.

90. Beck AT, Steer RA, Brown G. *Beck Depression Inventory*, 2nd ed.. San Antonio, TX: The Psychological Corporation, 1996.

91. Rush AJ, Gullion CM, Basco MR, et al. The Inventory of Depressive Symptomatology (IDS): Psychometric properties. *Psychol Med* 1996; 26(3):477–486.

92. Rush AJ, Trivedi MH, Ibrahim HM, et al. The 16-Item Quick Inventory of Depressive Symptomatology (QIDS), clinician rating (QIDS-C), and self-report (QIDS-SR): A psychometric evaluation in patients with chronic major depression. *Biol Psychiatry* 2003;54(5):573–583.

93. Trivedi MH, Rush AJ, Ibrahim HM, et al. The Inventory of Depressive Symptomatology, Clinician Rating (IDS-C) and Self-Report (IDS-SR), and the Quick Inventory of Depressive Symptomatology, Clinician Rating (QIDS-C) and Self-Report (QIDS-SR) in public sector patients with mood disorders: A psychometric evaluation. *Psychol Med* 2004;34(1):73–82.

94. Kroenke K, Spitzer RL, Williams JB. The PHQ-15: Validity of a new measure for evaluating the severity of somatic symptoms. *Psychosom Med* 2002;64(2):258–266.

95. Rush AJ, Bernstein IH, Trivedi MH et al. An evaluation of the Quick Inventory of Depressive Symptomatology and the Hamilton Rating Scale for Depression: a STAR*D report. *Biol Psychiatry* 2005;in press.

96. Rush AJ, Thase ME, Dube S. Research issues in the study of difficult-to-treat depression. *Biol Psychiatry* 2003;53(8):743–753.

97. Sackeim HA. The definition and meaning of treatment-resistant depression. *J Clin Psychiatry* 2001;62(Suppl 16):10–17.

98. Thase ME, Rush AJ. When at first you don't succeed: Sequential strategies for antidepressant nonresponders. *J Clin Psychiatry* 1997;58(Suppl 13):23–29.

99. Sackeim HA, Haskett RF, Mulsant BH, et al. Continuation pharmacotherapy in the prevention of relapse following electroconvulsive therapy: A randomized controlled trial. *JAMA* 2001;285(10): 1299–1307.

100. Souery D, Amsterdam J, de Montigny C, et al. Treatment resistant depression: Methodological overview and operational criteria. *Eur Neuropsychopharmacol* 1999;9(1–2):83–91.

101. Quitkin FM, Rabkin JG, Ross D, et al. Duration of antidepressant drug treatment. What is an adequate trial? *Arch Gen Psychiatry* 1984;41: 238–245.

102. Fava M. Diagnosis and definition of treatment-resistant depression. *Biol Psychiatry* 2003;53(8): 649–659.

103. Fava M, Rush AJ, Trivedi MH, et al. Background and rationale for the sequenced treatment alternatives to relieve depression (STAR*D) study. *Psychiatr Clin North Am* 2003;26(2):457–494.

104. Rush AJ, Crismon ML, Kashner TM, et al. Texas Medication Algorithm Project, phase 3 (TMAP-3): Rationale and study design. *J Clin Psychiatry* 2003;64(4):357–369.

105. Bakish D. New standard of depression treatment: Remission and full recovery. *J Clin Psychiatry* 2001;62 (Suppl 26):5–9.

106. Brown WA, Harrison W. Are patients who are intolerant to one serotonin selective reuptake inhibitor intolerant to another? *J Clin Psychiatry* 1995;56(1):30–34.

107. Zarate CA, Kando JC, Tohen M, et al. Does intolerance or lack of response with fluoxetine predict the same will happen with sertraline? *J Clin Psychiatry* 1996;57(2):67–71.

108. Thase ME, Blomgren SL, Birkett MA, et al. Fluoxetine treatment of patients with major depressive disorder who failed initial treatment with sertraline. *J Clin Psychiatry* 1997;58(1): 16–21.

109. Joffe RT, Levitt AJ, Sokolov ST, et al. Response to an open trial of a second SSRI in major depression. *J Clin Psychiatry* 1996;57(3):114–115.

110. Charney DS. Monoamine dysfunction and the pathophysiology and treatment of depression. *J Clin Psychiatry* 1998;59 (Suppl 14):11–14.

111. McGrath PJ, Stewart JW, Nunes EV, et al. A double-blind crossover trial of imipramine and phenelzine for outpatients with treatment-refractory depression. *Am J Psychiatry* 1993;150: 118–123.

112. McGrath PJ, Stewart JW, Nunes EN, et al. Treatment response of depressed outpatients unresponsive to both a tricyclic and a monoamine oxidase inhibitor antidepressant. *J Clin Psychiatry* 1994;55(8):336–339.

113. Thase ME, Mallinger AG, McKnight D, et al. Treatment of imipramine-resistant recurrent depression, IV: A double-blind crossover study of tranylcypromine for anergic bipolar depression. *Am J Psychiatry* 1992;149(2):195–198.

114. Beasley CM Jr., Sayler ME, Cunningham GE, et al. Fluoxetine in tricyclic refractory major depression. *J Affect Disord* 1990;20:193–200.

115. Fava M. Management of nonresponse and intolerance: Switching strategies. *J Clin Psychiatry* 2000;61 (Suppl 2):10–12.

116. Poirier MF, Boyer P. Venlafaxine and paroxetine in treatment-resistant depression. Double-blind, randomised comparison. *Br J Psychiatry* 1999; 175:12–16.

117. Thase ME, Feighner JP, Lydiard RB. Citalopram treatment of fluoxetine nonresponders. *J Clin Psychiatry* 2001;62:683–687.

118. Thase ME, Ferguson JM, Lydiard RB, et al. Citalopram treatment of paroxetine-intolerant depressed patients. *Depress Anxiety* 2002;16: 128–133.

119. Thase ME, Rush AJ, Howland RH, et al. Double-blind switch study of imipramine or sertraline treatment of antidepressant-resistant chronic depression. *Arch Gen Psychiatry* 2002;59(3): 233–239.

120. Fredman SJ, Fava M, Kienke AS, et al. Partial response, nonresponse, and relapse with selective serotonin reuptake inhibitors in major depression: A survey of current "next-step" practices. *J Clin Psychiatry* 2000;61(6):403–408.

121. Lam RW, Hossie H, Solomons K, et al. Citalopram and bupropion-SR: Combining versus switching in patients with treatment-resistant depression. *J Clin Psychiatry* 2004;65(3):337–340.

122. Fava M, Papakostas GI, Petersen T, et al. Switching to bupropion in fluoxetine-resistant major depressive disorder. *Ann Clin Psychiatry* 2003; 15(1):17–22.

123. de Montigny C, Silverstone PH, Debonnel G, et al. Venlafaxine in treatment-resistant major

depression: A Canadian multicenter, open-label trial. *J Clin Psychopharmacol* 1999;19(5):401–406.

124. Fava M, Dunner DL, Greist JH, et al. Efficacy and safety of mirtazapine in major depressive disorder patients after SSRI treatment failure: An open-label trial. *J Clin Psychiatry* 2001;62(6): 413–420.

125. de Montigny C, Grunberg F, Mayer A, et al. Lithium induces rapid relief of depression in tricyclic antidepressant drug non-responders. *Br J Psychiatry* 1981;138:252–256.

126. Rouillon F, Gorwood P. The use of lithium to augment antidepressant medication. *J Clin Psychiatry* 1998;59 (Suppl 5):32–39.

127. Bauer M, Adli M, Baethge C, et al. Lithium augmentation therapy in refractory depression: Clinical evidence and neurobiological mechanisms. *Can J Psychiatry* 2003;48(7):440–448.

128. Bauer M, Dopfmer S. Lithium augmentation in treatment-resistant depression: Meta-analysis of placebo-controlled studies. *J Clin Psychopharmacol* 1999;19(5):427–434.

129. Price LH, Charney DS, Heninger GR. Variability of response to lithium augmentation in refractory depression. *Am J Psychiatry* 1986;143(11): 1387–1392.

130. Bauer M, Bschor T, Kunz D, et al. Double-blind, placebo-controlled trial of the use of lithium to augment antidepressant medication in continuation treatment of unipolar major depression. *Am J Psychiatry* 2000;157(9):1429–1435.

131. Baumann P, Nil R, Souche A, et al. A double-blind, placebo-controlled study of citalopram with and without lithium in the treatment of therapy-resistant depressive patients: A clinical, pharmacokinetic, and pharmacogenetic investigation. *J Clin Psychopharmacol* 1996;16(4): 307–314.

132. Katona CL, Abou-Saleh MT, Harrison DA, et al. Placebo-controlled trial of lithium augmentation of fluoxetine and Lofepramine. *Br J Psychiatry* 1995;166:80–86.

133. Zullino D, Baumann P. Lithium augmentation in depressive patients not responding to selective serotonin reuptake inhibitors. *Pharmacopsychiatry* 2001;34(4):119–127.

134. Nierenberg AA, Papakostas GI, Petersen T, et al. Lithium augmentation of nortriptyline for subjects resistant to multiple antidepressants. *J Clin Psychopharmacol* 2003;23(1):92–95.

135. Aronson R, Offman HJ, Joffe RT, et al. Triiodothyronine augmentation in the treatment of refractory depression. A meta-analysis. *Arch Gen Psychiatry* 1996;53(9):842–848.

136. Joffe RT. The use of thyroid supplements to augment antidepressant medication. *J Clin Psychiatry* 1998;59(Suppl 5):26–29.

137. Gitlin MJ, Weiner H, Fairbanks L, et al. Failure of T3 to potentiate tricyclic antidepressant response. *J Affect Disord* 1987;13:267–272.

138. Thase ME, Kupfer DJ, Jarrett DB. Treatment of imipramine-resistant recurrent depression: I. An open clinical trial of adjunctive L-triiodothyronine. *J Clin Psychiatry* 1989;50(10): 385–388.

139. Joffe RT, Singer W. A comparison of triiodothyronine and thyroxine in the potentiation of tricyclic antidepressants. *Psychiatry Res* 1990; 32(3):241–251.

140. Joffe RT, Marriott M. Thyroid hormone levels and recurrence of major depression. *Am J Psychiatry* 2000;157(10):1689–1691.

141. Joffe RT, Singer W, Levitt AJ, et al. A placebo-controlled comparison of lithium and triiodothyronine augmentation of tricyclic antidepressants in unipolar refractory depression. *Arch Gen Psychiatry* 1993;50(5):387–393.

142. Joffe RT. Triiodothyronine potentiation of fluoxetine in depressed patients. *Can J Psychiatry* 1992;37(1):48–50.

143. Blier P, Bergeron R. Effectiveness of pindolol with selected antidepressant drugs in the treatment of major depression. *J Clin Psychopharmacol* 1995;15(3):217–222.

144. Vinar O, Vinarova E, Horacek J. Pindolol accelerates the therapeutic action of selective serotonin reuptake inhibitors (SSRIs) in depression. *Homeostatis* 1996;37:93–95.

145. Berman RM, Darnell AM, Miller HL, et al. Effect of pindolol in hastening response to fluoxetine in the treatment of major depression: A double-blind, placebo-controlled trial. *Am J Psychiatry* 1997;154(1):37–43.

146. Moreno FA, Gelenberg AJ, Bachar K, et al. Pindolol augmentation of treatment-resistant depressed patients. *J Clin Psychiatry* 1997; 58(10):437–439.

147. Perez V, Soler J, Puigdemont D, et al. A double-blind, randomized, placebo-controlled trial of pindolol augmentation in depressive patients resistant to serotonin reuptake inhibitors. Grup de Recerca en Trastorns Afectius. *Arch Gen Psychiatry* 1999;56(4):375–379.

148. Perry EB, Berman RM, Sanacora G, et al. Pindolol augmentation in depressed patients resistant to selective serotonin reuptake inhibitors: A double-blind, randomized, controlled trial *J Clin Psychiatry* 2004;65(2):238–243.

149. Artigas F, Perez V, Alvarez E. Pindolol induces a rapid improvement of depressed patients treated with serotonin reuptake inhibitors. *Arch Gen Psychiatry* 1994;51(3):248–251.

150. Martinez D, Broft A, Laruelle M. Pindolol augmentation of antidepressant treatment: Recent contributions from brain imaging studies. *Biol Psychiatry* 2000;48(8):844–853.

151. Rabiner EA, Bhagwagar Z, Gunn RN, et al. Pindolol augmentation of selective serotonin reuptake inhibitors: PET evidence that the dose used in clinical trials is too low. *Am J Psychiatry* 2001;158(12):2080–2082.

152. Blier P, Bergeron R. Effectiveness of pindolol with selected antidepressant drugs in the treatment of major depression. *J Clin Psychopharmacol* 1995;15(3):217–222.

153. Fabre LF. Buspirone in the management of major depression: A placebo-controlled comparison. *J Clin Psychiatry* 1990;51(9 Suppl):55–61.

154. Rickels K, Amsterdam J, Clary C, et al. Buspirone in depressed outpatients: A controlled study. *Psychopharmacol Bull* 1990;26(2):163–167.

155. Rickels K, Amsterdam JD, Clary C, et al. Buspirone in major depression: A controlled study. *J Clin Psychiatry* 1991;52:34–38.

156. Robinson DS, Rickels K, Feighner J, et al. Clinical effects of the 5-HT1A partial agonists in depression: A composite analysis of buspirone in the treatment of depression. *J Clin Psychopharmacol* 1990;10:67S–76S.

157. Bakish D. Fluoxetine potentiation by buspirone: Three case histories. *Can J Psychiatry* 1991;36:749–750.

158. Bouwer C, Stein DJ. Buspirone is an effective augmenting agent of serotonin selective re-uptake inhibitors in severe treatment-refractory depression. *S Afr Med J* 1997;87(4, Suppl):534–537, 540.

159. Dimitriou EC, Dimitriou CE. Buspirone augmentation of antidepressant therapy. *J Clin Psychopharmacol* 1998;18(6):465–469.

160. Harvey KV, Balon R. Augmentation with buspirone: A review. *Ann Clin Psychiatry* 1995;7:143–147.

161. Jacobsen FM. Possible augmentation of antidepressant response by buspirone. *J Clin Psychiatry* 1991;52(5):217–220.

162. Joffe RT, Schuller DR. An open study of buspirone augmentation of serotonin reuptake inhibitors in refractory depression. *J Clin Psychiatry* 1993;54(7):269–271.

163. Appelberg BG, Syvalahti EK, Koskinen TE, et al. Patients with severe depression may benefit from buspirone augmentation of selective serotonin reuptake inhibitors: Results from a placebo-controlled, randomized, double-blind, placebo wash-in study. *J Clin Psychiatry* 2001;62(6):448–452.

164. Landen M, Bjorling G, Agren H, et al. A randomized, double-blind, placebo-controlled trial of buspirone in combination with an SSRI in patients with treatment-refractory depression. *J Clin Psychiatry* 1998;59(12):664–668.

165. Nelson JC. Managing treatment-resistant major depression *J Clin Psychiatry* 2003;64(Suppl 1):5–12.

166. Fawcett J, Kravitz HM, Zajecka JM, et al. CNS stimulant potentiation of monoamine oxidase inhibitors in treatment-refractory depression. *J Clin Psychopharmacol* 1991;11(2):127–132.

167. Feighner JP, Herbstein J, Damlouji N. Combined MAOI, TCA, and direct stimulant therapy of treatment-resistant depression. *J Clin Psychiatry* 1985;46(6):206–209.

168. Linet LS. Treatment of a refractory depression with a combination of fluoxetine and d-amphetamine [letter]. *Am J Psychiatry* 1989;146:803–804.

169. Masand PS, Anand VS, Tanquary JF. Psychostimulant augmentation of second generation antidepressants: A case series. *Depress Anxiety* 1998;7(2):89–91.

170. Metz A, Shader RI. Combination of fluoxetine with pemoline in the treatment of major depressive disorder. *Int Clin Psychopharmacol* 1991;6(2):93–96.

171. Stoll AL, Pillay SS, Diamond L, et al. Methylphenidate augmentation of serotonin selective reuptake inhibitors: A case series. *J Clin Psychiatry* 1996;57(2):72–76.

172. Wharton RN, Perel JM, Dayton PG, et al. A potential clinical use for methylphenidate with tricyclic antidepressants. *Am J Psychiatry* 1971; 127(12):1619–1625.

173. Menza MA, Kaufman KR, Castellanos A. Modafinil augmentation of antidepressant treatment in depression *J Clin Psychiatry* 2000;61:378–381.

174. Markovitz PJ, Wagner S: An open-label trial of modafinil augmentation in patients with partial response to antidepressant therapy *J Clin Psychopharmacol* 2003;23(2):207–209.

175. DeBattista C, Doghramji K, Menza MA, et al. Adjunct modafinil for the short-term treatment of fatigue and sleepiness in patients with major depressive disorder: A preliminary double-blind, placebo-controlled study. *J Clin Psychiatry* 2003; 64(9):1057–1064.

176. Ostroff RB, Nelson JC. Risperidone augmentation of selective serotonin reuptake inhibitors in major depression. *J Clin Psychiatry* 1999;60: 256–259.

177. Pitchot W, Ansseau M. Addition of olanzapine for treatment-resistant depression. *Am J Psychiatry* 2001;158(10):1737–1738.

178. Shelton RC, Tollefson GD, Tohen M, et al. A novel augmentation strategy for treating resistant major depression. *Am J Psychiatry* 2001; 158:131–134.

179. Zhang W, Perry KW, Wong DT, et al. Synergistic effects of olanzapine and other antipsychotic agents in combination with fluoxetine on norepinephrine and dopamine release in rat prefrontal cortex. *Neuropsychopharmacology* 2000; 23:250–262.

180. O'Connor M, Silver H. Adding risperidone to selective serotonin reuptake inhibitor improves chronic depression. *J Clin Psychopharmacol* 1998;18(1):89–91.

181. Viner MW, Chen Y, Bakshi I, et al. Low-dose risperidone augmentation of antidepressants in nonpsychotic depressive disorders with suicidal ideation. *J Clin Psychopharmacol* 2003;23(1): 104–106.

182. Dube S, Andersen S, Paul S. Meta-analysis of olanzapine-fluoxetine use in treatment-resistant depression (Abstract p. 1.021). *J Eur Coll Neuropsychopharmacol* 2002;12(Suppl 3):S182,

183. Papakostas GI, Petersen TJ, Nierenberg AA, et al. Ziprasidone augmentation of selective serotonin reuptake inhibitors (SSRIs) for SSRI-resistant major depressive disorder. *J Clin Psychiatry* 2004;65(2):217–221.

184. Ascher JA, Cole JO, Colin JN, et al. Bupropion: A review of its mechanism of antidepressant activity. *J Clin Psychiatry* 1995;56:395–401.

185. Bodkin JA, Lasser RA, Wines JD Jr., et al. Combining serotonin reuptake inhibitors and bupropion in partial responders to antidepressant monotherapy. *J Clin Psychiatry* 1997;58: 137–145.

186. DeBattista C, Solvason HB, Poirier J, et al. A prospective trial of bupropion SR augmentation of partial and non-responders to serotonergic antidepressants. *J Clin Psychopharmacol* 2003; 23(1):27–30.

187. Fatemi SH, Emamian ES, Kist DA. Venlafaxine and bupropion combination therapy in a case of treatment-resistant depression. *Ann Pharmacother* 1999;33(6):701–703.

188. Spier SA. Use of bupropion with SRIs and venlafaxine. *Depress Anxiety* 1998;7(2):73–75.

189. Mischoulon D, Nierenberg AA, Kizilbash L, et al. Strategies for managing depression refractory to selective serotonin reuptake inhibitor treatment: A survey of clinicians. *Can J Psychiatry* 2000; 45(5):476–481.

190. Ashton AK, Rosen RC: Bupropion as an antidote for serotonin reuptake inhibitor-induced sexual dysfunction. *J Clin Psychiatry* 1998;59(3): 112–115.

191. Walker PW, Cole JO, Gardner EA, et al. Improvement in fluoxetine-associated sexual dysfunction in patients switched to bupropion. *J Clin Psychiatry* 1993;54:459–465.

192. Grigoriadis S, Kennedy SH. Role of estrogen in the treatment of depression. *Am J Ther* 2002;9(6): 503–509.

193. Shapira B, Oppenheim G, Zohar J, et al. Lack of efficacy of estrogen supplementation to imipramine in resistant female depressives. *Biol Psychiatry* 1985;20(5):576–579.

194. Zohar J, Shapira B, Oppenheim G, et al. Addition of estrogen to imipramine in female-resistant depressives. *Psychopharmacol Bull* 1985; 21(3):705–706.

195. Amsterdam J, Garcia-Espana F, Fawcett J, et al. Fluoxetine efficacy in menopausal women with and without estrogen replacement. *J Affect Disord* 1999;55(1):11–17.

196. Rasgon NL, Altshuler LL, Fairbanks LA, et al. Estrogen replacement therapy in the treatment of major depressive disorder in perimenopausal women. *J Clin Psychiatry* 2002;63(Suppl 7):45–48.

197. Schneider LS, Small GW, Hamilton SH, et al. Estrogen replacement and response to fluoxetine in a multicenter geriatric depression trial. *Am J Geriatr Psychiatry* 1997;5:97–106.

198. Schneider LS, Small GW, Clary CM. Estrogen replacement therapy and antidepressant response

to sertraline in older depressed women. *Am J Geriatr Psychiatry* 2001;9(4):393–399.

199. Abou-Saleh MT, Coppen A. The biology of folate in depression: Implications for nutritional hypotheses of the psychoses. *J Psychiatr Res* 1986;20(2):91–101.

200. Abou-Saleh MT, Coppen A. Serum and red blood cell folate in depression. *Acta Psychiatr Scand* 1989;80(1):78–82.

201. Carney MW, Chary TK, Laundy M, et al. Red cell folate concentrations in psychiatric patients. *J Affect Disord* 1990;19(3):207–213.

202. Fava M, Borus JS, Alpert JE, et al. Folate, vitamin B12, and homocysteine in major depressive disorder. *Am J Psychiatry* 1997;154(3):426–428.

203. Taylor MJ, Carney S, Geddes J, et al. Folate for depressive disorders. *Coch Database Syst Rev* 2003;(2):CD003390.

204. Coppen A, Bailey J. Enhancement of the antidepressant action of fluoxetine by folic acid: A randomised, placebo controlled trial. *J Affect Disord* 2000;60:121–130.

205. Haddjeri N, Blier P, de Montigny C. Noradrenergic modulation of central serotonergic neurotransmission: Acute and long-term actions of mirtazapine. *Int Clin Psychopharmacol* 1995;10 (Suppl 4):11–17.

206. Carpenter LL, Yasmin S, Price LH. A double-blind, placebo-controlled study of antidepressant augmentation with mirtazapine. *Biol Psychiatry* 2002;51(2):183–188.

207. Nelson JC, Mazure CM, Bowers MB, et al. A preliminary open study of the combination of fluoxetine and desipramine for rapid treatment of major depression. *Arch Gen Psychiatry* 1991;48: 303–307.

208. Fava M, Alpert J, Nierenberg A, et al. Double-blind study of high-dose fluoxetine versus lithium or desipramine augmentation of fluoxetine in partial responders and nonresponders to fluoxetine. *J Clin Psychopharmacol* 2002;22(4): 379–387.

209. Kapur S, Mann JJ. Role of the dopaminergic system in depression. [Review]. *Biol Psychiatry* 1992;32:1–17.

210. Corrigan MH, Denahan AQ, Wright CE, et al. Comparison of pramipexole, fluoxetine, and placebo in patients with major depression. *Depress Anxiety* 2000;11(2):58–65.

211. Rektorova I, Rektor I, Bares M, et al. Pramipexole and pergolide in the treatment of depression in Parkinson's disease: A national multicentre prospective randomized study. *Eur J Neurol* 2003;10(4):399–406.

212. Sporn J, Ghaemi SN, Sambur MR, et al. Pramipexole augmentation in the treatment of unipolar and bipolar depression: A retrospective chart review. *Ann Clin Psychiatry* 2000;12(3): 137–140.

213. Lattanzi L, Dell'Osso L, Cassano P, et al. Pramipexole in treatment-resistant depression: A 16-week naturalistic study. *Bipolar Disord* 2002;4(5):307–314.

214. Goldberg JF, Burdick KE, Endick CJ. Preliminary randomized, double-blind, placebo-controlled trial of pramipexole added to mood stabilizers for treatment-resistant bipolar depression. *Am J Psychiatry* 2004;161(3):564–566.

215. Izumi T, Inoue T, Kitagawa N, et al. Open pergolide treatment of tricyclic and heterocyclic antidepressant-resistant depression. *J Affect Disord* 2000;61(1–2):127–132.

216. Calabrese JR, Bowden CL, Sachs GS, et al. A double-blind placebo-controlled study of lamotrigine monotherapy in outpatients with bipolar I depression. Lamictal 602 Study Group. *J Clin Psychiatry* 1999;60:79–88.

217. Normann C, Hummel B, Scharer LO, et al. Lamotrigine as adjunct to paroxetine in acute depression: A placebo-controlled, double-blind study. *J Clin Psychiatry* 2002;63(4):337–344.

218. Barbosa L, Berk M, Vorster M. A double-blind, randomized, placebo-controlled trial of augmentation with lamotrigine or placebo in patients concomitantly treated with fluoxetine for resistant major depressive episodes. *J Clin Psychiatry* 2003;64(4):403–407.

219. Fava GA. Well-Being Therapy: Conceptual and technical issues. *Psychother Psychosom* 1999;68: 171–179.

220. Scott J, Teasdale JD, Paykel ES, et al. Effects of cognitive therapy on psychological symptoms and social functioning in residual depression. *Br J Psychiatry* 2000;177:440–446.

221. Ward E, King M, Lloyd M, et al. Randomised controlled trial of non-directive counselling, cognitive-behaviour therapy, and usual general practitioner care for patients with depression. I: Clinical effectiveness. *Br Med J* 2000;321(7273): 1383–1388.

222. Paffenbarger RS Jr, Lee IM, Leung R. Physical activity and personal characteristics associated

with depression and suicide in American college men. *Acta Psychiatr Scand* 1994;(Suppl 377):16–22.

223. Ruuskanen JM, Ruoppila I. Physical activity and psychological well-being among people aged 65 to 84 years. *Age Ageing* 1995;24(4):292–296.

224. Lee IM, Hsieh CC, Paffenbarger RS Jr. Exercise intensity and longevity in men. The Harvard Alumni Health Study. *JAMA* 1995;273(15):1179–1184.

225. Lee IM, Paffenbarger RS Jr. Associations of light, moderate, and vigorous intensity physical activity with longevity. The Harvard Alumni Health Study. *Am J Epidemiol* 2000;151(3):293–299.

226. Berlin JA, Colditz GA. A meta-analysis of physical activity in the prevention of coronary heart disease. *Am J Epidemiol* 1990;132(4):612–628.

227. Wannamethee SG, Shaper AG. Physical activity and the prevention of stroke. *J Cardiovasc Risk* 1999;6(4):213–216.

228. Chipkin SR, Klugh SA, Chasan-Taber L. Exercise and diabetes. *Cardiol Clin* 2001;19(3):489–505.

229. Lee IM, Paffenbarger RS Jr., Hsieh C. Physical activity and risk of developing colorectal cancer among college alumni. *J Natl Cancer Inst* 1991;83(18):1324–1329.

230. Lee IM, Paffenbarger RS Jr., Hsieh CC. Physical activity and risk of prostatic cancer among college alumni. *Am J Epidemiol* 1992;135(2):169–179.

231. Craft LL, Landers DM. The effects of exercise on clinical depression and depression resulting from mental illness: A meta-regression analysis. *J Sport Exerc Psychol* 2005;20:339–357.

232. North TC, McCullagh P, Tran ZV. Effect of exercise on depression. *Exerc Sport Sci Rev* 1990;18:379–415.

233. Lawlor DA, Hopker SW. The effectiveness of exercise as an intervention in the management of depression: Systematic review and meta-regression analysis of randomised controlled trials. *Br Med J* 2001;322(7289):763–767.

234. Blumenthal JA, Babyak MA, Moore KA, et al. Effects of exercise training on older patients with major depression. *Arch Intern Med* 1999;159(19):2349–2356.

235. Babyak M, Blumenthal JA, Herman S, et al. Exercise treatment for major depression: Maintenance of therapeutic benefit at 10 months. *Psychosom Med* 2000;62(5):633–638.

236. Dunn AL, Trivedi MH, Kampert JB, et al. The DOSE study: A clinical trial to examine efficacy and dose response of exercise as treatment for depression. *Control Clin Trials* 2002;23(5):584–603.

237. Mather AS, Rodriguez C, Guthrie MF, et al. Effects of exercise on depressive symptoms in older adults with poorly responsive depressive disorder: Randomised controlled trial. *Br J Psychiatry* 2002;180:411–415.

238. Thase ME, Friedman ES, Howland RH. Management of treatment-resistant depression: Psychotherapeutic perspectives. *J Clin Psychiatry* 2001;62 (Suppl 18):18–24.

239. Dobson KS. A meta-analysis of the efficacy of cognitive therapy for depression. *J Consult Clin Psychol* 1989;57:414–419.

240. Schatzberg AF, Rush AJ, Arnow BA, et al. Chronic depression: medication (nefazodone) or psychotherapy (CBASP) is effective when the other is not. *Arch Gen Psychiatry* 2005;62:513–520.

241. Thase ME, Greenhouse JB, Frank E, et al. Treatment of major depression with psychotherapy or psychotherapy-pharmacotherapy combinations. *Arch Gen Psychiatry* 1997;54(11):1009–1015.

242. Thase ME. When are psychotherapy and pharmacotherapy combinations the treatment of choice for major depressive disorder? *Psychiatr Q* 1999;70(4):333–346.

243. McCullough JP Jr. *Treatment for Chronic depression: Cognitive-behavioral Analysis System of Psychotherapy.* New York: Guilford; 2000.

244. de Jonghe F, Kool S, van Aalst G, et al. Combining psychotherapy and antidepressants in the treatment of depression. *J Affect Disord* 2001;64:217–229.

245. Rush AJ. Strategies and tactics in the management of maintenance treatment for depressed patients. *J Clin Psychiatry* 1999;60(Suppl 14):21–26.

246. Rosenbaum JF, Fava M, Hoog SL, et al. Selective serotonin reuptake inhibitor discontinuation syndrome: A randomized clinical trial. *Biol Psychiatry* 1998;44:77–87.

247. Mueller TI, Keller MB, Leon AC, et al. Recovery after 5 years of unremitting major depressive disorder. *Arch Gen Psychiatry* 1996;53(9):794–799.

248. Thase ME, Howland RH. Refractory depression: Relevance of psychosocial factors and therapies. *Psychiatr Ann* 1994;24:232–240.

249. Greden JF. Clinical prevention of recurrent depression. The need for paradigm shifts. In:

Greden JF (ed.), *Treatment of Recurrent Depression,* 5th ed. Washington, DC: American Psychitric Press, Vol. 20, 2001, pp. 143–170.

250. Greden JF. Recurrent depression—its overwhelming burden. In: Greden JF (ed.), *Treatment of Recurrent Depression,* 5th ed. Washington, DC: American Psychiatric Press, Vol. 20: 2001, pp. 1–18.

251. Frank E, Kupfer DJ, Perel JM, et al. Three-year outcomes for maintenance therapies in recurrent depression. *Arch Gen Psychiatry* 1990;47: 1093–1099.

252. Kupfer DJ, Frank E, Perel JM, et al. Five-year outcome for maintenance therapies in recurrent depression. *Arch Gen Psychiatry* 1992;49: 769–773.

253. Klerman GL, Weissman MM, Rounsaville BJ, et al. *Interpersonal Psychotherapy of Depression.* New York: Basic Books, 1984.

254. Kramer TL, Daniels AS, Zieman GL, et al. Psychiatric practice variations in the diagnosis and treatment of major depression. *Psychiatr Serv* 2000;51(3):336–340.

255. Ornstein S, Stuart G, Jenkins R. Depression diagnoses and antidepressant use in primary care practices: A study from the Practice Partner Research Network (PPRNet). *J Fam Pract* 2000; 49(1):68–72.

256. Institute of Medicine Committee to Advise the Public Health Service on Clinical Practice Guidelines: *Clinical Practice Guidelines. Directions for a New Program.* Washington, DC: National Academy Press, 1990.

257. American Psychiatric Association. Practice guideline for major depressive disorder in adults. *Am J Psychiatry* 1993;150(Suppl 4):1–26.

258. Jobson K. International Psychopharmacology Algorithm Project: Algorithms in psychopharmacology. *Int J Psychiatry Clin Pract* 1997;1(Suppl 1):S3–S4.

259. Kasper S, Jobson K. First European meeting for algorithms on the psychopharmacology of psychiatric disorders. *Int J Psychiatry Clin Pract* 1997;1(Suppl 1):S1.

260. Russell JM, Hawkins K, Ozminkowski RJ, et al. The Cost Consequences of Treatment-Resistant Depression. *J Clin Psychiatry* 2004;65(3): 341–347.

261. Rush AJ, Fava M, Wisniewski SR, et al. Sequenced treatment alternatives to relieve depression (STAR*D): Rationale and design. *Control Clin Trials* 2004;25(1):119–142.

262. Rush AJ, Ryan ND. Current and emerging therapeutics for depression. In: Davis KL, Charney D, Coyle JT, (eds.), *Neuropsychopharmacology. The Fifth Generation of Progress.* Philadelphia, PA: Lippincott Williams & Wilkins, 2002, pp. 1081–1095.

263. Gilbert DA, Altshuler KZ, Rago WV, et al. Texas Medication Algorithm Project: Definitions, rationale, and methods to develop medication algorithms. *J Clin Psychiatry* 1998;59(7):345–351.

264. Rush AJ, Rago WV, Crismon ML, et al. Medication treatment for the severely and persistently mentally ill: The Texas Medication Algorithm Project. *J Clin Psychiatry* 1999;60(5):284–291.

265. Rush AJ, Crismon ML, Toprac MG, et al. Implementing guidelines and systems of care: Experiences with the Texas Medication Algorithm Project (TMAP). *J Pract Psychiatry Behav Health* 1999;5:75–86.

266. Katon W, Von Korff M, Lin E, et al. Population-based care of depression: Effective disease management strategies to decrease prevalence. *Gen Hosp Psychiatry* 1997;19:169–178.

267. Von Korff M, Katon W, Bush T, et al. Treatment costs, cost offset, and cost-effectiveness of collaborative management of depression. *Psychosom Med* 1998;60(2):143–149.

268. Katon W, Von Korff M, Lin E, et al. Collaborative management to achieve treatment guidelines. Impact on depression in primary care. *JAMA* 1995;273:1026–1031.

269. Katon W, Robinson P, Von Korff M, et al. A multifaceted intervention to improve treatment of depression in primary care. *Arch Gen Psychiatry* 1996;53:924–932.

270. Katon W, Von Korff M, Lin E, et al. Stepped collaborative care for primary care patients with persistent symptoms of depression: A randomized trial. *Arch Gen Psychiatry* 1999;56:1109–1115.

271. Unützer J, Katon W, Callahan CM, et al. Collaborative care management of late-life depression in the primary care setting: A randomized controlled trial. *JAMA* 2002;288(22):2836–2845.

272. Adli M, Berghofer A, Linden M, et al. Effectiveness and feasibility of a standardized stepwise drug treatment regimen algorithm for inpatients with depressive disorders: Results of a 2-year observational algorithm study. *J Clin Psychiatry* 2002;63(9):782–790.

273. Katon W, Russo J, Von Korff M, et al. Long-term effects of a collaborative care intervention in

persistently depressed primary care patients. *J Gen Intern Med* 2002;17(10):741–748.

274. Kroenke K, Spitzer RL, Williams JBW. The PHQ-9. Validity of a brief depression severity measure. *J Gen Intern Med* 2001;16:606–613.

275. Nezu AM, Nezu CM, Perri MG. *Problem-Solving Therapy for Depression: Theory, Research, and Clinical Guidelines.* New York: Wiley, 1989.

276. Miller AL, Chiles JA, Chiles JK, et al. The Texas Medication Algorithm Project (TMAP) schizophrenia algorithms. *J Clin Psychiatry* 1999; 60(10):649–657.

277. Suppes T, Swann AC, Dennehy EB, et al. Texas Medication Algorithm Project: Development and feasibility testing of a treatment algorithm for patients with bipolar disorder. *J Clin Psychiatry* 2001;62(6):439–447.

278. Suppes T, Rush AJ, Dennehy EB, et al. Texas Medication Algorithm Project, phase 3 (TMAP-3): Clinical results for patients with a history of mania. *J Clin Psychiatry* 2003;64(4):370–382.

279. Toprac MG, Rush AJ, Conner TM, et al. The Texas Medication Algorithm Project Patient and Family Education Program: A consumer-guided initiative. *J Clin Psychiatry* 2000;61(7):477–486.

280. Rush AJ, Carmody TJ, Reimitz PE. The Inventory of Depressive Symptomatology (IDS): Clinician (IDS-C) and self-report (IDS-SR) ratings of depressive symptoms. *Int J Methods Psychiatr Res* 2000;9:45–59.

281. McCall WV, Reboussin DM, Weiner RD, et al. Titrated moderately suprathreshold vs fixed high-dose right unilateral electroconvulsive therapy: Acute antidepressant and cognitive effects. *Arch Gen Psychiatry* 2000;57:438–444.

282. Sackeim HA, Prudic J, Devanand DP, et al. A prospective, randomized, double-blind comparison of bilateral and right unilateral electroconvulsive therapy at different stimulus intensities. *Arch Gen Psychiatry* 2000;57:425–434.

283. Klein E, Kreinin I, Chistyakov A, et al. Therapeutic efficacy of right prefrontal slow repetitive transcranial magnetic stimulation in major depression: A double-blind controlled study. *Arch Gen Psychiatry* 1999;56(4):315–320.

284. Pascual-Leone A, Rubio B, Pallardo F, et al. Rapid-rate transcranial magnetic stimulation of left dorsolateral prefrontal cortex in drug-resistant depression. *Lancet* 1996;348:233–237.

285. Lisanby SH, Luber B, Schlaepfer TE, et al. Safety and feasibility of magnetic seizure therapy (MST) in major depression: Randomized within-subject comparison with electroconvulsive therapy. *Neuropsychopharmacology* 2003;28(10): 1852–1865.

286. Marangell LB, Rush AJ, George MS, et al. Vagus nerve stimulation (VNS) for major depressive episodes: One year outcomes. *Biol Psychiatry* 2002;51(4):280–287.

287. Rush AJ, George MS, Sackeim HA, et al. Vagus nerve stimulation (VNS) for treatment-resistant depressions: A multicenter study. *Biol Psychiatry* 2000;47(4):276–286.

288. Sackeim HA, Rush AJ, George MS, et al. Vagus nerve stimulation (VNS) for treatment-resistant depression: Efficacy, side effects, and predictors of outcome. *Neuropsychopharmacology* 2001; 25(5):713–728.

289. Rush AJ, Marangell LB, Sackeim HA, et al. Vagus nerve stimulation (VNS) for treatment-resistant depression: A randomized, controlled acute phase trial. *Biol Psychiatry* 2005;in press.

290. Rush AJ, Sackeim HA, Marangell LB, et al. Effects of 12 months of vagus nerve stimulation in treatment-resistant depression: A naturalistic study. *Biol Psychiatry* 2005;in press.

CHAPTER 3

Psychotherapeutic Treatment of Depression and Bipolar Disorder

BRAD A. ALFORD AND AARON T. BECK

In addition to pharmacotherapy, psychologic approaches have been validated in the treatment of clinical depression. The depression-focused psychotherapies that have been subjected to empirical examination include behavior therapy, interpersonal therapy (IPT), and cognitive therapy (CT).[1] In the sections to follow, we briefly describe each of these approaches, as well as consider general psychotherapeutic strategies. A concluding section presents the controlled trials of psychologic versus pharmacologic treatments.

▶ BEHAVIORAL THEORIES AND METHODS

Several behavioral theories of depression have been advanced. Among the early theorists are Ferster,[2] Seligman,[3,4] and Lewinsohn.[5] More recently, McCullough[6] developed a "Cognitive Behavioral Analysis System of Psychotherapy (CBASP)."

Seligman suggested that the phenomena of "learned helplessness" in animal models might be analogous to clinical depression in humans.

Briefly, Seligman found that when a normal dog receives escape-avoidance training, it quickly learns to avoid a shock by moving to the safe side of a shuttle box. However, dogs given inescapable shocks before avoidance training were found to act quite differently. Instead of attempting to escape, they would give up, and passively accept the shock.

Seligman reviewed similar studies with a variety of animals, and observed "learned helplessness" in ". . . rats, cats, dogs, fish, mice, and men."[4] Based on this, he hypothesized a specific reinforcement contingency, i.e., inescapable punishment, to be a causative factor in people who become clinically depressed.

The concepts of Ferster[2] and Lewinsohn[5] likewise make reference to basic behavioral principles to account for clinical depression. Ferster[2] theorizes that depression may be a reduced frequency of "adjustive behavior," or behavior that maximizes reinforcing outcomes. Put simply, the person engages in avoidance and escape behavior in situations where positive reinforcement would be obtained. Conversely, the depressed person develops a passive behavioral repertoire in circumstances where escape would be reinforcing, thus (as in the learned helplessness model) failing to escape punishment.

Like Ferster's theory, Lewinsohn[5] suggested the operant behavioral theoretical concept "reinforcement" to explain the origins of clinical depression. He conceptualized depression as due to (or constituted by) "low rate response-contingent positive reinforcement." He used this basic construct to elucidate other aspects of clinical depression, such as low rates of behavior.

Limitations of the behavioral theories include the observation that behavioral factors alone have not been shown to induce clinical depression. Also, some have concluded that pure behavioral interventions have not been found to be effective treatments for clinically significant depression.[7] Consistent with this, some comprehensive volumes on depression no longer include pure behavioral theories among the significant approaches to etiology and treatment.[8]

When more purely behavioral interventions have been evaluated (and they have not been extensively tested), they typically have done well in controlled trials.[9] In components analysis research, one element of CT of depression, "behavioral activation," has generated some renewed theoretical interest. However, problems remain in trying to disentangle the cognitive from the noncognitive processes (for a review, see Hollon[9]). We further consider the important topic of behavioral activation in the section "General Psychotherapeutic Strategies."

Interpersonal Therapy

In discussing the development of depression, Beck[10] theorized a "circular feedback model" between thoughts and emotions. In this theory, an unpleasant life situation triggers schemas relevant to loss and negative expectancies. Such expectancies, in turn, become activated and stimulate affective structures that are responsible for the subjective feeling of depression. The affective structures further innervate the schemas to which they are connected, reinforcing

the activity of such. Thus, the interaction schemas ↔ affective structures constitutes a reciprocal determinism in generating the depressive syndrome.[10]

Similar to this formulation, Interpersonal Psychotherapy is based on the idea that negative life events can lead to disturbed mood, and vice versa.[11] An interpersonal history is taken (using the *interpersonal inventory*), and the therapist explains the depressive episode in one of two ways: (1) connecting a recent life event to the acute depressive episode or (2) linking a mood episode to a negative impact on the person's interpersonal competence, thus generating problems and distressing life events.[11–13]

Manualized treatment consists of 12–16 weekly sessions that center on solving an interpersonal crisis, such as complicated bereavement, role dispute, role transition, or deficits in relationship skills. The sessions discuss associations between the patient's depressive mood state and relevant life events. The therapist provides social approval for incidents where the patient succeeds in interpersonal encounters. If such an encounter goes badly, the therapist explores with the patient alternative ways to handle future similar interpersonal situations.[11]

IPT for Chronic Depression

Markowitz[12] suggests the adaptation of IPT to chronic forms of unipolar depression. To do so, the identification of recent interpersonal life events is replaced by the recognition and resolution of chronic social skills deficits. The emphasis is on building interpersonal function.

However, according to the few studies conducted to date, the advantages of such an adaptation of IPT appear modest.[12] This is consistent with the opinion of other experts. For example, Eugene S. Paykel, one of the key participants in the original Yale-Boston collaborative trial, reports that the precursor of IPT did not prevent relapse, though continuation of antidepressants did.[14]

A study on the prophylaxis of future depressive episodes using IPT was conducted by Frank et al.[15] They studied 128 patients with recurrent depression in a randomized 3-year maintenance trial. The study site was a specialty clinic with over 10 years' experience in treating recurrent affective disorders.

All participants had previously responded to combined treatment with imipramine and IPT. Active imipramine at an average dose of 200 mg reduced recurrence to only about 22% over the following 3-year period. A maintenance form of IPT alone resulted in a recurrence rate of about 61% over the subsequent 3-year period. Combined active imipramine and maintenance IPT resulted in a recurrence rate of about 24% over 3 years. In patients who did not receive active medication, continued monthly IPT maintenance sessions extended "survival time," or time without recurrence, to greater than 1 year. They concluded that there is a highly significant prophylactic effect for active imipramine therapy, and a modest preventative effect for monthly interpersonal psychotherapy.[15]

IPT for Elderly Populations

Hinrichsen[16] writes on how psychiatric illness strains family relations, and notes that interpersonal factors can influence remission and relapse rates. He suggests that IPT holds promise as a treatment for late-life depression.

Elaborating a treatment rationale for the use of IPT in elderly patient populations, Hinrichsen cites findings of a strong association between expressed emotion (EE) (e.g., expressions of criticism) and psychiatric outcome. Specifically, he notes that sociologists focus on the "rolelessness" and "normlessness" often associated with late life. This is said to parallel IPT's attention to role transitions. In his geriatric psychiatry clinic, IPT is used to focus on the problem of role transitions and interpersonal difficulties. Hinrichsen[16] reports reductions in depressive symptoms in several patients treated with this adaptation of IPT for the elderly.

▶ EXPRESSED EMOTION PREDICTS RELAPSE

Consistent with interpersonal theory, an interpersonal stress hypothesis of depression relapse has been conjectured.[17] The effects of interpersonal stress over time were subjected to empirical scrutiny in a clinical population.

Hayhurst et al.[17] noted that of the four studies on the effects of EE (criticism by significant others within the family), two found a positive association between EE and relapse during acute depressive illness. In their more long-term study, 39 depressed patients and their partners were interviewed individually at 3 monthly intervals for about 1 year.

Patients who fully recovered had partners who were consistently uncritical. Those with residual symptoms during remission had more continuously critical partners. However, the causal sequence of events was questioned.

Rather than criticism leading to depression, Hayhurst et al.[17] concluded that " . . . continuing criticism was a result of continuing depression" (p. 442). As in discussing the development of depression, the idea of a "circular feedback model" might fit here.[10]

The interaction between the negative effects of depressed mood on significant others, and in turn increased criticism from those significant others directed toward the patient, may be the best model of the interpersonal interactions identified in this study. Thus, the interaction would be depressed symptoms ↔ EE (criticism) by family members.

▶ COGNITIVE THERAPY

Beck described the theoretically integrative nature of CT in the following manner: "By working within the framework of the cognitive model, the therapist formulates his therapeutic approach according to the specific needs of a given patient at a particular time. Thus, the therapist may be modifying cognitive processes and/or structure even though he is utilizing predominantly behavioral or abreactive (emotion releasing) techniques."[18]

The technically eclectic procedures used in the standard practice of CT are chosen only when the following criteria are met: (1) the procedures are not inconsistent with cognitive theory; (2) a comprehensive cognitive conceptualization is undertaken in order to match treatment to the patient's introspective limitations, problem solving abilities, and so on; (3) the principles of guided discovery and collaborative empiricism are utilized; and (4) the standard structure of sessions is followed unless there are reasons to deviate from the standard format.[19]

Basic Elements of Cognitive Therapy

Cognitive therapy is the application of cognitive theory to the individual case. In general, the cognitive therapist modifies current thinking to reduce symptoms, and corrects beliefs in order to prevent relapse.

The application to the individual case includes the following basic elements: (1) cognitive assessment, (2) case formulation, (3) treatment goals, (4) educating the patient, (5) identifying negative automatic thoughts and beliefs, (6) logical analysis, (7) testing automatic thoughts and dysfunctional beliefs, (8) homework development, and (9) treatment evaluation. Following a brief consideration of each of these components, we consider how the theory of CT is applied to modify aspects of clinical depression.

There are many related conceptual ingredients to CT, including the breakdown of problems into resolvable units of analysis. The Socratic method and problem definition facilitate the achievement of therapeutic goals, including (1) identifying negative attitudes, (2) pinpointing the most urgent and accessible problem, (3) developing homework strategies, (4) monitoring (recording) homework strategies between therapy sessions, and (5) reviewing problems and accomplishments since the previous session.[18]

The latent cognitive structures/processes implicated in clinical depression are activated through exposure to stressful conditions. These elements are targeted for correction in various ways, as follows:

First, cognitive assessment is carried out in order to obtain baseline information concerning the nature of disordered cognitions that are in need of correction. An individual case formulation is developed that identifies the historical antecedents that are related to the current dysfunction. In providing a case formulation, the cognitive therapist explores with the patient the ideas that could interact with negative events to elicit depressive symptoms.

Next, treatment goals are set in collaboration with the patient. Educating the patient is an essential component of treatment. Indeed, the educative component of a number of diverse psychotherapies may result in reducing a patient's concerns about the meaning of depressive symptoms, thus reducing "depression about depression."

Other essential constituents include identifying negative automatic thoughts and beliefs. The depressed individual will hold absolute and pervasive negative self-referent thinking about the self, world, and future.

Positive self-referent information is often excluded. These basic cognitive processes are identified and individualized as the therapist and the patient work together to identify negative thinking and beliefs, typically using a Daily Record of Dysfunctional Thoughts.

Logical analysis is needed to evaluate the results of "personal experiments." These experiments are designed to test/examine specific negative automatic thoughts identified by means of the thought recordings.

Homework development follows each problem focus in treatment, so that the patient learns the procedures of CT independently. Homework exercises facilitate learning new skills at both the intellectual (rational) and the experiential (automatic processing) level. Patients are taught to disrupt the negatively biased automatic processing and to generate "controlled processing."

Finally, treatment evaluation occurs during and following CT through the use of standardized tests such as the Beck Depression/Hopelessness Scales and a variety of other psychometric devices.

Theorized Processes of Change

In CT, the patient is assisted to develop alternative perspectives and new conceptualizations of personally relevant life events. The intractability with which such biased conceptualizations are often held can be best overcome through *collaborative empiricism*. The patient is guided to actively engage in hypothesis testing. Homework activities are essential to the empirical testing of negative thoughts and beliefs.

Controlled processing may be activated by certain beliefs (e.g., *I don't know, I'm not sure about this*). Like a personal scientist, the depressed patient is guided (through the therapeutic relationship) to question and explore aspects of reality previously subjected to biased processing. In psychotherapy, "distancing" from dysfunctional concept(s) is facilitated. This involves ". . . being able to make the distinction between "I believe" (an opinion that is subject to validation) and "I know" (an irrefutable fact)."[20] Through the process of CT, patients learn that, by changing the content of thoughts, feeling states (depressed mood) may be altered.

All cognitive techniques are designed to directly or indirectly identify, test, and correct dysfunctional thoughts and beliefs. This overall strategy of CT has been summarized as follows: ". . . (CT emphasizes) the *empirical investigation* of the patient's automatic thoughts, inferences, conclusions, and assumptions. We formulate the patient's dysfunctional idea and beliefs about himself, his experiences, and his future into hypotheses and then attempt to test the validity of these hypotheses in a systematic way."[18]

Behavioral Aspects of Cognitive Therapy

From its beginning, CT incorporated the established behavioral principles of operant and classical conditioning.[21] This is probably most apparent in the use of clinical techniques to facilitate engagement with the environment, such as activity schedules and graded task assignment.

One of the core processes of clinical depression is the negative perspectives of self. The depressed person is often quick to accept blame or responsibility for adverse events. Negative events are blamed on the person's imagined lack of effort, talent, or abilities. The technique of reattribution focuses the depressed person's attention on alternative explanations for failure experiences, and tests the negative formulations both through homework assignments (*behavioral* tests) and prior and subsequent logical analysis.

Activity Scheduling

There are many techniques available to increase behavioral activation, and to modify the negative self-concept. Early in therapy, negative cognition content can be modified through encouraging the patient to become involved in constructive activities. *Activity schedules* counter the patient's loss of motivation, fixation on depressive ideas, and negative concepts regarding personal capability.

The specific technique of scheduling the patient's time can facilitate momentum and prevent slipping back into inactivity. The activity schedule focuses on specific goal-directed tasks and furnishes the patient and therapist with specific data on which to realistically evaluate the patient's functional abilities.[18]

Prior to utilizing activity scheduling, several principles should be clear to the patient. These include (1) the idea that no one can accomplish all of their plans; (2) one's goals should be in terms of what kind of actions to take rather than on how much should be accomplished; (3) acceptance of the fact that external uncontrollable factors (interruptions, computer/mechanical failures) and subjective factors (fatigue, motivation) can interfere with progress; and (4) the need to set aside time to plan for the next day. These ideas are intended to counteract negative thoughts about attempting the scheduling task. In scheduling activities, "... the therapist clearly states that the initial purpose of the program is to *observe* and not to *evaluate* how well or how much the patient does each day."[18]

Graded Task Assignment

Activities are categorized as either "mastery" (accomplishment) or "pleasure" (pleasant feelings). These dimensions are rated on a 5-point scale with 0 being no mastery (pleasure), and 5 maximum mastery (pleasure). Graded task assignment modifies schematic content by inducing the patient to recognize *partial successes* and *small degrees* of pleasure, and counteracts dichotomous (all-or-nothing) thinking.[18]

As with activity scheduling, there are several principles of graded task assignment, including: (1) problem definition; (2) formulation of a task; (3) stepwise assignment of activities from simpler to more complex; (4) immediate and direct observation of success experiences; (5) verbalization of the patient's doubts and negative reactions, and minimization of achievements; (6) encouragement of realistic evaluation of performance; (7) emphasis on goal achievement as a result of the patient's own efforts; and (8) the collaborative development of new, more complex goals.[18] All these procedures weaken the patient's beliefs regarding personal inadequacies by providing corrective experiences that, with the therapist's assistance, can form the basis for more realistic interpretations on the part of the patient.

▶ GENERAL PSYCHOTHERAPEUTIC STRATEGIES

Thase et al.[22] suggest several general guidelines or principles for psychotherapeutic intervention, based on their review of depression-focused therapies (cognitive, interpersonal, and behav-

ioral). Among their suggested guidelines are the following: (1) use a collaborative therapy relationship centered on the goal of developing new coping skills; (2) incorporate from other medical models examples of treating chronic disorders; (3) elicit feedback about what has failed to work in the past, while remaining cautiously optimistic about the possibility of improvement; (4) establish stepwise, short-term goals with graded task assignments; (5) have frequent meetings with short sessions, if necessary; (6) use homework and rehearsal to develop skills; (7) meet with and involve significant others in order to enhance alliance and provide psychoeducation; (8) as short-term goals are reached, establish intermediate and long-term ones; and (9) keep the patient in therapy for 4–6 months following therapeutic response.

The modification of cognitive structures is central to the human change process. However, multiple intervention levels (e.g., cognitive, behavioral, experiential, interpersonal, or pharmacologic therapies) may be utilized in order to change the faulty information processing system that theoretically underlies the characteristics of depression. Sustained recovery will occur when the underlying beliefs are corrected, rather than only the negative thinking.

In this section, we elucidate the general cognitive, interpersonal, and behavioral pathways to correct biased information processing. In the present context, "information processing" refers broadly to the interpretation (and concepts) of one's self and one's experiences. We consider the interpersonal, cognitive, and behavioral aspects of change.

One distinguishing characteristic of the examination of one's beliefs is the active monitoring of conscious experience. The "intentional," deliberative control function of conscious experience is accentuated.[20,23,24] This mode is characterized by an increased cognizance of one's experiences and of the manner in which experience is organized or conceptually structured, and stands in contrast to the automatic level in which the person acts with less conscious mediation.

The correction of distressful/dysfunctional emotional states and syndromes can occur through the "reinterpretation" process. This information processing is characterized by an increased cognizance of one's experiences and of the manner in which experience is organized (conceptually structured), and stands in contrast to the automatic level in which the person acts without intentional elaboration.

Beck et al.[18] identified several ways in which this is facilitated, including the observation of negative, automatic thoughts; recognizing correlations between cognition, affect, and behavior; examining evidence for and against specific thoughts; exchanging realistic interpretations for biased cognitions; and learning to identify and modify the predisposing dysfunctional beliefs. However, the correction of distressful and dysfunctional emotional states and syndromes may be activated through diverse routes (e.g., cognitive, behavioral, interpersonal). We next consider the cognification of interpersonal dysfunctions in treating clinical depression.

Modification of Interpersonal Dysfunctions

Thase et al.[22] offer a review of the psychosocial factors that may adversely impact treatment of depression. They note that many of the relevant psychosocial factors that predict poor response to pharmacologic interventions are amenable to psychotherapeutic solutions. These include cognitive or personality factors like neuroticism or pessimism. Other aspects may also be ameliorated through psychologic therapies, but to a smaller degree, factors like low social support, life stress, and chronic adversity.[22]

Interpersonal behaviors associated with a transient dysthymic mood can potentially escalate in a "vicious cycle." Beck[25] cited Bandura's work and the concept *reciprocal determinism* in explicating this phenomenon.

A person's behavior can influence others' behavior toward that person. Negative actions associated with the onset of depression can result in negative interpersonal interactions that then exacerbate the depressed mood.

The first link in the chain leading to depression can be either negative reactions from others, such as rejection, or negative actions on the part of the depressed person toward others, such as withdrawal from social interaction with significant others.

To take the latter as an example, one natural consequence of a depressed person withdrawing from friends and relatives is criticism or rejection by those significant other people. This may exacerbate the depressed person's self-criticism and negative conceptualizations of others, thus leading to further impairment in interpersonal functioning, and thereby to additional negative cognitive processing. This vicious interpersonal-cognitive cycle can deepen the person's depression to the point that intervention by significant others becomes fruitless, thereby necessitating professional treatment.

Of course, such a negative cycle probably accounts for only some cases of clinical depression, since there is individual variation in the impact of interpersonal factors on functioning. Also, for many individuals precipitating social-environmental events appear to play a minimal role in the development and maintenance of depression.[25]

When the individual case formulation suggests a significant role for behavioral/interpersonal dysfunctions, the cognitive therapist works with the patient to (1) increase the patient's cognizance of this phenomenon, (2) incorporate tests of this conceptualization into homework assignments, and (3) provide guidance in the development of more functional conceptualizations as to the meanings attributed to the interpersonal difficulties experienced by the depressed patient. Homework can consist, for example, of relatively simple "behavioral" experiments, such as approaching others and engaging in brief conversations.

As in the standard practice of CT, such exercises are posed as graded tasks so that the likelihood of success is maximized. If the therapist is careful to explain and convey the conceptualization, as elaborated above, then the depressed individual will be better able to understand the treatment rationale, and thereby have reason to persist in correcting the "vicious interpersonal cycle" that can exacerbate the depression. Thus, the cognitive therapist utilizes behavioral and interpersonal techniques in cases that suggest social factors to be implicated in the disorder.

Behavioral Activation

Jacobson et al.[26] found that using only one component of CT, "behavioral activation," was as effective as their application of all the other techniques of CT in terms of altering negative thinking, as well as modifying dysfunctional attributional styles. This would appear to be an important finding, and one that deserves theoretical comment.

A process closely related to facilitating coping, success, and mastery is to reactivate the interest in the person's prior intrinsic life goals (or to develop such goals, if absent). One central aspect of clinical depression is its negative effect on goal-relevant actions. It attenuates motivation to achieve previously valued goals and ambitions.

In order to reactivate the depressed person's interest in persisting toward goals, the therapist and patient list and discuss the actions that were previously "reinforcing" (or valued) but are now latent due to the depressive state. The myriad goals that are typically no longer salient are then arranged in order of priority. These interactions between therapist and patient help to refocus on positive goal-directed activities that the depressed person may (incorrectly) believe are no longer possible. Concrete methods to hypothesis-test the negative predictions in this regard—along with between-session practice of such skills—can help develop a sense of hope and resourcefulness in overcoming one's depressive state.

At times and with certain patients it may be possible, through the influence of the thera-peutic relationship, to make specific suggestions for activity scheduling that patients may carry out, even though they may not yet be convinced such actions will lead to alleviation of depression. In such cases, the process of therapeutic change may properly be conceptualized as an interpersonal influence process whereby the patient agrees to test the cognitive model as suggested by the therapist.

In other words, to facilitate (or *activate*) a depressed person's goal-directed behaviors, the therapist in some cases must engage in a collaborative interpersonal influence process with the patient. If the patient is agreeable, and carries out actions that have in the past brought satisfaction and pride in accomplishment, then the consequences may serve to disconfirm (or deactivate) the negative schematic processing, and thus facilitate the remission of the depressed mode.

An analogy to the scientific method as such provides an effective model of behavioral activation as a method to facilitate empirical tests of thoughts/beliefs in CT. In the initial sessions of CT, a conceptualization of the patient's presenting problem(s) is developed. The most salient questions and focus must be identified. At this point in therapy—as in the "Introduction" sections of scientific reports—clear and *operational* questions are developed.

Operationalization of relevant hypotheses may be brief, a few minutes only, or may take much longer. In either case, the process must set the stage is being set to devise appropriate methods to test out specific hypothesis. The actual test requires something similar to what Jacobson et al.[26] call behavioral activation.

In the case of both the scientific investigator, as well as in the collaborative relationship between cognitive therapist and patient, the crucial test of successful process at this stage is whether reasonable hypotheses are developed which may be tested through the next logical process to be carried out, i.e., developing appropriate methods to evaluate the questions.

In summary, to test beliefs or hypotheses, behavioral actions (*experiments*) are required.[21]

It is made clear to the patient that hypotheses are taken to be neither "true" nor "false," and that, in the absence of proof, it is advantageous to doubt one's preconceived ideas. In this manner, the value of maintaining openness to observation is imparted to the patient. The adaptive value of leaving oneself open to the accommodation of new information (rather than fitting observations exclusively into preexisting molds) is discussed. The patient learns that behavioral experiments are necessary to test ideas.

Modification of Cognitive Functioning

Hartlage et al.[27] identified a number of theorized processes by which negative automatic cognitions can be corrected. They include changing automatically processed self-referent content from negative to positive, deactivation of negative self-referent content by the alleviation of stress, and teaching compensatory skills. They point out that changing automatically processed self-referent content from negative to positive may not be easily accomplished, and suggested specific ideas for techniques to accomplish this.

In order to deactivate negative self-referent content through stress reduction, they suggest the use of organizing skills, problem solving, and discriminating past from present situations (so as to reduce overgeneralization), and the focusing of attention on others in order to reduce negative self-focused attention. In reviewing how to train compensatory skills, they include evaluation of automatic thoughts, the correction of biases in information processing, use of adaptive reattributions, and training to recognize the automatic (and hence recurring) nature of biases.[27]

All of these methods (above) may be of utility in the modification of biased cognitive processing. In the sections to follow, we focus on the following: (1) deactivating hypervalent schemas, (2) modifying schematic content, and (3) reactivating compensatory schemas.

Deactivating Hypervalent Schemas

Schemas developed from previous experience function to organize incoming information about self and context. These cognitions, manifested as verbal or pictorial "events" within the stream of consciousness, influence the person's affect and behavior.

In clinical depression, persons experience biased cognitive processing in a manner that maintains the dysfunctional mode. One basic strategy for the correction of such biases is to deactivate the specific schemas associated with the manifest syndrome.

The personalized concepts that are activated in depression include the following thematic content: low self-regard, ideas of deprivation, self-criticisms and self-blame, overwhelming problems and duties, self-commands and injunctions, and escapist and suicidal wishes. The cognitive processing biases include (among others) arbitrary inference, selective abstraction, overgeneralization, magnification and minimization, and inexact labeling.[10]

Schemas have a number of properties, including (1) breath, (2) flexibility or rigidity, and (3) density.[28] They also differ in the tendency to be active versus latent, and it is this characteristic that is of interest in the process of deactivating dysfunctional schemas.

The practice of CT involves the use of controlled strategic processes to counteract primal negative automatic processing. In deactivating schemas, one method used is the redirection of attentional resources (refocusing). In deactivating a schema, the patient refocuses attention from a particular interpretation. By "allocating" attentional processes to a different task or focus, the overactive schema is terminated.

In addition, biased schematic processing may be deactivated through "behavioral" methods, such as changing the context (environment) so that other more adaptive cognitive processes are activated. However, for sustained improvement it is necessary to directly modify or "restructure" schematic content, which we consider next.

Modifying Schematic Content

One of the ways in which psychologic treatments are theorized to produce change is through the modification of the content of schemas. The therapist focuses on the patient's thoughts and images. Typically, these include low self-concept, deprivation, self-criticism and blame, the perception of overwhelming problems and duties, self-commands and injunctions, escapist thoughts, and sometimes thoughts of suicide.

The thoughts associated with depression generally reflect the patient's beliefs of incompetence, unattractiveness, failure to meet obligations, or social disconnection. These stereotyped responses must be eliminated in order to reduce the intense negative affect, and to allow the patient to focus on his actual, reality-based problems.

Modifying such schematic content requires skilled intervention. The relevant thoughts and beliefs must first be identified. However, since the depressed person's cognitions are automatic, habitual, and plausible, the individual seldom questions the validity of these thoughts.[18]

Negative Cognitive Processing

The cognitive process in clinical depression is relatively undifferentiated. Beck et al.[18] observed that, in depression, the cognitive mode of organizing reality is "primitive." Judgments of life events are broad and global. Meanings are extreme, negative, categorical, absolute, and judgmental, leading to an emotional response that is negative and extreme.

By contrast, more mature thinking harmonizes life situations into multidimensions or qualities rather than a single category. Mature processing is generally quantitative, rather than exclusively in qualitative terms, and standards are relative rather than absolute. Adaptive thinking is characterized by its greater complexity and variability, whereas primal thinking reduces the diversity of human experiences into a few crude categories.[18]

Ideas are seen as "facts" more so in clinical depression than in the nondepressed state. The negative bias becomes exacerbated when the patient behaves in a manner that conforms with the biased thinking. In modifying the negative cognitive processing, the patient learns relevant attentional and recording skills, and comes to recognize the links among certain cognitions and painful affects.

Two standard CT techniques have been designed to increase the patient's objectivity. These involve *reattribution* and *alternative conceptualization*. These techniques teach skills of empirical hypothesis testing so the patient learns to "distance" from thoughts, or to see thoughts as psychologic events.[18,29] The initial focus is the correction of the present thinking in order to provide immediate relief from symptoms. Then the therapist works with the patient to reexamine dysfunctional beliefs in order to prevent relapse.

Reactivating Compensatory Schemas

In this section, we consider ways in which CT can be employed to reactivate compensatory (positive) schemas.

One hypothesis that has been subjected to empirical scrutiny is whether depression is characterized by the exclusion of positive self-referent thinking. Another is that depression is characterized by a selective bias for mood-congruent negative self-referent information that is linked to one's current life concerns. Here we consider ways that cognitive therapists typically treat this aspect of depressive phenomena.

The following are homework experiences that are useful for the activation or development of compensatory schemas: (1) disconfirming the patient's negative predictions; (2) specific coping, success, or mastery experiences; (3) extricating himself or herself from negative circumstances; (4) positive self-focused attention, (5) modification of behavioral/interpersonal dysfunctions. We elaborate how the process of therapy can activate compensatory schemas in each of these specific deficit areas.

Disconfirming Negative Predictions

Consistent with the cognitive negativity hypothesis, depressed persons have been found to make negative predictions about the future.[30] Therefore, one standard CT strategy for facilitating change is to strengthen compensatory conceptual skills in this important area.

The cognitive deficit in question is the inability to conceive or imagine positive outcomes. The depressed individual typically makes negative predictions that then preclude or discourage engagement in the activities in question.

For example, a person may predict rejection in initiating romantic involvement. This prediction then serves to reduce the likelihood the person will (a) initiate conversations, (b) progress to intimate topics of conversation in those cases where contact may be made, and (c) reveal personal romantic interest in potential partners.

To activate compensatory schemas that may already be present (but latent), the cognitive therapist has any number of possible strategies available. For example, a Socratic dialogue can be used to explore previous relationships (if they in fact exist). The therapist prompts memories of reactions to previous efforts to initiate conversations. The memories so prompted, of course, would be quite select memories limited to any previous cases where romantic involvement had been successfully initiated. The therapist is quite directive in this regard, quickly guiding the patient away from irrelevant memories, and toward those of utility.

If this line of questioning is successful (i.e., if it yields outcomes to disconfirm the patient's "overgeneralized" negative predictions), then attention is directed to this specific example from the patient's history. Similar techniques would focus on the outcomes of increased intimacy in conversations, and the patient's revealing personal romantic interest.

In cases where no such positive experiences exist, the therapist aims to develop compensatory schemas. Continuing with the prior example, a depressed patient who predicts rejection and has no positive specific memories may be given directed positive imagery, both within sessions as well as for homework exercises. Such imagery could make use of recalling scenes that the patient has actually observed in real life, at the theater, or in movies (as examples). Thus, compensatory schemas can be developed through vicarious means, or by employing personal specific imagery of desired outcomes.

Coping, Success, and Mastery Experiences

The therapist and patient work together to increase the number and quality of coping, success, and mastery experiences in the patient's everyday life. The interrelated processes of (1) deactivating dysfunctional modes, (2) modifying schematic content, as well as (3) the activation of compensatory schemas may be simultaneously accomplished through this strategy.

Of course, there are as many ways of creatively enhancing positive experiences as there are therapist and patient situations and characteristics. The application of psychotherapy is properly unique to each patient and therapist enterprise.

Despite the above points, one way that cognitive therapists (in particular) have discovered to enhance coping, success, and mastery experiences is *activity scheduling using graded task assignments*. This classic approach simply identifies with the patient those actions that have in the past resulted in a sense of accomplishment and pride on the part of the patient. These activities are then explicitly scheduled for specific days and times during the week, following the strategy of assigning such activities from easy to most difficult. Time spent in each activity should also be considered, calibrated from more time in early assignments to a fading of homework assignments toward the end of therapy. Tasks are organized so the patient does not experience them as overwhelming, since this could be discouraging.

Modifying Negative Circumstances

Persons suffering from clinical depression typically report being the victims of various negative circumstances, which are often blamed for the depressed symptoms. In many cases, such patients are correct in these appraisals. The depressive mode is theorized to be an atavistic survival mechanism that is activated in current environments where its previous adaptive purpose (conservation of resources) is now more counterproductive than useful.

It follows from this that the cognitive therapist and patient must examine the extent to which situations are inevitably negative, versus the degree to which such circumstances may be exaggerated, or otherwise constructed in a negatively biased manner. For example, the breakup of a relationship generally results not only in losses, but also in opportunities for alternative (perhaps more agreeable) relationships. In some cases, exploring new ways of understanding can remove the depressed person from personally devastating negative circumstances that elicited a depressogenic response or interpretation.

Of course, in other cases the depressed person is in a genuinely negative situation. In these cases, the cognitive therapist and patient must work together toward coping. The therapeutic work will generally emphasize the process of learning to accept the imperfections of one's life context, redirection of attention to past or present positive aspects of one's life, and coping behaviors appropriate to the specifics of the stresses experienced.

Positive Self-focused Attention

A core etiologic process in depression is negative perceptions or constructions of the self. The correction of negativity regarding the self is an important part of therapy. One approach to accomplish this is to increase the frequency and duration of positive self-focused attention.

Various strategies may be employed by the therapist and patient to enhance attention to positive aspects of the self. This serves to counteract the tendency of depressed individuals to seek information that depicts the self in an unfavorable manner.

The "behavioral" exercises delineated in the sections above offer clients opportunities to view themselves in a more positive light, thereby modifying negative views of the self. For this reason, such action-oriented strategies are an integral part of therapy with depressed individuals.

▶ INTERPERSONAL ASPECTS OF CHANGE

Several aspects of relationship between therapist and patient have been identified as important in predicting therapy outcome, including alliance, empathy, agreement on goals, and collaboration.[31]

The therapeutic interaction (cognitive, behavioral, emotional exchanges) between the therapist and the patient is the "therapeutic relationship."[32] The idiosyncratic, relatively autonomous nature of the depressed person's biased cognitions can make establishing a therapeutic relationship difficult. Beck et al.[18] explained this disengagement by comparing the depressed person to a purely "cerebral" being; seeing the point of a joke but not being amused; describing positive aspects of significant others without a sense of satisfaction; detecting the appeal of a favored foods or music, but with no sense of enjoyment.[18]

In order to better penetrate the biases, Beck et al.[18] suggested that the therapist keep certain principles in mind during treatment. One of these is that the depressed patient's personal world view (negative ideas and beliefs) appear sensible to the patient, though they may be quite unbelievable to the therapist.

The fact that biased perceptions are plausible to the patient has implications for the manner in which clinical treatment should proceed, in order to better modify the predisposing beliefs. Specifically, steps must be taken to activate the patient's own evaluative processes (processes of critical thought).

The radically different constructions of personal meaning of the therapist and patient can place considerable strain on the interpersonal interactions, making it difficult to establish a collaborative, trusting, and empathic therapeutic context. Thus before an effective psychologic intervention can be introduced, the therapist must nurture a healthy therapeutic relationship, despite holding an opposing perspective to that of the patient.

▶ A COLLABORATIVE CONTEXT

The patient and therapist must assume responsibilities in the development of a therapeutic relationship.[32] To facilitate this relationship, the respective responsibilities must be made clear. The patient's expectations must be articulated, and corrected as needed.

Among the essential areas of agreement are the patient's candid reactions (positive or negative) to treatment. On the part of the therapist, the following: (1) to provide the best treatment possible, and to help the patient apply the principles of therapy; (2) an authentic attempt to understand the patient from the patient's viewpoint; (3) to help develop homework assignments that are agreeable to the patient (i.e., that the patient agrees to carry out); and (4) to take the initiative to direct and guide the development of interventions.

Parallel to the therapist's responsibilities, the patient must accept the following: (1) to provide a good faith effort to master the strategies of clinical treatment; (2) candor in revealing symptoms, thoughts, and the reasons for seeking CT; (3) to fulfill the homework exercises that are necessary for understanding specific problems, and that are essential for the successful implementation of therapy; and (4) to follow the therapist's lead in problem solving by cooperating and assisting with the development of homework experiences. In addition, the patient must accept that effort and personal risk are often required in order to correct longstanding problems.

▶ THERAPIST AS EDUCATOR

All three of the empirically tested therapies for depression are directive, focused, structured approaches.[22] A large part of such guidance by the therapist involves educating the patient regarding the nature and treatment of depression. Thus, part of the interpersonal relationship between the therapist and the patient will include the therapist playing the role of "educator" concerning the application of therapy.

The therapeutic relationship in treatment of depression is highly structured, and specific responsibilities are assumed by therapist and patient.[32] One primary responsibility of the therapist is to develop an accurate understanding of the patient, and of unique aspects of the particular therapeutic relationship. The therapist must understand the patient's view of the therapist and of therapy, and how this changes over time. Also, the therapist must apprehend any errors in the patient's idea of the collaborative therapy process. To take one example of a common misconception, homework is not to be taken as "directions from an expert," but rather as a structured opportunity to test one's thoughts and beliefs.

Homework empowers the patient, since only the patient can determine (and report on) the impact of the various therapeutic techniques utilized outside the therapy sessions. By collaboratively developing homework assignments, and by discussing the outcomes of these activities, the patient learns skills that are generalized to new problem situations that will inevitably arise in the future. This equips the patient to independently resolve problems by applying principles that are learned through repeated applications in homework.

Dependency in psychotherapy can be categorized as either therapeutic or nontherapeutic. *Therapeutic dependency* has been described as an interpersonal position of the patient toward the therapist in which the patient endeavors to learn the cognitive theory (and techniques) as explained by the therapist. *Nontherapeutic dependency* designates an interpersonal stance in which the patient resists the collaborative empirical approach, and persists in relying completely on the therapist (rather than his/her own experience) as an arbiter or source of information.[32]

▶ MAINTAINING A THERAPEUTIC RELATIONSHIP

Safran and Segal[33] coined the term "ruptures" in the therapeutic relationship, referring to problems in working collaboratively with patients in therapy. There are a number of ways in which the working alliance may go awry. In this section, we consider the sources of these difficulties.

Ruptures in the therapeutic relationship are times in therapy when therapist and patient are not working together on common therapeutic goals. This failure can be caused by several factors, such as (1) lapses in effective communication, (2) differences in interpretations or values between therapist and patient concerning the nature of the presenting problems and the actions that might correct such problems, and/or (3) dysfunctional personality strategies (or disorders) that frequently are present along with the depressed mood.

One source is the patient not understanding the rationale of therapy, and/or thinking that the therapist does not understand his or her perspective. In such cases, the therapist must demonstrate an understanding of the patient's perspective. Using the patient's own words can sometimes assist in this regard. The therapist must go back and review any aspects that have been misunderstood, in order to repair the relationship.

Another potential problem stems from the patient's emotional turmoil associated with the depressed state. If the patient is overwhelmed by affect, and can focus only on how bad s/he feels, then the therapist will have difficulty in educating the patient and in providing the other components of effective CT. If the therapist suspects that emotions are so overwhelming that the therapeutic relationship has been damaged, or that establishing such a relationship is problematic, then this issue must be directly discussed with the patient in order to properly understand the cause(s) of the rupture.

Some patients do not carry out the homework assignments that are necessary to obtain information on their negative interpretations. Other patients are very sensitive to criticism, and prone to interpret the therapist's focus as blaming them for their problems. Others fail to self-disclose, keep therapy at a distance, and treat it as an intellectual exercise. Still others may have a hidden agenda (the patient is in therapy to please someone else, e.g., wife or employer), and really does not believe therapy is needed. In all these cases, the therapist must utilize effective listening skills and empathic response to repair the interpersonal difficulties.

▶ PSYCHOTHERAPY VERSUS PHARMACOTHERAPY

The focus of this section is outcome studies of comparing psychologic to pharmacologic treatments. Studies will be considered from more recent to earlier trials, recognizing that (in general) the more recent studies offer more rigorous experimental design and controls.

A number of comprehensive reviews have been written.[34–39] We have limited this review to those studies that provide (1) a convincing basis for the diagnosis of major depression, (2) a comparison to clinical pharmacotherapy, (3) the source of patients treated, (4) the length of therapy, (5) completion rates, and (6) the percentage of patients that recovered following treatment.

Ecologic Validity and Randomized Clinical Trials

The use of randomized-controlled trials (RCTs) to determine the empirically validated (supported) therapies has generated much attention (Kendall, 1998). Chambless and Hollon[40] noted that the term "empirically validated" may suggest that the results of research are definitive in cases where this may not be true, and that using the term "empirically supported" is probably better. Also, randomized clinical trials may differ in several ways from clinical practice.[41] Jonas[42] has identified and responded to several issues in the use of clinical trials: (1) limited numbers and homogeneous groups, (2) short duration, (3) no individualization of therapy, (4) use of surrogate endpoints, (5) significance and usefulness, (6) relevance, (7) data interpretation, and (8) adverse effects.

Chambless and Hollon[40] used the term *efficacy* to refer to the performance of a psychologic treatment in a randomized trial, and *effectiveness* to designate the utility of the treatment in actual clinical practice. For example, a study by Persons et al.[43] have provided empirical support for the clinical *effectiveness* of CT of depression. They compared the outcome of 45 depressed patients treated in a private practice to patients in two RCTs. They found that the private practice patients had more psychiatric and medical comorbidities and a wider range of initial depression severity, but that Beck Depression Inventory (BDI) scores at posttreatment were not different between the private practice and research settings.[43]

The Randomized Clinical Trials

Table 3-1 summarizes the RCTs. Hollon et al.[44] reported on a comparison between CT and imipramine hydrochloride tricyclic pharmacotherapy, singly and in combination. Patients were 107 nonpsychotic, nonbipolar depressed outpatients who were randomly assigned to treatment. Sixty-four percent of patients met criteria for recurrent depression. Of these, 27% had no previous major depressive episodes, whereas 37% did. Of the 107 patients assigned to treatment conditions, 43 (40%) dropped out before completing the 12-week protocol. Thirty-eight (35%) began but did not complete treatment, and five (5%) failed to begin treatment. These rates of drop out did not differ significantly across the treatments. However, medications were more likely to result in problem reactions that prevented continuation. Two participants died by suicide, using study medication.[37,44]

The Hollon et al.[44] study found no differences of symptom measures between the treatment groups (CT vs. drugs). Also, the sample as a whole was rated to be at least as severely depressed as the National Institute of Mental Health-Treatment of Depression Collaborative Research Project (NIMH-TDCRP)[45] as well as other comparable studies. Results found all three groups (drug, CT, and combined drug and CT) improved substantially from pretreatment to midtreatment (first 6 weeks). Greater than 90% of clinical improvement was found to occur within the first 6 weeks of treatment compared to the next 6 weeks, and only the combined CT + drugs group continued to improve between 6 weeks (midtreatment) and 12 weeks (posttreatment).

Bowers[46] evaluated the treatment of 33 inpatients who were divided into three groups, including (1) CT plus medication, (2) medication (nortriptyline) alone, and (3) relaxation therapy plus medication. All patients received "ward milieu." At sessions 1, 6, 12, and at discharge, symptoms of depression and related cognitive variables (automatic thoughts and dysfunctional attitudes) were assessed. It was found that, in all groups, depressed symptoms and cognitive variables improved as a result of treatment. However, the group receiving CT plus ward milieu improved the most by the time of discharge.

The NIMH Collaborative study[45] is among the many studies that have addressed the question of effectiveness. Elkin et al.[45] compared the

► TABLE 3-1 TRIALS OF COGNITIVE THERAPY OF DEPRESSION

Study	Overall Conclusions	Patients Entering Treatment	Source(s) of Patients	Basis for Depression Diagnosis	Length of Therapy	Treatment Comparisons	Treatment Completion Rates	% Recovered	% Remaining well After Recovery
Hollon et al. (1992)	CT is as effective as drugs or combined cognitive drug treatment	107: M = 20%, F = 80%	(1) Psychiatric treatment facility, (2) mental health center	Research Diagnostic Criteria, BDI, GAS, HRSD, MMPI, MMPI-D, RDS	12 weeks	(1) CT (n = 16), (2) PH (n = 32), (3) CT + PH (n =16)	(1) CT = 64%, (2) PH = 56%, (3) CT + PH = 64%	(1) CT = 50%, (2) PH = 53%, (3) CT + PH = 75%	Not reported
Bowers (1990)	CT + drugs is more effective than drugs alone or drugs and relaxation	33: M = 20%, F = 80%	Psychiatric hospital inpatients	ATQ, BDI, DAS, HRSD, HS	(1) CT + PH = 29 days, (2) PH = 32 days, (3) PH + relaxation = 27 days	(1) CT + PH (n =10), (2) PH (n = 10), (3) PH + relaxation (n =10)	(1) CT + PH = 91%, (2) PH = 91%, (3) PH + relaxation = 91%	(1) CT + PH = 80%, (2) PH = 20%, (3) PH + relaxation = 10%	Not reported
Elkin et al. (1989)	CT is as effective as drug treatment	239: M = 30%, F = 70%	(1) Psychiatric outpatients, (2) self-referrals, (3) mental health facilities	Research Diagnostic Criteria, BDI, GAS, HRSD, HSCL	16 weeks	(1) CT (n = 37), (2) IPT (n = 47), (3) IMI-CM (n = 37), (4) PLA-CM (n = 34)	(1) CT = 68%, (2) IPT = 77%, (3) IMI-CM = 67%, (4) PLA-CM = 60%	(1) CT = 51%, (2) IPT = 55%, (3) IMI-CM = 57%, (4) PLA-CM = 29%	Not reported
Miller et al. (1989)	CT adds to the effectiveness of pharmaco-therapy for severely depressed patients	46: M = 26%, F = 74%	Psychiatric hospital inpatients	Diagnostic Interview Schedule, BDI, HRSD	During hospita-lization + 20 weeks	(1) CT (n = 15), (2) PH (n = 17), (3) Social skills training (n = 14)	(1) CT = 67%, (2) PH = 59%, (3) social skills training = 86%	(1) CT = 80%, (2) PH = 41%, (3) social skills training = 50%	Not reported
Covi and Lipman (1987)	CT and CT + PH are more effective than traditional therapy	70: M = 40%, F = 60%	Newspaper ads	Research Diagnostic Criteria, BDI, HRSD	14 weeks of individual and group therapy	(1) CT (n = 27), (2) CT + PH (n = 23), (3) traditional group psychotherapy (n = 20)	(1) CT = 84%, (2) CT + IMI = 68%, (3) TRAD = 83%	(1) CT = 52%, (2) CT + IMI = 61%, (3) traditional therapy = 5%	Not reported

Study	Finding	Sample	Setting	Criteria/Measures	Duration	Treatment groups			
Beck et al. (1985)	CT alone is as effective as combined cognitive-drug treatment	33: M = 27%, F = 73%	(1) Self-referrals, (2) professional referrals	Feighner's Diagnostic Criteria, BDI, HRSD	12 weeks, 20 sessions	(1) CT (n = 18), (2) CT + PH (n = 15)	(1) CT = 78%, (2) CT + PH = 73%	(1) CT = 71%, (2) CT + PH = 36%	(1) CT = 58%, (2) CT + PH = 82%
Murphy et al. (1984)	CT alone is as effective as combined cognitive-drug treatment	87: M = 26%, F = 74%	Psychiatric outpatient hospital	Research Diagnostic Criteria, BDI, HRSD	12 weeks	(1) CT (n = 24), (2) PH (n = 24), (3) CT + PH (n = 22), (4) CT + active placebo (n = 17)	(1) CT = 79%, (2) PH = 67%, (3) CT + PH = 82%, (4) CT + active placebo = 100%	(1) CT = 53%, (2) PH = 56%, (3) CT + PH = 78%, CT + active placebo = 65%	Not reported
Blackburn et al. (1981)	While CT + drugs was most effective, CT alone was more effective than drugs alone	88: M = 28%, F = 72%	(1) Hospital outpatient clinics, (2) a general practice clinic	Research Diagnostic Criteria, BDI	12–15 weeks	(1) CT (n = 22), (2) PH (n = 20), (3) CT + PH (n = 22)	(1) CT = 73%, (2) PH = 71%, (3) CT + PH = 73%	(1) CT = 77%, (2) PH = 60%, (3) CT + PH = 86%	Not reported
Rush et al. (1977)	CT was more effective than drugs	41: M = 37%, F = 63%	Moderate and severe hospital outpatients	Feighner's Diagnostic Criteria, BDI, HRSD	12 weeks, 20 sessions	(1) CT (n = 19), (2) PH (n = 22)	(1) CT = 95%, (2) PH = 64%	(1) CT = 79%, (2) PH = 22%	(1) CT = 67%, (2) PH = 38%

Abbreviations: 1. Measures used—ATQ = automatic thoughts questionnaire; BDI = Beck depression inventory; CRT = cognitive response test; DAS = dysfunctional attitudes scale; GAS = global assessment scale; GIS = global improvement scale; HRSD = Hamilton rating scale for depression; IDA = irritability, depression & anxiety (mood rating scale); LIFE-II-II = longitudinal interval follow-up evaluation II; MADS = Montgomery & Asberg depression scale; PSR = psychiatric status ratings; RDS = Raskin depression scale; SCL-90 = Hopkins symptom checklist; VAS = visual analogue scale.

2. Treatment comparisons—CT = cognitive therapy; PH = pharmacotherapy; IPT = interpersonal therapy; PLA-CM = placebo + clinical management; IMI-CM = IMI-CM + clinical management; TAU = treatment as usual.

effectiveness of CT to that of IPT, imipramine hydrochloride plus "clinical management (CM)," and placebo plus CM (see Table 3-1). The experimenters randomly assigned 250 patients to the respective treatments. Of this number, 239 patients ($M = 30\%$; $F = 70\%$) actually entered treatment. The diagnosis of major depression was obtained by utilizing Research Diagnostic Criteria. The overall conclusions of Elkin et al.[45] were stated as follows: "In analyses carried out on the total samples without regard to initial severity of illness (the primary analyses), there was no evidence of greater effectiveness of one of the psychotherapies as compared with the other and no evidence that either of the psychotherapies was significantly less effective than the standard reference treatment, imipramine plus clinical management."[45] Patients showed significant reduction in measures of depression across treatments. Table 3-1 shows completion rates and percentage of patients recovering for each of the four treatment comparisons.

Among the group of patients in Elkin et al.[45] who were more severely depressed, differences in favor of drug treatment were found on a minority of relevant comparisons.[45] However, research site differences were found in the more severely depressed patients.[47] More specifically, differential effects of specific treatments were observed between sites. The authors concluded: "Until we unravel these findings, final judgment must be withheld about the specific effectiveness of the two psychotherapies with more severely depressed and impaired patients."[45] Several other important issues concerning this study were reviewed by Jacobson and Hollon,[47,48] and interested readers may refer directly to their critique.

Miller et al.[49] were interested in the question of whether CT might produce additional improvement in patients who were provided a standard regime of "hospital milieu," pharmacotherapy, and brief supportive psychotherapy (Table 3-1). Patients were recruited from the inpatient units at Butler Hospital, a private psychiatric hospital in Rhode Island. To study the possible incremental efficacy of CT, they ran-

domly assigned 47 depressed inpatients to one of three conditions. (Of these 47 patients, 46 actually entered treatment.) The patients in this study generally had an early onset, chronic course (mean of 6.7 previous depressive episodes), and 44% had a concurrent diagnosis of dysthymia. Treatments included (1) a "standard treatment" of hospital milieu, pharmacotherapy, medication, and management sessions; (2) CT + standard treatment; and (3) social skills training + standard treatment. The hospital milieu treatment component consisted of several hospital activities that were standard treatment for all inpatients, such as meetings with nurses, occupational therapy, social work evaluations. In order to provide the best possible pharmacotherapy, the usual procedure of increasing dosages of a single medication was replaced by utilizing at least 150 mg/day of two different medications thought to work through modification of different neurotransmitters. The medication protocol allowed much flexibility on the part of treating physicians, including the use of other types of agents such as neuroleptics and antianxiety drugs.

Both the CT and social skills training treatments began after the second week of hospitalization and continued for a 20-week outpatient period. In both therapies, flexibility was allowed in the frequency of sessions provided. The three treatments began during hospitalization and continued after discharge for a period of 20 weeks. Categorical analyses of outcomes defined "responders" in three ways: (1) a BDI score of 9 or less; (2) a modified Hamilton Rating Scale for Depression (HRSD) score of less than 7; and (3) a SCL-90 General Symptom Index of at least 50% improvement from pretreatment symptom levels. Results across the three definitions were fairly consistent. Table 3-1 shows the percentage of responders as defined by HRSD scores at the end of outpatient treatment to be 805 response rate for CT, 41% response rate for standard treatment, and 50% response rate for social skills training. The CT and social skills training groups were significantly lower than the standard treatment group at the end of outpatient treatment, but not at the time of discharge from the hospital. Compared to pretreatment symptom levels, all treatment groups showed significant improvement both at the time of discharge from the hospital and at the end of outpatient treatment.

Covi and Lipman[50] evaluated whether the addition of drug treatment to CT would result in greater clinical improvement than CT alone (Table 3-1). Participants were 70 individuals ($M = 40\%$; $F = 60\%$) recruited from advertisements placed in daily newspapers. Participants met criteria for primary major depression based on Research Diagnostic Criteria. Those selected had depression of at least 1-month duration, cutoff scores of 20 on the BDI, and 14 on the HRSD. These criteria were reviewed by an independent evaluator, a highly experienced psychiatrist who did not have access to the initial ratings. The independent evaluator was blind to the treatment conditions throughout treatment, and provided follow-up evaluations. Treatment was conducted both in individual sessions and in group sessions, 15 patients per group. Therapists were a psychiatrist and a psychologist who had 2 years' training in CT. The treatment comparisons were CT ($n = 27$), CT + imipramine treatment ($n = 23$), and traditional psychotherapy ($n = 20$), which was based on "interpersonal-psychoanalytic" theories and provided a credible (placebo) control treatment. Results showed that end-point remission rates were 52% for CT alone, 61% for CT plus imipramine treatment, and 5% for interpersonal-psychoanalytic (traditional) psychotherapy. These differences were statistically significant at the end of therapy, and at 3- and 9-month follow-up, both for the independent physician-rated Global Improvement Scale (GIS) and the BDI. Data were not reported on the percentage of each group remaining well after recovery.

Beck et al.[51] tested whether the combination of drugs and CT improve the efficacy of either treatment alone in outpatients with nonbipolar depression (see Table 3-1). Prior knowledge of CT and potential expectation biases were similar for the two groups. The research protocol was 20 sessions over a 12-week period.

Therapists were three psychiatrists and six psychologists who had at least 6 months of experience prior to seeing their first study patient. Results showed comparable therapy completion rates for the two groups, both groups improved substantially during therapy, and there were no differences between the two groups in the magnitude of the improvement of depressive symptoms. During the short-term treatment phase, the use of tricyclic antidepressant medication along with CT did not improve the response obtained by CT alone. Seventy-one percent of those patients treated with CT markedly or completely recovered, compared to 36% of those treated with CT plus pharmacotherapy.

At 12 months following treatment, the findings were that 58% remained well for the group that received CT alone, and 82% for the combined treatment. This might suggest a nonsignificant trend of greater stability of gains for the combined treatment. However, this difference at 12 months is probably the result of the patients in the combined group receiving more therapy during the follow-up period compared to the CT group alone. Ninety-one percent of patients in the combined treatment group received additional therapy during the 12-month follow-up period, whereas only 71% of those who received CT alone sought additional treatment. Those receiving combined treatment had more CT sessions (14.81 additional sessions) during follow-up period compared the CT alone group (5.93 sessions).[51]

Murphy et al.[52] assigned 87 moderately to severely depressed psychiatric outpatients to 12 weeks of CT ($n = 24$), pharmacotherapy ($n = 24$), CT plus pharmacotherapy ($n = 22$), or CT plus active placebo ($n = 17$) (Table 3-1). The Diagnostic Interview Schedule, BDI, and HRSD were among the instruments used as the basis for the depression diagnosis. Seventy patients (18 males, 52 females) completed the 12-week treatment protocol. CT consisted of 50-min sessions twice weekly for 8 weeks, then weekly, for the remaining 4 weeks. Those receiving combined cognitive and pharmacotherapy were seen on this same schedule but for 60 min per session. The group that received pharmacotherapy alone was seen for 20 min weekly. The CT plus active placebo group was given placebo capsules that had a mild sedative and anticholinergic effects similar to actual medication. The completion rates were 79% for CT, 67% for pharmacotherapy, 82% for combined treatment, and 100% for CT plus active placebo. Thus, 70 of the original group of 87 patients continued in therapy to the end of treatment, and dropout rates did not differ statistically among the four treatment groups.

Those participants who completed treatment showed significant improvement from initial evaluation to termination on BDI and the HRSD. The differing treatments did not produce significantly different improvement rates. The percentage of patients who recovered in each treatment modality were calculated using diverse cutoff scores of the BDI and HRSD. Using BDI scores of less than or equal to 9, the percentages of each group that recovered were 53% for CT, 56% for drugs, 78% for CT plus drugs, and 65% for CT plus active placebo. Overall conclusions were that CT alone is as effective as combined cognitive-drug treatment. Either CT or antidepressant drug treatment was effective with nonbipolar moderate to severe depression. Gains in all groups were continued 1 month after treatment termination.

Blackburn et al.[53] found CT alone to be more effective than drugs alone, while CT plus drugs was most effective (Table 3-1). There were two selection criteria for the study participants: (1) Research Diagnostic Criteria and (2) at least mild depressive symptoms as measured by BDI scores (greater than or equal to 14 according to British norms). One-hundred and forty patients were screened, and eighty-eight were selected, from teaching hospital outpatient clinics and a general practice clinic. They were randomly assigned to CT, antidepressant drugs, and a combination of these two treatments. Sixty-four patients completed the trial. Attrition rates were equal across the three groups, with completion rates being 73% for CT, 71% for antidepressant drugs, and 73% for the combination of both treatments.

Overall recovery rates were 73% for patients treated with CT, 55% for those treated with pharmacotherapy, and 82% for combined CT and drugs. The antidepressant drug group (typically 150 mg/day of amitriptyline or clomipramine) responded more poorly in both hospital and general practice. In both settings, the combination treatment was superior on seven mood measures to drug treatment alone. In general practice, CT alone was superior to drug treatment alone. The response of endogenous and nonendogenous subgroups was equivalent across treatments.

Rush et al.[54] randomly assigned a sample of 15 males and 26 females to either CT or antidepressant medication (imipramine hydrochloride) (see Table 3-1). The patients were moderately to severely depressed hospital outpatients, and the majority of whom had previously been treated with psychotherapy and/or antidepressant medications. Twenty-two percent had been previously hospitalized, 12% had a previous suicide attempt, and 75% reported suicidal ideation. The sample had a median of 2 previous therapists, 2.9 previous episodes of depression, and 39% had been depressed for longer than 1 year at the time of the study.

Both CT and drugs were provided over a 12-week period, with a maximum of 20 sessions for CT or 12 sessions of pharmacotherapy. Completion rates were significantly lower for pharmacotherapy (64% completion rate) as compared with CT (95% completion rate). On both clinical ratings as well as self-report measures, CT was found to be more effective than pharmacotherapy. This finding was true both for patients who completed treatment and for the entire sample admitted to treatment. Recovery rates (BDI < 10) were 79% for CT, and 22% for pharmacologic treatment.

Overall Conclusions

As concluded by the Task Force on Promotion and Dissemination of Psychologic Procedures,[55]

CT of depression has been found to be an effective treatment for clinical depression. Chambless and Hollon[40] have suggested that a more appropriate term is "empirically supported" to make clear the point that research continues, rather than being entirely conclusive. For example, one important unresolved issue in need of further research is whether the combination of CT with pharmacotherapy is better than either alone.

Three of the RCTs reviewed here[53,46,56] suggest there might be an advantage to the combined treatments (see Table 3-1). Also, a meta-analysis by Thase et al.[57] suggest that combined therapy may be superior to either CT alone or IPT alone in treating more severe recurrent depressions. Their data analysis included 595 patients with major depressive disorder (MDD) who were treated in six standardized protocols. [57]

CT has generally proven to be a superior treatment for depression when compared to minimal treatment controls and alternative interventions.[58] Studies have demonstrated its efficacy in comparisons with no treatment or wait-list in college students, adult outpatients, community volunteers, geriatric populations.[58] In addition, it has been found effective compared with behavioral interventions, and dynamic, interpersonal, and nondirective therapies.[34,58]

Using the BDI in computing effect sizes, a meta-analysis of 56 studies (all studies published before January, 1991) found CT to be at least as effective as drug therapy, combined therapies, or other diverse psychotherapies in the treatment of depression.[34,59] Greater efficacy for CT is found on the BDI but not on the HSRD (perhaps because the BDI is more sensitive in detecting levels of depression, or maybe because the BDI detects cognitive changes specifically). At the same time, the follow-up BDI scores in Dobson et al.[58] showed that CT was no better than pharmacotherapy, combination therapy, or "other" therapies. This was said to be equivocal, however, because (1) subjects who relapse were usually not included in follow-up data which gives more favorable results than may

actually be the case, (2) variables between treatment termination and follow-up may account for differences between groups, and (3) follow-up varied among studies.[58]

Aspects of the NIMH-TDCRP study remain puzzling. The CM plus placebo condition showed as much improvement as active treatments in previous studies. CM included the provision of support, encouragement, and direct advice that perhaps resulted in greater engagement in activities and a sense of mastery and pleasure.[60] Concerning the treatment of more severe depression, research site differences were found.[47] McLean and Taylor[61] examined treatment-by-severity interactions with depressed outpatients, and concluded the NIMH trial findings could not be replicated, and that this failure to replicate was not due to treatment differences, populations, or statistical power.[61] Ahmed et al.[62] critique the status of RCTs in the psychiatric literature, and suggest that a single such trial is not sufficient to guide clinical practice.

The TDCRP is also inconsistent with findings of Jarrett et al.[63] Jarrett et al. conducted a 10-week, double-blind, randomized-controlled trial comparing CT or CM plus either phenelzine or placebo. Response rates on 21-item HRSD were 58% for CT, 58% for phenelzine, and 28% for placebo. This study suggests that CT is equally as effective as monoamine oxidase inhibitors (MAOIs).[64,65] Given all these questions and anomalies, we agree with the following conclusion on the TDCRP: "Until we unravel these findings, final judgment must be withheld about the specific effectiveness of the two psychotherapies with more severely depressed and impaired patients."[45]

▶ RELAPSE PREVENTION

Major depressive disorders are now understood to be chronic rather than an acute illness.[66] There are reasons to believe that CT prevents relapse.[36] Table 3-2 summarizes the randomized clinical trials that provide data on relapse prevention.

► **TABLE 3-2** PERCENTAGE OF PATIENTS REMAINING WELL

Study	Source(s) of Patients	Treatment Comparisons	% Recovered	% Remaining well after Recovery	Definition of "Remaining well"	Follow-up Period	Follow-up Conclusions
Evans et al. (1992) [follow-up on Hollon et al. (1992)]	(1) Psychiatric treatment facility (2) mental health center	(1) CT (n = 10), (2) PH (n = 10), (3) CT + PH (n = 13), (4) PH continuation (n = 11)	(1) CT = 70%, (2) PH =20%, (3) CT + PH = 55%, (4) PH continuation = 77%	(1) CT = 79%, (2) PH =50%, (3) CT + PH = 85%, (4) PH continuation = 68%	No two consecutive BDI scores of 16 or above	4,8,12, 16, 20, and 24 months	CT alone or with drugs reduces relapse rates by >50%
Shea et al. (1992) [follow-up on Elkin et al. (1989)]	(1) Psychiatric outpatients, (2) self-referrals, (3) mental health facilities	(1) CT (n = 59), (2) IPT (n = 61), (3) IMI-CM (n = 57), (4) PLA-CM (n = 62)	(1) CT = 49%, (2) IPT = 40%, (3) IMI-CM = 38%, (4) PLA-CM = 31%	(1) CT = 28%, (2) IPT = 17%, (3) IMI-CM = 15%, (4) PLA-CM = 18%	Absence of MDD criteria and receiving no treatment	6, 12, and 18 months	Though not statistically significant, the results favored cognitive therapy
Blackburn et al. (1986) [follow-up on Blackburn et al. (1981)]	(1) Hospital outpatient clinics, (2) a general practice clinic	(1) CT (n = 22), (2) PH (n = 20), (3) CT + PH (n = 22)	(1) CT = 77%, (2) PH = 60%, (3) CT + PH = 86%	(1) CT = 77%, (2) PH = 22%, (3) CT + PH = 79%	BDI of 8 or less and HRSD of 7 or less	2 years	CT alone or with PH was more effective than drugs alone
Simons et al. (1986) [follow-up on Murphy et al. (1984)]	Psychiatric outpatient hospital	(1) CT (n = 24), (2) PH (n = 24) (3) CT + PH (n = 22), (4) CT + active placebo (n = 17)	(1) CT = 53%, (2) PH = 56%, (3) CT + PH = 78%, (4) CT + active placebo = 65%	(1) CT = 100%, (2) PH = 33%, (3) CT + PH = 83%, (4) CT + active	BDI of 15 or lower and not reentering treatment	1 year	CT is more effective for preventing relapse than drugs
Kovacs et al (1981) [follow-up on Rush et al. (1977)]	Moderate and severe hospital outpatients	(1) CT (n = 19), (2) PH (n = 25)	(1) CT = 83%, (2) PH = 29%	(1) CT = 67%, (2) PH = 35%	BDI of 9 or lower	1 year	CT is more effective than drugs

84

To review individual studies, Evans et al.,[67] a follow-up on Hollon et al.,[36] monitored patients who were successfully treated during a 3-month period with either imipramine hydrochloride pharmacotherapy, CT, or combined cognitive-pharmacotherapy. The initial sample included 107 nonbipolar, nonpsychotic outpatients from a psychiatric treatment facility and a mental health center. To be included in the follow-up, patients had to both complete and respond to treatment. Of the 64 patients who completed treatment, 50 showed at least partial treatment response and were found to be sufficiently remitted to be considered as part of the post-treatment follow-up. Of these, 44 participated in the follow-up. Participants were observed during a 2-year posttreatment follow-up period, during which half of the patients treated with pharmacotherapy alone were continued on study medications for the first year of the follow-up. This medication-continuation condition included 11 participants, and there were 10 in the medication, no continuation group, 10 in the CT group, and 13 in the combined cognitive-pharmacotherapy group. Except for the medication-continuation participants, patients continued treatment only through the termination of the acute treatment phase. Findings showed that those treated with CT (alone or in combination with drugs) were only half as likely to relapse as those patients placed in the "medication-no continuation" condition. Moreover, the rate of relapse for those treated with CT was no greater than patients who were provided with continuation medication. Conclusions were that relapse may be prevented by using CT during acute treatment.

Similar findings come from Shea et al.[68] who conducted a naturalistic 18-month follow-up of outpatients with MDD treated in the NIMH-TDCRP (see Table 3-2). The treatments tested in the NIMH-TDCRP included 16 weeks of CT, IPT, imipramine hydrochloride plus CM, or placebo plus CM. The follow-up assessments were conducted at 6, 12, and 18 months. With relapse defined as either major depressive disorder or additional treatment, the following rates of "recovery and remained well" were found for each of the four treatments: 28% (13 patients out of 46) for CT group, 17% (9 of 53) for IPT, 15% (7 of 48) for imipramine plus CM group, and 18% (9 of 51) for placebo plus CM. Though not reaching statistical significance, as in Evans et al.[67] the results favored CT.

Blackburn et al.[69] addressed the question of the prophylactic effect of CT using a naturalistic follow-up period of 2 years (see Table 3-2). Participants were those patients who had responded to CT, pharmacotherapy, or combined CT plus drug therapy (see Blackburn et al.[70]). The researchers adopted Klerman's definition for relapse, which is the return of symptoms within 6–9 months of treatment. A naturalistic methodology was adopted, meaning that in the follow-up period (as in the treatment period, Blackburn et al.[70]) physicians followed their normal practice with regard to the medications prescribed. Maintenance medications were stipulated to continue for at least 6 months. Sixty-four patients who had completed treatment and responded to treatment were included in the study. Positive response rates were 77% for CT (across referral sources), 60% for pharmacotherapy, and 86% for combined CT and drugs. Patients in the pharmacotherapy treatment group experienced greater relapse rates at 6 months, and more recurrences over the 2-year follow-up, compared to the combined or CT treatment groups. Recurrence rates were as follows: 17% for CT; 75% for pharmacotherapy, and 33% for combined CT and drugs. Thus, the percentage of patients who remained well over follow-up differed substantially between the CT groups compared to pharmacotherapy alone (see Table 3-1).

Simons et al.[71] compared the relapse rates of 70 patients with nonbipolar affective disorder who had previously completed a 12-week course of either CT, pharmacotherapy, CT plus active placebo, or CT plus pharmacotherapy.[72] Assessment was conducted 1 month, 6 months, and 1 year after termination of active treatment.

In the original study,[72] 70 patients completed treatment, and 44 responded as defined by BDI scores of less than 10 at termination of therapy. Twenty-eight of these 44 responders remained well, and 16 relapsed. When the researchers defined "responders" as those patients who had BDI scores of less than 4 at termination, 26 remained well.[71] Using these 26 patients, statistical tests of remission rates between groups found that CT and CT + active placebo were significantly more like to remain well for the 1-year follow-up period (CT vs. PH: generalized Wilcoxon = 4.12, $P = 0.04$; CT + active placebo vs. PH: generalized Wilcoxon = 5.42, $P = 0.02$).[71] Percentage of patients remaining well was 100% for CT, 100% for CT + active placebo, 33% for pharmacotherapy, and 83% for CT + pharmacotherapy. Those patients who had relatively high levels of remaining depressive symptoms following treatment relapsed more often than those who showed no residual depression (BDI scores of less than 10 following treatment). Relapse was also related to higher scores on a measure of dysfunctional attitudes.

Kovacs et al.[73] provided a follow-up of Rush et al.[54] (see Table 3-2). This study used Feighner's Diagnostic Criteria, the Hamilton Rating Scale, and the BDI to select 44 hospital clinic outpatients suffering from at least a moderate level of clinical depression. Seventeen men and 27 women were assigned randomly to either CT or imipramine hydrochloride. The average length of treatment was 11 weeks and 20 sessions. Completion rates were 95% for the CT patients, and 64% for the pharmacotherapy group. The clinical status was compared between groups at 1-year posttreatment. Results found no significant between-groups differences, although the trends favored CT. Self-ratings of depressive symptoms on the BDI showed 67% of those treated with CT remained free of symptoms at 1-year follow-up, compared to 35% of those treated with imipramine.

Averaging across studies, the patients treated with CT had a relapse rate of only 30% compared to a relapse rate of 69% for those patients treated with pharmacotherapy alone. The definition of "relapse" differed across these five studies (see Table 3-2). Also, note that the percentages reported here differ slightly from those cited in Hollon et al.[36] This is because here we are including Shea et al.[68] which was not available earlier. Hollon et al.[36] reported a relapse rate of 26% for patients treated to remission with CT versus 64% for pharmacotherapy. Thus, data so far indicate that, compared to drug therapy, there may be a relapse preventative effect resulting from the application of CT top clinical depression. In addition, one study has shown that continuation phase CT may reduce depressive relapse/recurrence.[65]

There is some evidence to support the possibility that by modifying cognition, control over other symptoms follows. Rush et al.[73] conducted an analysis of the data collected by Rush et al.[74] to evaluate the temporal order of changes in views of the self, hopelessness, mood, motivation, and vegetative symptoms. Findings of the study were that patients improved first on measures of hopelessness, followed by improvement in self-view, motivation, mood, and vegetative symptoms. This was not found to be true for drug treatment.

A number of other methodological issues remain. Therapy outcomes are better when conducted by therapists who are committed to a particular approach to treatment, and the mechanisms of this effect are not known.[47,48] Treatment integrity is also an issue for future research. The effective application of therapy depends upon considering unique patient characteristics, the context of the depressive episode, and the case formulation.

Outcome measures must be designed to detect treatment effects, such as the modification of cognitive, behavioral, and interpersonal factors that may relate to relapse prevention. Individual-subject analyses are needed in order to better identify individual differences in the speed of response, course of response, direction of response (improvement or deterioration), and degree of end-point improvement. Dropout rates must be understood both in terms of the interpersonal processes that may be implicated in such outcomes, as well as in terms of patient characteristics that may predict dropout.

▶ BIPOLAR DISORDER: PSYCHOTHERAPY PREVENTS RELAPSE

Since the time of Campbell's *Manic-Depressive Disease* (1953), the treatment of bipolar disorder has undergone great innovation. This is especially true in the last decade.[71]

For mania, at least five placebo-controlled studies show that lithium produces short-term recovery rates twice as high as the 25–35% found with placebo and nonspecific management. In bipolar disorder, a review of 28 studies with a total of 2985 participants found recurrence risk to be 3.2-fold lower during lithium treatment. None of the clinical factors thought to contradict the utility of lithium were supported, including (1) mixed manic-depressive states, (2) multiple episodes, (3) long history of untreated disorder, and (3) rapid cycling.[71]

The question of the possible utility of psychotherapies for relapse prevention is especially relevant, given the natural course of bipolar affective disorder. Despite the value of lithium in long-term prevention of relapse, full protection (zero recurrences) over 1 year is obtained in only about one-third of patients.[71] A randomized trial in bipolar patients by Colom et al.[75] tested whether psychologic-educational intervention can reduce relapse when added to standard pharmacotherapy.

Study participants included 120 bipolar outpatients matched for age and sex (Young Mania Rating Scale score <6, HDRCScale 17 score <8). All had been in remission for at least 6 months prior to the study, and all were receiving standard pharmacologic treatment. Subjects received standard psychiatric care, plus either 21 sessions of group psychoeducation or 21 nonstructured group meetings. Assessment was conducted monthly during the treatment period and throughout the 2-year follow-up.

By the use of group psychoeducational procedures, they found that only 38% of those in the educational group relapsed, compared to 60% in the control group, during the 21-week treatment period. At the end of a 2-year follow-up period, 92% of those receiving only standard psychiatric care (pharmacologic treatment) had experienced relapse compared to 67% of those in whom a psychoeducational component was added. By excluding mild episodes (hypomania) from the data analysis, recurrence rates were found to be 87% for standard drug therapy versus 63% in the psychoeducational group approach.[75]

Citing two promising pilot studies, Lam et al.[76] used a randomized-controlled design to study the effects of CT for relapse prevention for bipolar affective disorder. In conjunction with mood stabilizers, they hypothesized CT might be well suited to teaching patients to cope with bipolar illness.

A treatment-manual based CT was devised which added to the standard approach used in treating depression. New elements included the following specific areas of focus: (1) teaching the diathesis-stress model, and the need for combining psychologic and medical approaches; (2) monitoring mood, especially prodromal symptoms, and developing skills to obviate expansion of the full-blown syndrome; (3) in order to avoid sleep deprivation acting as a trigger for a bipolar episode, the value of sleep and routine were addressed; and (4) treatment of compensatory behaviors, or extreme striving, which patients sometimes use to make up for time perceived to have been lost during previous periods of illness.

The study design included 103 patients with bipolar 1 disorder. All had relapsed frequently, despite being treated with mood stabilizers. Subjects were randomized into a CT group or control group, with both groups receiving mood stabilizers and regular psychiatric follow-up. The CT group received an average of 14 sessions of CT during the first 6 months and 2 booster sessions in the second 6 months.

Results found an overall relapse rate of 53% during the 12-month treatment period. Relapse rate for the CT group was 28% at month 6, and

44% at month 12. Relapse rate for the control group was 50% at month 6, and 75% at month 12. In addition, the CT group had significantly fewer days in a bipolar episode, and a smaller number of admissions for bipolar episode. Moreover, they showed significantly higher social functioning, less mood symptoms on the monthly mood questionnaires, and significantly less fluctuation in manic symptoms.

Compared to the use of psychoeducational procedures, reviewed above[75] it might be noted that CT produced a lower relapse rate (28%) compared to educational therapy (38%) at a comparable time in treatment (month 6). Moreover, the CT group relapse rate of only 44% at month 12 (vs. 75% for the control group) appears substantially less than the 67% rate found using lithium alone for long-term relapse prevention.[77] Limitations of this study were said to include the absence of controls for sleep routine, and better medication compliance in the patients receiving CT.[76]

▶ TESTING COGNITIVE THEORY: PROCESSES OF CHANGE

Several studies have addressed the process of CT within randomized clinical trials. Simons et al.[78] tested the lasting benefit of CT compared to a 3-month treatment of antidepressant medication (without medication continuation). The authors, based on their findings, concluded that CT and pharmacotherapy may differ in how they lead patients to consider their depressive symptoms.

In CT, patients come to view their symptoms as "cues for hope," or as reminders to strive to use the various cognitive and behavioral strategies they have learned from their therapist. Such learned coping skills may account for the differential effects between CT and pharmacotherapy that were observed in this study.[78]

Robins and Hayes[38] concluded that studies support specific components of CT to be associated with change: ". . . interventions designed to identify, reality test, and correct distorted conceptualizations and the dysfunctional schemata that underlie them."[38] Teaching hypothesis-testing by means of concrete methods and between-session practice of such skills appear to be active ingredients of CT, but ". . . further research is clearly warranted."[38]

Rush et al.[73] conducted an analysis of the data collected by Rush et al.[74] which compared 35 patients treated with CT ($n = 18$) or pharmacotherapy (imipramine HCl) ($n = 17$). Patients were unipolar depressed outpatients. Rush et al.[73] used cross-legged panel analyses to evaluate the temporal order of changes in views of the self, hopelessness, mood, motivation, and vegetative symptoms. Findings of the study were that, during weeks 1–2 of treatment, patients improved first on measures of hopelessness, followed by improvement in self-view, motivation, mood, and vegetative symptoms. During weeks 2–3, hopelessness preceded improvement in mood. Finally, from weeks 3 to 4 self-view and mood improved before motivation, and mood changed prior to vegetative symptoms. Overall conclusions were that CT may lead to therapeutic changes in cognitive factors (view of self and future), and thereafter to improvements in other symptoms. This was not found to be true for drug treatment. Findings are consistent with the hypothesis that alterations in negative thinking and mood leads to improvements in other depressive symptoms.

For relapse prevention, change may be necessary at the "structural" or schematic level. If a schema is sufficiently permeable, then it should be possible to modify its content, or "beliefs." For example, a schema—that is, its content—can be modified from dysfunctional to functional. A person may have a low-level schema "I am a failure," or even more dysfunctional, "Since I am a failure, I am worthless." These beliefs could be modified to the following, "I have failed at some things and succeeded at others so its a trade-off." Also, "Even if I am a failure, it does not mean I am worthless."

The dysfunctional schemas become prepotent when they are activated, usually through a congruent external stimulus, but possibly also through some internal, endocrine, or other biologic derangement. Consistent with this, Segal and Ingram[79] reviewed the issue of the activation of schemas, and concluded that those studies that have ensured the activation of the cognitive constructs to be tested have been supportive of cognitive theory. They suggest that future studies must do a better job of triggering diathesis-stress processes in order to test the causal role of theorized constructs.

Finally, Oei and Free[80] reviewed 44 outcome or process studies of therapy with depression. The categories of treatment included CT, drug therapy, other-psychologic therapy, and wait-list controls. They concluded that cognitive change occurs in all treatments, and that the relationship between cognitive change and depression is not unique to CT. Cognitive change may be the final pathway to change across diverse systems of therapy.

▶ ISSUES FOR FURTHER STUDY

One of the most important questions for continuing research is the preventative effect of the psychotherapeutic treatments. For example, CT is theorized to achieve a prophylactic action through modification of the depressotypic schemas.[81] As a collaborative endeavor, CT enhances self-knowledge and personal responsibility. The depressed individual views self, world, and future as bleak, hopeless, and without personal meaning or control. Through CT, personal control is restored, and the negativity is undermined. The patient learns to be "realistically optimistic" that, regardless of the perceived and/or objective difficulties, some degree of personal control over symptoms can be achieved. Further studies are needed to determine whether any or all of these components contribute to relapse prevention.

The modification of schematic content—or the correction of negative thinking and beliefs—are the central therapeutic processes of CT of depression. One speculative theoretical issue is whether depression is best understood as a deficit of positive schemas, or as an overabundance of negative ones. Also, is it the relative presence of each of these categories of cognitive processing/structure that characterizes the depressive disorders, or is it, rather, some absolute quantity of either deficit or excess that activates the depressive mode? In any case, the development, activation, or reactivation of positive or compensatory schemas is another (perhaps equivalent) method to treat negative cognitive processing, and needs further examination.

DeRubeis et al.[82] studied the issue of whether pharmacotherapy or CT works better for severe depression. They compared the outcomes of antidepressant medication and cognitive behavior therapy in the severely depressed outpatient subgroups of four major randomized trials. Also, they evaluated the results obtained in the NIMH-TDCRP with the other three studies. Their analysis of effect sizes showed no advantage of antidepressant medication over CT with severely depressed outpatients.[82] This finding is in need of further empirical validation.

Jacobson and Hollon[47] have written on how difficult it is to adequately determine competence in the application of CT. The competent therapist response at any given point in treatment is determined by (1) idiosyncratic patient characteristics, (2) the issues that are the focus of treatment, (3) the specific issues that have already been dealt with, and (4) the overall case conceptualization. Thus, to rate the competence of a given therapist response requires a knowledge of the entire context of therapy, rather than merely asking raters to rate a specific session without the benefit of what came before and the case formulation guiding CT with a specific case. Thus, assessing therapist competence is in need of further refinement.

Thase et al.[22] suggest the inability to adhere to treatment is responsible for as many as one-third of antidepressant nonresponders. Better medication compliance has been found in patients receiving CT.[76] This is an important discovery. Research should attempt to identify the robustness of this finding, as well as the mechanisms of action (if replication is obtained).

A further question that must be addressed is how to handle the fact that there are technical and conceptual overlaps between CT and other therapies (e.g., IPT), and that these are sometimes eliminated in the interest of therapy differentiation in clinical trials. As one example, a comparison among CT, IPT, and supportive psychotherapy (with and without imipramine) described IPT as follows: "interpersonal psychotherapy connects life events to mood episodes (1) to help patients mourn life upheavals while (2) pragmatically and optimistically encouraging them to find new life goals and adjustments."[83] Yet, CT likewise could be described in this manner, and as typically practiced in clinical settings (as reviewed above) would incorporate the "interpersonal" pragmatic goals.

Finally, Teasdale[84] advanced the idea that the educative component of a number of diverse psychotherapies may reduce a patient's concerns about the depressive symptoms. Through providing information and guidance to patients, and helping them to see the symptoms of depression as normal features of a well-defined psychologic state, there may be a reduction in "depression about depression." This educative aspect of CT has been hypothesized as an important source of clinical improvement, and has been discussed in detail elsewhere.[29] Process-oriented clinical research is needed to examine this cognitive thesis.

REFERENCES

1. Chambless DL, Ollendick TH. Empirically supported psychological interventions: Controversies and evidence. *Ann Rev Psychol* 2001;52:685–716.
2. Ferster CB. Behavioral approaches to depression. In: Friedman RJ, Katz MM (eds.), *The Psychology of Depression: Contemporary Theory and Research*. New York: Wiley, 1974, pp. 29–45.
3. Seligman MEP, Groves D. Non-transient learned helplessness. *Psychon Sci* 1970;19:191–192.
4. Seligman MEP. Depression and learned helplessness. In: Friedman RJ, Katz MM (eds.), *The Psychology of Depression: Contemporary Theory and Research*. Washington, DC: Hemisphere, 1974, pp. 29–45.
5. Lewinson PM. A behavioural approach to depression. In: Friedman RJ, Katz MM (eds.), *The Psychology of Depression*. Washington, DC: Winston & Sons, 1974.
6. McCullough JP. *Treatment for Chronic Depression*. New York: Guilford, 2000.
7. Dubovsky SL, Buzan R. Mood disorders. In: Hales RE, Yudofsky SC, Talbott JA (eds.), *Textbook of Psychiatry*. Washington, DC: American Psychiatric Press, 1999, pp. 479–565.
8. Gotlib IH, Hammen CL (eds.), *Handbook of Depression*. New York: Guilford, 2002.
9. Hollon SD, Haman KL, Brown LL. Cognitive behavioral treatment of depression. In: Gotlib IH, Hammen CL (eds.), *Handbook of Depression*. New York: Guilford, 2002, pp. 383–403.
10. Beck AT. *Depression: Causes and Treatment*. Philadelphia, PA: University of Pennsylvania Press, 1967.
11. Markowitz JC. Learning the new psychotherapies. In: Weissman MM (ed.), *Treatment of Depression: Bridging the 21st Century*. Washington, DC: American Psychiatric Press, 2001, pp. 135–149.
12. Markowitz JC. Interpersonal psychotherapy for chronic depression. *J Clin Psychol* 2003;59(8): 847–858.
13. Weissman MM, Markowitz JC, Klerman GL. *Comprehensive Guide to Interpersonal Psychotherapy*. New York: Basic Books, 2000.
14. Paykel ES. Treatment of depression in the United Kingdom. In: Weissman MM (ed.), *Treatment of Depression: Bridging the 21st Century*. Washington, DC: American Psychiatric Press, 2001, pp. 135–149.
15. Frank E, Kupfer DJ, Perel JM, et al. Three-year outcomes for maintenance therapies in recurrent depression. *Arch Gen Psychiatry* 1990;47:1093–1099.
16. Hinrichsen GA. Interpersonal psychotherapy for depressed older adults. *J Geriatr Psychiatry* 1997;30:239–257.
17. Hayhurst H, Cooper Z, Paykel ES, et al. Expressed emotion and depression: A longitudinal study. *Br J Psychiatr* 1997;171:439–443.
18. Beck AT, Rush JA, Shaw BF, et al. *Cognitive Therapy of Depression*. New York: Guilford, 1979.
19. Beck AT. Cognitive therapy: A 30-year retrospective. *Am Psychol* 1991;46:368–375.
20. Beck AT. *Cognitive Therapy and the Emotional Disorders*. New York: International Universities Press, 1976.

21. Beck AT. Role of fantasies in psychotherapy and psychopathology. *J Nervous Mental Dis* 1970; 150(1):3–17.

22. Thase ME, Friedman ES, Howland RH. Management of treatment-resistant depression: Psychotherapeutic perspectives. *J Clin Psychiatr* 2001;62(18):18–24.

23. Moore RG. It's the thought that counts: The role of intentions and meta-awareness in cognitive therapy. *J Cogn Psychother Int Quart*, 1996;10:255–269.

24. Reisberg D. *Cognition: Exploring the Science of Mind*. New York: Norton, 1997.

25. Beck AT. Cognitive therapy of depression: New perspectives. In: Clayton PJ, Barrett JE (eds.), *Treatment of Depression: Old Controversies and New Approaches*. New York: Raven Press, 1982, pp. 265–290.

26. Jacobson NS, Dobson KS, Truax PA, et al. A component analysis of cognitive-behavioral treatment for depression. *J Consult Clin Psychol* 1996;64: 295–304.

27. Hartlage S, Alloy LB, Vazquez C, et al. Automatic and effortful processing in depression. *Psychol Bull* 1993;113:247–278.

28. Beck AT, Freeman A, Davis D, et al. *Cognitive Therapy of Personality Disorders*. New York: Guilford, 1990.

29. Beck JS. *Cognitive Therapy: Basics and Beyond*. New York: Guilford, 1995.

30. Haaga DAF, Dyck MJ, Ernst D. Empirical status of cognitive theory of depression. *Psychol Bull* 1991;110:215–236.

31. Norcross JC (ed.). *Psychotherapy Relationships that Work: Therapist Contributions and Responsiveness to Patients*. Oxford: Oxford University Press, 2002.

32. Alford BA, Beck AT. Therapeutic interpersonal support in cognitive therapy. *J Psychother Integr* 1997;7:275–289.

33. Safran JD, Segal ZV. *Interpersonal Process in Cognitive Therapy*. New York: Basic Books, 1990.

34. Dobson KS. A meta-analysis of the efficacy of cognitive therapy for depression. *J Consult Clin Psychol* 1989;57(3):414–419.

35. Hollon SD, Beck AT. Cognitive and cognitive-behavioral therapies. In: Garfield SL, Bergin AE (eds.), *Handbook of Psychotherapy and Behavior Change*, 4th ed. New York: Wiley, 1994, pp. 428–466.

36. Hollon SD, DeRubeis RJ, Seligman MEP. Cognitive therapy and the prevention of depression. *Appl Prevent Psychol* 1992;1:89–95.

37. Hollon SD, DeRubeis RJ, Evans MD. Cognitive therapy in the treatment and prevention of depression. In: Salkovskis PM (ed.), *Frontiers of Cognitive Therapy*. New York: Guilford, 1996, pp. 293–317.

38. Robins CJ, Hayes AM. An appraisal of cognitive therapy. *J Consult Clin Psychol* 1993;61:205–214..

39. Sacco WP, Beck AT. Cognitive theory and therapy. In: Beckham EE, Leber WR (eds.), *Handbook of Depression*. New York: Guilford, 1995, pp. 329–351.

40. Chambless DL, Hollon SD. Defining empirically supported therapies. *J Consult Clin Psychol* 1998;66:7–18.

41. Goldfried MR, Wolfe BE. Psychotherapy practice and research: Repairing a strained alliance. *Am Psychol* 1996;51:1007–1016.

42. Jonas WB. Clinical trials for chronic disease: Randomized, controlled clinical trials are essential. *J NIH Res* 1997;9:33–39.

43. Persons JB, Bostrom A, Bertagnolli A. *Results of Randomized Controlled Trials of Cognitive Therapy for Depression Generalize to Private Practice*. Paper Presented at the 30th Annual Convention of the Association for the Advancement of Behavior Therapy, New York, 1996.

44. Hollon SD, DeRubeis RJ, Evans MD, et al. Cognitive therapy and pharmacotherapy for depression: Singly and in combination. *Arch Gen Psychiatry* 1992;49:774–781.

45. Elkin I, Shea MT, Watkins JT, et al. National Institute of Mental Health Treatment of Depression Collaborative Research Program: General effectiveness of treatments. *Arch Gen Psychiatry* 1989;46:971–982.

46. Bowers WA. Treatment of depressed in-patients: Cognitive therapy plus medication, relaxation plus medication, and medication alone. *Br J Psychiatr* 1990;156:73–78.

47. Jacobson NS, Hollon SD. Cognitive behavior therapy vs pharmacotherapy: Now that the jury's returned its verdict, it's time to present the rest of the evidence. *J Consult Clin Psychol* 1996;64: 74–80.

48. Jacobson NS, Hollon SD. Prospects for future comparisons between drugs and psychotherapy: Lessons from the CBT versus pharmacotherapy exchange. *J Consult Clin Psychol* 1996;64:104–108.

49. Miller IW, Norman WH, Keitner GI, et al. Cognitive-behavioral treatment of depressed inpatients. *Behav Therap* 1989;20:25–47.

50. Covi L, Lipman RS. Cognitive behavioral group psychotherapy combined with imipramine in major depression. *Psychopharmacol Bull* 1987;23: 173–176.

51. Beck AT, Hollon SD, Young JE, et al. Treatment of depression with cognitive therapy and amitriptyline. *Arch Gen Psychiatry* 1985;42: 142–148.

52. Murphy GE, Simons AD, Wetzel RD, et al. Cognitive therapy and pharmacotherapy: Singly and together in the treatment of depression. *Arch Gen Psychiatry* 1984;41:33–41.

53. Blackburn IM, Bishop S, Glen AIM, et al. The efficacy of cognitive therapy in depression: A treatment trial using cognitive therapy and pharmacotherapy, each alone and in combination. *Br J Psychiatr* 1981;139:181–189.

54. Rush AJ, Beck AT, Kovacs M, et al. Comparative efficacy of cognitive therapy and pharmacotherapy in the treatment of depressed outpatients. *Cogn Therap Res* 1977;1:17–37.

55. Task Force on Promotion and Dissemination of Psychological Procedures, Division of Clinical Psychology. Training in and dissemination of empirically-validated psychological treatments: Report and recommendations. *Clin Psychol*, 1995;48:3–23.

56. Miller IW, Norman WH, Keitner GI, et al. Cognitive-behavioral treatment of depressed inpatients. *Behav Therap* 1989;20:25–47.

57. Thase ME, Greenhouse JB, Frank E, et al. Treatment of major depression with psychotherapy or psychotherapy-pharmacotherapy combinations. *Arch Gen Psychiatry* 1997;54:1009–1015.

58. Hollon SD, Shelton RC, Davis DD. Cognitive therapy for depression: Conceptual issues and clinical efficacy. *J Consult Clin Psychol* 1993;61: 270–275.

59. Dobson KS, Pusch D, Jackman-Cram S. Further evidence for the efficacy of cognitive therapy for depression: Multiple outcome measures and long-term effects. Paper presented at the 25th Annual Convention of the Association for the Advancement of Behavior Therapy, New York, 1991. Fink M. ECT has proved effective in treating depression. *Nature* 2000;403:826.

60. Williams JMG. *Depression*. In: Clark DM, Fairburn CA (eds.), *Science and Practice of Cognitive Behaviour Therapy*. Oxford: Oxford University Press, 1997, pp. 259–283.

61. McLean P, Taylor S. Severity of unipolar depression and choice of treatment. *Behav Res Therap* 1992;30(5):443–451.

62. Ahmed I, Soares KVS, Seifas R, et al. Randomized controlled trials in Archives of General Psychiatry (1959-1995): A prevalence study. *Arch Gen Psychiatry* 1998;55:754–755.

63. Jarrett RB, Schaffer M, McIntire D, et al. Treatment of atypical depression with cognitive therapy or phenelzine: A double-blind, placebo-controlled trial. *Arch Gen Psychiatry* 1999;56:431–437.

64. Sherman C. Psychotherapy works in atypical depression. *Clin Psychiatry News* 1998;26:1–2.

65. Jarrett RB, Basco MR, Risser RC, et al. Is there a role for continuation phase cognitive therapy for depressed outpatients? *J Consul Clin Psychol* 1998;66:1036–1040.

66. Judd LL. The clinical course of unipolar major depressive disorders. *Arch Gen Psychiatry* 1988;55:989–991.

67. Evans MD, Hollon SD, DeRubeis RJ, et al. Differential relapse following cognitive therapy and pharmacotherapy for depression. *Arch Gen Psychiatry* 1992;49:802–808.

68. Shea MT, Elkin I, Imber SD, et al. Course of depressive symptoms over follow-up: Findings from the National Institute of Mental Health Treatment of Depression Collaborative Research Program. *Arch Gen Psychiatry* 1992;49:782–787.

69. Blackburn IM, Eunson KM, Bishop S. A two-year naturalistic follow-up of depressed patients treated with cognitive therapy, pharmacotherapy and a combination of both. *J Affect Disord* 1986;10:67–75.

70. Blackburn IM, Bishop S, Glen AIM, et al. The efficacy of cognitive therapy in depression: A treatment trial using cognitive therapy and pharmacotherapy, each alone and in combination. *Br J Psychiatry* 1981;139:181–189.

71. Simons AD, Murphy, GE, Levine JL, et al. Cognitive therapy and pharmacotherapy for depression: Sustained improvement over one year. *Arch Gen Psychiatry* 1986;43:43–48.

72. Murphy GE, Simons AD, Wetzel RD, et al. Cognitive therapy and pharmacotherapy: Singly and together in the treatment of depression. *Arch Gen Psychiatry* 1984;41:33–41.

73. Kovacs M, Rush AJ, Beck AT, et al. Depressed outpatients treated with cognitive therapy or pharmacotherapy: A one-year follow-up. *Arch Gen Psychiatry* 1981;38:33–39.

74. Rush AJ, Beck AT, Kovacs M, et al. Comparative efficacy of cognitive therapy and pharmacotherapy in the treatment of depressed outpatients. *Cogn Therap Res* 1977;1:17–37.

75. Colom F, Vieta E, Martinez-Aran A, et al. A randomized trial on the efficacy of group psychoeducation in the prophylaxis of recurrences in bipolar patients whose disease is in remission. *Arch Gen Psychiatry* 2003;60:402–407.

76. Lam DH, Watkins ER, Hayward P, et al. A randomized controlled study of cognitive therapy for relapse prevention for bipolar affective disorder. *Arch Gen Psychiatry* 2003;60:145–152.

77. Baldessarini RJ, Tonodo L, Hennen J, et al. Is lithium still worth using? An update of selected recent research. *Harv Rev Psychiatry* 2002;10:59–75.

78. Simons AD, Murphy GE, Levine JL, et al. Cognitive therapy and pharmacotherapy for depression: Sustained improvement over one year. *Arch Gen Psychiatry* 1986;43:43–48.

79. Segal ZV, Ingram RE. Mood priming and construct activation in tests of cognitive vulnerability to unipolar depression. *Clin Psychol Rev* 1994;14: 663–695.

80. Oei TPS, Free ML. Do cognitive behaviour therapies validate cognitive models of mood disorders? A review of the empirical evidence. *Int J Psychol* 1995;30:145–179.

81. Segal ZV, Gemar M, Williams S. Differential cognitive response to a mood induction following successful cognitive therapy and pharmacotherapy for depression. *J Abnorm Psychol* 1999;108: 3–10.

82. DeRubeis RJ, Gelfand LA, Tang TZ, et al. Medications versus cognitive behavior therapy for severely depressed outpatients: Mega-analysis of four randomized comparisons. *Am J Psychiatry* 1999;156:1007–1013.

83. Markowitz JC. *Interpersonal Psychotherapy for Dysthymic Disorder.* Washington, DC: American Psychiatric Press, 1998.

84. Teasdale JD, Segal Z, Mark J, et al. How does cognitive therapy prevent depressive relapse and why should attentional control (mindfulness) training help? *Behav Res Therap* 1995;33:25–39.

CHAPTER 4

Diagnosis and Treatment of Depression (MDD) and Bipolar Disorder (BPD) in Children and Adolescents

DANIEL P. DICKSTEIN, DANIEL S. PINE, AND ELLEN LEIBENLUFT*

▶ INTRODUCTION

Depression and bipolar disorder (BPD) represent major health concerns for all those involved in the care of children and adolescents. The magnitude of this problem derives both from the prevalence of these conditions as well as their potential to dramatically impact the lives of children and their families. Childhood depression and BPD have been relatively neglected until recently, due to the stigmatization about mental illnesses, misconceptions about the nature of psychopathology during childhood, and disagreements concerning the most appropriate techniques for diagnosing mental disorders in children and adolescents.[219] The degree to which recent advances have increased focus on the problem of pediatric mental disorders is reflected in a recent government report (Mental Health: A Report of the Surgeon General, 1999).[257]

The diagnostic criteria for depression and BPD, mostly informed by research on adults with psychiatric disorders, are codified in the latest edition of the Diagnostic and Statistical Manual Text Revision (DSM-IVTR).[2] Both disorders require the presence of distinct mood episodes different from the person's normal, baseline mood. The diagnosis of major depressive disorder (MDD) requires that the patient experience a major depressive episode (MDE) defined by the presence of three key features: (1) either depressed/irritable mood or a loss of interest in pleasure (anhedonia), (2) neurovegetative symptoms (i.e., changes in sleep, appetite, concentration, interest, and so on), (3) and resultant functional impairment for most of the day, every day, for 2 or more weeks (Table 4-1).

The diagnosis of BPD requires an episode, distinctly different from baseline, of: (1) hypomania (≥4 days) or mania (≥7 days), characterized by a persistently elevated, expansive, or irritable mood, and (2) neurovegetative symptoms unique to mania (Tables 4-2 and 4-3). Clinicians caring for children should be aware that while current DSM criteria for depression contain

*The views expressed in this book do not necessarily represent the views of the National Institutes of Health or the U.S. Govt.

▶ **TABLE 4-1** MAJOR DEPRESSIVE DISORDER (MDD) DIAGNOSTIC CRITERIA

(A) Presence of a major depressive episode (MDE) as defined by:
   ≥5 of the following symptoms (with AT LEAST 1 being depressed mood OR loss of interest/pleasure) for most of the day, on more days than not, during the SAME 2-week period AND represent a change from previous functioning
      Depressed OR irritable mood as indicated by subjective account or others' observation
      Markedly diminished interest OR pleasure in almost all activities
      Significant (more than 5%/month) weight loss OR decrease/increase in appetite
      Insomnia OR hypersomnia
      Psychomotor agitation OR retardation observed by others (NOT merely subjective report)
      Low energy or fatigue
      Feelings of worthlessness OR excessive/inappropriate guilt
      Poor concentration OR difficulty making decisions
      Recurrent thoughts of death, suicidal ideation, or suicide attempt.
(B) The MDE is not better accounted for by schizophrenia, schizoaffective disorder, delusional disorder, or psychotic disorder not otherwise specified
(C) No prior history of manic, hypomanic, or mixed episodes
(D) The disturbance is not exclusively part of a chronic psychotic disorder, such as schizophrenia
(E) The disturbance is not due to the direct effects of a substance or general medical condition
(F) The symptoms cause clinically significant impairment in social, occupational, or other area of function

▶ **TABLE 4-2** MANIC EPISODE DIAGNOSTIC CRITERIA*

(A) A distinct period of abnormally AND persistently elevated, expansive, OR irritable mood, lasting AT LEAST 1 week
(B) During the mood disturbance, ≥3 have PERSISTED (≥4 if mood is only IRRITABLE) and have been present to a significant degree:
      Inflated self-esteem or grandiosity
      Decreased need for sleep (e.g., feels rested after <3 h of sleep)
      Pressured speech
      Flight of ideas (subjective experience that thoughts are racing)
      Distractibility (attention too easily drawn to unimportant external stimuli)
      Increased goal-directed activity OR psychomotor agitation
      Excessive involvement in pleasurable activity with high potential for painful consequences (e.g., spending sprees, sexual activity)
(C) Symptoms are not part of a mixed episode (i.e., during the same 1-week period meets criteria for manic episode AND major depressive episode [including need for symptoms to be present for most of the day for the full week])
(D) Mood disturbance causes functional impairment
(E) Symptoms are not due to physiologic effect of substance OR medical condition

*"Hypomanic episode" is defined by the same diagnostic features of a manic episode EXCEPT the duration is ≥4 days AND the mood change results in observable functional change but not severe enough to cause marked impairment (i.e., not severe enough to require psychiatric hospitalization).

▶ **TABLE 4-3** BIPOLAR DISORDER (BPD) DIAGNOSTIC CRITERIA

- BPD type I: presence of 1 manic episode (not requirement to have had a major depressive episode).
- BPD type II: presence of >1 major depressive episode AND presence of >1 hypomanic episode WITHOUT history of manic episodes.
- Cyclothymic disorder: for at least 1 full year, presence of numerous periods with hypomanic symptoms and numerous periods with depressive symptoms that do NOT meet criteria for MDE. No symptom-free period longer than 2 months.

Note: For all, not better accounted for by schizoaffective disorder, schizophrenia, delusional disorder, or psychotic disorder not otherwise specified.

developementally informed modifications, DSM criteria for BPD do not.

In children and adolescents, mood disorders, meaning depression and BPD, are common, and they extort a heavy toll on developing youth. The resultant functional role impairment is manifest as reduced performance in school, disruption in social relationships with peers, and perturbations in family cohesion. Not only do mood disorders exert concurrent dysfunction in children and adolescents, but also their effects can propagate in time. Longitudinal studies of children and adolescents find that depression predicts a high risk for various adverse outcomes over time. This includes an increased risk for morbidity associated with other mental disorders as well as an increased mortality, primarily from suicide. Those with prepubertal depression have increased risk of suicide into adulthood (nearly three times the risk of healthy and three times the risk of those with prepubertal anxiety), substance abuse, conduct disorders (CD), and long-term, recurrent use of both medical and psychiatric services.[270] Finally, as the general consensus that pediatric BPD is a more serious, impairing condition, these findings suggest that the long-term impact of this condition on the lives of children and adolescents is likely to be even more severe.

Given the magnitude of the problem, it is not surprising that treatment of pediatric depression and BPD is no longer the exclusive concern of child and adolescent psychiatrists and psychologists. Rather, treatment of pediatric MDD and BPD is increasingly becoming part of primary care pediatrics. Several studies have demonstrated markedly increasing rates of prescriptions for psychotropic medications, including antidepressants, with the majority of these prescriptions being written by general practitioners and pediatricians.[114,206,238,284] A national study of pediatricians in the mid-1990s demonstrated that while many physicians working with children and adolescents considered it their responsibility to recognize depression (90%), only about one-third felt comfortable treating depression. Given the complexity in treating BPD, even greater numbers of primary care physicians are likely to feel uncomfortable in managing children with this condition. Major reasons cited for this lack of comfort included lack of time and training.[207]

The purpose of this chapter is to address these concerns among primary care pediatricians by providing a current review of the treatment of depression and BPD in children and adolescents. For the purposes of this chapter, we will discuss primarily medication treatment of these disorders, but we will also present important information about psychotherapy. We will first discuss unipolar depression and then BPD.

▶ DEPRESSION/MAJOR DEPRESSIVE DISORDER

Introduction

Depression, in all of its subtypes, is a significant concern for all health professionals involved with the care of children and adolescents. Both from research reports as well as popular press, currently there is a sense that the problem is growing. Yet, this was not always the case. In fact, it was only in the 1970s that professionals began to believe that depression in children was a diagnosable and treatable entity.[50,54,226,269]

Epidemiologic studies have shown, through both community-based or epidemiologic sampling frames, that MDD is a relatively rare problem before puberty, with a prevalence in children of no greater than 0.4–2%.[62–64] However, rates of MDD increase steadily with age, to become an unfortunately common problem in adolescence, affecting somewhere in the range of 2–10% of all adolescents.[25,62,136,164,165] A particularly marked increase in prevalence is observed in later puberty, around age 14–15 years. With respect to gender, MDD occurs at same rate in boys and girls, but in adolescents, female-to-male ratio approximates 2:1, which is the same as in adults.[64,141] Given that this gender divergence occurs around the time of puberty, interest has been generated in the role of sex steroids in MDD.[10]

Not only is depression a prevalent disorder, but it is also a burgeoning problem for children and adolescents. Several studies, including those based in large epidemiologic samples, have demonstrated increased rates of depression in youth with successive generations during the twentieth century. This effect has been labeled as the "age-cohort effect" or the "rising secular trend" in pediatric depression.[67,158,166]

Several methodological issues regarding this trend are important for clinicians to understand in order to interpret these data. First, most of these estimates are based on retrospective data and generate comparable effects for other types of psychopathology besides depression. Thus, these findings may not reflect a specific increase in rates of depression, but rather may result from an artifact of reporting bias. Second, reductions in the stigma associated with mental illnesses and refinements in diagnostic interviews may result in more recent cohorts' data to more accurately reflect the genuine prevalence of MDD. Third, assessment methods contribute to variability of youth depression prevalence because, while the common DSM definition of depression is consistently used across studies, cross-study variability persists, in terms of sampling frames and the methods for applying these DSM criteria. For example, some studies rely primarily on information from children or adolescents themselves; other studies attempt to integrate these data with information from adults, e.g., parents. A fourth source of variability stems from the time frame of assessment. Some studies rely on cross-sectional data to generate estimates of current or "point" prevalence. Others rely on retrospective data to generate lifetime estimates. Still others rely on serial assessments in longitudinal designs to derive lifetime estimates. In general, the prevalence of MDD increases across these three types of studies. Despite these potential confounds, the data suggest that youth depression may truly represent a growing problem.

Probably the most persuasive data is derived from studying completed suicides. More than 10% of all deaths in those aged 10–24 years are the result of suicide, making it the fourth leading cause of death in this age group.[38] Depression and BPD are two of the most common mental disorders in cases of youth suicide.[40] Data on completed suicide are free of many biases and artifacts that plague epidemiologic self-report data on rates of depression. The data on completed suicide demonstrate robust increases in prevalence in the United States during the final half of the twentieth century, a trend that only leveled off in the final few years of the century. Thus, both epidemiologic data on prevalence of depression and data on youth suicide point to the fact that youth depression may represent an increasingly prevalent problem.

While the cause of this potential increase in youth depression is unclear, the potential impact on children's well-being is not, given the morbidity and mortality resulting from depression. Children and adolescents suffering from depression have an increased risk of school absenteeism, substance abuse, and suicide.[48] Also, child- and adolescent-onset depression is often a relapsing disorder, with increased risk of recurrence either in adolescence or early adulthood, with rates approximating 10–50%.[11,148,164,165,218,227] Consequently, all healthcare professionals, regardless of training specialty, need to have a familiarity with the diagnosis and treatment of depression in children and adolescents.

Toward this goal, the first half of this section reviews major diagnostic and treatment issues, respectively, about depression based upon a current review of research literature. Our intent is to provide a detailed entry point for practitioners to expand their knowledge.

Diagnosing Depression in Children and Adolescents

General Psychiatric Assessment of Children and Adolescents

Psychiatric evaluation of children and adolescents requires the same systematic approach, along with collaboration from others who know the child, which one would use to evaluate a primary physical complaint. Detailed explanations of how to conduct such an assessment are found in the practice parameters of the American Academy of Child and Adolescent Psychiatry (AACAP; www.AACAP.org).[145]

This general approach is used for all evaluations of pediatric psychiatric issues, including depression and BPD. It adopts principles of the theoretical school known as "developmental psychopathology." This school recognizes that children's behavior changes over time, as the child passes through successive phases of development. These developmental fluctuations in behavior represent normal maturational patterns. Changes in the expression, experience, and regulation of emotion represent a fundamental aspect of this developmental process. Given the robustness of these changes, the boundaries of normal behavior and emotional regulation also develop as children pass through various developmental phases. For example, it might be fully expected for a preschool child to respond with tears, irritable behavior, and protestations of despair when the child is not allowed to engage in one or another of his or her favorite activities. This type of reaction would be highly unusual in a 10-year-old. The framework of developmental psychopathology provides a vital backdrop against which to consider issues of assessment in children. However,

in practice, this school also creates some problems when considering issues of diagnosis and assessment in children. Specifically, the diagnostic criteria codified in DSM, the standard diagnostic nomenclature in the United States, places a higher priority on explicitly describing differences rather than on providing developmentally informed modifications for the pediatric psychiatric disorders. This disconnect between the DSM and the school of developmental psychopathology has led to some criticism of the DSM as not being developmentally informed.[219]

Beyond theory, the psychiatric evaluation in pediatric patients begins with interviewing the parent and child, usually both together and separately. Open-ended questions are followed by closed-ended questions to trace the features of the presenting complaint of depression. While older children and adolescents are engageable in this more straightforward verbal interview, younger children often require practitioners to use more creative techniques, such as drawing or playing while talking. With respect to a developmentally informed assessment, the way in which young children express depression is often not as straightforward as in adolescents and adults. For example, young children may not directly acknowledge feeling sad or depressed, though they may show it through behavior that is distinctly different than their usual baseline—e.g., a child who no longer likes to play as enthusiastically as s/he did in the past.

The results from the in-office assessment of the child typically are summarized in the report of the mental status examination (Table 4-4). Based on the nature of presenting problem, specific aspects of the mental status should be explored in more or less detail. An accurate assessment of the child's current mood, meaning the sustained subjective sense of emotional state, is essential to evaluating a patient for the diagnosis of depression or BPD. As part of this assessment, it might be valuable to engage the child in discussions concerning aspects of his or her life that the child typically finds to be enjoyable. Evidence that the child is capable of

▶ **TABLE 4-4** MENTAL STATUS EXAMINATION (MSE)

- Manner: cooperative, guarded, hostile appearance: neat/well-kempt or disheveled. Distinguishing features (glasses, tattoos, piercings)
- Orientation: level of awareness/alertness to person, place, time, and why they are present in a clinical setting
- Mood: self-report of emotional state
- Affect: observed emotional state (i.e., depressed, euthymic, manic), including range (i.e., full-range, restricted, flat)
- Speech: rate, volume, prosody (musical quality of normal speech vs. monotone)
- Motor behavior: quality (i.e., coordination, motor/vocal tics, stereotypy [flapping/rocking]) and quantity (i.e., agitated, fidgety, listless)
- Thought process: linear (patient able to organize and convey thoughts clearly), tangential (patient wanders off topic without returning), circumstantial (subject wanders off topic but eventually returns to the original topic), flight of ideas (feature of mania; patient jumps from topic to disconnected topic)
- Thought content: major focus of patient's thoughts (i.e., self-esteem, peer/parent relationships, depressed/anxious/psychotic, and so on thoughts—includes assessment for suicidality [presence/absence of suicidal ideation/thoughts, plans, and attempts])
- Insight: patient's self-awareness of strengths/ongoing illness
- Judgment: patient's ability to make appropriate decisions and predict her/his own behavior in hypothetical social situations (i.e., *If you felt more depressed tonight, what would you do?*)

enjoying these activities should be weighed as suggesting that the diagnosis of an MDE may not be appropriate, whereas clear signs that the child is not capable of this suggest that the diagnosis of MDE may be appropriate. Depending on the nature of the differential diagnosis, other aspects of the mental status examination should be probed in more or less detail. For example, aspects of language and thought processes exhibited during the mental status examination can be important clues in differentiating an MDE from a manic episode.

Collaboration is essential in the psychiatric assessment of children. This often includes speaking with teachers, daycare, or after-school activity staff once appropriate releases of information have been obtained. Though difficult in a busy pediatric outpatient setting, these brief conversations yield vital information regarding the child's functioning in each of these settings which is essential to proper diagnosis: depression is characterized not just by mood symptoms but also by functional impairment at home, school, or both. Consid-

ering the degree to which children's lives are spent in various contexts outside the home, clinicians could not possibly determine if this criterion is indeed met without some information from parallel historians besides a parent, either directly from such informants or indirectly, as conveyed by the parent. Discussing the child's progress with adults observing the child in various settings is essential to establishing the proper diagnosis. Moreover, these collaborations will also yield key information once treatment is initiated, if indicated, for depression or other disorders.

Mental health practitioners have used the term "parallel" history to describe information about a child's symptoms of mental illness acquired from such collaborations. A few types of parallel history information are vital in terms of making an appropriate diagnosis. For example, the diagnosis of pediatric MDD can be differentiated from other mental disorders based on the duration and quality or type of symptoms. Parallel history provides invaluable information in clarifying the clinical picture.

Diagnostic Features of Pediatric Depression

Evaluating youth for depression requires specific information to make the diagnosis. Several psychiatric disorders share the common feature of depressed mood, though they represent different diagnoses, with different prognostic and treatment implications. As noted previously, duration of the depressed mood is essential information. A MDE requires the presence of three key features: (1) either depressed/irritable mood or a loss of interest in pleasure (anhedonia), (2) neurovegetative symptoms (i.e., changes in sleep, appetite, concentration, interest, and so on) symptoms, (3) and resultant functional impairment for most of the day, every day, for 2 or more weeks. DSM-IV recognizes nine potential symptoms, including depressed or irritable mood as well as the neurovegetative symptoms, which occur during an MDE, each of which must be manifest during the 2-week period. To qualify for the diagnosis of an MDE, five of these nine symptoms must be present, one of which must be either a perturbation in mood or a loss of interest in pleasure. More chronic depression may be consistent with dysthymic disorder, which requires the child's mood to be aberrantly depressed or irritable for 1 year, with a maximum of 2 months in a row of normal mood (Table 4-5). However, the perturbation of mood in dysthymia is less persistent, occurring only most but not every day during this year long period.

Impairment and distress represent a key aspect of all diagnoses, including MDD. The clinician should recognize these symptoms to either cause considerable upset in the child or to directly interfere with the child's efforts to function. In practice, however, it is very rare to see a child or adolescent who exhibits five symptoms of an MDE for 2 weeks and does not clearly exhibit signs of significant distress or impairment. Interestingly, this is not true for all mental conditions. For example, it is not unusual for children to manifest symptoms of an anxiety disorder but

▶ **TABLE 4-5** DYSTHYMIC DISORDER DIAGNOSTIC CRITERIA

(A) Depressed or irritable mood for most of the day, more days than not, as indicated by subjective account or others' observation for at least 1 year[*]

(B) Presence, while depressed of ≥2:
  Poor appetite OR overeating
  Insomnia OR hypersomnia
  Low energy or fatigue
  Low self-esteem
  Poor concentration OR difficulty making decisions
  Hopelessness

(C) During the 1-year period, the child/adolescent is not without the symptoms for more than 2 months at a time

(D) No major depressive episode during the first year of the disturbance—i.e., the disturbance is not better accounted for by MDD. However, there may have been a previous MDE provided there was a full remission (no symptoms for 2 months) BEFORE development of dysthymic disorder. Also, if both dysthymic disorder and MDD are present, both can be diagnosed

(E) No prior manic, hypomanic, or mixed episodes

(F) The disturbance is not exclusively part of a chronic psychotic disorder, such as schizophrenia

(G) The disturbance is not due to the direct effects of a substance or general medical condition

(H) The symptoms cause clinically significant impairment in social, occupational, or other area of function

[*]In adults, this criterion is 2 years and only depressed (not irritable) mood.

not exhibit sufficient distress or impairment to qualify for the diagnosis. If a child exhibits problematic depressive symptoms but they are not felt to be present on a daily basis or on every single day for a 2-week period, this does not suggest that the symptoms are meaningless. Rather, this suggests that the child meets criteria for a distinct syndrome besides MDD. This is important, however, since most of the data on therapeutics, especially for pharmacologic agents, apply to children with MDD in particular.

Parallel history is very important when specifically considering the diagnosis of depression. Through such history, clinicians can identify the temporal fluctuation of symptoms, including the presence or absence of discrete mood episodes, which provides vital information concerning the most appropriate diagnosis. At least according to some experts, differentiating MDD from related affective syndromes, such as BPD, rests on the identification of "distinct" or episodic periods during which a characteristic pattern of affective disturbance emerges relatively abruptly (see below for full description of a "manic episode," as occurs in BPD). Parallel history provides vital information when attempting to make this distinction. Additionally, pediatric mental disorders in general, and MDD in particular, are tightly linked to the occurrence of stressful life events. The occurrence of such an event can catalyze the onset of an episode, and the presence of such events can disrupt efforts to reduce symptoms of depression. Parallel historians can provide vital information that may be unavailable to parents in terms of potential covert stressful events that impact on children and adolescents.

Considerable controversy remains concerning the symptom of irritability as it relates to the specific diagnosis of pediatric depression. DSM recognizes irritability as a unique symptom in pediatric as opposed to adult MDD. This symptom "qualifies" as a manifestation of an MDE in children and adolescents, but not in adults. This difference is thought to reflect developmental differences in the manifestation of an MDE. While this recognition represents an important

observation, it has also generated considerable confusion. Episodes of mania also involve the symptom of irritability, both in children and adolescents as well as adults (see below). Moreover, DSM provides relatively little guidance in terms of differentiating irritability that represents a manifestation of an MDE in a child as opposed to a manic episode. Given that irritability might represent a manifestation of either such episode, this convention complicates the differential diagnosis of pediatric MDD.

Clinicians often evaluate pediatric depression in relation to specific events. For example, with the death of a loved one, it is normal for children to experience bereavement. Though the symptoms, including mood and neurovegetative symptoms, are often the same, the diagnosis of MDD is more appropriate than bereavement if the following are present: symptoms present more than 2 months after the loss, suicidal ideation, or developmentally inappropriate perceptual experiences consistent with psychosis (i.e., recurrent or command auditory hallucinations of the deceased telling the child to harm her/himself). Such a distinction is quite complicated, and it may often require consultation with a child psychiatrist. Another example is when a particular stressor results in the development of symptoms, such as depressed or irritable mood. The term "adjustment disorder" is used to describe such situations, and these conditions may involve depressed or anxious mood changes, behavior or conduct changes, or combinations of the two (Table 4-6). As with bereavement, the diagnostic distinction between adjustment disorders and MDD is quite important for prognosis and treatment.

Two special pediatric populations deserve specific mention with regard to assessment. First, symptoms of depression represent a common problem in children and adolescents who suffer from various developmental disabilities, including mental retardation, static encephalopathy, and learning or language-related disabilities. In general, the assessment of MDD in these individuals is thought to involve similar procedures as in individuals free of such problems. However,

▶ **TABLE 4-6** ADJUSTMENT DISORDER
DIAGNOSTIC CRITERIA*

- Development of emotional or behavioral symptoms in response to an identifiable stressor within 3 months of the stressor's onset
- Symptoms are clinically significant with either: (1) excess distress than expected to the stressor OR (2) significant social/occupational (academic) functional impairment
- Not consistent with prior or other major depressive episode, manic episode, or other axis I disorder
- Not bereavement
- Once the stressor has terminated, the symptoms do not persist for more than 6 months

Subtypes: with depressed mood; with anxiety; with mixed anxiety and depressed mood; with disturbance of conduct; with mixed disturbance of emotions and conduct.

in practice, the assessment of MDD in children with significant developmental delay is often not straightforward. Second, considerable debate has emerged on the degree to which preschool children manifest symptoms of MDD. While consensus has emerged on the view of MDD as a disorder primarily of adolescents as opposed to children, some have suggested that MDD is more common in preschoolers than previously recognized. As with the diagnosis in developmental disabilities, the diagnosis of MDD in preschoolers remains an area where more information is needed before firm guidelines can be provided. In both areas, primary care physicians confronted with diagnostic questions concerning mood disorders in such children and adolescents should seek the assistance of an expert in one or the other of these areas.

Differential Diagnosis

The differential diagnosis of depression in children and adolescents includes careful evaluation of the type of depression, medical conditions causing symptoms of depression, substance use,

and other psychiatric diagnoses. A systematic, methodical approach to evaluate these issues improves diagnostic certainty. In turn, this leads to more appropriate therapy, and ideally improved outcomes. As with all medical diagnoses, this is a process, requiring continuous hypothesis testing to see if diagnostic and therapeutic choices are correct and adequately meeting the patient's needs. If the child is not doing well, providers should reexamine their diagnostic or therapeutic choices and seek consultation with another practitioner.

The clinician should be aware of two general aspects of differential diagnosis when preparing a diagnostic formulation in children and adolescents presenting with depressive symptoms. First, symptoms resembling a MDE can be produced by a number of medical conditions. When this occurs, the diagnosis of MDD should not be given, but the depressive symptoms should be considered to represent a "phenocopy" or a "medical mimic." From the technical perspective, in this situation, the DSM diagnosis "mood disorder due to a general medical condition" is the most appropriate category within which to place such symptoms. From the clinical perspective, such categorization is important when considering aspects of therapeutics. When depressive symptoms occur in the context of a medical condition, the first priority should be to comprehensively evaluate the magnitude of the medical problem and stabilize the clinical state of the patients. This intervention can dramatically alter ongoing mood symptoms, to the point where no other treatments are indicated.

Second, symptoms of other mental disorders can complicate symptoms of depression. When this occurs, clinicians and epidemiologists appropriately consider the child to suffer both from an MDE as well as another, "comorbid" mental syndrome. Some controversy remains concerning the validity of this approach. This controversy reflects the very high rates of comorbidity that arise in psychiatric epidemiology, relative to other branches of medicine. This likely reflects fundamental differences in the nosology of mental disorders and other mental conditions.

For example, in a child who presents with otitis media, one would never consider this child to suffer from "fever" that is comorbid with "erythema" of the middle ear. The controversy surrounding comorbidity reflects the fact that current nosologic categories in psychiatry remain relatively removed from the underlying perturbations in physiology that generate the symptoms. Until pathophysiologic understandings of brain function can be integrated into nosology, diagnosis of mental disorders will necessarily involve classification systems that produce imperfect categorizations, as reflected in the very high rates of "comorbidity."

PHENOCOPIES AND MEDICAL MIMICS

Several medical conditions may produce symptoms resembling those of primary depression. Table 4-7 lists several conditions occurring in childhood causing depressed mood and/or

▶ **TABLE 4-7** MEDICAL CONDITIONS ON THE DIFFERENTIAL DIAGNOSIS OF DEPRESSION

- Neurologic disorders: CNS infections (meningitis, encephalitis), epilepsy/seizures, cerebral neoplasms, migraine, hydrocephalus, sleep apnea
- Infectious disease: human immuno-deficiency virus/acquired immunodeficiency syndrome (HIV/AIDS)
- Metabolic disorders: Wilson disease, porphyria
- Endocrine disorders: thyroid (hypo- or hyper-), parathyroid (hypo- or hyper-), adrenal (Cushing or Addison disease), hyperaldosteronism, postpartum
- Vitamin deficiency: folate, B_{12}, niacin, vitamin C, thiamine
- Rheumatologic: systemic lupus erythematosus, rheumatoid arthritis, temporal arteritis, fibromyalgia, Sjögren syndrome
- Medications: steroids, antineoplasia treatment, oral contraceptives, opiates, antibiotics
- Other: cancer (all types, solid organ and lymphoma/leukemia), cardiopulmonary disease, renal disease/failure/uremia

neurovegetative dysfunction; however, it is by no means an exhaustive list given the constraints of this chapter. This table further suggests the need for collaboration between health workers, regardless of professional training, united for the health of their pediatric patients. If a patient has depression plus other symptoms of one or more of these disorders, an appropriate investigation, including physical examination, laboratory studies, or ancillary tests should be performed as indicated. However, physicians do not need to perform unnecessary tests or procedures when children do not have symptoms or stigmata of these disorders. As with most aspects of psychiatric assessments, the mental status examination can be a key component in detecting signs of an underlying phenocopy. For example, children with MDE should exhibit an intact sensorium with no sign of disorientation. Similarly, while subtle cognitive impairment can accompany an MDE, the degree of impairment relative to a child's baseline should be relatively mild. In contrast, dramatic alterations in alertness or cognitive capacity should alert the clinician to potential underlying medical factors that might complicate the clinical picture, such as an intracranial neoplasm or toxidrome. Finally, if a child initially thought to have depression without physical illness has inadequate or atypical response to treatment, physicians should reconsider the diagnosis and revisit the possibility of primary medical condition with depression as a symptom.

SUBSTANCE USE

Clinicians need to assess all children and adolescents presenting with psychiatric or behavioral complaint for substance use for two reasons. First, high rates of substance use have been demonstrated in children and adolescents with depression.[15,151] Second, virtually any substance of abuse may have depressed mood as a symptom of either intoxication or withdrawal. This includes traditional substances of abuse, such as alcohol, cannabis, cocaine, sedatives, but also novel drugs, such as ecstasy or ketamine, or other household items, such as inhalants (e.g., paint or paint thinner) or hygiene items (e.g., mouthwash often has a high alcohol content). Studies have shown youth with both substance use disorders and mood disorders, such as depression, are more likely to commit suicide.[42]

Screening for substance use begins with a thorough history. Surprisingly, clinicians' lack of inquiry is often the biggest obstacle to determining if a patient is abusing substances.[169] The added utility of urine toxicologic screens is much debated; some substances are not detected at all or eliminated from the body rapidly so as to give a false negative result.[128,216,268] Studies have shown that a good substance use history taken by a clinician can often provide as many clues as a urine toxicologic screen in detecting substance use.

As with all aspects of psychiatric assessment in children, unique complications arise when attempting to assess symptoms that either would embarrass a child or cause significant distress in a parent. Hence, one must carefully communicate to the child or adolescent the degree to which admissions about substance use will or will not be kept confidential. Ideally, the clinician will consider carefully, prior to the initiation of the assessment, the ramifications of either disclosing or failing to disclose to the parent previously unsuspected substance use in a patient. Moreover, the clinician should directly ask about use of illicit substances, and the clinician should take quite seriously any reports of such use. However, denials of use should be weighed with at least a mild degree of skepticism in children or adolescents who deny such use but present with features that raise suspicion. Such features include the presence of ongoing conduct disturbance, a history of substance abuse, and the participation in peer groups where substance use is endemic.

COMORBID ANXIETY DISORDERS

The most common group of psychiatric diagnoses comorbid to depression in children and adolescents are anxiety disorders. Numerous studies have shown that the rate of anxiety disorders in children with depression is between 25 and 75%.[9,16] Moreover, the combination of depression and comorbid anxiety is often a substantially more impairing condition than either alone.[21,136] When present, anxiety disorders often predate the development of depression; furthermore, anxiety often persists after depression remits.[149]

Given their prevalence and prognostic impact, practitioners should seek out comorbid anxiety in children and adolescents presenting with depression. Interventions, whether medication or psychotherapy, must incorporate considerations of anxiety comorbidity.

EATING DISORDERS

Eating disorders, as with substance use disorders, can both produce symptoms of depression and also be highly comorbid, especially in girls, with depression.[150,195] Screening for eating disorders starts with a thorough history of restrictive or binge eating, inquiry about body self-image, asking about attempts at weight loss, and asking about menstrual history. Additionally, a physical examination for signs of eating disorders, such as bruised knuckles or tooth erosions from self-induced vomiting, alopecia, or abnormal body mass index (BMI).[121–123] Children and adolescents suffering from eating disorders often require treatment from an integrated, multispecialty group or clinic combining mental and physical health providers along with nutritionists and therapists.

Pathophysiology

In general, the current summary focuses most explicitly on issues of diagnosis and therapeutics, given the focus of this volume on these issues in primary care settings. However, as noted above in the discussion on comorbidity and differential diagnosis, limitations in the current diagnostic approach to pediatric mental disorders, in general, and pediatric MDD in particular largely reflect the limited understanding of the disorders' pathophysiology. Similarly, deficiencies in the therapeutic armamentarium also reflect the limited understanding of pathophysiology. Since future advances in diagnosis and treatment are likely to derive from advances in understandings of pathophysiology, the current section does summarize current research in this area.

Pathophysiologic understandings of mental disorders have developed markedly over the past 30 years. These advances have been particularly marked for pediatric MDD, given that many questioned whether children were even capable of manifesting this syndrome as recently as 25 years ago. Moreover, as understandings of mental disorders has evolved, investigators increasingly recognize the degree to which current nosology must remain tentative. As pathophysiologic understandings increase, the current nosologic boundaries of MDD and other syndromes may change. By analogy, as the understanding of blood pressure regulation and the long-term effects of mild elevations in blood pressure increased, the range of blood pressure values considered "normal" has changed.

MDD is recognized to be a "complex" disorder from the standpoint of pathophysiology. The term "complex" has been taken to have various meanings. The disorder is complex in that it can be produced by multiple risk factors, each exerting relatively small effects on risk. Alternatively, the disorder is considered "complex" in that it probably includes a family of syndromes that have both shared and discrepant underlying pathophysiology, comprising an etiologically heterogeneous collection of specific disease entities. To the extent that MDD involves a common underlying pathophysiology, this core is thought to be reflected in perturbation in a common, underlying brain circuit.

From the standpoint of genetics, virtually all of the research on MDD examines adults. Information on genetic contributions to MDD derives from both behavioral and molecular genetic studies. Both sets of studies support the view of MDD as etiologically complex. Behavioral genetic studies have partitioned variance in the risk for MDD into genetic and environmental factors using the classic methods of the twin or adoption study design. Using these methods, studies in adults demonstrate that the patho-

physiology of MDD involves moderate effects of both genetics and nonshared environment, with genetic factors accounting for about 40% of the variance and nonshared environment accounting for slightly more variance than this. These adult studies also suggest that developmental factors impact on the risk for MDD, in that retrospective reports of some childhood symptoms, such as anxiety, exhibit strong genetic correlation with the underlying genetics of adult MDD.

Far fewer studies examine children and adolescents. Family studies clearly establish the fact that MDD is a familial disorder: offspring of MDD parents exhibit higher rates of MDD than offspring of healthy parents. Nevertheless, significant questions arise from these data. For example, the association extends beyond MDD per se. Not only do children of MDD parents exhibit high rates of MDD, but they also exhibit high rates of anxiety disorders. As with findings from adult twin studies, these findings linking childhood anxiety to adult MDD raise questions on the nature of the pathophysiologic relationship anxiety and MDD. Moreover, the degree to which familial associations derive from genetic as opposed to environmental factors also remains unclear. The few available twin studies of MDD symptoms or diagnosis in children and adolescents implicate both genetic and nonshared environmental factors in MDD.

In terms of molecular genetic studies of MDD, research among adults remains in relatively early stages. Virtually no research examines the molecular genetics of pediatric MDD. In general, some of the most exciting results in both children and adults attempt to delineate the manner in which genetic and environmental factors interact. Studies attempting to examine this issue have typically relied upon association designs, whereupon specific candidate genes are targeted. For example, a recent study focused on the serotonin transporter gene, given considerable research reviewed below examining the role of serotongeric dysfunction in both adult and pediatric MDD. This study demonstrated that a specific polymorphism in this gene increased the degree to which adverse environmental events were capable of provoking an MDE.

Recent research in both behavioral and molecular genetics has attempted to define the interaction between genes and the child's environment in the pathophysiology of depression. Such an emphasis reflects the wealth of evidence from genetically oriented studies implicating environmental factors, coupled with evidence of studies directly examining the impact of stress on MDD susceptibility. For example, the studies of a prospective birth cohort demonstrated that a functional polymorphism in the promoter region of the serotonin transporter (5-HT T) gene moderated the influence of stressful life events on depression. Specifically, individuals with one or two copies of the short allele of this gene had more depressive symptoms, diagnosable depression, and suicidality in association with stressful life events than individuals who were homozygous for the long allele of the 5-HT T gene.[285] An overwhelming series of findings document abnormalities in stress responsivity among children as well as adults, with MDD. Stressful life events have been shown to represent particularly potent triggers of an MDE episode, with some evidence suggesting that this relationship appears particularly strong either early in life or for the first episode of MDD.

From the psychobiology perspective, a wealth of data in adults with MDD documents relatively robust perturbations in stress response systems. These perturbations are manifest in measures of sleep or arousal, hypothalamic-pituitary-adrenal (HPA) axis regulation, and neural dysfunction. Some retrospective data suggest that these stress-related deficiencies reflect the long-term impact of stressors operating during development. Studies directly in children and adolescents provide some evidence to support these views, in that pediatric MDD is also associated with perturbations in stress physiology. Nevertheless, the consistency and magnitude of such abnormalities appear less robust in pediatric relative to adult MDD.

Both genetic and environmental factors are hypothesized to produce MDD by altering functional aspects of an underlying brain circuit. This circuit encompasses a diverse collection of brain regions, though the circuit is focused on the prefrontal cortex (PFC) and medial temporal lobe (MTL). Data implicating this circuit in MDD derive from a range of studies using diverse methodologies. These include molecular or basic physiologic studies in rodents and nonhuman primates, postmortem studies in adult humans, and brain-imaging studies in both children and adults with MDD. In terms of specific brain regions, three structures have been the most intensive focus of ongoing neuroimaging studies: (1) the amygdala, (2) medial PFC encompassing the cingulate gyrus, and finally (3) ventrolateral PFC encompassing the orbitofrontal cortex (OFC).

Treatments for MDD are thought to exert their effects by altering activity in this circuit. This might be possible either through pharmacologic or psychotherapeutic means. Particular interest has focused on the role of serotonin (5HT) in MDD, through effects on the underlying brain circuitry. Five sets of studies implicate 5HT in MDD. First, research in animal models strongly implicates 5HT in core aspects of MDD, including hedonic regulation, anxiety, and mechanism of antidepressant response.[26,27,72,88,89,189] Second, postmortem studies document abnormal densities of 5HT-related proteins among suicide completers, the majority of whom have a history of MDD.[13,14,174,175] Third, neuroimaging studies document similar 5HT abnormalities in adults who are acutely symptomatic with MDD.[72,84,139,208] Fourth, treatments effective for MDD exert strong modulatory influences on the human 5HT system.[56,90] Selective serotonin reuptake inhibitors (SSRIs) have emerged as the first-line pharmacologic treatment for adult and pediatric MDD.[96] These agents are thought to treat MDD by improving the 5HT raphe neuron's ability to regulate the PFC, hypothalamus, and MTL.[28,56] Finally, clinical psychobiology studies show that acute manipulations of the 5HT system produce distinct changes in symptoms, chemistry, cognition, and activity in specific brain regions among individuals with MDD, relative to comparison individuals.[20,37,61,85,137,146]

Acute pharmacologic manipulations of 5HT have been used to examine perturbations in 5HT regulation of the PFC, hypothalamus, and MTL. Some studies have increased 5HT activity via 5HT agonists. Following agonist administration, adult MDD patients exhibit abnormalities in PFC and MTL function as well as abnormal secretions of hypothalamic hormones.[84,174,208] Other studies have decreased 5HT activity through dietary manipulation, using the tryptophan depletion paradigm (TDP).[20,92,146] This reduces the levels of serum tryptophan, decreasing its availability for central nervous system (CNS) 5HT synthesis. As reviewed elsewhere, in 10 of 14 studies, the procedure has been shown to induce a significantly greater increase in MDD symptoms among medicated, remitted formerly depressed adults, relative to never-depressed, nonmedicated comparisons.[259]

Treatment of Depression

Pharmacotherapy of Depression
CURRENT CONTROVERSY HERALDS NEED TO CONDUCT RANDOMIZED-CONTROLLED TRIALS
At present, much attention has been directed at evidence-based pharmacotherapy of depression in children and adolescents. In particular, this concern has focused on SSRIs, a category of medications used to treat a wide variety of psychiatric disorders, including depression and anxiety, in adults, adolescents, and children. The era of SSRIs began in the United States in the 1980s with the release of fluoxetine (Prozac). Numerous other SSRIs have been developed and are in use worldwide.

In the summer of 2003, the British government announced an investigation into the use of paroxetine (Paxil) to treat childhood depression. Subsequently, concern has been raised that SSRIs may not only be ineffective but also more dangerous than previously recognized.[132] Some contend that confusion has been increased

by industry funding of three-fourths of the large SSRI trials in adolescents. This assertion is based upon a meta-analysis of randomized-controlled trials (RCT) using SSRI in subjects 5–18 years conducted by the British Committee on Safety of Medicines, which showed a discrepancy between published and unpublished risk/benefit profiles of several SSRIs, including paroxetine, sertraline, citalopram, and venlafaxine.[274] This meta-analysis suggested that the risks outweigh benefits overall in treating depression in children and adolescents with SSRIs.

In February 2004, the Food and Drug Administration (FDA) required a change in the labeling of antidepressant medication based upon their inquiry into the safety of these medications in children and adolescents. This so-called *black box warning* consisted of the following warning "Antidepressants increased the risk of suicidal thinking and behavior (suicidality) in short-term studies in children and adolescents with Major Depressive Disorder (MDD) and other psychiatric disorders. Anyone considering the use of . . . antidepressant in a child or adolescent must balance this risk with the clinical need. Patients who are started on therapy should be observed closely for clinical worsening, suicidality, or unusual changes in behavior. Families and caregivers should be advised of the need for close observation and communication with the prescriber (Source: www.fda.gov)." The FDA warning briefly summarizes the data upon which this recommendation was based "Pooled analyses of short-term (4 to 16 weeks) placebo-controlled trials of 9 antidepressant drugs (SSRIs and others) in children and adolescents with major depressive disorder (MDD), obsessive compulsive disorder (OCD), or other psychiatric disorders (a total of 24 trials involving over 4400 patients) have revealed a greater risk of adverse events representing suicidal thinking or behavior (suicidality) during the first few months of treatment in those receiving antidepressants. The average risk of such events in patients receiving antidepressants was 4%, twice the placebo risk of 2%. No suicides occurred in these trials." Finally, the FDA added to the package insert, but not in the *black box*, a warning that clinicians should carefully screen patients for BPD, because a "major depressive episode may be the initial presentation of BPD." Following this action, clinicians must have (1) increased vigilance in their evaluation of pediatric patients for both MDD and BPD; (2) greater communication of potential risks, benefits, and alternatives of antidepressant medication with their pediatric patients and their families; and (3) enhanced monitoring, meaning greater quality and quantity of contact, for potential side effects, safety, and benefits for all patients taking antidepressant medication. Given the burden of disease from depression in children and adolescents, further study is necessary. This includes larger studies, free from potential pharmaceutical industry bias, to determine the safety and efficacy of pharmacologic treatments for all childhood disorders, including psychiatric illnesses.[180] Additionally, due to public and legal pressure, pharmaceutical companies are disclosing previously unreleased data. Finally, the National Institute of Mental Health (NIMH) strategic roadmap is committed to create large research networks to conduct studies of sufficient sample size to determine which treatments for childhood psychopathology are effective and safe.

PREGNANCY: NEED TO CONSIDER WHEN TREATING DEPRESSION OR BIPOLAR DISORDER

For all of these medications discussed for both depression and BPD, clinicians should be aware of the unique treatment implications of pregnancy. Specifically, consultation and collaboration with specialists, including child and adolescent psychiatrists and obstetrician/gynecologists, is essential to help female patients with mood disorders make informed decisions about medication. This often requires balancing the need to discontinue or reduce psychiatric medications during pregnancy due to concerns about the effects on the fetus or newborn child with the potential resulting harm of treatment changes, including risk of precipitating a major depressive or manic episode. The latter's impact would not only be on the fetus or child, but also on the mother and all involved caregivers. Ideally, discussion about the impact of pregnancy on treatment should be held prior to conceiving.[43,280]

Selective Serotonin Reuptake Inhibitors
EVIDENCE-BASED REVIEW

While controversy exists about the use of SSRIs to treat children and adolescents with depression, as evidenced by Table 4-8, several double-blind placebo-controlled randomized trials have been conducted to evaluate their safety and efficacy. Nine RCTs have been published to date evaluating SSRIs in pediatric depression. Of these, three out of four trials have shown that flouxetine is more effective than placebo in treating children and adolescents with depression.[95,97,179,244] Of note, only one of these three trials was sponsored by a pharmaceutical company whereas the other three were sponsored by the NIMH. The authors of one RCT each of paroxetine and sertraline reported their studies as demonstrating safe and effective treatment of depression, though the investigations of the FDA and British government's investigation have questioned these findings.[140,262] One published RCT of venlafaxine plus psychotherapy did not find benefit over placebo plus psychotherapy.[170] However, other negative venlafaxine trials have been implemented, though these remain unpublished. The pharmaceutical company that marketed venlafaxine advised physicians not to use the medication for pediatric mood and anxiety disorders in 2003. Citalopram is another SSRI that a recent RCT in children and adolescents with depression showed superiority over a placebo, though another unpublished trial failed to show such effect,[286] which is currently marketed in the United States under a different trade name. Given the inconsistency of the findings and the potential that a sizable number of unreported, negative studies exist, current consensus suggests that only fluoxetine should definitively be considered an effective SSRI. As such, this medication usually should be considered the first-line medication in pediatric MDD. Nevertheless, given that data in adults do not document

▶ **TABLE 4-8** SSRI TRIALS IN DEPRESSED YOUTH

	Wagner et al. (2004)	Emslie et al. (2004)	March et al. (2003)	Wagner et al. (2002)	Emslie et al. (2001)	Keller et al. (1997)	Emslie et al. (1997)	Mandoki et al. (1990)	Simeon et al. (2004)
Funding source	Forest Pharmaceuticals	Eli Lilly and Company	NIMH (medication provided by Eli Lilly)	Pfizer	Eli Lilly	Glaxo Smith Kline	NIMH and Eli Lilly	Unknown	Unknown
Sample	MDD children and adolescents	MDD adolescents stabilized on fluoxetine N = 20 continued fluoxetine while N = 20 were switched to placebo	N = 439 MDD adolescents. Randomized to 4 groups: (1) CBT + fluoxetine (N = 107); (2) fluoxetine alone (N = 109); (3) CBT alone (N = 111); (4) placebo (N = 112)	N = 376 MDD moderate; exclusion: prior suicide attempt, significant suicidal or homicidal risk, or history of bipolar disorder	N = 119 MDD; excluded BPD and those with serious risk for suicide	N = 275 adolescents with MDD excluded history of suicidality	N = 96 MDD without psychosis; excludes any with family history of bipolar disorder in first-degree relative	N = 40 MDD; excludes suicidal patients (N = 20 venlafaxine + CBT; N = 20 placebo + CBT)	N = 40
Medication	Citalopram 20–40 mg (mean dose in sample 24 m/day). 8 weeks	Fluoxetine 20 to 60 mg	Fluoxetine 10–40 mg	Sertraline 50–200 mg	Fluoxetine 10–20 mg	Paroxetine 20–40 mg, imipramine 200–300 mg placebo	Fluoxetine 20 mg	Venlafaxine 12.5 mg qd-tid (8–12 years old) or 25 mg qd-tid (13–17 years old)	Fluoxetine
Duration		32-week relapse-prevention phase of a double-blind, multi-center, placebo-controlled 51-week study	12 weeks	10 weeks	9 weeks (1 week 10 mg, then 8 at 20 mg)	8 weeks	8 weeks	6 weeks	8 weeks
Outcome measure	Children's Depression Rating Scale-Revised; the response criterion was defined as a score of ≤ 28	Children's Depression Rating Scale, Revised score of >40	Total Child Depression Rating Scale (CDRS) score	>40% change from baseline CDRS	CDRS	Hamilton Depression Rating (HAM-D) <8 or 50% HAM-D reduction	Clinician's global impression (CGI), CDRS	CDRS, HAM-D, Children's depression inventory (CDI), child behavior checklist (CBCL)	
Author's conclusion	Citalopram reduced depressive symptoms to a significantly greater extent than placebo treatment and was well tolerated.	Fluoxetine was well tolerated and can significantly delay relapse of major depressive symptoms in children and adolescents.	Combination fluoxetine plus CBT offered most favorable outcome	Sertraline is an effective and well-tolerated short-term treatment for MDD	Fluoxetine 20 mg daily is well-tolerated effective acute treatment for depression	Paroxetine is safe and effective treatment for depression	Fluoxetine better than placebo in acute depression treatment	Venlafaxine not significantly more helpful than placebo when combined with psychotherapy	Fluoxetine is helpful

	Col 1	Col 2	Col 3	Col 4	Col 5	Col 6	Col 7	Col 8
Outcome	Mean Children's Depression Rating Scale-Revised scores decreased significantly more from baseline in the citalopram treatment group than in the placebo treatment group, beginning at week 1 and continuing at every observation point to the end of the study (effect size = 2.9). The difference in response rate at week 8 between placebo (24%) and citalopram (36%) also was statistically significant.	Mean time to relapse was longer in those continuing to receive fluoxetine compared to those switched to placebo. Relapse occurred in an estimated 34% of those continuing to receive fluoxetine and in 60% of those switched to placebo.	Response rate: (1) CBT + fluoxetine 71%; (2) fluoxetine 60.6%; (3) CBT alone 43.2%; (4) placebo 34.8%	69% on sertraline and 59% on placebo were considered responders ($P = 0.05$)	41% on fluoxetine and 20% on placebo met outcome criteria ($P < 0.01$); 65% fluoxetine and 53% placebo with >30% decrease in CDRS ($P = 0.09$)	Paroxetine better than placebo in HAM-D response; imipramine not better than placebo; no difference in self or parent report of symptom reduction	56% on fluoxetine and 33% on placebo acutely respond; no significant difference in full remission	N = 30/40 completed study. Two-thirds of each group had marked/moderate improvement
Adverse events	Rates of discontinuation due to adverse events were comparable in the placebo and citalopram groups (5.9% versus 5.6%, respectively). Rhinitis, nausea, and abdominal pain were the only adverse events to occur with a frequency exceeding 10% in either treatment group	No "serious adverse events." 1/20 fluoxetine patients discontinued due to agitation. 2/20 placebo patients discontinued due to hyperkinesias (one) and infection (one).	7/439 patients attempted suicide. No completed suicides	17/189 sertraline and 9/187 placebo discontinued study. Suicide attempts: 2 sertraline, 1 placebo; suicidal ideation (3 sertraline), aggression (1 sertraline); medical hospitalization (1 sertraline, 4 placebo)	No significant group difference in adverse events; 5/(4.6%) fluoxetine (rash, agitation, constipation, hyperkinesias, mania) and 9/(8.2%) placebo (rash, abdominal pain, alopecia, anxiety, dizziness, headache) discontinue due to adverse events	Paroxetine: 11 (1 headache, 2 depression, 5 suicidal ideation, 2 conduct problems, 1 manic symptoms); imipramine: 5 (1 each—chest pain and dyspnea, rash, emotional lability, hostility, hallucinations); (2) placebo: 2	7 fluoxetine subjects dropped out for lack of efficacy; 4 for side effects (1 = rash, 3 = manic symptoms); 19 placebo subjects dropped out for lack of efficacy and 1 for unspecified side effects	6/40 dropped out of study on their own; 1 in venlafaxine group was hospitalized for mania

consistent therapeutic differences between fluox-etine and other SSRIs, this perspective generates many questions. For example, this might suggest that other SSRIs beyond fluoxetine actually are effective, but available studies fail to demonstrate this effect. Alternatively, this might suggest that the therapeutics of pediatric MDD clearly differ from that of adult MDD.

Proposed Mechanism

Selective serotonin reuptake inhibitors are believed to treat depression by decreasing their transport from the synapse to inside neurons, thus increas-ing synaptic levels of serotonin. Besides clinical response, the role of serotonin in the patho-physiology of depression is supported by the induction of depression by agents that deplete serotonin.[204,246] Also, studies have found decreased serotonin in victims of suicide.[228] While SSRIs increase synaptic serotonin quickly, the clinical response often requires several weeks. Recent studies have suggested that this may be due to the fact that SSRIs' clinical effect may be the result of increased neurogenesis from chroni-cally increased serotonin.[239]

Monitoring/Side Effects

Selective serotonin reuptake inhibitors are hepat-ically metabolized. Most SSRIs have a half-life of approximately 24 hours, making once per day dosing the norm. Fluoxetine has the longest half-life, averaging 72–96 hours in adults, not to mention the active metabolite norfluoxetine which has a similar half-life. Therefore, clini-cians should carefully examine all medications that their patients are taking for drug-drug interactions, including herbals, over-the-counter medications, and supplements.

Common side effects of SSRIs include gas-trointestinal complaints (nausea, vomiting, diar-rhea, and constipation), headache, and sexual dysfunction.

Serotonin Syndrome

Patients taking serotonergic medications, includ-ing SSRIs, need to be aware of and monitored for the serotonin syndrome (Table 4-9). This syn-drome is thought to be the result of excess synap-tic serotonin. The clinical picture includes the following: altered mental status (including delir-ium and coma), autonomic dysfunction (e.g., hyperthermia, tachycardia, labile blood pressure), salivation, diaphoresis, dilated pupils, and neuro-muscular abnormalities (including rigidity, tremor, myoclonus, and seizures). Given the shared symp-toms of autonomic instability and neuromuscular dysfunction, clinicians may need to differentiate serotonin syndrome from neuroleptic malignant syndrome (NMS) (discussed further in atypical neuroleptic use in pediatric BPD; Table 4-11) in patients treated with atypical neuroleptics, as these medications target both dopamine (NMS) and serotonin (serotonin syndrome) receptors. Treatment of serotonin syndrome includes stop-ping the offending agent, maintaining hydration, and supportive care to handle autonomic insta-bility, altered mental status, and patient safety. Typically, once recognized and properly treated, serotonin syndrome resolves in 1–3 days.

Contraindications

Use of SSRIs or monoamine oxidase inhibitors (MAOIs) within 2 weeks of one another should never occur due to the high resultant risk of serotonin syndrome. Due to their hepatic metab-olism, patients should be cautioned about con-suming alcohol. Finally, careful examination of drug interactions is urged, since SSRIs may alter the pharmacodynamics of other hepatically metabolized agents.

▶ **TABLE 4-9** SEROTONIN SYNDROME

- Altered mental status (including delirium and coma)
- Autonomic dysfunction (e.g., hyperthermia, tachycardia, labile blood pressure)
- Salivation
- Diaphoresis
- Dilated pupils
- Neuromuscular abnormalities (including rigidity, tremor, myoclonus, and seizures)

Tricyclic Antidepressants

EVIDENCE-BASED REVIEW

Tricyclic antidepressants (TCAs) are a group of medications predating the SSRIs named for their chemical structure consisting of three connected rings. The few RCTs of TCAs that have been conducted have demonstrated mixed efficacy in treating children and adolescents with depression.[107,157,249,271]

PROPOSED MECHANISM

The antidepressant property of TCAs is thought to result from their ability to inhibit the reuptake of serotonin and norepinephrine, thus increasing the relative concentration of both within the synapse.

MONITORING/SIDE EFFECTS

Common side effects from TCAs include dry mouth, constipation, drowsiness, orthostatic hypotension, weight gain, and sexual dysfunction. These effects are medicated via TCAs' antagonism of muscarinic acetylcholine and histamine receptors. TCAs are hepatically metabolized, and therefore clinicians need to be careful for multidrug interactions. Serum drug levels are available and should be monitored routinely.[224,225]

Clinicians need to be aware of TCAs potential for cardiac toxicity, especially in an overdose. Studies have shown conflicting results regarding whether or not TCAs cause significant ECG changes at therapeutic levels, including potentially tachycardia, flattened T waves, prolonged QT intervals, and depressed ST segments.[129,275] In overdose, this has led some to suggest that TCAs should not be used in treating children or adolescents for depression.[272]

CONTRAINDICATIONS

Pediatric patients with preexisting cardiac arrhythmias should not take TCAs for depression due to exacerbated prolonged conduction time. Patients taking oral contraceptive pills may have decreased TCA serum levels due to hepatic enzyme induction. Patients taking SSRIs concomitantly may have increased TCA serum levels due to inhibition of TCA hepatic metabolism.

Psychotherapy of Depression

Besides medication, psychotherapy is often an important part of the treatment of child and adolescent depression. While a complete discussion of therapy is beyond the scope of this chapter, nonpsychiatrist physicians should have an awareness of the basics. Also, as has been emphasized throughout this chapter, optimal care of the child or adolescent with psychiatric issues requires the close collaboration between all involved practitioners. Though difficult, it is crucial in those receiving "split treatment," meaning someone going to a physician for medication and either a psychiatrist, psychologist, or social worker for therapy.

There are many types of therapy used to treat pediatric depression. Each has its idea of the etiology of depression and the theory of change required to eliminate it. Systematic study of therapy is difficult due to the need to create a placebo therapy, which would be exactly like the study therapy except it must lack the active ingredient.

Cognitive-behavioral therapy (CBT) has become one of the most studied treatments for depression across the lifespan. CBT focuses on dysfunctional beliefs, called cognitive distortions, which cause people to feel depressed.[18] Also, people's actions and behaviors often lead to further depression. In CBT, the therapist works to help patients become aware of and then change self-defeating patterns of automatic thoughts and behaviors. Some of this change comes through the therapist's challenging the patient to examine the evidence for attitudes, beliefs, and actions to determine if they are helpful or, instead, if they are unsubstantiated and contribute to exacerbated depression. Data comparing the efficacy of CBT to wait-list conditions document clear benefits over "no treatment." This represents a relatively "low bar" to consider a treatment as effective, given the possible aversive effects of a no treatment condition in a randomized-controlled trial. The beneficial effects of CBT may derive more from nonspecific aspects of contacts with therapists, as opposed to the specific aspects of CBT.

However, data from a recent trial demonstrated that treatment of depressed adolescents with CBT combined with fluoxetine was superior to treatment with fluoxetine alone.[179] Interpersonal therapy (IPT) is one type of therapy used to treat depression across the lifespan. IPT focuses on the present, without dwelling in the past, and holds that depression is often the result of relationship difficulties between the patient and others. In IPT, the therapist's intervention is to help the patient become aware of these interpersonal problems leading to depression. The four areas focused upon are grief, interpersonal role disputes, role transitions, and interpersonal deficits. Three RCTs of IPT showed feasibility and efficacy of IPT for treating depressed adolescents.[196,198,199]

Family therapy is also often used to treat pediatric depression. There are numerous models of family therapy, but most involve bringing families together to examine their contribution to depression. Family therapy does not seek to blame anyone for causing psychopathology. Evidence in support of family therapy for depression comes from long-term follow-up studies demonstrating the importance of a depressed patient's family functioning in relapse prevention.[190,191] However, available data suggest that this treatment does not offer many advantages over traditional CBT.[39]

► PEDIATRIC BIPOLAR DISORDER

Introduction

Our understanding of pediatric BPD is much more limited than that of unipolar depression. Just as with MDD, there once was a wide spread belief that children could not have manic episodes. While this sentiment continues for some, current research indicates that BPD can and does occur in children. Pediatric BPD is among the most active and controversial areas of child and adolescent psychiatry research, particularly with regard to the appropriate limits of the diagnosis.[106,111,278] This section of the chapter will focus clinicians' attention on current diagnostic and therapeutic issues in pediatric BPD.

Research on pediatric BPD has lagged behind that on pediatric depression. One cause for this relates to disagreement about diagnosis. While consensus has emerged on the appropriate modifications of DSM criteria for depression and its subtypes for children and adolescents, debate continues about diagnostic criteria for BPD to children and adolescents. Some suggest that the same criteria used for adults should be applied to children and adolescents. Others suggest that pediatric BPD presents with a fundamentally different picture in children than it does in older individuals. Without consensus on diagnostic criteria, it is difficult to study key clinical features of the disorder. For example, few data exist concerning the prevalence of pediatric BPD in the community. While initial epidemiologic studies indicates that the disorder is considerably rarer than MDD or anxiety disorders in children and adolescents, some researchers suggest that such figures are inaccurate because they apply criteria to children and adolescents that are more appropriate for adults. Regardless, general consensus has emerged that pediatric BPD is a very serious condition that exerts at least as disruptive of an effect on the lives of children and adolescents as MDD. In fact, most clinicians working with pediatric mental disorders recognize BPD as the more serious condition.

Diagnostic Dilemmas in Pediatric BPD: Elation versus Irritability, Manic Episode Duration, and Comorbidity

Three issues contribute to the difficulty diagnosing mania, and in turn BPD, in children: (1) whether elevated versus irritable mood is essential for the diagnosis and, if not, how to differentiate the irritability of mania from that of other illnesses; (2) the minimum duration of a manic episode; (3) comorbid diagnoses. Clinicians who understand these issues are better prepared to appropriately diagnose and treat pediatric BPD. The diagnostic procedure for BPD is the same as outlined earlier for MDD, though clinicians must, obviously, determine if a manic or hypo-manic episode has occurred.[1]

ELEVATED, EXPANSIVE MOOD VERSUS IRRITABILITY?

As shown in Table 4-2, the (A) criterion from the DSM-IV-TR definition of a manic episode requires the presence of an elevated, expansive, or irrita-ble mood which represents a change from base-line, lasting >7 days for a manic episode or >4 days (but <7 days) for a hypomanic episode. Elevated/expansive mood is rarely seen outside of mania, whereas irritability is fairly ubiquitous in child psychopathology. Investigators disagree about whether elevated mood should be required for the diagnosis of mania, but differ-ent number of (B) symptoms are required based upon which mood is present (>3 if elevated/expansive or >4 if only irritable mood). Differ-entiating irritability due to BPD, rather than to depression or other psychopathology, requires that the irritability be accompanied by other fea-tures of a manic or hypomanic episode. That is, the irritability should follow an episodic course and be accompanied by other neurovegetative symptoms, such as decreased need for sleep, grandiosity, flight of ideas, and so on. Moreover, irritability must be noticeable to others for a diag-nosis of hypomania and severely impairing for a diagnosis of mania

EPISODES: HOW LONG?

The second, related issue is minimum symptom duration of a mood episode or cycle. DSM-IVTR clearly defines manic episodes as periods aber-rant mood, different from that individual's normal, baseline mood, with associated symp-toms lasting a minimum of 4 days for a hypo-manic or 7 days for manic episode. Also DSM-IVTR states that the term "rapid cycling" may be used to indicate someone who has at least 4 mood episodes per year. However, some have blurred these definitions of "cycle" and "episode" to enable children with extremely brief mood changes to fit these DSM-IVTR defi-nitions. These truncated episodes, which are not found in DSM-IV-TR, are commonly known

as (1) "ultra-rapid cycling" describing those with mood changes every few days, and (2) "ultra-dian cycling" referring to those with episodes lasting minutes occurring four or more times per day.[154] Nevertheless, only those children and adolescents who meet DSM-IV-TR criteria for episode duration—i.e. 4 or more days (hypo-manic episode) or 7 or more days (manic episode)—can be diagnosed with confidence as having BPD."

COMORBIDITY: DIAGNOSTIC CONFOUND OR COOCCURRING DISORDER?

Comorbidity is the third issue contributing to the difficulty diagnosing BPD in children in two respects. First, an individual child rarely has only BPD; rather, most children with BPD have other comorbid, meaning co-occurring, psychiatric dis-orders. These comorbid disorders include, but are not limited to anxiety disorders, attention deficit hyperactivity disorder (ADHD), conduct disorder, and substance use disorders. Thus, the diagnostic dilemma is often not "either BPD or one of those comorbid disorders" but both—e.g., BPD plus comorbid condition(s). Second, the DSM-IV-TR definitions of these comorbid psychi-atric disorders have considerable overlap with the definition of BPD. This problem has been most evident in the case of ADHD, where the hyper-activity and distractibility of an irritable child with ADHD can be mistaken for symptoms of mania. Sorting out these diagnostic issues is not trivial, as they have serious treatment and prognostic implications.

STEPWISE GUIDANCE FOR CLINICIANS IN DIAGNOSING BPD

Having spelled out the three dilemmas in diag-nosing BPD in children and adolescents, namely (1) elevated, expansive mood versus irritability, (2) episode duration, and (3) comorbidity, how should clinicians properly evaluate and diag-nose individual patients?

The process of evaluating a child or adoles-cent for BPD should utilize the same approach outlined in the section on MDD. This should include (1) the use of multiple informants, including the pediatric patient, parents, and teachers (the latter once releases of information have been obtained); (2) interviewing the pediatric patient and parents both together and separately to obtain a detailed account of both the present and past psychiatric and medical history; and (3) review of relevant evaluations that may have been obtained before the clinician was consulted about possible BPD diagnosis, including recent school, psychological, educational, and medical/neurologic evaluations.

Simultaneously, the content of the evaluation of a child or adolescent for BPD must focus on determining whether or not the pediatric patient's symptoms are consistent with a diagnosis of BPD. Of necessity, clinicians must consider the alternative—e.g., that the child's symptoms are not BPD, but rather due to a different condition. The differential diagnosis of pediatric BPD includes: (1) psychiatric conditions that are either frequently comorbid (co-occuring) with BPD or frequently have overlapping diagnostic symptoms; (2) nonpsychiatric medical disorders causing symptoms resembling those of mania (see table 4-10); and (3) substance use disorders.

Before considering each of these categories of disorders in the differential diagnosis of BPD, several caveats should be mentioned. First and foremost, clinicians should be aware that diagnosis is an ongoing process, not just an end.

This diagnostic process requires constant hypothesis testing to ensure that, as the child develops, changes in symptoms and functional impairment incorporated into her/his diagnosis. Put another way, just because a child does not have BPD when evaluated at 7 years does not mean that he/she may not have BPD when evaluated at 12 years. Second, some children and adolescents do not neatly fit into a single DSM-IV-TR diagnosis—of BPD or others. In this situation, clinicians should seek consultation with a child/adolescent psychiatrist, step back to consider a broader differential diagnosis of their patient's symptoms, and treat conditions—i.e., ADHD, depression—whose diagnosis the child fully meets.

Differential Diagnosis of Pediatric BPD
OTHER PSYCHIATRIC CONDITIONS

As previously mentioned, a number of psychiatric conditions are in the differential diagnosis of BPD in children and adolescents. Some of these conditions have overlapping diagnostic criteria with BPD, most notably ADHD. Others share core traits of affect dysregulation, including anxiety disorders, externalizing disorders (such as CD or oppositional defiant disorder [ODD]), and substance use disorders. Complicating matters further, all of these disorders can be comorbid with BPD.

▶ **TABLE 4-10** MEDICAL CONDITIONS IN THE DIFFERENTIAL DIAGNOSIS OF BIPOLAR DISORDER

- Neurologic disorders: CNS infections (meningitis, encephalitis), epilepsy/seizures (temporal lobe epilepsy), cerebral neoplasms, cerebrovascular accident/stroke, multiple sclerosis, cerebral trauma, Klein-Levin syndrome
- Infectious disease: human immunodeficiency virus/acquired immunodeficiency syndrome (HIV/AIDS)
- Metabolic disorders: Wilson disease, porphyria, Kleinfelter syndrome
- Endocrine disorders: hyperthyroidism, carcinoid syndrome, postpartum
- Vitamin deficiency: B_{12}, niacin (pellagra)
- Rheumatologic: systemic lupus erythematosus
- Medications: corticosteroids, cyclosporine, baclofen, isoniazid, drugs of abuse (amphetamines, cocaine, hallucinogens, opiates, phencyclidine), psychotropic medications (including SSRIs, TCAs, MAOIs, carbamazepine, methlphenidate/psychostimulants)
- Other: renal disease/failure/uremia

Clinicians need to carefully determine if any of these diagnoses more accurately fits a particular patient as the primary presenting condition, or if a child or adolescent with BPD has any of these diagnoses as a comorbid problem. With respect to ADHD, much work has focused on differentiating it from BPD.[24,47,109] Both ADHD and the manic phase of BPD share features of inattention, excess physical activity and energy, rapid speech, and impaired concentration. However, BPD as in DSM-IV-TR, first and foremost requires an elevated, expansive, or irritable mood, readily differentiable from the child's normal mood, lasting most of the day for at least 4 (hypomanic episode) to 7 (manic episode) days. Distractibility that follows an episodic course, fluctuating with simultaneous mood changes, might be part of a manic episode of BPD. In contrast, nonepisodic distractibility would be more likely to be ADHD. Clinicians may refer patients for psycho-educational testing, including measures of attention and intelligence, to more fully evaluate children in whom both ADHD and BPD are suspected, as well as to determine if other learning disorders are present and needing treatment. However, the diagnosis of ADHD in BPD rests on a comprehensive psychiatric evaluation, not on the results of these tests alone. Information gained from clinician's consultation with other significant people in the patient's life, including parents, teachers, after-school staff, often helps clinicians to evaluate psychiatric comorbidity in pediatric patients possibly with BPD.

The term "externalizing behavior disorders" has been applied to the diagnosis of ADHD as well as ODD and CD. These conditions frequently complicate the diagnosis of BPD in children and adolescents. As with ADHD, clinicians should carefully assess for the mood criteria of a hypo/manic episode—i.e. 4–7 day period of aberrant mood that is either elevated/expansive or irritable—in order to differentiate BPD from either CD or ODD.

Clinicians should also consider unipolar depression in the differential diagnosis of BPD. Specifically, data suggest more cautious, judicious use of antidepressant medication in children or adolescents presenting with depression that is very severe, marked by extreme psychomotor retardation or hypersomnia, is accompanied by psychosis, or occurs in an individual with first-degree relatives with BPD. Importantly, this does not mean that pediatric patients with depression plus any of those three features are necessarily bipolar or that they should be treated as though they are bipolar. Rather particularly close supervision of such patients is warranted.

MEDICAL MIMICS

Table 4-10 lists the medical conditions known to cause mania. As with depression, clinicians need not perform laboratory testing to evaluate all of these conditions. However, it is vitally important that clinicians consider, based on their evaluation of the pediatric patient, whether one or more of these medical conditions might possibly be causing the symptoms of mania in a particular patient. If so, appropriate evaluation, including physical examination, laboratory or other testing, or consultation with other specialists is warranted.

Numerous medications, herbals, and dietary supplements may cause symptoms mirroring mania. Clinicians should take a thorough history of recent substances used by the child. This includes an open, developmentally appropriate history with parent and patient together and separately, inquiring not only about prescribed medications, but also over the counter, herbal, and supplement preparations. Both psychotropic medications, such as SSRIs and psychostimulants, as well as nonpsychiatric medications, such as steroids, are well known to cause mania.[65,83,112,147,215]

In particular, clinicians should remain vigilant for the onset of extreme irritability or mania following initiation of psychiatric medications, including antidepressants—e.g. SSRIs—and stimulants—e.g. methylphenidate or dextroamphetamine. Also, as discussed above, irritability is not a specific symptom of BPD in children; rather, irritability may be a diagnostic feature of MDD and anxiety disorders in pediatric patients.

Under these circumstances, the clinican usually should seek consultation immediately from an expert in pediatric mental illness. While awaiting consultation, a potential offending agents should be stopped, and the patient monitored for reduction in manic symptoms. Drug- or substance-induced mania is not the same diagnostic entity as BPD, whose diagnosis explicitly requires that the symptoms are not due to the ingestion of any substance, legal or illicit.

SUBSTANCE USE

Numerous substances of abuse can cause disinhibition or mood alterations consistent with mania. Clinicians should have a high index of suspicion for substance abuse in pediatric patients that they are evaluating for psychiatric disorders. As in MDD, this evaluation starts by taking an open, nonjudgmental history with patient and parents separately. Studies have shown increased risk for substance use disorders in adolescents with BPD, in comparison to children with BPD.[276] Treatment of youth with BPD and substance use disorders requires a collaborative team approach, as the two disorders together cause more morbidity, mortality, and health care utilization than either alone.[125]

Pathophysiology of Pediatric Bipolar Disorder

What causes BPD in children and adolescents? The simple answer is that researchers have not yet identified any single cause. Like MDD, BPD is a multifactorial disease process. Furthermore, as already discussed, investigations of BPD are more complicated than those of MDD for several reasons, including the fact that the field of research is younger and debates about developmentally informed diagnostic phenotypes are more unsettled in BPD.

Nevertheless, research into the cause of BPD is, in some ways, easier than unipolar depression because true manic episodes are a homogeneous entity, easily recognized, especially in adults. This is not the case of MDE, which are often marked by the previously discussed issues of less overt, manifest symptoms and frequent comorbidity with anxiety.

Studies of BPD patients and their families across the lifespan have in the past, and continue in the present, to advance our understanding of the pathophysiology of BPD in children and adolescents. The chief foci of such research include neural circuitry, intracellular mechanisms, genetics, and sleep physiology.

Brain Circuitry

CONNECTING BEHAVIOR WITH NEUROIMAGING

The goal of neuropsychiatric research in BPD is that by studying the brains of people with BPD, we will identify brain circuits that are specifically aberrant, so that targeted treatments can be designed to repair such changes. There are three methods of studying brain function in people with BPD. First, researchers have evaluated people whose brain lesions, such as following brain surgery, cause behavioral symptoms resembling mania. Second, neuroimaging techniques, including magnetic resonance imaging (MRI) and positron emission tomography (PET; generally used only in adults due to radiation exposure), make it possible to evaluate brain changes in BPD patients. Third, behavioral measures, such as neuropsychologic testing, enable us to test for cognitive impairments in BPD subjects. When taken as a whole, these results suggest that impairment in the frontal and temporal lobes is at the heart of BPD.

Frontal lobe structures involved in BPD include the orbitofrontal cortex (OFC) and the dorsolateral prefrontal cortex (DLPFC). As its name suggests, the orbitofrontal cortex OFC is part of the frontal lobes immediately above the eyes. The OFC's role in emotion regulation was identified by studies of people suffering brain lesions long before brain-imaging technology existed. Perhaps the most famous case is that of Phineas Gage, a railroad worker who survived an iron rod being driven through his skull, from below his eye through the top of his skull, during an accident in the 1800s. Afterward, Gage was not his even-tempered self. Instead, he was volatile, labile, and prone to rage—in short, Gage had symptoms similar to those of BPD. Modern scientists have used neuroimaging of Gage's skull to determine that the iron rod injured his OFC.[68] Functional MRI of BPD adults has shown impairment in the OFC during the Stroop cognitive interference task.[30] These and other studies have led to the hypothesis that the OFC plays a role in cognitive and emotional inflexibility in BPD.[232,233]

The DLPFC is the second region in the frontal lobes hypothesized to be involved in BPD. The DLPFC, as its name suggests, is located in the rostral area of the frontal lobes (toward the top of the skull). The DLPFC is involved in a number of functions, including shifting attention from one stimulus to the next. Numerous studies, including several in adults and one in children and adolescents, have shown impaired attention in BPD across mood states, including mania, depression, and euthymia.[59,60,82,200,234,235] Corroborating evidence of DLPFC dysfunction in BPD emanates from MRI studies which have found decreased volume and density.[81,86,168,240]

Recent data has also implicated the striatum in the pathophysiology of BPD. Four functional MRI studies in patients with BPD (two of adults and two of youth) have reported increased neural activation in patients vs. controls. These studies have used paradigms involving emotional faces or pictures[288,289] an interference task[290] a spatial working memory task[289], or a task designed to generate affect.[291] Blumberg et al.[292] have suggested that striatal abnormalities are present in adolescents with BPD, with PFC deficits developing later."

Temporal lobe structures demonstrated to be involved in pediatric BPD include the amygdala and hippocampus. Although small in size, the amygdala is great in its functional connections with other brain regions, including the OFC and hippocampus, and is hypothesized to be at the center of emotional regulation, including learning from reward and punishment conditions.[71,73,115,135,160] MRI studies in adults appear inconsistent regarding amygdala volume,

finding increased, decreased, or no change. Those in pediatric BPD have found decreased amygdala volume, suggesting that pediatric BPD may have neurodevelopmental differences from adult-onset BPD.[5,6,29,36,79,214] The hippocampus is another temporal lobe structure, involved in memory, which is putatively involved in BPD. Although most adult BPD studies have not found hippocampal volume differences in comparison to healthy controls, one study of adolescents with BPD did show hippocampal volume reduction.[5–7,29,36,120,240,251] Thus, studies of temporal lobe structures, including the amygdala and hippocampus, provide evidence that pediatric-onset BPD may be neurodevelopmentally different than more typical adult-onset BPD.

Thus, ongoing work uniting brain and behavioral changes characteristic in children and adolescents holds the potential to identify the core pathophysiology responsible for BPD. At present, fronto-temporal structures are the major areas of research emphasis.

INTRACELLULAR CLUES

We have learned much about the potential cause of BPD from the pharmacology of the medications used to treat the disorder. Studies have shown that lithium and valproate, two of the most common medications used to treat BPD, exert their effect on intracellular second messenger cascades, rather than on the neuronal synapse. Second messenger systems are responsible for amplifying signals from outside the cell to within the cell, resulting in chemical cascades modifying DNA and RNA translation, and regulating protein synthesis. Thus, a small change in a chemical messenger can result in large alterations in cell function. Lithium is hypothesized to exert its mood stabilizing effect by reducing concentrations of myoinositol through inhibition of inositol monophosphatase.[174] At therapeutically relevant levels, this results in the reduction of the concentration of myoinositol, whose effects continue to trickle down to reduced protein synthesis.[193] However, just as with antidepressants used to treat depression, there is a time lag between this biochemical alteration and the clinical effect.

Lithium and valproate also work to inhibit the protein kinase C pathway, another second messenger cascade.[171,174] In the future, scientists hope that by studying the intracellular effects of current medications used to treat BPD, we will accomplish two things. First, we will understand potential biologic changes responsible for BPD. Second, we will be able to design specific interventions, including novel medications, to treat or even prevent the morbidity and mortality from BPD.

GENETICS

In the future, scientists will hopefully identify the gene or genes responsible for BPD. At present unfortunately, there is no single gene or genetic test available for BPD. There are several candidate genes that have been identified, largely through studies of adults, which include areas of the following chromosomes: 6p, 6q, 10p, 11p, 13q, 20p, 22p.[58,184,242] Moreover, studies have not demonstrated mitochondrial inheritance of BPD.[188]

There is cause for optimism about the identification of the genes responsible for pediatric BPD. For example, evidence suggests that the earlier onset of one's BPD symptoms, the greater the amount of genetic "loading" one has.[253] Also, several ongoing studies are using linkage analysis to evaluate triads (a BPD child plus two parents) for genetic markers of BPD; this technique is more powerful and efficient than simply searching affected individuals for genetic markers.[243]

SLEEP/CIRCADIAN RHYTHMS

Changes in sleep rhythm are diagnostic features of both depression and BPD. In the context of a manic episode, BPD patients have insomnia without the usually accompanying symptom of fatigue. Studies have shown that abnormal circadian rhythms are present in adults with BPD.[267] Moreover, sleep deprivation may trigger a manic episode in those with BPD.[266] Decreased sleep duration on previous nights may be predictive of impending manic episodes.[161] Sleep studies of young adults (age 18–35) have demonstrated that adults with either BPD or depression have similar polysomnographic abnormalities in comparison to healthy controls, possibly suggesting that the two patient groups share a common alteration in sleep dysfunction.[126] When it comes to children with BPD, decreased need for sleep is one of the most useful symptoms for discriminating BPD from other conditions, especially ADHD.[110] Further study will reveal what central mechanism is responsible for the sleep changes characteristic of mania, and in turn, what these mechanisms reveal about BPD itself.

Treatment of BPD

Treatment of BPD in children and adolescents is complicated not only by the diagnostic issues already discussed, but also by lack of RCT. This holds for both medication and psychotherapy interventions. However, trials of both are underway and will hopefully yield useful information on which to base clinical decisions. In the interim, clinicians on the front lines must make informed decisions when attempted to help children and families struggling with BPD. Clinicians should be open to consultation with child and adolescent psychiatrists when considering the treatment of a pediatric patient with BPD, especially if that child is a preadolescent, as these patients require complex and comprehensive treatment planning.

What is a "mood stabilizer?" The term "mood stabilizer" is frequently used to describe medications used to treat BPD. This term has been used by both clinicians and the pharmaceutical industry since the 1980s to describe medications that may reduce mood variability, including reducing both manic and depressive episodes.[138] However, clinicians need to be aware that this term does not connote a specific pharmacologic property or definition of a medication.[282] In fact, the 2002 American Psychiatric Association's practice guideline for BPD specifically refrains from using the term mood stabilizer because of its lack of pharmacologic precision.[4] We are awaiting further pharmacologic research to determine the mechanism by which current and future medications reduce mood variability. In the interim, clinicians must weigh the potential risks and benefits of initiating or changing therapeutic interventions, both medications and therapies, for children and adolescents with BPD.

Given the lack of data in pediatric patients, clinicians must often use treatments studied only or primarily in adults with BPD. At present, the following list represents the medications and indications approved by the Food and Drug Administration (FDA): (1) lithium is approved to age 12 years for acute mania and maintenance therapy of BPD; (2) valproate is approved for adults with acute mania; (3) lamotrigine is a novel atypical antiepileptic drug (AED) approved for maintenance treatment; (4) olanzapine, risperidone, and quetiapine are atypical neuroleptics approved in adults for acute mania; (5) lamotrigine and the combination of fluoxetine plus olanzapine are approved for depressed adults with BPD.

What follows is an evidence-based discussion of the major pharmacologic agents used to treat BPD. Where possible, pediatric studies are referenced; otherwise, important findings from adult patients are discussed.[23] Psychopharmacologic treatment for a child or adolescent with BPD is complicated because the following factors must be considered: (1) treatment of mania and/or potential to develop mania; (2) treatment of comorbid psychiatric conditions, including depression, anxiety, ADHD, and so forth; (3) education of patients and their parents about, and active monitoring of, side effects, including physical symptoms, agitation, suicidality, and medication-specific syndromes (e.g., serotonin syndrome [SSRIs and atypical antipsychotics], metabolic syndrome, neuroleptic malignant syndrome, and dystonic reactions [typical and atypical antipsychotics]). Practice parameters by Kowatch et al. suggest that first-line treatment for pediatric BPD should include an anti-manic agent, including one of the following: lithium, valproate, carbamazepine, or an atypical antipsychotic medication (e.g., risperidone, olanzapine, or quetiapine). While medication treatment starts as monotherapy, an individual patient's needs, including the abovementioned factors, may necessitate cautious use of more than one psychotropic agent. In this situation,

clinicians should be cautioned to *start low and go slow* with respect to dose, to avoid adding/adjusting too many medications simultaneously (to avoid confusion about which agent is improving/worsening a patient's functioning), and finally to seek consultation with an experienced child/adolescent psychiatrist when contemplating polypharmacy.[293]

Lithium
EVIDENCE-BASED REVIEW
Lithium is an ionic salt used to treat both depression and mania since the late nineteenth century. Studies in BPD adults have shown that those who discontinue lithium have a threefold increase in relapse and a 7.5-fold increase in suicide attempts.[254,256] Importantly, the risk for relapse is increased if lithium is discontinued rapidly, i.e., within 3 weeks. Several open-label prospective case series as well as retrospective chart reviews in children and adolescents with severe emotional dysregulation and BPD indicate lithium's therapeutic benefit.[12,23,41,53,116,134,187,260,281] An open-label study determined that lithium had a 38% response rate in children and adolescents with BPD.[153] A large double-blind placebo-controlled study found lithium to be efficacious for adolescents with BPD and secondary substance use disorders.[109]

PROPOSED MECHANISM
Lithium's proposed mechanism of action is on second-messenger pathways with cells. This is relatively novel as most other psychopharmacologic agents act on the synapse. The inositol phosphate pathway has been demonstrated to be an important second-messenger system, transmitting signals from outside cells to intracellular organelles, which in turn activate an amplified response cascade. Both in vivo and in vitro work suggest that lithium may reduce mania by reducing abnormally elevated myoinositol, a metabolite part of the inositol phosphate pathway.[171,192–194,229] This has been shown in BPD children as well.[69] Also, several studies have shown that chronic lithium increases levels of the neuroprotective

protein BCL-2.[173] Thus, lithium's role in reducing mania and treating depression may result from its neuroprotective actions.

MONITORING/SIDE EFFECTS

Despite numerous studies demonstrating its efficacy and tolerability, concern about side effects has made clinicians wary of using lithium in BPD youth. Nonetheles, awareness of and monitoring for side effects makes lithium a safe, effective treatment for children and adolescents with BPD. Kidney and thyroid function are the two primary systems which may be impaired from long-term lithium treatment and thus require active monitoring before and during treatment. Lithium undergoes renal excretion, therefore the need to ensure adequate kidney function prior to its use. Also, chronic lithium treatment may result in renal dysfunction, and possibly failure, in some individuals. Clinicians should, therefore, routinely monitor kidney function including serum BUN and creatinine levels, in children undergoing lithium treatment. Vitiello et al. showed that children taking lithium had a shorter elimination half-life and a higher total lithium clearance than adults.[261] As with renal function, clinicians should monitor thyroid function thyroid function, including serum thyroid stimulating hormone (TSH) and free thyroxine (Free T4) levels, both before and during lithium treatment. How lithium causes thyroid dysfunction is not known, though some have suggested increased antithyroid antibodies as one possible mechanism.[159] Clinicians should seek consultation if their pediatric patient's renal or thyroid function, as assessed by the above-mentioned screening tests, is abnormal, as judged by appropriate pediatric reference values.

In addition to monitoring kidney and thyroid function, clinicians should monitor lithium levels for two reasons. First, some have suggested that a serum lithium level between 0.6 and 1.0 meq/L provides optimum reduction of manic symptoms. Second, studies have shown that side effects are more likely to occur at serum concentrations in excess of 1.5 meq/L. This is especially relevant for children and adolescents, due to their increased body surface area and vulnerability to dehydration in comparison to adults.

Studies have shown that serum lithium levels in adults are closely related to side-effect symptom clusters. At therapeutic levels less than 1.2 meq/L, patients may experience side effects, such as gastrointestinal symptoms (nausea, vomiting, diarrhea, anorexia, dry mouth), fatigue, drowsiness, tremor, or blurred vision. At levels between 1.5 and 2.0 meq/L, patients may experience dry mouth, upper extremity fine tremor, stomach upset, decreased concentration or memory, leukocytosis, muscle weakness, polyuria, or polydipsia. Levels between 2.0 and 2.5 meq/L are toxic, representing a medical emergency, and may result in the additional symptoms of cogwheel rigidity, acne, psoriasis, alopecia, rash, weight gain, metallic taste, non-specific T-wave changes, decreased libido, and hypothyroidism. Levels exceeding 2.5 meq/L may result in the following impairing symptoms: ataxia, coarse upper extremity tremor, severe stomach upset (nausea/vomiting), nephrotoxicity, muscle weakness, seizures or muscle twitches, dysarthria, lethargy, coma or confusion, hyperreflexia, and nystagmus. Markedly elevated lithium levels, for example from delayed care seeking in an overdose, may result in the need for hemodialysis for levels greater than 4.0 meq/L or for anyone having serious signs and symptoms of lithium toxicity.

CONTRADINDICATIONS

Caution is urged in using lithium during pregnancy, especially during the first trimester, due to fetal anomalies, including Ebstein's anomaly (malformed tricuspid cardiac valve; 1/1000 risk with lithium exposure). Lithium is excreted in breast milk.

ANTIEPILEPTIC DRUGS

Medications used to treat seizures, often referred to as AEDs, are commonly used to treat BPD in adults and children. This is based upon the suggestion that manic-depression resembles temporal lobe seizures.[223]

While no data have shown increased seizure activity in BPD, physicians have studied the efficacy of AEDs in treating BPD. The first two AEDs used to treat BPD were valproate and carbamazepine. Given their different mechanism of action and side-effect profile, we will separate the AEDs into three categories: valproate, carbamazepine, and novel AEDs.

Valproate
EVIDENCE-BASED REVIEW
Valproate is frequently used to treat people of all ages with BPD. In adults, valproate was demonstrated to be superior to placebo and as effective as lithium in treating hospitalized manic adults.[33,34] As with most medications, fewer studies exist in children and adolescents. Several published case reports and open trials of valproate have shown reduced mania in children and adolescents.[197,210,211,273] More structured open-label trials have demonstrated safety in treating adolescents with BPD.[263] A randomized open trial of lithium, valproate, and carbamazepine for BPD adolescents showed large effect size for all three agents, though that for valproate was greater than the other two agents.[153] Many pediatric patients with BPD require the use of two or more psychotropic agents, and an open-label study of combined valproate and lithium showed significant symptom reduction in a sample of BPD adolescents.[99] At present, no double-blind randomized placebo-controlled studies exist for the treatment of pediatric BPD with valproate.

PROPOSED MECHANISM
As with other AEDs, the use of valproate to treat BPD is based upon its efficacy in treating various types of seizure disorder. On a neurochemical level, the theoretical underpinning behind its use is that valproate increases levels of γ-aminobutyric acid (GABA), the major inhibitory neurotransmitter. More inhibition is thought to, in turn, result in less excitation, as evidenced by less mania, much as one would apply a brake to a car.[93,94]

MONITORING/SIDE EFFECTS
Valproate undergoes hepatic metabolism. Serum levels are readily obtainable for valproate, with literature supporting a therapeutic range of 50–100 µg/mL.[31,35] Common side effects include nausea, vomiting, diarrhea, sedation, ataxia, tremor, and sedation. Regular use of valproate has also been associated with alopecia, weight gain, and menstrual irregularities.[186,205] With regard to the latter, controversial evidence exists regarding the association between valproate use and polycystic ovary disease (PCO). PCO refers to hyperandrogenism and chronic anovulation in the absence of pituitary or adrenal pathology. Open-label studies have shown higher rates of menstrual irregularities in women treated for BPD with valproate than lithium; this same study found valproate associated with significantly higher follicular phase androgen concentration.[43,185]

Two acutely life-threatening side effects are hepatic failure and pancreatitis. There are case reports of both in children and adolescents in the literature.[117] Clinicians should monitor valproate levels and hepatic function both before and during treatment with valproate. Additionally, the sudden onset of gastrointestinal symptoms, including nausea, vomiting, and abdominal pain, in a child or adolescent taking valproate should result in a thorough medical evaluation, including evaluation of liver transaminases and pancreatic function. Given its hepatic metabolism, clinicians should also be mindful of medication interactions with other hepatically metabolized agents, including antidepressant or antipsychotic medications.

CONTRAINDICATIONS
Pregnant women should not take valproate due to increased risk of neural tube defects, including spinal bifida. This risk, about 1–2% of those taking it during the first trimester, may be slightly reduced if valproate must be continued due to lack of alternatives by taking 1–4 mg of folate daily. Valproate is secreted in breast milk. Finally, patients with preexisting hepatic failure should not take valproate.

Carbamazepine
EVIDENCE-BASED REVIEW

Carbamazepine is the second common AED used to treat BPD. In BPD adolescents, open-label studies have demonstrated symptom reduction and functional improvement with carbamazepine.[66,153,277]

PROPOSED MECHANISM

As described above, carbamazepine was the first AED proposed to reduce mania.[223] Chemically, it is similar in structure to the TCA imipramine. At the neuronal level, carbamazepine binds to voltage-dependent sodium channels, rendering them inactive, which in turn reduces voltage-dependent calcium channel activation, ultimately reducing synaptic transmission. Carbamaezpine also inhibits N-methyl-D-aspartate glutamate inhibitors (NMDA-gluatmate). Since these receptors are normally excitatory, inhibiting them reduces excitation, thus theoretically reducing mania.

MONITORING/SIDE EFFECTS

Serum levels of carbamazepine should be kept between 4 and 12 µg/mL. Common side effects include benign/transient leukopenia (white blood counts usually remain >3000), hyponatremia (via vasopressin-like activity on vasopressin receptor), and rash. More serious side effects include agranulocytosis, pancytopenia, aplastic anemia, lupus-like allergic reaction, and decreased atrioventricular (AV) block. Additionally, several case reports have been published about children having manic-like symptoms when placed on carbamazepine.[201,220]

Carbamazepine is hepatically metabolized. With daily use, carbamazepine induces hepatic enzyme function. This means that other hepatically metabolized medications, such as SSRIs or oral contraceptive medications, will be metabolized faster (resulting in decreased effective serum concentration—e g if carbamazepine is added to an oral contraceptive, the dose of oral contraceptive may need to be increased. Since carbamazepine induces its own metabolism, clinicians must regularly monitor carbamazepine levels, especially early in treatment, as serum levels will drop with longer exposure to the same dose of carbamazepine.

CONTRAINDICATIONS

Given its effect on AV conduction, subjects with preexisting AV block should not take carbamazepine.

Novel AEDs
EVIDENCE-BASED REVIEW

In recent years, novel AEDs have rapidly been developed and approved for treating seizures. Uses of valproate and carbamazepine have paved the way for these novel AEDs to be used to treat BPD in adults, adolescents, and children. At present, these medications include topiramate, gabapentin, oxcarbamazepine, lamotrigine, tiagabine. A complete discussion of the pharmacology for all of these individual agents is beyond the scope of this chapter.

At present, no double-blind randomized placebo-controlled trials exist of novel AEDs as primary pharmacotherapy for pediatric BPD. A retrospective evaluation of topiramate has shown some success in open adjunctive treatment trial with mania symptom reduction and functional improvement.[76] Case reports exist documenting the benefit of novel AEDs in treating pediatric BPD. For example, topiramate as an augmenting agent may reduce risperidone-induced weight gain in pediatric patients.[213] There are several reports of gabapentin and lamotrigine in treating BPD adolescents.[46,119,247] At present, there are no published case reports (by PUBMED search) in children or adolescents with BPD for gabatril, oxcarbamazepine, or tiagabine.

The adult BPD literature offers more data about novel AEDs. Three studies of gabapentin as an adjunctive treatment failed to show efficacy in treating mixed/manic state BPD adults.[209,217,264] Lamotrigine has been shown to be effective in treating BPD adults, possibly only for the depressive phase of the illness, with both double-blind placebo-controlled and open-label trials.[32,45,113,183] Several studies of topiramate have demonstrated efficacy as an adjunctive agent for BPD adults.[186]

Also, topiramate appears to have a potentially beneficial side effect of decreased weight, given the issue of weight gain associated with other psychopharmacologic agents.[118,163] Oxcarbazapine has also shown promise as an adjunctive therapy for mania in BPD adults.[19,127]

PROPOSED MECHANISM

As with other AEDs, reduced neural excitation as a means of reducing mood fluctuation is the proposed rationale for their use in pediatric BPD. However, studies documenting this effect in vivo have not been done.

Antipsychotics
EVIDENCE-BASED REVIEW

Antipsychotic medications have been used to treat BPD in adults for quite some time. Since the late 1980s, a new era of antipsychotic medications was heralded by the introduction of clozaril as the first so-called atypical antipsychotic. Unlike previous medications, such as thorazine or haloperidol, whose potency was based on dopamine receptor antagonism, atypical antipsychotics are both dopamine and serotonin-2A antagonists. This dual action may result in reduced risk for the side effects seen in older "typical" antipsychotics, including extrapyramidal side effects, such as akithesia (uncomfortable sense of inner restlessness) or dystonic reactions (painful or uncomfortable prolonged muscle contractions, such as tongue or neck). Additionally, manufacturers also suggest a decreased risk for tardive dyskinesia, the systemic condition from prolonged neuroleptic treatment resulting in repetitive, involuntary, and purposeless movements, such as lip smacking and rapid eye blinking. However, the evidence supporting this claim remains sparse.

Since clozaril, a number of atypical antipsychotics are currently available in the United States, including risperidone, olanzapine, ziprasidone, aripiprazole. Several case reports using atypical antipsychotics to treat adolescents with BPD have been published, including using clozaril, olanzapine, and risperidone.[80,104,143,248] A retrospective chart review showed risperidone's efficacy in treating preadolescents with BPD.[101] Open treatment trials using olanzapine as primary or augmenting agent in preadolescents and adolescents with severe psychiatric disorders, including BPD, have shown symptom reduction.[55,155] Antipsychotic augmentation of lithium in adolescents with psychotic mania resulted in a two-thirds response rate; however, once antipsychotics were discontinued, significant numbers had symptom return.[133] At present, there is only one double-blind randomized placebo-controlled study of atypical antipsychotic medications in pediatric BPD. In that study, quetiapine was found to be more effective than placebo as an adjunctive treatment to a primary mood stabilizer in manic adolescents.[77]

PROPOSED MECHANISM

The exact mechanism of atypical antipsychotics in BPD have not been determined at present. However, speculation is that it is via their dual action blocking dopamine receptors (associated with aggression and psychosis) and serotonin receptors (associated with depression and anxiety).

MONITORING/SIDE EFFECTS

Atypical neuroleptics are hepatically metabolized; therefore, caution regarding interactions with psychotropic and other hepatically metabolized medications is warranted. No serum levels need be monitored with their use. Side effects from this category of medications include sedation, constipation and other gastrointestinal disturbance, and weight gain.

Concern has been raised about extreme weight gain from these agents causing a so-called "metabolic syndrome" involving weight gain and diabetes mellitus.[44] An open trial of olanzapine found evidence supporting the potential for this to occur in children and adolescents, with average weight gain of 5 kg in 8 weeks.[100] Routine measurement of weight and height is urged to ensure that children are growing according to sex/age appropriate curves.

METABOLIC SYNDROME

Concern has been raised about extreme weight gain and endocrine abnormalities, including diabetes mellitus, from atypical antipsychotic agents.[44] Knowledge about the pathophysiology, treatment, and surveillance for metabolic syndrome is an area of rapid change, so clinicians are urged to have an awareness of emerging studies in this field. An open trial of olanzapine found evidence supporting the potential for this to occur in children and adolescents, with average weight gain of 5 kg in 8 weeks. Ref 100 Routine measurement of weight, height, and body mass index (BMI) is urged to ensure that children are growing according to age/sex specific data—e.g., pediatric growth charts.

NEUROLEPTIC MALIGNANT SYNDROME

Neuroleptic malignant syndrome is an acutely life-threatening potential side effect of atypical neuroleptics (Table 4-11). According to DSM-IV, symptoms of NMS include the development of severe muscle rigidity and elevated body temperature, while taking a neuroleptic medication, plus >2 of the following: diaphoresis, dysphagia, tremor, incontinence, altered mental status, mutism, tachycardia, elevated/labile blood pressure, leukocytosis, or laboratory evidence of muscle injury (increased creatinine phosphokinase [CPK]).[2] Mortality from NMS is estimated at 20%. NMS has been reported in adolescents treated with risperidone and olanzapine.[22,230] Treatment of NMS requires, first and foremost, that clinicians be aware of it as a possible side effect of neuroleptics. After making the diagnosis, treatment involves stopping the neuroleptic, supportive care to restore normal blood pressure and hydration, closely monitoring the patient for mental status changes and safety, and possible treatment with dantrolene or bromocriptine.

Close monitoring for changes in psychiatric symptoms, for efficacy or lack thereof, is important. Even though atypical neuroleptics are intended to help BPD, there are case reports of mania induced in children on these medications.[167]

CONTRAINDICATIONS

While there are no general contraindications to atypical antipsychotic medications, clinicians should be cautious in pediatric patients with pre-existing hepatic dysfunction, given the hepatic metabolism of these medications, or obesity/diabetes, given the risk of metabolic syndrome with these medications. However, treatment with clozapine requires participation in the national clozapine registry, with weekly blood draws due to the life-threatening side effect of agranulocytosis. Additional side effects from clozapine are seizures (5% of adults taking >600 mg/day; 1–2% of adults taking <300 mg/day) and cardiovascular effects (ECG changes, tachycardia, hypotension, syncope).

Treatment of Comorbid Conditions
ADHD AND STIMULANTS

There are two important and related issues in the treatment of ADHD with stimulants. First, how do you treat a child with BPD who also has comorbid ADHD? Second, is it safe to treat a child with ADHD, accompanied by irritability, with a stimulant? Controversy surrounds the

▶ **TABLE 4-11** NEUROLEPTIC MALIGNANT SYNDROME (NMS)

(A) Development of severe muscle rigidity and elevated body temperature, while taking a neuroleptic medication
(B) Plus >2 of the following: 　　Diaphoresis 　　Dysphagia 　　Tremor 　　Incontinence 　　Altered mental status 　　Mutism 　　Tachycardia 　　Elevated/labile blood pressure 　　Leukocytosis 　　Laboratory evidence of muscle injury (increased CPK)

potential for stimulants to induce irritability and frank mania in pediatric subjects either already diagnosed as bipolar or in those at risk of developing BPD.[51,75,78] Little evidence exists to support the notion that children with ADHD who become irritable when taking psychostimulants are, by definition bipolar.[49] Moreover, data from the multimodal treatment of ADHD (MTA) study, perhaps the largest study of stimulants in children for ADHD, found that youth with ADHD and manic-like symptoms, such as severe irritability accompanied by being more happy, excited, energetic, or confident than usual, actually had a robust response to methylphenidate, without an increase in adverse outcome.[105] In the end, clinicians must be mindful that ADHD is highly comorbid in pediatric BPD, that it often requires use of psychostimulants in the context of first using medication to address primary mood symptoms, such as lithium, valproate, or carbamazepine.[221] If a child seems to be having unintended side effects upon initiation of a medication, clinicians should consider expert consultation.

ANXIETY/DEPRESSION AND SSRIs

Mania is not the only impairing condition or mood state experienced by children, as previously discussed. Both adolescent and adult studies have demonstrated that more time and functional morbidity results from the depressive phase of the illness than from frank mania.[108,131] However, this has not been shown in children with BPD. Anxiety is also commonly comorbid with primary BPD in children, adolescents, and adults (Dickstein, in press).[181,245] Moreover, response to medication treatment is greatly reduced in subjects with comorbid anxiety.[98,102,182]

There are no RCT investigating the treatment of anxiety or depression in children or adolescents with BPD. Clinicians who contemplate using anti-depressant/anti-anxiety medications in pediatric patients with BPD may feel stuck between two unsavory options—i.e. either use these medications to treat anxiety or depression and run the risk of inducing mania, or do not use

these medications and run the risk of increased morbidity and mortality in a child with BPD and untreated comorbid anxiety or depression.

By medication category, the following rates of medication-induced mania have been reported in adults with BPD: TCAs (i.e., desipramine, imipramine) 25–50%; SSRIs (i.e., paroxetine) 0–3.7%[202,215,283]; MAOIs (i.e., tranylcypromine) 7%[124]; buproprion 11%[237]; and venlafaxine 33%.[222] However, these results vary in duration of follow up and scientific rigor.[8] To place these results in context, these studies' placebo arms had mania rates between 2.3 and 4.2%.[202,215] Taken as a whole, investigators have shown that serotonergic agents, especially SSRIs, can be used safely and effectively in adults with BPD in combination with a "mood stabilizer." However, the safety of psychotropic medication use by children and adolescents is a rapidly changing issue, as evidenced by the previously discussed FDA black box warning on SSRIs, about which clinicians must remain current.

The few studies that do exist in children and adolescents with BPD support the careful, judicious use of SSRIs in pediatric BPD. For example, children hospitalized for MDD with psychotic features treated with antidepressants experienced four times less mania and hypomania after 1–2 years of follow up than did similarly ill children not treated with antidepressants.[74] Moreover, combination pharmacotherapy with "mood stabilizers" plus additional agents, including serotonergic antidepressants, may significantly reduce functional impairment in pediatric BPD.[152] Finally, given current knowledge, it is unclear what treatment emergent side effects, such as SSRI-induced mania, reveal about an individual child's diagnosis.[52] However, to reiterate a major point from this chapter: medication-induced mania is not sufficient to diagnose a child with BPD.

In short, clinicians treating children and adolescents with BPD should consider consultation with child or adolescent psychiatrists when treating depression or comorbid anxiety in children with BPD. This is especially true given current concern about the use of SSRIs in children and adolescents with unipolar depression. Also, practice guidelines suggest initially treating manic symptoms and then progressing to symptoms of depression.

Psychotherapy of BPD

Major types of therapy in use for BPD are the same as for MDD. At present, published psychotherapy studies specific to pediatric BPD are limited to three. In the first, Fristad et al. have shown in pilot data that family psychoeducation improves overall functioning in pediatric BPD.[103] The second study from a family therapy perspective, showed subjective self-report of family functioning in interepisode BPD adolescents was not different from that of control adolescents.[231] Finally, Pavuluri et al. found that CBT combined with medication treatment resulted in significant improvement in comparison to pretherapy function.[212]

Complementary and Alternative Medicine in the Treatment of Depression and Bipolar Disorder

As defined by the National Center for Complementary and Alternative Medicine (NCCAM), one of the National Institutes of Health, the terms "complementary and alternative medicine" refers to medical and health care systems, practices, and products that are not presently considered part of conventional medicine. This group of practice is quite diverse, consisting of treatments used in addition to (complementary) or in place of (alternative) conventional medicine. A partial list of these types of treatments includes: alternative health care systems (i.e., Chinese traditional medicine or homeopathy); mind-body interventions (i.e., yoga, hypnosis); biologically based therapies (i.e., herbals or supplements); manipulatives (i.e., massage or chiropractic manipulation); energy therapies (i.e., therapeutic touch).

A complete discussion of these potential interventions, their theoretical mechanism of action, and the research to investigate their efficacy in treating psychiatric disorders, is beyond the scope of this chapter. However, clinicians need to be aware that their patients are likely using these complementary and/or alternative therapies. For example, a large study found more than half of all adults suffering from depression or anxiety were likely to utilize complementary or alternative medicine.[142] Patients suffering from a wide range of conditions use the therapies.[70,236]

Patients and physicians share the responsibility for communicating about the use of such therapies. Unfortunately, often a "don't ask, don't tell" approach is used by both parties. However, this is a lost opportunity by clinicians to begin an open dialogue into what is becoming standard health practice among people worldwide. Furthermore, natural remedies should not be construed as side-effect free, as demonstrated by ephedra, which gained initial popularity because it was a "natural" appetite suppressant but was then found to be associated with life-threatening side effects, including dangerously increased risk of stroke and heart attack.[57] Through open, nonjudgmental dialogue with patients, clinicians can inquire about complementary and alternative treatments in use for psychiatric and nonpsychiatric conditions, share current research about such treatments, and check for possible adverse interactions between alternative treatments and traditional treatments.

Numerous complementary and alternative treatments for depression and BPD are currently being studied. Useful sources of information about these ongoing studies include the NCCAM (http://nccam.nih.gov), the NIH Office of Dietary Supplements (http://ods.od.nih.gov), and U.S. FDA Center for Food Safety and Applied Nutrition (http://cfsan.fda.gov). With time, more of these treatments will be evaluated with the same unbiased scientific rigor as other, traditional treatments.

One such alternative therapy is omega-3-fatty acids. These essential fatty acids are derived from naturally occurring fish oils and are used by many for the treatment of mood disorders. Several studies have shown that omega-3 supplementation may help augment primary antidepressant medication therapy for major depression in comparison to placebo augmentation.[177,203,255] However, studies for use of omega-3 fatty acids as primary treatment for depression did not find any improvement in comparison to placebo.[178] With regard to BPD, studies have not shown a clear benefit to their use.[250]

Mind/Body Interactions: Role of Physical Exercise in the Treatment of Depression and Bipolar Disorder

Mind/body interactions in the treatment of mood disorders, including depression and BPD, are an important area of both clinical and research attention. As previously described, the diagnostic criteria for both disorders involve alterations in neurovegetative functions. Numerous studies have documented that patients suffering from psychiatric disorders are not immune from also having physical maladies. In fact, quite the opposite is true, with an unfortunate increase in morbidity and mortality from medical conditions in those with psychiatric disorders.[294-297]

The etiology of the morbidity and mortality from physical diseases in those suffering from psychiatric conditions is multifactorial. Studies have demonstrated association between depression, BPD, and other psychiatric disorders and numerous physical conditions, including cardiovascular (hypertension, myocardial infarction), neurologic (stroke), and immunologic (increased autoimmune and infectious diseases).[144,265,279] This may be the result of health care provider bias—e.g., too readily dismissing physical complaints by psychiatric patients.[87] Another reason may be increased risk factors in those with psychiatric disorders, such as increased tobacco or substance abuse or dependency. Research is beginning to detect underlying metabolic abnormalities, such as aberrant serotonin receptors, which may play a role in both mood and medical maladies.[241] Finally, some of the increased morbidity and mortality may be iatrogenic due to the consequences of psychotropic medication, such as weight gain from antidepressants or atypical neuroleptics.

Beyond causation of morbidity and mortality from physical ailments in those with psychiatric conditions, clinicians of all disciplines should be aware of the positive benefits of regular physical exercise in improving the overall health of their patients, including those with depression and BPD. Several studies in adults have evaluated the role of physical exercise in the comprehensive treatment of patients with psychiatric disorders. Regular aerobic exercise combined with medication treatment has been shown to improve executive function in depressed adults.[156] This is important given the cognitive impairments in depression and BPD. Furthermore, long-term follow up demonstrates that depressed subjects who maintain an exercise routine are less likely to have recurrence of depression.[177] Moreover, children and adolescents, regardless of presence or absence of psychiatric disorders, have increased self-esteem, self-worth, and creativity from participating in regular aerobic physical activity.[91,252] As with any treatment, practitioners need to consider potential side effects of exercise. Health status needs to be taken into account when prescribing physical exercise. This is especially true in children and adolescents, who may be more vulnerable to injury. This includes the possibility of dehydration due to increased body surface area and also ligamentous inury due to developing joint structures. However, when properly monitored by a health care team, exercise is important for all people, as further evidenced by the Surgeon General's statement (2001) "Call to Action Prevent and Decrease Overweight and Obesity."[258]

In short, ample evidence exists for clinicians of all disciplines to encourage regular aerobic physical activity in all patients, especially those with psychiatric conditions, to improve mood and self-esteem and to reduce medical and psychiatric morbidity and mortality.

► CONCLUSION: PEDIATRIC DEPRESSION AND BIPOLAR DISORDER

Clinicians treating children and adolescents need to evaluate the emotional health and development of their patients, just as they do so for their physical development. While depression is more common in pediatric patients than BPD, if unrecognized these disorders extort a heavy toll in morbidity and mortality. The effective diagnosis and treatment of both disorders often requires a primary care provider to spearhead a collaborative approach and to carefully screen for distinct, functionally impairing mood episodes of depression or mania. Child and adolescent psychiatric consultation should not be reserved until late in treatment. Finally, comprehensive care with both medication and psychotherapy offers effective treatment for children and adolescents suffering from depression and BPD.

REFERENCES

1. AACAP official action. Practice parameters for the assessment and treatment of children and adolescents with bipolar disorder. *J Am Acad Child Adolesc Psychiatry* 1997;36:138–157.
   Beyer J, Kuchibhatla M, Gersing K, Krishnan KR. Neuropsychopharmacology. 2005 Feb;30(2): 401–4.

2. *Diagnostic and Statistical Manual of Mental Disorders*, 4th ed., Text Revision. Washington, DC: American Psychiatric Association, 2000.

3. National Institute of Mental Health research roundtable on prepubertal bipolar disorder. *J Am Acad Child Adolesc Psychiatry* 2001;40: 871–878.

4. Practice guideline for the treatment of patients with bipolar disorder (revision). *Am J Psychiatry* 2002;159:1–50.

5. Altshuler LL, Bartzokis G, Grieder T, et al. An MRI study of temporal lobe structures in men with bipolar disorder or schizophrenia. *Biol Psychiatry* 2000;48:147–162.

6. Altshuler LL, Bartzokis G, Grieder T, et al. Amygdala enlargement in bipolar disorder and hippocampal reduction in schizophrenia: An MRI study demonstrating neuroanatomic specificity. *Arch Gen Psychiatry* 1998;55:663–664.

7. Altshuler LL, Conrad A, Hauser P, et al. Reduction of temporal lobe volume in bipolar disorder: A preliminary report of magnetic resonance imaging. *Arch Gen Psychiatry* 1991;48: 482–483.

8. Altshuler LL, Frye MA, Gitlin MJ. Acceleration and augmentation strategies for treating bipolar depression. *Biol Psychiatry* 2003;53:691–700.

9. Angold A, Costello EJ. Depressive comorbidity in children and adolescents: Empirical, theoretical, and methodological issues. *Am J Psychiatry* 1993;150:1779–1791.

10. Angold A, Costello EJ, Erkanli A, et al. Pubertal changes in hormone levels and depression in girls. *Psychol Med* 1999;29:1043–1053.

11. Angst J, Merikangas K, Scheidegger P, et al. Recurrent brief depression: A new subtype of affective disorder. *J Affect Disord* 1990;19: 87–98.

12. Annell AL. Manic–depressive illness in children and effect of treatment with lithium carbonate. *Acta Paedopsychiatr* 1969;36:292–301.

13. Arango V, Underwood MD, Boldrini M, et al. Serotonin 1A receptors, serotonin transporter binding and serotonin transporter mRNA expression in the brainstem of depressed suicide victims. *Neuropsychopharmacology* 2001;25:892–903.

14. Arango V, Underwood MD, Mann JJ. Serotonin brain circuits involved in major depression and suicide. *Prog Brain Res* 2002;136:443–453.

15. Armstrong TD, Costello EJ. Community studies on adolescent substance use, abuse, or dependence and psychiatric comorbidity. *J Consult Clin Psychol* 2002;70:1224–1239.

16. Axelson DA, Birmaher B. Relation between anxiety and depressive disorders in childhood and adolescence. *Depress Anxiety* 2001;14:67–78.

17. Babyak M, Blumenthal JA, Herman S, et al. Exercise treatment for major depression: Maintenance of therapeutic benefit at 10 months. *Psychosom Med* 2000;62:633–638.

18. Beck AT. Cognition, affect, and psychopathology. *Arch Gen Psychiatry* 1971;24:495–500.

19. Benedetti A, Lattanzi L, Pini S, et al. Oxcarbazepine as add-on treatment in patients with bipolar manic, mixed or depressive episode. *J Affect Disord* 2004;79:273–277.

20. Benkelfat C, Ellenbogen MA, Dean P, et al. Mood-lowering effect of tryptophan depletion. Enhanced susceptibility in young men at genetic risk for major affective disorders. *Arch Gen Psychiatry* 1994;51:687–697.

21. Bernstein GA. Comorbidity and severity of anxiety and depressive disorders in a clinic sample. *J Am Acad Child Adolesc Psychiatry* 1991;30:43–50.

22. Berry N, Pradhan S, Sagar R, et al. Neuroleptic malignant syndrome in an adolescent receiving olanzapine-lithium combination therapy. *Pharmacotherapy* 2003;23:255–259.

23. Bhangoo RK, Lowe CH, Myers FS, et al. Medication use in children and adolescents treated in the community for bipolar disorder. *J Child Adolesc Psychopharmacol* 2003;13:515–522.

24. Biederman J, Klein RG, Pine DS, et al. Resolved: Mania is mistaken for ADHD in prepubertal children. *J Am Acad Child Adolesc Psychiatry* 1998; 37:1091–1096.

25. Birmaher B, Ryan ND, Williamson DE, et al. Childhood and adolescent depression: A review of the past 10 years. Part I. *J Am Acad Child Adolesc Psychiatry* 1996;35:1427–1439.

26. Blanchard CD, Hynd AL, Minke KA, et al. Human defensive behaviors to threat scenarios show parallels to fear- and anxiety-related defense patterns of non-human mammals. *Neurosci Biobehav Rev* 2001;25:761–770.

27. Blanchard C, Blanchard R, Fellous JM, et al. The brain decade in debate: III. Neurobiology of emotion. *Braz J Med Biol Res* 2001;34:283–293.

28. Blier P. The pharmacology of putative early-onset antidepressant strategies. *Eur Neuropsychopharmacol* 2003;13:57–66.

29. Blumberg HP, Kaufman J, Martin A, et al. Amygdala and hippocampal volumes in adolescents and adults with bipolar disorder. *Arch Gen Psychiatry* 2003;60:1201–1208.

30. Blumberg HP, Martin A, Kaufman J, et al. Frontostriatal abnormalities in adolescents with bipolar disorder: Preliminary observations from functional MRI. *Am J Psychiatry* 2003;160:1345–1347.

31. Bowden CL. Valproate. *Bipolar Disord* 2003;5: 189–202.

32. Bowden CL, Asnis GM, Ginsberg LD, et al. Safety and tolerability of lamotrigine for bipolar disorder. *Drug Saf* 2004;27:173–184.

33. Bowden CL, Brugger AM, Swann AC, et al. Efficacy of divalproex vs lithium and placebo in the treatment of mania. The Depakote Mania Study Group. *JAMA* 1994;271:918–924.

34. Bowden CL, Davis J, Morris D, et al. Effect size of efficacy measures comparing divalproex, lithium and placebo in acute mania. *Depress Anxiety* 1997;6:26–30.

35. Bowden CL, Janicak PG, Orsulak P, et al. Relation of serum valproate concentration to response in mania. *Am J Psychiatry* 1996;153:765–770.

36. Brambilla P, Harenski K, Nicoletti M, et al. MRI investigation of temporal lobe structures in bipolar patients. *J Psychiatr Res* 2003;37:287–295.

37. Bremner JD, Innis RB, Salomon RM, et al. Positron emission tomography measurement of cerebral metabolic correlates of tryptophan depletion-induced depressive relapse. *Arch Gen Psychiatry* 1997;54:364–374.

38. Brent DA. Assessment and treatment of the youthful suicidal patient. *Ann NY Acad Sci* 2001;932:106–128.

39. Brent DA, Kolko DJ, Birmaher B, et al. Predictors of treatment efficacy in a clinical trial of three psychosocial treatments for adolescent depression. *J Am Acad Child Adolesc Psychiatry* 1998;37:906–914.

40. Brent DA, Perper JA, Moritz G, et al. Suicide in affectively ill adolescents: A case-control study. *J Affect Disord* 1994;31:193–202.

41. Brumback RA, Weiberg WA. Mania in childhood. II. Therapeutic trial of lithium carbonate and further description of manic-depressive illness in children. *Am J Dis Child* 1977;131: 1122–1126.

42. Bukstein O. Practice parameters for the assessment and treatment of children and adolescents with substance use disorders. *J Am Acad Child Adolesc Psychiatry* 1997;36:140S–156S.

43. Burt VK, Rasgon N. Special considerations in treating bipolar disorder in women. *Bipolar Disord* 2004;6:2–13.

44. Caballero E. Obesity, diabetes, and the metabolic syndrome: New challenges in antipsychotic drug therapy. *CNS Spectr* 2003;8:19–22.

45. Calabrese JR, Suppes T, Bowden CL, et al. A double-blind, placebo-controlled, prophylaxis study of lamotrigine in rapid-cycling bipolar disorder. Lamictal 614 Study Group. *J Clin Psychiatry* 2000;61:841–850.

46. Carandang CG, Maxwell DJ, Robbins DR, et al. Lamotrigine in adolescent mood disorders. *J Am Acad Child Adolesc Psychiatry* 2003;42:750–751.

47. Carlson GA: Mania and ADHD: Comorbidity or confusion. *J Affect Disord* 1998;51:177–187.

48. Carlson GA. The challenge of diagnosing depression in childhood and adolescence. *J Affect Disord* 2000;61(Suppl 1):3–8.

49. Carlson GA. The bottom line. *J Child Adolesc Psychopharmacol* 2003;13:115–118.

50. Carlson GA, Cantwell DP. A survey of depressive symptoms in a child and adolescent psychiatric population: Interview data. *J Am Acad Child Psychiatry* 1979;18:587–599.

51. Carlson GA, Kelly KL. Stimulant rebound: How common is it and what does it mean? *J Child Adolesc Psychopharmacol* 2003;13:137–142.

52. Carlson GA, Mick E. Drug-induced disinhibition in psychiatrically hospitalized children. *J Child Adolesc Psychopharmacol* 2003;13:153–163.

53. Carlson GA, Rapport MD, Pataki CS, et al. Lithium in hospitalized children at 4 and 8 weeks: Mood, behavior and cognitive effects. *J Child Psychol Psychiatry* 1992;33:411–425.

54. Carlson GA, Strober M. Affective disorder in adolescence: Issues in misdiagnosis. *J Clin Psychiatry* 1978;39:59–66.

55. Chang KD, Ketter TA. Mood stabilizer augmentation with olanzapine in acutely manic children. *J Child Adolesc Psychopharmacol* 2000;10:45–49.

56. Charney DS, Grothe DR, Smith SL, et al. Overview of psychiatric disorders and the role of newer antidepressants. *J Clin Psychiatry* 2002; 63(Suppl 1):3–9.

57. Chen C, Biller J, Willing SJ, et al. Ischemic stroke after using over the counter products containing ephedra. *J Neurol Sci* 2004;217:55–60.

58. Chen YS, Akula N, Detera-Wadleigh SD, et al. Findings in an independent sample support an association between bipolar affective disorder and the G72/G30 locus on chromosome 13q33. *Mol Psychiatry* 2004;9:87–92.

59. Clark L, Iversen SD, Goodwin GM. A neuropsychological investigation of prefrontal cortex involvement in acute mania. *Am J Psychiatry* 2001;158:1605–1611.

60. Clark L, Iversen SD, Goodwin GM. Sustained attention deficit in bipolar disorder. *Br J Psychiatry* 2002;180:313–319.

61. Coccaro EF, Silverman JM, Klar HM, et al. Familial correlates of reduced central serotonergic system function in patients with personality disorders. *Arch Gen Psychiatry* 1994;51: 318–324.

62. Cohen P, Cohen J, Kasen S, et al. An epidemiological study of disorders in late childhood and adolescence. I. Age- and gender-specific prevalence. *J Child Psychol Psychiatry* 1993;34: 851–867.

63. Costello EJ. Child psychiatric disorders and their correlates: A primary care pediatric sample. *J Am Acad Child Adolesc Psychiatry* 1989;28: 851–855.

64. Costello EJ, Pine DS, Hammen C, et al. Development and natural history of mood disorders. *Biol Psychiatry* 2002;52:529–542.

65. Couturier J, Steele M, Hussey L, et al. Steroid-induced mania in an adolescent: Risk factors and management. *Can J Clin Pharmacol* 2001;8: 109–112.

66. Craven C, Murphy M. Carbamazepine treatment of bipolar disorder in an adolescent with cerebral palsy. *J Am Acad Child Adolesc Psychiatry* 2000;39:680–681.

67. Crow TJ. Secular changes in affective disorder and variations in the psychosis gene. *Arch Gen Psychiatry* 1986;43:1013–1014.

68. Damasio H, Grabowski T, Frank R, et al. The return of Phineas Gage: Clues about the brain from the skull of a famous patient. *Science* 1994;264:1102–1105.

69. Davanzo P, Thomas MA, Yue K, et al. Decreased anterior cingulate myo-inositol/creatine spectroscopy resonance with lithium treatment in children with bipolar disorder. *Neuropsychopharmacology* 2001;24:359–369.

70. Davidson JR, Morrison RM, Shore J, et al. Homeopathic treatment of depression and anxiety. *Altern Ther Health Med* 1997;3:46–49.

71. Davidson RJ. Anxiety and affective style: Role of prefrontal cortex and amygdala. *Biol Psychiatry* 2002;51:68–80.

72. Davidson RJ, Lewis DA, Alloy LB, et al. Neural and behavioral substrates of mood and mood regulation. *Biol Psychiatry* 2002;52:478–502.

73. Davis M, Whalen PJ. The amygdala: Vigilance and emotion. *Mol Psychiatry* 2001;6:13–34.

74. DelBello MP, Carlson GA, Tohen M, et al. Rates and predictors of developing a manic or hypomanic episode 1 to 2 years following a first hospitalization for major depression with psychotic features. *J Child Adolesc Psychopharmacol* 2003; 13:173–185.

75. DelBello MP, Geller B. Review of studies of child and adolescent offspring of bipolar parents. *Bipolar Disord* 2001;3:325–334.

76. DelBello MP, Kowatch RA, Warner J, et al. Adjunctive topiramate treatment for pediatric bipolar disorder: A retrospective chart review. *J Child Adolesc Psychopharmacol* 2002;12:323–330.

77. DelBello MP, Schwiers ML, Rosenberg HL, et al. A double-blind, randomized, placebo-controlled study of quetiapine as adjunctive treatment for adolescent mania. *J Am Acad Child Adolesc Psychiatry* 2002;41:1216–1223.

78. DelBello MP, Soutullo CA, Hendricks W, et al. Prior stimulant treatment in adolescents with

bipolar disorder: Association with age at onset. *Bipolar Disord* 2001;3:53–57.

79. DelBello MP, Zimmerman ME, Mills NP, et al. Magnetic resonance imaging analysis of amygdala and other subcortical brain regions in adolescents with bipolar disorder. *Bipolar Disord* 2004;6:43–52.

80. Dicker R, Solis S. Risperidone treatment of a psychotic adolescent. *Am J Psychiatry* 1996;153: 441–442.

81. Dickstein DP, Milham MP, Nugent AC, Drevets WC, Charney DS, Pine DS, Leibenluft E. Frontotemporal alterations in pediatric bipolar disorder: results of a voxel-based morphometry study. *Arch Gen Psychiatry* 2005;62:734–741.

82. Dickstein DP, Treland JE, Snow J, et al. Neuropsychological performance in pediatric bipolar disorder. *Biol Psychiatry* 2004;55:32–39.

83. Diler RS, Avci A. SSRI-induced mania in obsessive-compulsive disorder. *J Am Acad Child Adolesc Psychiatry* 1999;38:6–7.

84. Drevets WC. Neuroimaging studies of mood disorders. *Biol Psychiatry* 2000;48:813–829.

85. Drevets WC. Neuroimaging and neuropathological studies of depression: Implications for the cognitive-emotional features of mood disorders. *Curr Opin Neurobiol* 2001;11:240–249.

86. Drevets WC, Price JL, Simpson JR Jr., et al. Subgenual prefrontal cortex abnormalities in mood disorders. *Nature* 1997;386:824–827.

87. Druss BG, Bradford WD, Rosenheck RA, et al. Quality of medical care and excess mortality in older patients with mental disorders. *Arch Gen Psychiatry* 2001;58:565–572.

88. Duman RS. Novel therapeutic approaches beyond the serotonin receptor. *Biol Psychiatry* 1998;44:324–335.

89. Duman RS. Synaptic plasticity and mood disorders. *Mol Psychiatry* 2002;7(Suppl 1):S29–S34.

90. Duman RS. Windows on the human brain and the neurobiology of psychiatric illness. *Neuropsychopharmacology* 2002;26:141–142.

91. Ekeland E, Heian F, Hagen KB, et al. Exercise to improve self-esteem in children and young people. *Cochrane Database Syst Rev* 2004;CD003683.

92. Ellenbogen MA, Young SN, Dean P, et al. Acute tryptophan depletion in healthy young women with a family history of major affective disorder. *Psychol Med* 1999;29:35–46.

93. Emrich HM, Altmann H, Dose M, et al. Therapeutic effects of GABA-ergic drugs in affective disorders. A preliminary report. *Pharmacol Biochem Behav* 1983;19:369–372.

94. Emrich HM, von Zerssen D, Kissling W, et al. Effect of sodium valproate on mania. The GABA-hypothesis of affective disorders. *Arch Psychiatr Nervenkr* 1980;229:1–16.

95. Emslie GJ, Heiligenstein JH, Wagner KD, et al. Fluoxetine for acute treatment of depression in children and adolescents: A placebo-controlled, randomized clinical trial. *J Am Acad Child Adolesc Psychiatry* 2002;41:1205–1215.

96. Emslie GJ, Mayes TL. Mood disorders in children and adolescents: Psychopharmacological treatment. *Biol Psychiatry* 2001;49:1082–1090.

97. Emslie GJ, Rush AJ, Weinberg WA, et al. A double-blind, randomized, placebo-controlled trial of fluoxetine in children and adolescents with depression. *Arch Gen Psychiatry* 1997;54: 1031–1037.

98. Feske U, Frank E, Mallinger AG, et al. Anxiety as a correlate of response to the acute treatment of bipolar I disorder. *Am J Psychiatry* 2000;157: 956–962.

99. Findling RL, McNamara NK, Gracious BL, et al. Combination lithium and divalproex sodium in pediatric bipolarity. *J Am Acad Child Adolesc Psychiatry* 2003;42:895–901.

Frayne SM, Seaver MR, Loveland S, Christiansen SL, Spiro A III, Parker VA, Skinner KM. Burden of medical illness in women with depression and posttraumatic stress disorder. Archives of Internal Medicine. 2004; 164(12): 1306–1312.

100. Frazier JA, Biederman J, Tohen M, et al. A prospective open-label treatment trial of olanzapine monotherapy in children and adolescents with bipolar disorder. *J Child Adolesc Psychopharmacol* 2001;11:239–250.

101. Frazier JA, Meyer MC, Biederman J, et al. Risperidone treatment for juvenile bipolar disorder: A retrospective chart review. *J Am Acad Child Adolesc Psychiatry* 1999;38:960–965.

102. Freeman MP, Freeman SA, McElroy SL. The comorbidity of bipolar and anxiety disorders: Prevalence, psychobiology, and treatment issues. *J Affect Disord* 2002;68:1–23.

103. Fristad MA, Gavazzi SM, Mackinaw-Koons B. Family psychoeducation: An adjunctive intervention for children with bipolar disorder. *Biol Psychiatry* 2003;53:1000–1008.

104. Fuchs DC. Clozapine treatment of bipolar disorder in a young adolescent. *J Am Acad Child Adolesc Psychiatry* 1994;33:1299–1302.

105. Galanter CA, Carlson GA, Jensen PS, et al. Response to methylphenidate in children with attention deficit hyperactivity disorder and manic symptoms in the multimodal treatment study of children with attention deficit hyperactivity disorder titration trial. *J Child Adolesc Psychopharmacol* 2003;13:123–136.

106. Geller B, Craney JL, Bolhofner K, et al. Two-year prospective follow-up of children with a prepubertal and early adolescent bipolar disorder phenotype. *Am J Psychiatry* 2002;159:927–933.

107. Geller B, Reising D, Leonard HL, et al. Critical review of tricyclic antidepressant use in children and adolescents. *J Am Acad Child Adolesc Psychiatry* 1999;38:513–516.

108. Geller B, Tillman R, Craney JL, et al. Four-year prospective outcome and natural history of mania in children with a prepubertal and early adolescent bipolar disorder phenotype. *Arch Gen Psychiatry* 2004;61:459–467.

109. Geller B, Williams M, Zimerman B, et al. Prepubertal and early adolescent bipolarity differentiate from ADHD by manic symptoms, grandiose delusions, ultra-rapid or ultradian cycling. *J Affect Disord* 1998;51:81–91.

110. Geller B, Zimerman B, Williams M, et al. DSM-IV mania symptoms in a prepubertal and early adolescent bipolar disorder phenotype compared to attention-deficit hyperactive and normal controls. *J Child Adolesc Psychopharmacol* 2002;12:11–25.

111. Geller B, Zimerman B, Williams M, et al. Phenomenology of prepubertal and early adolescent bipolar disorder: Examples of elated mood, grandiose behaviors, decreased need for sleep, racing thoughts and hypersexuality. *J Child Adolesc Psychopharmacol* 2002;12:3–9.

112. Ghaziuddin M. Mania induced by sertraline in a prepubertal child. *Am J Psychiatry* 1994;151:944.

113. Goodwin GM, Bowden CL, Calabrese JR, et al. A pooled analysis of 2 placebo-controlled 18-month trials of lamotrigine and lithium maintenance in bipolar I disorder. *J Clin Psychiatry* 2004;65:432–441.

114. Goodwin R, Gould MS, Blanco C, et al. Prescription of psychotropic medications to youths in office-based practice. *Psychiatr Serv* 2001;52:1081–1087.

115. Gottfried JA, O'Doherty J, Dolan RJ. Encoding predictive reward value in human amygdala and orbitofrontal cortex. *Science* 2003;301:1104–1107.

116. Gram LF, Rafaelsen OJ. Lithium treatment of psychotic children and adolescents. A controlled clinical trial. *Acta Psychiatr Scand* 1972;48: 253–260.

117. Grauso-Eby NL, Goldfarb O, Feldman-Winter LB, et al. Acute pancreatitis in children from Valproic acid: Case series and review. *Pediatr Neurol* 2003;28:145–148.

118. Gupta S, Masand PS, Frank BL, et al. Topiramate in bipolar and schizoaffective disorders: Weight loss and efficacy. *Prim Care Companion J Clin Psychiatry* 2000;2:96–100.

119. Hamrin V, Bailey K. Gabapentin and methylphenidate treatment of a preadolescent with attention deficit hyperactivity disorder and bipolar disorder. *J Child Adolesc Psychopharmacol* 2001;11:301–309.

120. Hauser P, Matochik J, Altshuler LL, et al. MRI-based measurements of temporal lobe and ventricular structures in patients with bipolar I and bipolar II disorders. *J Affect Disord* 2000;60: 25–32.

121. Herzog DB, Dorer DJ, Keel PK, et al. Recovery and relapse in anorexia and bulimia nervosa: A 7.5-year follow-up study. *J Am Acad Child Adolesc Psychiatry* 1999;38:829–837.

122. Herzog DB, Keller MB, Sacks NR, et al. Psychiatric comorbidity in treatment-seeking anorexics and bulimics. *J Am Acad Child Adolesc Psychiatry* 1992;31:810–818.

123. Herzog DB, Nussbaum KM, Marmor AK. Comorbidity and outcome in eating disorders. *Psychiatr Clin North Am* 1996;19:843–859.

124. Himmelhoch JM, Thase ME, Mallinger AG, et al. Tranylcypromine versus imipramine in anergic bipolar depression. *Am J Psychiatry* 1991;148: 910–916.

125. Hoff RA, Rosenheck RA. The cost of treating substance abuse patients with and without comorbid psychiatric disorders. *Psychiatr Serv* 1999;50:1309–1315.

126. Hudson JI, Lipinski JF, Keck PE Jr. et al. Polysomnographic characteristics of young manic patients. Comparison with unipolar depressed patients and normal control subjects. *Arch Gen Psychiatry* 1992;49:378–383.

127. Hummel B, Walden J, Stampfer R, et al. Acute antimanic efficacy and safety of oxcarbazepine in an open trial with an on-off-on design. *Bipolar Disord* 2002;4:412–417.

128. Jain R, Tripathi BM, Singh R. Comparison of reported drug use and urinalysis in the

assessment of drug use. *Natl Med J India* 2001; .14: 315–316.

129. Johnson A, Giuffre RM, O'Malley K. ECG changes in pediatric patients on tricyclic antidepressants, desipramine, and imipramine. *Can J Psychiatry* 1996;41:102–106.

130. Johnson JG, Cohen P, Brook JS. Associations between bipolar disorder and other psychiatric disorders during adolescence and early adulthood: A community-based longitudinal investigation. *Am J Psychiatry* 2000;157:1679–1681.

131. Judd LL, Akiskal HS, Schettler PJ, et al. The long-term natural history of the weekly symptomatic status of bipolar I disorder. *Arch Gen Psychiatry* 2002;59:530–537.

132. Jureidini JN, Doecke CJ, Mansfield PR, et al. Efficacy and safety of antidepressants for children and adolescents. *Br Med J* 2004;328:879–883.

133. Kafantaris V, Coletti DJ, Dicker R, et al. Adjunctive antipsychotic treatment of adolescents with bipolar psychosis. *J Am Acad Child Adolesc Psychiatry* 2001;40:1448–1456.

134. Kafantaris V, Coletti DJ, Dicker R, et al. Lithium treatment of acute mania in adolescents: A large open trial. *J Am Acad Child Adolesc Psychiatry* 2003;42:1038–1045.

135. Kalin NH, Shelton SE, Davidson RJ, et al. The primate amygdala mediates acute fear but not the behavioral and physiological components of anxious temperament. *J Neurosci* 2001;21:2067–2074.

136. Kashani JH, Carlson GA, Beck NC, et al. Depression, depressive symptoms, and depressed mood among a community sample of adolescents. *Am J Psychiatry* 1987;144:931–934.

137. Kaufman J, Martin A, King RA, et al. Are child-, adolescent-, and adult-onset depression one and the same disorder? *Biol Psychiatry* 2001;49: 980–1001.

138. Keck PE Jr., McElroy SL, Richtand N, et al. What makes a drug a primary mood stabilizer? *Mol Psychiatry* 2002;7(Suppl 1):S8–S14.

139. Kegeles LS, Malone KM, Slifstein M, et al. Response of cortical metabolic deficits to serotonergic challenge in familial mood disorders. *Am J Psychiatry* 2003;160:76–82.

140. Keller MB, Ryan ND, Strober M, et al. Efficacy of paroxetine in the treatment of adolescent major depression: A randomized, controlled trial. *J Am Acad Child Adolesc Psychiatry* 2001;40:762–772.

141. Kessler RC, McGonagle KA, Zhao S, et al. Lifetime and 12-month prevalence of DSM-III-R psychiatric disorders in the United States. Results from the National Comorbidity Survey. *Arch Gen Psychiatry* 1994;51:8–19.

142. Kessler RC, Soukup J, Davis RB, et al. The use of complementary and alternative therapies to treat anxiety and depression in the United States. *Am J Psychiatry* 2001;158:289–294.

143. Khouzam HR, El Gabalawi F. Treatment of bipolar I disorder in an adolescent with olanzapine. *J Child Adolesc Psychopharmacol* 2000;10:147–151.

144. Kiecolt-Glaser JK, Glaser R. Depression and immune function: Central pathways to morbidity and mortality. *J Psychosom Res* 2002;53:873–876.

145. King RA. Practice parameters for the psychiatric assessment of children and adolescents. *J Am Acad Child Adolesc Psychiatry* 1997;36:4S–20S.

146. Klaassen T, Riedel WJ, van Someren A, et al. Mood effects of 24-hour tryptophan depletion in healthy first-degree relatives of patients with affective disorders. *Biol Psychiatry* 1999;46:489–497.

147. Koehler-Troy C, Strober M, Malenbaum R. Methylphenidate-induced mania in a prepubertal child. *J Clin Psychiatry* 1986;47:566–567.

148. Kovacs M, Akiskal HS, Gatsonis C, et al. Childhood-onset dysthymic disorder. Clinical features and prospective naturalistic outcome. *Arch Gen Psychiatry* 1994;51:365–374.

149. Kovacs M, Gatsonis C, Paulauskas SL, et al. Depressive disorders in childhood. IV. A longitudinal study of comorbidity with and risk for anxiety disorders. *Arch Gen Psychiatry* 1989;46: 776–782.

150. Kovacs M, Obrosky DS, Sherrill J. Developmental changes in the phenomenology of depression in girls compared to boys from childhood onward. *J Affect Disord* 2003;74:33–48.

151. Kovacs M, Obrosky DS, Sherrill J. Developmental changes in the phenomenology of depression in girls compared to boys from childhood onward. *J Affect Disord* 2003;74:33–48.

152. Kowatch RA, Sethuraman G, Hume JH, et al. Combination pharmacotherapy in children and adolescents with bipolar disorder. *Biol Psychiatry* 2003;53:978–984.

153. Kowatch RA, Suppes T, Carmody TJ, et al. Effect size of lithium, divalproex sodium, and carbamazepine in children and adolescents with bipolar disorder. *J Am Acad Child Adolesc Psychiatry* 2000;39:713–720.

Kilbourne AM, Cornelius JR, Han X, et al. Burden of general medical conditions among individuals with bipolar disorder. Bipolar Disord. 2004;6: 368–373.

154. Kramlinger KG, Post RM. Ultra-rapid and ultra-dian cycling in bipolar affective illness. *Br J Psychiatry* 1996;168:314–323.

155. Krishnamoorthy J, King BH. Open-label olanzapine treatment in five preadolescent children. *J Child Adolesc Psychopharmacol* 1998;8:107–113.

156. Kubesch S, Bretschneider V, Freudenmann R, et al. Aerobic endurance exercise improves executive functions in depressed patients. *J Clin Psychiatry* 2003;64:1005–1012.
    Kupfer DJ. The increasing medical burden in bipolar disorder. JAMA. 2005 May 25;293(20): 2528–30.

157. Kye CH, Waterman GS, Ryan ND, et al. A randomized, controlled trial of amitriptyline in the acute treatment of adolescent major depression. *J Am Acad Child Adolesc Psychiatry* 1996;35:1139–1144.

158. Lavori PW, Klerman GL, Keller MB, et al. Age-period-cohort analysis of secular trends in onset of major depression: Findings in siblings of patients with major affective disorder. *J Psychiatr Res* 1987;21:23–35.

159. Lazarus JH, John R, Bennie EH, et al. Lithium therapy and thyroid function: A long-term study. *Psychol Med* 1981;11:85–92.

160. LeDoux J. The emotional brain, fear, and the amygdala. *Cell Mol Neurobiol* 2003;23:727–738.

161. Leibenluft E, Albert PS, Rosenthal NE, et al. Relationship between sleep and mood in patients with rapid-cycling bipolar disorder. *Psychiatry Res* 1996;63:161–168.

162. Leibenluft E, Charney DS, Towbin KE, et al. Defining clinical phenotypes of juvenile mania. *Am J Psychiatry* 2003;160:430–437.

163. Levy E, Margolese HC, Chouinard G. Topiramate produced weight loss following olanzapine-induced weight gain in schizophrenia. *J Clin Psychiatry* 2002;63:1045.

164. Lewinsohn PM, Clarke GN, Seeley JR, et al. Major depression in community adolescents: Age at onset, episode duration, and time to recurrence. *J Am Acad Child Adolesc Psychiatry* 1994;33:809–818.

165. Lewinsohn PM, Hops H, Roberts RE, et al. Adolescent psychopathology: I. Prevalence and incidence of depression and other DSM-III-R disorders in high school students. *J Abnorm Psychol* 1993;102:133–144.

166. Lewinsohn PM, Rohde P, Seeley JR, et al. Age-cohort changes in the lifetime occurrence of depression and other mental disorders. *J Abnorm Psychol* 1993;102:110–120.

167. London JA. Mania associated with olanzapine. *J Am Acad Child Adolesc Psychiatry* 1998;37: 135–136.

168. Lyoo IK, Kim MJ, Stoll AL, et al. Frontal lobe gray matter density decreases in bipolar I disorder. *Biol Psychiatry* 2004;55:648–651.

169. Mallin R, Slott K, Tumblin M, et al. Detection of substance use disorders in patients presenting with depression. *Subst Abus* 2002;23:115–120.

170. Mandoki MW, Tapia MR, Tapia MA, et al. Venlafaxine in the treatment of children and adolescents with major depression. *Psychopharmacol Bull* 1997;33:149–154.

171. Manji HK, Chen G. PKC, MAP kinases and the bcl-2 family of proteins as long-term targets for mood stabilizers. *Mol Psychiatry* 2002;7(Suppl 1): S46–S56.

172. Manji HK, Hsiao JK, Risby ED, et al. The mechanisms of action of lithium. I. Effects on serotoninergic and noradrenergic systems in normal subjects. *Arch Gen Psychiatry* 1991;48:505–512.

173. Manji HK, Moore GJ, Chen G. Lithium up-regulates the cytoprotective protein Bcl-2 in the CNS in vivo: A role for neurotrophic and neuroprotective effects in manic depressive illness. *J Clin Psychiatry* 2000;61(Suppl 9):82–96.

174. Manji HK, Moore GJ, Chen G. Bipolar disorder: Leads from the molecular and cellular mechanisms of action of mood stabilizers. *Br J Psychiatry* 2001;41:s107–s119.

175. Mann JJ, Brent DA, Arango V. The neurobiology and genetics of suicide and attempted suicide: A focus on the serotonergic system. *Neuropsychopharmacology* 2001;24:467–477.

176. Mann JJ, Huang YY, Underwood MD, et al. A serotonin transporter gene promoter polymorphism (5-HTTLPR) and prefrontal cortical binding in major depression and suicide. *Arch Gen Psychiatry* 2000;57:729–738.

177. Marangell LB, Martinez JM, Zboyan HA, et al. Omega-3 fatty acids for the prevention of postpartum depression: Negative data from a preliminary, open-label pilot study. *Depress Anxiety* 2004;19:20–23.

178. Marangell LB, Martinez JM, Zboyan HA, et al. A double-blind, placebo-controlled study of the omega-3 fatty acid docosahexaenoic acid in the treatment of major depression. *Am J Psychiatry* 2003;160:996–998.

179. March J, Silva S, Petrycki S, et al. Fluoxetine, cognitive-behavioral therapy, and their combination for adolescents with depression: Treatment for Adolescents With Depression Study (TADS) randomized controlled trial. *JAMA* 2004;292:807–820.

180. March J, Silva S, Petrycki S, et al. Fluoxetine, cognitive-behavioral therapy, and their combination for adolescents with depression: Treatment for Adolescents With Depression Study (TADS) randomized controlled trial. *JAMA* 2004;292:807–820.

181. Masi G, Toni C, Perugi G, et al. Anxiety disorders in children and adolescents with bipolar disorder: A neglected comorbidity. *Can J Psychiatry* 2001;46:797–802.

182. McElroy SL, Altshuler LL, Suppes T, et al. Axis I psychiatric comorbidity and its relationship to historical illness variables in 288 patients with bipolar disorder. *Am J Psychiatry* 2001;158:420–426.

183. McElroy SL, Zarate CA, Cookson J, et al. A 52-week, open-label continuation study of lamotrigine in the treatment of bipolar depression. *J Clin Psychiatry* 2004;65:204–210.

184. McInnis MG, Dick DM, Willour VL, et al. Genome-wide scan and conditional analysis in bipolar disorder: Evidence for genomic interaction in the National Institute of Mental Health genetics initiative bipolar pedigrees. *Biol Psychiatry* 2003;54:1265–1273.

185. McIntyre RS, Mancini DA, McCann S, et al. Valproate, bipolar disorder and polycystic ovarian syndrome. *Bipolar Disord* 2003;5:28–35.

186. McIntyre RS, Mancini DA, McCann S, et al. Topiramate versus bupropion SR when added to mood stabilizer therapy for the depressive phase of bipolar disorder: A preliminary single-blind study. *Bipolar Disord* 2002;4:207–213.

187. McKnew DH, Cytryn L, Buchsbaum MS, et al. Lithium in children of lithium-responding parents. *Psychiatry Res* 1981;4:171–180.

188. McMahon FJ, Chen YS, Patel S, et al. Mitochondrial DNA sequence diversity in bipolar affective disorder. *Am J Psychiatry* 2000;157:1058–1064.

189. Meaney MJ. Maternal care, gene expression, and the transmission of individual differences in stress reactivity across generations. *Annu Rev Neurosci* 2001;24:1161–1192.

190. Miller IW, Kabacoff RI, Epstein NB, et al. The development of a clinical rating scale for the McMaster model of family functioning. *Fam Process* 1994;33:53–69.

191. Miller IW, McDermut W, Gordon KC, et al. Personality and family functioning in families of depressed patients. *J Abnorm Psychol* 2000;109:539–545.

192. Moore GJ, Bebchuk JM, Hasanat K, et al. Lithium increases N-acetyl-aspartate in the human brain: In vivo evidence in support of bcl-2's neurotrophic effects? *Biol Psychiatry* 2000;48:1–8.

193. Moore GJ, Bebchuk JM, Parrish JK, et al. Temporal dissociation between lithium-induced changes in frontal lobe myo-inositol and clinical response in manic-depressive illness. *Am J Psychiatry* 1999;156:1902–1908.

194. Moore GJ, Bebchuk JM, Wilds IB, et al. Lithium-induced increase in human brain grey matter. *Lancet* 2000;356:1241–1242.

195. Moorhead DJ, Stashwick CK, Reinherz HZ, et al. Child and adolescent predictors for eating disorders in a community population of young adult women. *Int J Eat Disord* 2003;33:1–9.

196. Moreau D, Mufson L, Weissman MM, et al. Interpersonal psychotherapy for adolescent depression: Description of modification and preliminary application. *J Am Acad Child Adolesc Psychiatry* 1991;30:642–651.

197. Mota-Castillo M, Torruella A, Engels B, et al. Valproate in very young children: An open case series with a brief follow-up. *J Affect Disord* 2001;67:193–197.

198. Mufson L, Dorta KP, Wickramaratne P, et al. A randomized effectiveness trial of interpersonal psychotherapy for depressed adolescents. *Arch Gen Psychiatry* 2004;61:577–584.

199. Mufson L, Weissman MM, Moreau D, et al. Efficacy of interpersonal psychotherapy for depressed adolescents. *Arch Gen Psychiatry* 1999;56: 573–579.

200. Murphy FC, Sahakian BJ. Neuropsychology of bipolar disorder. *Br J Psychiatry* 2001;41: s120–s127.

201. Myers WC, Carrera F III. Carbamazepine-induced mania with hypersexuality in a 9-year-old boy. *Am J Psychiatry* 1989;146:400.

202. Nemeroff CB, Evans DL, Gyulai L, et al. Double-blind, placebo-controlled comparison of imipramine and paroxetine in the treatment of bipolar depression. *Am J Psychiatry* 2001;158:906–912.

203. Nemets B, Stahl Z, Belmaker RH. Addition of omega-3 fatty acid to maintenance medication treatment for recurrent unipolar depressive disorder. *Am J Psychiatry* 2002;159:477–479.

204. Neumeister A. Tryptophan depletion, serotonin, and depression: Where do we stand? *Psychopharmacol Bull* 2003;37:99–115.

205. O'Donovan C, Kusumakar V, Graves GR, et al. Menstrual abnormalities and polycystic ovary syndrome in women taking valproate for bipolar mood disorder. *J Clin Psychiatry* 2002;63:322–330.

206. Olfson M, Marcus SC, Weissman MM, et al. National trends in the use of psychotropic medications by children. *J Am Acad Child Adolesc Psychiatry* 2002;41:514–521.

207. Olson AL, Kelleher KJ, Kemper KJ, et al. Primary care pediatricians' roles and perceived responsibilities in the identification and management of depression in children and adolescents. *Ambul Pediatr* 2001;1:91–98.

208. Oquendo MA, Placidi GP, Malone KM, et al. Positron emission tomography of regional brain metabolic responses to a serotonergic challenge and lethality of suicide attempts in major depression. *Arch Gen Psychiatry* 2003;60:14–22.

209. Pande AC, Crockatt JG, Janney CA, et al. Gabapentin in bipolar disorder: A placebo-controlled trial of adjunctive therapy. Gabapentin Bipolar Disorder Study Group. *Bipolar Disord* 2000;2:249–255.

210. Papatheodorou G, Kutcher SP. Divalproex sodium treatment in late adolescent and young adult acute mania. *Psychopharmacol Bull* 1993; 29:213–219.

211. Papatheodorou G, Kutcher SP, Katic M, et al. The efficacy and safety of divalproex sodium in the treatment of acute mania in adolescents and young adults: An open clinical trial. *J Clin Psychopharmacol* 1995;15:110–116.

212. Pavuluri MN, Graczyk PA, Henry DB, et al. Child- and family-focused cognitive-behavioral therapy for pediatric bipolar disorder: Development and preliminary results. *J Am Acad Child Adolesc Psychiatry* 2004;43:528–537.

213. Pavuluri MN, Janicak PG, Carbray J. Topiramate plus risperidone for controlling weight gain and symptoms in preschool mania. *J Child Adolesc Psychopharmacol* 2002;12:271–273.

214. Pearlson GD, Barta PE, Powers RE, et al. Ziskind-Somerfeld Research Award 1996. Medial and superior temporal gyral volumes and cerebral asymmetry in schizophrenia versus bipolar disorder. *Biol Psychiatry* 1997;41:1–14.

215. Peet M. Induction of mania with selective serotonin re-uptake inhibitors and tricyclic antidepressants. *Br J Psychiatry* 1994;164:549–550.

216. Perrone J, De Roos F, Jayaraman S, et al. Drug screening versus history in detection of substance use in ED psychiatric patients. *Am J Emerg Med* 2001;19:49–51.

217. Perugi G, Toni C, Ruffolo G, et al. Clinical experience using adjunctive gabapentin in treatment-resistant bipolar mixed states. *Pharmacopsychiatry* 1999;32:136–141.

218. Pine DS, Cohen E, Cohen P, et al. Adolescent depressive symptoms as predictors of adult depression: Moodiness or mood disorder? *Am J Psychiatry* 1999;156:133–135.

219. Pine DS, Cooke EH, Costello EJ, et al. Advances in developmental science and DSM-V. In: Kupfer DJ, Regier DA (eds.), *A Research Agenda for DSM-V*. Washington, DC: American Psychiatric Association Press, 2002.

220. Pleak RR, Birmaher B, Gavrilescu A, et al. Mania and neuropsychiatric excitation following carbamazepine. *J Am Acad Child Adolesc Psychiatry* 1988;27:500–503.

221. Pliszka SR. Comorbidity of attention-deficit/hyperactivity disorder with psychiatric disorder: An overview. *J Clin Psychiatry* 1998;59(Suppl 7): 50–58.

222. Post RM, Altshuler LL, Frye MA, et al. Rate of switch in bipolar patients prospectively treated with second-generation antidepressants as augmentation to mood stabilizers. *Bipolar Disord* 2001;3:259–265.

223. Post RM, Uhde TW, Putnam FW, et al. Kindling and carbamazepine in affective illness. *J Nerv Ment Dis* 1982;170:717–731.

224. Preskorn SH, Weller E, Hughes C, et al. Plasma monitoring of tricyclic antidepressants: Defining the therapeutic range for imipramine in depressed children. *Clin Neuropharmacol* 1986;9(Suppl 4): 265–267.

225. Preskorn SH, Weller E, Jerkovich G, et al. Depression in children: Concentration-dependent CNS toxicity of tricyclic antidepressants. *Psychopharmacol Bull* 1988;24:140–142.

226. Puig-Antich J, Blau S, Marx N, et al. Prepubertal major depressive disorder: A pilot study. *J Am Acad Child Psychiatry* 1978;17: 695–707.

227. Rao U, Ryan ND, Birmaher B, et al. Unipolar depression in adolescents: Clinical outcome in adulthood. *J Am Acad Child Adolesc Psychiatry* 1995;34:566–578.

228. Rilke O, Safar C, Israel M, et al. Differences in whole blood serotonin levels based on a typology of parasuicide. *Neuropsychobiology* 1998;38:70–72.

229. Risby ED, Hsiao JK, Manji HK, et al. The mechanisms of action of lithium. II. Effects on adenylate cyclase activity and beta-adrenergic receptor binding in normal subjects. *Arch Gen Psychiatry* 1991;48:513–524.

230. Robb AS, Chang W, Lee HK, et al. Case study. Risperidone-Induced neuroleptic malignant syndrome in an adolescent. *J Child Adolesc Psychopharmacol* 2000;10:327–330.

231. Robertson HA, Kutcher SP, Bird D, et al. Impact of early onset bipolar disorder on family functioning: Adolescents' perceptions of family dynamics, communication, and problems. *J Affect Disord* 2001;66:25–37.

232. Rogers RD, Owen AM, Middleton HC, et al. Choosing between small, likely rewards and large, unlikely rewards activates inferior and orbital prefrontal cortex. *J Neurosci* 1999;19:9029–9038.

233. Rogers RD, Ramnani N, Mackay C, et al. Distinct portions of anterior cingulate cortex and medial prefrontal cortex are activated by reward processing in separable phases of decision-making cognition. *Biol Psychiatry* 2004;55:594–602.

234. Rubinsztein JS, Fletcher PC, Rogers RD, et al. Decision-making in mania: A PET study. *Brain* 2001;124:2550–2563.

235. Rubinsztein JS, Michael A, Paykel ES, et al. Cognitive impairment in remission in bipolar affective disorder. *Psychol Med* 2000;30:1025–1036.

236. Russinova Z, Wewiorski NJ, Cash D. Use of alternative health care practices by persons with serious mental illness: Perceived benefits. *Am J Public Health* 2002;92:1600–1603.

237. Sachs GS, Lafer B, Stoll AL, et al. A double-blind trial of bupropion versus desipramine for bipolar depression. *J Clin Psychiatry* 1994;55:391–393.

238. Safer DJ. Changing patterns of psychotropic medications prescribed by child psychiatrists in the 1990s. *J Child Adolesc Psychopharmacol* 1997;7:267–274.

239. Santarelli L, Saxe M, Gross C, et al. Requirement of hippocampal neurogenesis for the behavioral effects of antidepressants. *Science* 2003;301:805–809.

240. Sax KW, Strakowski SM, Zimmerman ME, et al. Frontosubcortical neuroanatomy and the continuous performance test in mania. *Am J Psychiatry* 1999;156:139–141.

241. Schins A, Honig A, Crijns H, et al. Increased coronary events in depressed cardiovascular patients: 5-HT2A receptor as missing link? *Psychosom Med* 2003;65:729–737.

242. Schulze TG, Buervenich S, Badner JA, et al. Loci on chromosomes 6q and 6p interact to increase susceptibility to bipolar affective disorder in the national institute of mental health genetics initiative pedigrees. *Biol Psychiatry* 2004;56:18–23.

243. Schulze TG, McMahon FJ. Genetic linkage and association studies in bipolar affective disorder: A time for optimism. *Am J Med Genet* 2003;123C:36–47.

244. Simeon JG, Dinicola VF, Ferguson HB, et al. Adolescent depression: A placebo-controlled fluoxetine treatment study and follow-up. *Prog Neuropsychopharmacol Biol Psychiatry* 1990;14:791–795.

245. Simon NM, Smoller JW, Fava M, et al. Comparing anxiety disorders and anxiety-related traits in bipolar disorder and unipolar depression. *J Psychiatr Res* 2003;37:187–192.

246. Smith SE, Pihl RO, Young SN, et al. A test of possible cognitive and environmental influences on the mood lowering effect of tryptophan depletion in normal males. *Psychopharmacology* (Berl) 1987;91:451–457.

247. Soutullo CA, Casuto LS, Keck PE Jr. Gabapentin in the treatment of adolescent mania: A case report. *J Child Adolesc Psychopharmacol* 1998;8:81–85.

248. Soutullo CA, Sorter MT, Foster KD, et al. Olanzapine in the treatment of adolescent acute mania: A report of seven cases. *J Affect Disord* 1999;53:279–283.

249. Staton RD, Wilson H, Brumback RA. Cognitive improvement associated with tricyclic antidepressant treatment of childhood major depressive illness. *Percept Mot Skills* 1981;53:219–234.

250. Stoll AL, Locke CA, Marangell LB, et al. Omega-3 fatty acids and bipolar disorder: A review. *Prostaglandins Leukot Essent Fatty Acids* 1999;60:329–337.

251. Strakowski SM, DelBello MP, Sax KW, et al. Brain magnetic resonance imaging of structural abnormalities in bipolar disorder. *Arch Gen Psychiatry* 1999;56:254–260.

252. Strauss RS, Rodzilsky D, Burack G, et al. Psychosocial correlates of physical activity in healthy children. *Arch Pediatr Adolesc Med* 2001;155:897–902.

253. Strober M. Relevance of early age-of-onset in genetic studies of bipolar affective disorder. *J Am Acad Child Adolesc Psychiatry* 1992;31:606–610.

254. Strober M, Morrell W, Lampert C, et al. Relapse following discontinuation of lithium maintenance therapy in adolescents with bipolar I illness: A naturalistic study. *Am J Psychiatry* 1990;147:457–461.

255. Su KP, Huang SY, Chiu CC, et al. Omega-3 fatty acids in major depressive disorder. A preliminary double-blind, placebo-controlled trial. *Eur Neuropsychopharmacol* 2003;13:267–271.

256. Tondo L, Baldessarini RJ, Hennen J, et al. Lithium treatment and risk of suicidal behavior in bipolar disorder patients. *J Clin Psychiatry* 1998; 59:405–414.

257. U.S. Department of Health & Human Services. Mental Health: A Report of the Surgeon General. Rockville, MD: U.S. Department of Health and Human Services, Substance Abuse and Mental Health Services Administration, Center for Mental Health Services, National Institutes of Health, National Institute of Mental Health, 1999.

258. U.S. Department of Health & Human Services. The Surgeon General's call to action to prevent and decrease overweight and obesity. Rockville, MD: U.S. Department of Health and Human Services, Public Health Service, Office of the Surgeon General, 2001.

259. Van der Does AJ. The effects of tryptophan depletion on mood and psychiatric symptoms. *J Affect Disord* 2001;64:107–119.

260. Varanka TM, Weller RA, Weller EB, et al. Lithium treatment of manic episodes with psychotic features in prepubertal children. *Am J Psychiatry* 1988;145:1557–1559.

261. Vitiello B, Behar D, Malone R, et al. Pharmacokinetics of lithium carbonate in children. *J Clin Psychopharmacol* 1988;8:355–359.

262. Wagner KD, Ambrosini P, Rynn M, et al. Efficacy of sertraline in the treatment of children and adolescents with major depressive disorder: Two randomized controlled trials. *JAMA* 2003;290: 1033–1041.

263. Wagner KD, Weller EB, Carlson GA, et al. An open-label trial of divalproex in children and adolescents with bipolar disorder. *J Am Acad Child Adolesc Psychiatry* 2002;41:1224–1230.

264. Wang PW, Santosa C, Schumacher M, et al. Gabapentin augmentation therapy in bipolar depression. *Bipolar Disord* 2002;4:296–301.

265. Wassertheil-Smoller S, Shumaker S, Ockene J, et al. Depression and cardiovascular sequelae in post-menopausal women. The Women's Health Initiative (WHI). *Arch Intern Med* 2004;164:289–298.

266. Wehr TA. Improvement of depression and triggering of mania by sleep deprivation. *JAMA* 1992;267:548–551.

267. Wehr TA, Wirz-Justice A, Goodwin FK, et al. Phase advance of the circadian sleep-wake cycle as an antidepressant. *Science* 1979;206:710–713.

268. Weiss RD, Greenfield SF, Griffin ML, et al. The use of collateral reports for patients with bipolar and substance use disorders. *Am J Drug Alcohol Abuse* 2000;26:369–378.

269. Weissman MM, Myers JK. Affective disorders in a US urban community: The use of research diagnostic criteria in an epidemiological survey. *Arch Gen Psychiatry* 1978;35:1304–1311.

270. Weissman MM, Wolk S, Wickramaratne P, et al. Children with prepubertal-onset major depressive disorder and anxiety grown up. *Arch Gen Psychiatry* 1999;56:794–801.

271. Weller RA, Weller EB. Tricyclic antidepressants in prepubertal depressed children: Review of the literature. *Hillside J Clin Psychiatry* 1986;8:46–55.

272. Werry JS, Biederman J, Thisted R, et al. Resolved: Cardiac arrhythmias make desipramine an unacceptable choice in children. *J Am Acad Child Adolesc Psychiatry* 1995;34:1239–1245.

273. Whittier MC, West SA, Galli VB, et al. Valproic acid for dysphoric mania in a mentally retarded adolescent. *J Clin Psychiatry* 1995;56:590–591.

274. Whittington CJ, Kendall T, Fonagy P, et al. Selective serotonin reuptake inhibitors in childhood depression: Systematic review of published versus unpublished data. *Lancet* 2004;363:1341–1345.

275. Wilens TE, Biederman J, Baldessarini RJ, et al. Electrocardiographic effects of desipramine and 2-hydroxydesipramine in children, adolescents, and adults treated with desipramine. *J Am Acad Child Adolesc Psychiatry* 1993;32:798–804.

276. Wilens TE, Biederman J, Millstein RB, et al. Risk for substance use disorders in youths with child- and adolescent-onset bipolar disorder. *J Am Acad Child Adolesc Psychiatry* 1999;38:680–685.

277. Woolston JL. Case study: Carbamazepine treatment of juvenile-onset bipolar disorder. *J Am Acad Child Adolesc Psychiatry* 1999;38: 335–338.

278. Wozniak J, Biederman J. Childhood mania: Insights into diagnostic and treatment issues. *J Assoc Acad Minor Phys* 1997;8:78–84.

279. Yates WR, Wallace R. Cardiovascular risk factors in affective disorder. *J Affect Disord* 1987;12: 129–134.

280. Yonkers KA, Wisner KL, Stowe Z, et al. Management of bipolar disorder during pregnancy and

the postpartum period. *Am J Psychiatry* 2004; 161:608–620.

281. Younes RP, DeLong GR, Neiman G, et al. Manic-depressive illness in children: Treatment with lithium carbonate. *J Child Neurol* 1986;1: 364–368.

282. Young LT. What exactly is a mood stabilizer? *J Psychiatry Neurosci* 2004;29:87–88.

283. Young LT, Joffe RT, Robb JC, et al. Double-blind comparison of addition of a second mood stabilizer versus an antidepressant to an initial mood stabilizer for treatment of patients with bipolar depression. *Am J Psychiatry* 2000;157: 124–126.

284. Zito JM, Safer DJ, dosReis S, et al. Trends in the prescribing of psychotropic medications to preschoolers. *JAMA* 2000;283:1025–1030.

285. Caspi A, Sugden K, Moffitt TE, Taylor A, Craig IW, Harrington H, McClay J, Mill J, Martin J, Braithwaite A, Poulton R. Influence of life stress on depression: moderation by a polymorphism in the 5-HTT gene. *Science* 2003;301:386–389.

286. Wagner KD, Robb AS, Findling RL, Jin J, Gutierrez MM, Heydorn WE. A randomized, placebo-controlled trial of citalopram for the treatment of major depression in children and adolescents. *Am J Psychiatry* 2004;161:1079–1083.

287. Emslie GJ, Heiligenstein JH, Hoog SL, Wagner KD, Findling RL, McCracken JT, Nilsson ME, Jacobson JG. Fluoxetine treatment for prevention of relapse of depression in children and adolescents: a double-blind, placebo-controlled study. *J Am Acad Child Adolesc Psychiatry* 2004;43:1397–1405.

288. Lawrence NS, Williams AM, Surguladze S, Giampietro V, Brammer MJ, Andrew C, Frangou S, Ecker C, Phillips ML. Subcortical and ventral prefrontal cortical neural responses to facial expressions distinguish patients with bipolar disorder and major depression. *Biol Psychiatry* 2004;55:578–587.

289. Chang K, Adleman NE, Dienes K, Simeonova DI, Menon V, Reiss A. Anomalous prefrontal-subcortical activation in familial pediatric bipolar disorder: a functional magnetic resonance imaging investigation. *Arch Gen Psychiatry* 2004;61:781–792.

290. Blumberg HP, Martin A, Kaufman J, Leung HC, Skudlarski P, Lacadie C, Fulbright RK, Gore JC, Charney DS, Krystal JH, Peterson BS. Frontostriatal abnormalities in adolescents with bipolar disorder: preliminary observations from functional MRI. *Am J Psychiatry* 2003;160:1345–1347.

291. Malhi GS, Lagopoulos J, Sachdev P, Mitchell PB, Ivanovski B, Parker GB. Cognitive generation of affect in hypomania: an fMRI study. *Bipolar Disord* 2004;6:271–285.

292. Blumberg HP, Kaufman J, Martin A, Charney DS, Krystal JH, Peterson BS. Significance of adolescent neurodevelopment for the neural circuitry of bipolar disorder. *Ann N Y Acad Sci.* 2004;1021:376–383.

293. Kowatch RA, Fristad M, Birmaher B, Wagner KD, Findling RL, Hellander M; Child Psychiatric Workgroup on Bipolar Disorder. *J Am Acad Child Adolesc Psychiatry* 2005 Mar;44(3): 213–35.

294. Frayne SM, Seaver MR, Loveland S, Christiansen SL, Spiro A III, Parker VA, Skinner KM. Burden of medical illness in women with depression and posttraumatic stress disorder. *Archives of Internal Medicine* 2004;164(12):1306–1312.

295. Kupfer DJ. The increasing medical burden in bipolar disorder. *JAMA* 2005 May 25;293(20): 2528–30.

296. Kilbourne AM, Cornelius JR, Han X, et al. Burden of general medical conditions among individuals with bipolar disorder. *Bipolar Disord* 2004;6:368–373.

297. Beyer J, Kuchibhatla M, Gersing K, Krishnan KR. Neuropsychopharmacology 2005 Feb;30(2): 401–4.

CHAPTER 5

Empowering Patients and Families to Achieve Lasting Wellness

LYDIA LEWIS AND LAURA HOOFNAGLE

To move the mental health care system from a focus on providers to a focus on consumers, future care systems and quality tools will need to reflect person-centered values.

SURGEON GENERAL'S REPORT ON MENTAL HEALTH – 2000

[An important] goal of a transformed mental health system is treatment that is consumer and family driven.

FINAL REPORT, PRESIDENT'S NEW FREEDOM COMMISSION ON MENTAL HEALTH – 2003

For patients with depression, bipolar disorder, and other mental illnesses, empowerment is a critical factor in treatment adherence, treatment effectiveness, and recovery. Despite the limitations and challenges imposed by managed care, physicians can play an important role in patient empowerment by educating patients and their families about mood disorders and treatment options, involving them in treatment planning, connecting them with understanding peers, encouraging them to self-manage and set life goals, and restoring their faith in their own ability to reach wellness.

Increased patient wellness means decreased devastation and death due to mood disorders. Depression and bipolar disorder continue to take an overwhelming toll on patients and families. Suicide claims the lives of over 30,000 people in the United States every year.[1] Untreated, under-treated, or incorrectly treated mood disorders also severely impact quality of life. By empowering patients and families, physicians take a preemptive strike against costly and traumatic hospitalizations, years of suffering with unsuccessful treatment and most importantly, suicide.

▶ THE EMPOWERED PATIENT: A PARTNER IN TREATMENT

I thank God to this day that I started seeing a psychiatrist and a therapist who listened to me and observed my actions. I went through various medications over a long period of time, trying to find what worked best for me. As time passed, we found the right combination of medications and I began to feel better with a new and clearer outlook on life.

DEPRESSION AND BIPOLAR SUPPORT ALLIANCE (DBSA) WEB SITE VISITOR

Empowered patients can make significant contributions to their treatment plans and become more than just passive receivers of services. They are more likely to describe their full range of symptoms, give complete family medical histories, and offer additional information that is critical to a correct diagnosis. Empowered patients are educated about available treatments and able to discuss their options and preferences with their physicians.

Patients who can speak openly and honestly with physicians and ask for what they need are likely to find effective treatments more quickly. Empowered patients may also be better able to overcome mistrust of the health care system. They can approach mental health care knowing they have options and are less likely to feel victimized. They are more likely to persevere with long-term treatment if they believe the professionals treating them consider patients' best interests. Consequently, working with empowered patients is more likely to be rewarding for physicians.

Patients who are empowered know what to expect from treatment and are able to evaluate their progress and wellness with their health care providers. Working with their doctors, they persevere beyond remission of symptoms to full wellness.

▶ EMPOWERMENT THROUGH EDUCATION: BEYOND STEREOTYPES

It is such a relief to know that I'm not broken or just insane. . . I know it's going to be a long road but now that I'm becoming better educated, it's not so scary.

E-MAIL RECEIVED BY DBSA

Two of the greatest obstacles to patient empowerment are fear and misunderstanding, which prevent many people with mood disorders from seeking and receiving the help they need. Education of patients, families, and the general public is necessary to increase acceptance and decrease stigma and misconceptions regarding depression and bipolar disorder.

One of the primary challenges in mood disorder treatment is helping patients understand that mood disorders are real illnesses, not character flaws or attempts to get attention. As recently as 2002, nearly one-fourth of Americans believed that people with mood disorders were weak or lazy, and 25% believed they were dangerous.[2] These beliefs can seriously impact treatment success. Patient and family education is the key to correcting them.

Another challenge is the ignorance and stigma surrounding psychiatric medications, which can play a large part in patient resistance to treatment. Nearly three-fourth of the public surveyed by Depression and Bipolar Support Alliance (DBSA) in 2002 believed mood disorder medications change a person's personality, and more than two-thirds believed that mood disorder medications are habit-forming.[3] Physicians must impress upon patients that medication is safe, and very different from street drugs. Patients need to know that medication treats illness but does not change personality. It is also crucial that dually diagnosed patients understand that taking medications for depression or bipolar disorder does not mean they are no longer clean and sober.

Physicians can improve patients' understanding of mental illness by offering reliable information on mood disorders to all of their patients. Literature explaining a variety of "physical" illnesses is available in doctors' offices, but information about mental illnesses is more difficult to find. Placing literature in waiting rooms, asking mental health questions on medical history forms, and inquiring about mental health during routine appointments can make people more willing to talk about their own symptoms and has the potential to change people's attitudes about mental illness over time.

▶ EMPOWERMENT THROUGH SYMPTOM RECOGNITION: TIMELY, CORRECT DIAGNOSIS

In 1992, I was finally diagnosed with bipolar II disorder. I can trace the roots of my illness back to 1974. Having taken almost every antidepressant available, I finally found relief with a combination of mood stabilizers. A correct diagnosis and an understanding of my illness and its treatment has helped me maintain a reasonable quality of life ever since.

DBSA SUPPORT GROUP LEADER

When patients can recognize and accurately describe their symptoms—and when they are aware of external factors that may exacerbate them—they are more likely to ask for medical help early when symptoms worsen or unexpected events occur.

Improved symptom recognition can lead to more timely and accurate diagnosis, an urgent need in light of the fact that people with mood disorders, especially bipolar disorder, are misdiagnosed with alarming frequency. A 2000 DBSA survey of patients with bipolar disorder found that nearly 7 out of 10 had been misdiagnosed an average of 3.5 times. Thirty-five percent waited 10 or more years to receive an accurate diagnosis, and nearly half were misdiagnosed by a primary care provider.[4]

Screening for mood disorders should be done as part of routine medical evaluations. Patients who present with sleep, pain, or gastrointestinal symptoms must be paid special attention, as these can be among the first noticeable symptoms of a mood disorder. It is also especially important for physicians to actively probe for symptoms of mania in patients presenting with depression to avoid a misdiagnosis of unipolar depression and the potential for later manic episodes. Primary care physicians report that mania is significantly more difficult to diagnose than depression; while 74% of them said depression was "somewhat/very easy" to diagnose, 73% found mania "somewhat/very difficult" to diagnose.[5]

Difficulty in diagnosis may be due in part to the fact that people with bipolar disorder may have difficulty recognizing their own mania or hypomania. Patients are far more likely to visit a physician when experiencing symptoms of depression. This makes it even more critical for physicians to ask about symptoms of mania. Direct questions such as "Have there been times when you spent a lot more money than usual?" "Have there been times when you were more interested in sex?" or "Do you ever have trouble sleeping or concentrating?" can uncover the need for referral to a psychiatrist for a full spectrum bipolar disorder evaluation.

In addition to helping patients become more familiar with their own symptoms and triggers, physicians should encourage their patients to keep records of treatment adherence, mood and lifestyle, chart their progress day-to-day, and look for patterns. Mood tracking helps patients become aware of their actions, motivations, and the way they react to the world around them. A simple words-and-numbers rating system (including mood level, hours of sleep, meals, and so on) works for many people and is easy to follow over the long term. Patients should also track excessive alcohol consumption, use of street drugs, and behaviors that are destructive to them or those around them. In addition, they should be encouraged to practice preventative maintenance by keeping regular health care appointments, continuing to learn about their illness and attending peer support groups.

▶ EMPOWERMENT THROUGH PARTICIPATION: THE IMPORTANCE OF THE PATIENT PERSPECTIVE

The probability of forming a decision-making partnership between the consumer and the [physician] increases when consumers gain knowledge and are able to take a participatory role in decisions regarding the course of treatment.

DIALOGUE BETWEEN CONSUMERS AND PROVIDERS CONDUCTED BY THE U.S. DEPARTMENT OF HEALTH AND HUMAN SERVICES, CENTER FOR MENTAL HEALTH SERVICES (CMHS) IN 1997

Patients and health care providers share the goals of symptom management, relapse prevention and ultimately, wellness. Patients need to hear from their physicians that it is possible for them to feel better, and be given the opportunity to work collaboratively with their physicians to develop action steps toward wellness.

It is critical that physicians develop an understanding of the patient perspective, and it is imperative that physicians communicate in ways patients with mood disorders can understand. A truly effective doctor not only understands the medical aspects of the depression or bipolar disorder, but also is able to empathize with a patient's feelings about having the disorder, and adjust interactions accordingly.

Because of widespread social stigma and the patient self-stigma that often comes with it, the best treatment for mood disorders must go beyond the strictly medical approach. A physician who simply hands the patient a prescription and tells him to come back in a few weeks must understand that a couple of weeks can seem like an eternity for someone with depression. A patient who does not believe medication will help, or who, because of symptoms, is unable to see the difference between "a couple of weeks" and "forever," is much less likely to follow his doctor's orders. A patient whose doctor explains that these feelings of hopelessness are symptoms of his illness and that medication can help him manage these symptoms is more likely to stick with treatment and experience mood improvement.

Figure 5-1[6] illustrates that treatment satisfaction increased as understanding of treatment issues increased. DBSA has found that many patients would prefer to be more involved in their treatment. For example, while 71% of physicians reported their patients participated in treatment planning, only 54% of patients agreed with this statement (Fig. 5-2).[7] This suggests that, although physicians may be talking to patients about their treatment options, patients do not feel they have choices. Patients may not be hearing or comprehending important information, due to communication gaps, cultural differences, or untreated symptoms. They need to be encouraged by their physicians to talk about their treatment needs and preferences, and to bring up concerns and ideas about things that may help them.

Less than 25% of the patients in the above survey who had less-than-adequate communication and understanding felt their depression

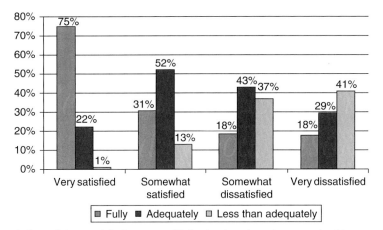

1. Overall, how satisfied are you with the treatment you have received for your depression from your current (or most recent) primary care doctor?
2. Do you usually come away from your primary care doctor feeling you have understood the important issues discussed about treatment of your depression—fully, adequately or less than adequately?

Figure 5-1. Treatment satisfaction can increase as understanding of treatment issues increases.

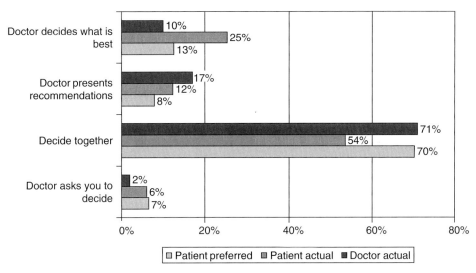

1. Which of the following statements best describes how decisions are actually made about the treatment of (patients with/your) depression?
2. Which of these same statements do you think is the best way to make treatment decisions about depression?

Figure 5-2. A communication disconnect exists between health care providers and patients as to whether the patient is an active partner in treatment planning.

had been completely controlled in the past 2 months. When patients are empowered, they can contribute substantially to their own wellness and are more likely to feel their illness is under control. Patients who know the facts about mood disorders are able to raise concerns based on their knowledge. They can get needed treatment earlier and significantly improve the possibility of full recovery. Education and empowerment can lead to successful management of symptoms, treatment adherence, and improvement in all areas of life. Every patient can play an active role in treatment, regardless of educational or socioeconomic status, age, gender, or symptom severity.

► EMPOWERMENT THROUGH CULTURAL AWARENESS: KNOWING WHERE PATIENTS COME FROM

Physicians must take into account an individual's cultural identity, cultural explanations of the individual's illness, cultural factors related to environment and functioning, and cultural elements of the doctor/patient relationship.

DSM-IV[8]

Physicians must be aware of their patients' cultures, beliefs, and experiences, and how these factors impact patients' reactions to diagnosis and treatment of mental illness. For example, in some cultures, people may believe they are hearing spirits, not voices; in others, people may believe their suffering is due to karma, not illness.

Patients who come from cultures in which mental illness is considered a failure of will, something caused by a lack of faith or an inability to live up to gender expectations need additional education as to the biologic nature of their illness. They should also be shown how determination, spirituality, and gender identity can play positive roles in their treatment. Patients must be able to reconcile their own long-held beliefs with the treatment they are receiving, and know that the things that give them strength will not be taken away or rendered useless if they receive mental health treatment. Physicians must communicate to them that treatment will not change who they are; it will help them to be themselves.

► EMPOWERMENT THROUGH COMMUNICATION: ASKING, LISTENING, AND HEARING

Trust is reinforced when the process of listening is formalized through the planned or mandated involvement of consumers at all levels of the system.

THE DIALOGUE BETWEEN CONSUMERS AND PROVIDERS CONDUCTED BY THE U.S. DEPARTMENT OF HEALTH AND HUMAN SERVICES, CENTER FOR MENTAL HEALTH SERVICES (CMHS), 1997

Patients with illnesses affecting their thinking and perception need empathy as much if not more than patients with other illnesses. A recent DBSA patient survey revealed that 67% of patients treated for mood disorders by primary care physicians wished their doctors would listen better and 65% wished their doctors would talk to them in a language they could understand.[9]

To ascertain patients' symptoms, experiences, and state of mind, physicians must ask direct questions. Mood disorders may not be easy to spot during routine, time restricted appointments. Rather than simply asking "How are you feeling?" (to which the answer is almost always, "Fine.") physicians might ask, "How are you sleeping?" "Have you had any racing thoughts lately?" or "Have you been crying a lot lately?" Patients are likely to welcome this opportunity if they are uneasy about raising their concerns or unaware of their own symptoms.

When patients with depression visited their primary care doctors for other health issues, only 42% reported that their doctors always asked about their depression.[10] Specific and direct questions addressing treatment adherence should be asked at every appointment. Rather than asking, "Have you been taking your medication?" physicians might consider asking, "Have you had any trouble remembering to take your medication?" or "Have you had problems with side effects?" If patients are not adhering to treatment, physicians should identify and address the reasons for nonadherence.

Medication side effects should be addressed early in treatment. Patients need to be reassured that there are many treatment options available, side effects can be alleviated, and their doctors are willing to work with them throughout the process. Side effects such as sexual dysfunction, weight gain, fatigue, or headaches often make patients reluctant to adhere to treatment. While it may appear obvious to a physician that weight gain is preferable to suicidal ideation or high-risk behavior, patients may not feel the same way. A patient's uncertain self-image may be further undermined by side effects like weight gain or sexual dysfunction. This patient might prefer to take chances with symptoms rather than risk having a socially undesirable appearance or being unable to perform sexually.

Only 36% of patients in DBSA's primary care survey[11] were asked what side effects they might be willing to tolerate when medications were prescribed (Fig. 5-3). Thirty-four percent said their doctor did not discuss side effects at all when prescribing antidepressants.

It is also important to make sure patients hear and understand all treatment instructions, regardless of how thoroughly they have been explained. Patients who are newly diagnosed and/or in the grip of acute manic or depressive symptoms may have trouble understanding or remembering what they have been told. Written information for all patients is preferable. Physicians should also encourage patients to write down treatment instructions so they can refer to the information at a later time.

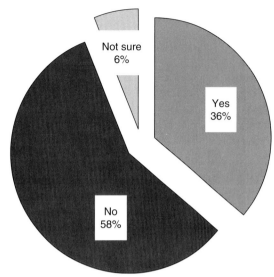

Did your primary care doctor ask you about your preferences or willingness to tolerate certain side effects related to antidepressant medications before making a decision about what to prescribe?

Figure 5-3. Only 36% of patients in DBSA's primary care survey were asked what side effects they might be willing to tolerate when medications were prescribed.

▶ EMPOWERMENT THROUGH FAMILY INVOLVEMENT: WELLNESS CAN BEGIN AT HOME

You will probably wonder if the whole thing was your fault. If wondering about it helps you correct mistakes and communicate better with your family member, good. But don't blame yourself. You can help your family member most if you keep yourself well and get the support you need.

MOTHER OF A YOUNG WOMAN WITH BIPOLAR DISORDER[12]

When someone has depression or bipolar disorder, the entire family can be affected. Patients may or may not choose to have their families involved in their recovery, but every patient should be given the option. However, DBSA's 2003 online survey found that while 65% of patients wanted their families involved in their treatment, only 27% of them said their primary care doctors suggested and facilitated family involvement.[13] Physicians should take the first step in recommending family involvement, since patients with mood disorders may be reluctant to suggest it.

Having a loved one with a mood disorder can be frightening, embarrassing, or frustrating. Families, whether or not they are involved in a relative's treatment, should have a place to go for support of their own. Families of people with mood disorders and families who have lost someone to suicide can be helped by giving and receiving support, insight, and guidance from one another. Physicians can help by referring all families to local support groups, and by posting support group information in waiting rooms where family members are likely to see it.

It is most important that families be educated about symptoms and treatments of mood disorders. Physicians should keep the same factors in mind when talking to families as they do when talking to patients: make sure explanations and instructions are heard and understood, provide written materials, pay attention to cultural factors, and take patients' and families' feelings and points of view into account.

▶ EMPOWERMENT THROUGH PEER SUPPORT: "WE'VE BEEN THERE. WE CAN HELP"

The people in my DBSA support group reached out to me and made me realize that I was not alone. If not for the support that I received from them, I probably wouldn't be here.

DBSA SUPPORT GROUP PARTICIPANT

Peer support groups connect patients with others living with depression and bipolar disorder. These groups can substantially help patients believe in their own resilience and commit to treatment. Yet DBSA's *Support Group Participation* survey of patients who had attended support groups for at least a year found that only one-third of them had been told about the groups by their health care providers. Nearly 6 out of 10 respondents had been diagnosed for over a year before they heard about DBSA support groups.[14]

It is imperative that physicians familiarize themselves with patient support groups and resources in their communities. Support groups can yield numerous benefits, the most important of which is a greater number of patients who are able to maintain their wellness. More than 1000 peer-led support groups are affiliated with DBSA. DBSA can also assist health care professionals in establishing new groups where they are needed.

Many patients have a list of painful issues too long and complex to address during a routine appointment. Some of these issues may be better addressed with a group of concerned peers who have "been there." Support groups can greatly aid in recovery by helping patients through difficult times. DBSA's research shows that participation in a support group makes patients more likely to adhere to treatment, less likely to be hospitalized, and more able to improve communication with their physicians.[15]

Patients with depression or bipolar disorder who have endured major life crises or periods of decreasing functionality may feel more discouraged than ever, especially when adjusting to life after hospitalization, trying new medications, coping with side effects, or stopping drinking, substance abuse, or other destructive behaviors. They may be left without much confidence or hope and feel they have no place to turn. They may question their own instincts, sanity, or ability to cope with life. Even if their families are sympathetic, they still need people with whom they can openly share their frustrations, fears, questions, and ultimately their victories and successes. Peers who have been through similarly harrowing experiences and are on their way toward lasting wellness can help those who are newly diagnosed truly find themselves and trust themselves again. By talking with experienced peers, patients can gain better understanding and acceptance of their illness and learn that they have the power to be equal partners in achieving their wellness goals, not just passive receivers of treatment.

Effective self-help groups do not focus solely on illness, but also on strategies for achieving wellness/recovery and fulfilling lives. They also foster fellowship and opportunities to build life-long friendships based on honesty and understanding. Participants find shared interests beyond their mental health and in doing so, come to understand that their illness does not define them and their abilities, talents, strengths, and unique personalities have not been lost.

▶ EMPOWERMENT THROUGH LIFE SKILL DEVELOPMENT: CERTIFIED PEER SPECIALISTS

Peers are ideally suited to deliver a message of hope and be role models for recovery, because they've walked the same path. When I help someone else in recovery, it strengthens my own recovery. It gives meaning to the hopelessness I once felt. [16]

LARRY FRICKS, DIRECTOR, OFFICE OF CONSUMER RELATIONS, GEORGIA DIVISION OF MENTAL HEALTH, DEVELOPMENTAL DISABILITIES AND ADDICTIVE DISEASES

While a physician can instill hope by educating patients and helping them develop treatment plans and a family can instill hope by being understanding and supportive, peers can instill a different and often more powerful kind of hope by sharing their own stories and showing by example that wellness is possible. An exciting and promising new addition to the treatment model is the training of Certified Peer Specialists, who are patients, to assist other patients in recovery and life skill development. At this time, peer specialists work primarily in the public sector, helping patients make the

most of their treatment choices and increase their chances of returning to productive lives. Even in its infancy, this approach has yielded encouraging results,[17] and plans are in progress to incorporate it into private sector care.

People recovering from manic or depressive episodes often need to be reeducated in living. They may have to learn entirely new sets of coping skills to replace old ones that no longer work. Continued dependence solely on medical treatment, with no reeducation in living, can keep patients from experiencing recovery beyond relief of symptoms. Without foundation and assistance in rebuilding a full life, patients have no reason to stop believing that they are helpless and worthless and will never amount to much. If health care providers, family, or the patient have low expectations, this can ultimately undermine a patient's recovery.

To have the best chance of staying on a recovery path, patients must believe they can be contributing members of their communities. Peer specialists help patients realize their own potential through self-directed recovery. They help patients discover they have power to move beyond their limitations. Peer specialists can teach patients that they are in charge of their recovery. They can help patients recognize their strengths, focus on those strengths, explore ways to find lasting recovery and create the lives they want.

Self-determination, with the help of a peer specialist, occurs in stages. A patient must first be willing to accept help and work toward mood stabilization. The next stage occurs as patients begin to accept that they have an illness that affects all areas of life. During this stage, the peer specialist helps instill hope and rebuild a positive self-image. The next stage occurs as patients realize that although their illness may change the course of their lives, it does not have to permanently marginalize or disable them. Peer specialists continue to encourage patients by showing them how to participate in their own recovery and reminding them how their lives can be different. Next, patients begin to explore the ways in which they can change their lives. With peer specialists' help, they identify their strengths and locate the resources they need to reach their goals. In the last stage of recovery, patients take concrete action steps toward the goals they have set. Peer specialists encourage them along the way and help them use the strengths they have identified.

Peer specialists can also help with crisis planning. When patients are well, they are advised to prepare advance directives that provide instructions for their care if they become too ill to care for themselves. It can be very reassuring for patients to know that if symptoms worsen, they will have their wishes honored, and that action can be taken before a crisis occurs.

While peer specialists do not provide psychotherapy, they can fill the gap that may be left when a patient cannot afford therapy or has a therapist with an approach that focuses on a patient's past. Peer specialists can also be effective educators, as they are able to speak to patients using terms and ideas they can easily understand.

Through work with peer specialists, patients can develop self-management skills. A patient who can self-manage has made an important and lasting change. Self-management not only enables people to live successfully on their own, but it also gives them power over their illness. They are prepared for unexpected mood changes; they can identify them and know what to expect. They also have a plan to address and treat mood switches and episodes when, and sometimes before, they happen.

▶ EMPOWERMENT THROUGH GOAL-SETTING: THE POWER OF POSSIBILITY

If there were two doors, one medication and symptom reduction and the other recovery and a meaningful, quality life in the community, which door do you think a person would pick? They want to go through the second door – recovery and a meaningful life.[18]

LARRY FRICKS

When patients believe their lives can and will change, they are ready to set life goals and outline actions they will take to reach them. During this process, peer specialists can assist them by pointing out strengths and improvements and providing resources and support. As patients progress, their goals become more specific and concrete.

Individual wellness goals must be developed by each patient and his physician in a partnership beginning at the time of diagnosis. Goals should be reviewed periodically throughout treatment. It is helpful to separate goals into short-term objectives (such as waking up and going to bed at the same time every day, being able to finish reading a book or news article, staying in school) and long-term objectives (such as finding a job or rebuilding family relationships). Physicians can assist patients in developing realistic wellness goals and help them believe their goals are reachable.

For example, a patient whose depression has prevented him from working for several years may believe he has no skills and will never hold a job. He must first want to change this belief and be willing to work with his physician, psychotherapist, and peer specialist toward a positive state of mind in which he can imagine himself working. He may not know what he will do, or how to do it, but he believes that he has a future. As this belief becomes more familiar, hope becomes stronger. He is now able to look at his skills. What is he good at? Are his skills verbal, mechanical, social? Where does he feel most comfortable? What can he offer an employer? Through this process he becomes ready to begin looking for a job. He can follow this same process with regard to his housing, relationships, and other life goals.

The entire process of patient empowerment will increase the quality of his wellness and his life. Becoming a secure, working member of the community can have powerful effects on his wellness. He is able to return to his physician appointments with more life experience, more coping skills, and a more enthusiastic attitude about treatment.

▶ EMPOWERMENT THROUGH HOPE: RECOVERY CAN BE A REALITY

How did I do it when there was no one to take care of me? Did I feel shaky? Yes. Was I scared out of my wits? Yes. Did I ever get fired because I could not do the work? You bet. But I kept on and kept on until I found something I could do. Even after all this time I have episodes and I know I must get help. But when I was told I had bipolar disorder, that was OK. And it's OK now.

DBSA WEB SITE VISITOR

When a person who is severely ill with depression or bipolar disorder regains the ability to hope, that person reaches a turning point in recovery. Because mood disorder symptoms can make patients believe that they will never be well again, patients must be encouraged to believe recovery is possible every step of the way. The goal for *all* patients must be full wellness, not just remission of symptoms.

Empowered patients who believe they can recover have improved self-esteem and are involved in their communities. They engage in activities that bring satisfaction and a sense of purpose, such as working, volunteering, caring for a family, being part of a social group, or pursuing other interests. They regain a sense of dignity. They are aware of their own unique strengths and how these assets can aid in their recovery. They no longer feel disabled or defined by their illness, and they are able to communicate a sense of hope to others.

Empowered patients know their goals for symptom reduction, wellness, and full recovery. They inform their health care providers when they believe they could be doing better. They seek optimal treatment and are willing to try new options if necessary. Patient empowerment also improves and strengthens patients' relationships,

particularly with their families, and helps them make informed choices about their loved ones' involvement in their treatment. Many loved ones are able to provide valuable support and understanding to patients with mood disorders if they, too, are educated. Empowered patients are able to prepare for the future and decide how their loved ones can assist them if they become too ill to care for themselves. Their illness does not own them or dictate their actions. Feelings of helplessness and hopelessness do not immobilize them. They trust their instincts and choices, and they can inspire others to trust them.

▶ CONCLUSION

Patient empowerment is a powerful force in recovery. The physician's role in empowering the patient cannot be overemphasized. Physicians must be patients' best source of information about their illness. The more information patients are given, and the more they are encouraged to participate in making treatment choices, the more likely they are to feel they can overcome the obstacles their illness presents. Patients must trust their health care providers and be confident in their providers' knowledge and interest in helping them. Cooperative, constructive relationships with physicians foster this trust. Participation in their treatment planning can help restore patients' faith in themselves, which, in turn, strengthens their recovery. When physicians acknowledge patients' feelings and show empathy, patients' satisfaction with treatment increases.

When patients are educated and empowered, they are more likely to stick with treatment and more willing to keep trying treatments until the best one is found. Knowledge about their symptoms and triggers empowers patients to seek help before symptoms worsen and crises occur. Improved confidence in their ability to get well helps them define their own wellness, and become better equipped to reach it.

Physicians must pay attention to their own communication styles and be sure patients are able to understand and use the information they are given. Direct questions during routine appointments can reveal hidden mood disorder symptoms and patient reservations about treatment, and enable physicians to treat patients more effectively. Patients' cultural backgrounds should be taken into account and treatment plans should be culturally relevant.

Physicians should assist patients in setting treatment and life goals. Families should be educated and, when appropriate, included in treatment. Patients should be encouraged to become part of support groups where they can share their experiences. Support groups can restore patients' sense of belonging and empower them to pursue life goals.

Low expectations erode recovery. Physicians must project an attitude of hope to every patient, no matter how ill. Certified peer specialists can help patients develop and maintain hope by guiding them in concrete goal setting and connecting them with the resources they need.

Depression and bipolar disorder are devastating and deadly, but full recovery is possible. The best recovery is achieved when physicians pay attention to patients' individual needs, communicate clearly and effectively, and empower patients to return to full wellness and productive lives in their communities.

REFERENCES

1. American Foundation for Suicide Prevention, www.afsp.org, Facts about Suicide, accessed 10/6/04.
2. Depression and Bipolar Support Alliance. *General Public Survey Findings*. Chicago, IL: Lipman Hearne, 2002, not published.
3. *Ibid.*
4. Depression and Bipolar Support Alliance. *Living with Bipolar Disorder: How Far Have We Really Come?* Chicago, IL: Depression and Bipolar Support Alliance, 2001.
5. Depression and Bipolar Support Alliance. *Beyond Diagnosis: A Landmark Survey of Patients, Partners and Health Professionals on Depression and Treatment*. Chicago, IL: Depression and Bipolar Support Alliance, 2000.
6. *Ibid.*, *Executive Summary, Graphs, Figure 14*, Chicago, IL.
7. *Ibid.*, Figure 12.
8. American Psychiatric Association. *Diagnostic and Statistical Manual of Mental Disorders*, 4th ed. Washington, DC: Outline for Cultural Formulation and Glossary of Culture-Bound Syndromes, 1994, p. 843.
9. Depression and Bipolar Support Alliance. *Treatment Satisfaction Online Survey*, 2002, not published.
10. See Ref. 5.
11. *Ibid.*
12. Depression and Bipolar Support Alliance. *Psychiatric Hospitalization, A Guide for Families*, 2004.
13. See Ref. 9.
14. Depression and Bipolar Support Alliance. National DMDA Support Group Survey of 2,049 people from 190 cities in 38 states. Presented at American Psychiatric Association Annual Meeting, 1999.
15. *Ibid.*
16. Depression and Bipolar Support Alliance. *Outreach* 2004.
17. Emerging New Practices in Organized Peer Support: Report from NTAC's National Experts Meeting on Emerging New Practices in Organized Peer Support, March 17-18, 2003, Alexandria, VA, 25 www.nasmhpd.org/publications.cfm, accessed 10/6/04.
18. See Ref. 16.

SECTION II

Disorders of Endocrinology and Metabolism

CHAPTER 6

Depression and Diabetes

Jeffrey P. Staab, Dwight L. Evans, and Dominique L. Musselman

▶ INTRODUCTION

Diabetes and depression are highly prevalent, chronic medical conditions that cause considerable emotional and physical suffering, lead to premature death, and consume substantial health care resources.[1–4] Over the last 25 years, clinical researchers have described high rates of comorbidity between diabetes and depression.[5–8] Additional studies investigated biologic[9–25] and psychosocial factors[8,26–35] that may explain the interrelationship of these illnesses.[36] Treatment research has lagged, but well-controlled intervention trials designed to improve both depressive symptoms and glycemic control are beginning to emerge.[37–41] This chapter will review the epidemiology of coexisting diabetes and depression, the multiple effects that each illness has on the other, potential pathophysiologic and psychosocial mechanisms linking them, and current data on the efficacy of various treatment interventions.

▶ EPIDEMIOLOGY

The prevalence of diabetes is increasing rapidly throughout the world. Using data from the World Health Organization (WHO), Wild and colleagues[7] estimated that 171 million people worldwide suffered from diabetes in 2000 and predicted that this number will more than double by the year 2030 due to sedentary lifestyles,

urbanization, increasing rates of obesity, and the effects of an aging population. Diabetes is one of the leading causes of death throughout the world[42] and contributes to the morbidity and mortality of cardiovascular and cerebrovascular diseases as a risk factor for these conditions.[43] Diabetes-related complications include foot ulceration,[44] loss of limbs,[45] peripheral neuropathy,[46] end-stage renal disease,[47] and blindness.[48]

Diabetes and depression cause considerable disability, lost work productivity, and economic burden.[2,49] In the 30,000 person National Health Interview Survey, patients with either diabetes or depression were 2.5–3 times more likely than healthy individuals to be functionally impaired, whereas those with coexisting conditions had a sevenfold increase in disability.[3] The economic costs of medical care for patients with diabetes are high and depression raises these expenditures even further. In a study of 1694 adults, the average 3-year cost of medical care for those with uncomplicated diabetes was $14,223. Comorbid depression increased these costs by 50%.[4] A separate investigation of older Medicare recipients found that total costs for inpatient and outpatient medical care were significantly higher for those with depression and diabetes than diabetes alone.[1]

Over the last 25 years, a large number of studies have investigated the prevalence of depression in patients with diabetes using clinician-administered diagnostic interviews and patient self-report instruments. Two meta-analyses summarized these efforts and found the prevalence of major depressive disorder in patients with diabetes to be 9–14% in studies using clinician-administered diagnostic interviews,[5,6] which is twice the prevalence of depression in the general population. Investigations that employed patient self-reports revealed higher rates of moderate to severe depressive symptoms, averaging 26 and 32% in the two meta-analyses, respectively. A recently completed public health survey of 10,000 New York City residents confirmed the twofold increase in depression among patients with diabetes.[8] Furthermore, patients with diabetes and depression were more likely to live in poverty, report poor health, have no access to health care, and have lost a partner. The high levels of depression and socioeconomic stressors are frequently not appreciated in diabetic patients.[50,51] For example, depression was recognized in only 51% of patients with diabetes in primary care practices associated with a large Health Maintenance Organization (HMO). Among the individuals whose depression was diagnosed, only 43% were prescribed an antidepressant and just 7% received more than three psychotherapy sessions.[51]

▶ PATHOPHYSIOLOGY

Effects of Diabetes on the Development of Depression

Diabetes may contribute to the developement of depressive disorders because of the burden of the medical illness.

Burden of Illness

Several researchers have studied the relationship between severity of depressive symptoms and diabetes in an effort to understand the medical factors that may cause psychiatric morbidity. Lustman and colleagues conducted a meta-analysis of well-controlled, cross-sectional studies of patients with type 1 and type 2 diabetes.[28] They found that the severity of depressive symptoms correlated modestly with gylcosylated hemoglobin

(HbA1C) levels ($r = 0.28$, 95% confidence interval: 0.2–0.36), suggesting that poor glycemic control may contribute to depressive symptoms. Other investigators worldwide found that patients with diabetic complications had higher levels of depression[30–33] and patients with depression perceived a greater burden of illness, reporting twice as many physical symptoms as those without depression.[34] Quality of life is also poorer among patients with coexisting diabetes and depression versus patients with either illness alone.[35] Prospective studies have investigated the temporal relationships between depressive symptoms and glycemic control. A large study of 569 patients with type 2 diabetes suggested that improvements in glycemic control may reduce psychiatric comorbidity.[52] In this randomized, placebo-controlled trial of glipizide, patients who achieved better glycemic control reported lower levels of depression and improved quality of life. However, neither of these changes reached statistical significance, possibly due to the fact that the short duration of the study (3 months) may not have allowed enough time for the patients' improved metabolic status to yield its full psychiatric benefits.

Not all studies have found an association between diabetes and depression. In a Dutch investigation, 2280 patients aged 55–85 were followed prospectively for 6 years with regular evaluations of their physical and mental health.[53] Lung disease, arthritis, cardiac disease, and cancer were associated with increasing levels of depression, but diabetes and atherosclerosis were not. Another study of 303 Blacks in a U.S. primary care setting found no excess prevalence of depression among those with diabetes.[54] However, diabetic patients with depression had three times more emergency department visits and three times more inpatient hospital days than those who were not depressed.

Social Factors

Socioeconomic factors affect the relationship between depression and diabetes. Patients with diabetes who are unmarried, poorly educated, have lower incomes, limited social supports, or experience negative life events are at greater risk of developing depression.[8,27,30,55] Women with diabetes are more likely to report psychologic distress than men. Gender and social factors may interact to further increase the psychologic vulnerability of socially disadvantaged women with diabetes.[26,30,56] These social risk factors are not unique to patients with diabetes. They also increase the risk of depression in medically healthy individuals. However, among patients with diabetes, social factors appear constitute the greatest risk for psychiatric morbidity early in the course of illness, whereas medical factors (e.g., diabetic complications) have a stronger influence in later years.[55]

Disease-Specific Biologic Factors

Alterations in glucose regulation have been reported in patients with major depression since the 1930s.[57–61] Early studies showed that depressed patients had a blunted hypoglycemic response during the insulin tolerance test (ITT).[58,62,63] In a similar vein, nondiabetic patients with major depression had lower glucose utilization and higher plasma insulin levels during glucose tolerance tests (GTT) than normal controls.[59,60,64]

More recent studies expanded this line of research. In a series of experiments, Amsterdam and colleagues reported a blunted glucose decrement in response to the ITT in men, but not women, with unipolar and bipolar depression and a trend toward insulin resistance in men with melancholic depression.[9–11] They also found higher basal glucose levels, a greater increase in serum glucose, a higher insulin response, and greater changes in glucagon during the GTT in 28 medically healthy, drug-free patients with major depression compared to 21 control subjects. The glucose and insulin utilization curves in the depressed patients resembled those seen in patients with non-insulin-dependent diabetes mellitus. Patients with melancholic features had the largest

abnormalities. These findings suggest that major depression produces a relatively insulin-resistant state, even in patients without diabetes. For patients with diabetes, serum glucose levels may increase during major depressive episodes[65–67] and successful treatment of major depression may improve glycemic control.[67–69]

The insulin-resistant state seen in patients with major depression may have several causes. In addition to evidence of an increased release of counter-regulatory hormones in the GTT studies, there is a substantial literature showing that patients with major depression produce excessive amounts of corticosteroid, which may approach that seen in Cushing syndrome.[70] The enhanced hypothalamus pituitary adrenal (HPA) axis activity may add another layer of metabolic abnormalities to the altered state of insulin and glucagon utilization.

Serotonin may have an important role in glycemic control. In animal studies, the serotonin precursor, 5-HTP, lowered blood glucose levels independent of insulin secretion. This effect was blocked by the serotonin antagonist, cyproheptadine.[71] Other animal studies showed that selective serotonin reuptake inhibitors (SSRIs) could significantly reduce plasma glucose levels.[72] In humans, fluoxetine improved glycemic control in obese, non-insulin-dependent patients without depression, reducing HbA1C levels and decreasing daily insulin requirements compared to placebo-treated subjects.[73,74] Fluoxetine also may increase glucose clearance.[75]

Another link between depression and diabetes may be the immune system. In patients with diabetes, adipose tissue secretes excessive amounts of the proinflammatory cytokines, interleukin (IL)-1, IL-6, and tumor necrosis factor-α (TNF-α).[12] Monocytes and macrophages may contribute to these elevated levels with advancing age.[13,14] Overexpression of these cytokines inhibits insulin action.[13,15–18] It also may generate a syndrome known as sickness behavior, a constellation of anorexia, anhedonia, fatigue, sluggishness, and poor self-care that closely resembles major depression.[19,20] Increased levels of IL-6 have been found in patients with major depression with and without comorbid medical illness.[21–25] The potential relationships among cytokine activation, diabetes, and depression are under investigation.

Effects of Depression on the Development of Diabetes

Inactivity and obesity are risk factors for the development of type 2 diabetes.[76] Patients with psychiatric illnesses, including depressive disorders, share these risk factors with the general population. However, data are accumulating from large epidemiologic studies that suggest that clinically significant depressive symptoms may contribute to the development of type 2 diabetes. Seven studies involving more than 100,000 subjects collectively and follow-up periods of 2–13 years yielded odds ratios of 1.13–2.81 for the risk of type 2 diabetes among individuals who were depressed at the baseline assessments versus those who were not.[77–83] These studies included young and old men and women from diverse ethnic backgrounds. The most detailed of these studies found a strong association between baseline depression and risk factors for diabetes such as higher body mass index, fasting insulin, caloric intake, and lower physical activity.[81] However, all seven studies found that depression was a significant risk factor for new-onset diabetes, even after controlling for demographics and diabetes risk factors. In contrast, a large Danish study that used hospitalization as its outcome measure found that 29,000 patients with unipolar depression and 6700 patients with bipolar disorder were no more likely to develop diabetes than 108,500 patients with osteoarthritis.[84] The U.S. National Health and Nutrition Examination Epidemiologic Study yielded mixed results. In the overall group of 8870 subjects, depression did not confer a higher risk for diabetes after accounting for diabetes risk factors.[85] However, in a subset of participants with less than a high school education and, presumably, a low socioeconomic status, depression was associated with a threefold increase in diabetes over 15 years.[86]

Among patients who have diabetes, the presence of comorbid depression is associated with lower levels of adherence to diabetes education programs, exercise, oral hypoglycemic medications and dietary interventions,[87–90] greater functional impairment, and increased health care costs.[3,87,91] A meta-analysis demonstrated that patients with coexisting diabetes and depression had poorer glycemic control and higher rates of diabetic complications, including peripheral neuropathy, retinopathy, nephropathy, vascular disease, and sexual dysfunction.[20] A subsequent study of 2830 elderly Mexican Americans confirmed the additive effects of depression on diabetes complications.[92] A prospective study of 117 adolescents found that those with clinically significant depressive symptoms at baseline had higher HbA1C levels at 2-year follow-up.[93] Comorbid depression and diabetes may carry particular risk for coronary artery disease. A 10-year, prospective study of 76 women with type 1 or type 2 diabetes showed an earlier onset of coronary artery disease in women with depression compared to their nondepressed counterparts, a difference that remained significant after controlling for other cardiac risk factors.[52] Patient with diabetes and depression are 1.5–2 times more likely to have three or more cardiac risk factors than those without depression, including smoking, sedentary lifestyles, and obesity.[94]

Thus, depression may represent a dual risk for diabetes, increasing the likelihood of developing type 2 diabetes in the first place, and then increasing the risks of medical complications in those who have the disease. The mechanisms underlying these potential increased risks are not certain. The biologic factors outlined in the previous section require rigorous prospective study. Behavioral factors almost certainly play an additional role. For example, one study found that more than half of patients with non-insulin-dependent diabetes and comorbid major depression failed to complete a weight-control program for their diabetes, while the dropout rate was <25% in patients without depression.[95]

► CLINICAL CARE

Diagnosis

Patients with chronic medical illnesses present special challenges in diagnosing major depression because the medical conditions may produce changes in sleep, appetite, and energy levels that mimic depression.[96] In addition, a certain amount of demoralization is expected in those afflicted with unremitting medical conditions.[97] Diabetes is no different than other chronic illnesses in this regard. However, identification of mood and cognitive symptoms can reliably lead to the diagnosis of depression in those with type 1 or type 2 diabetes. Intermittent demoralization may be common, but a persistently depressed mood, anhedonia, and loss of interest in usual activities indicate the presence of major depression. Similarly, excessive guilt, feelings of hopelessness or worthlessness, and any suicidal thoughts are not part of a healthy psychologic adaptation to diabetes, but symptoms of a depressive disorder.[98] "Symptom amplification" may be another clue to the presence of depression. Patients with diabetes and coexisting depression experience more physical symptoms than those without depression, including symptoms that may not be easily explained by their medical condition.[87]

Treatment

Successful treatment of major depression in patients with diabetes holds the promise of better outcomes by enhancing patient compliance, promoting glycemic control, and improving quality of life. The alternative may be particularly devastating. After following patients with diabetes and depression through a 5-year prospective study in 1988, Lustman and colleagues characterized the natural course of depression in patients with diabetes as "malevolent," more serious than in medically healthy individuals.[99]

Despite this, only five controlled clinical trials of antidepressive treatments have been published in patients with diabetes, one psychotherapy trial,[38] two antidepressant medication trials,[37,39] and two intervention trials comparing enhanced depression disease management to usual care.[40,41] In the first study,[37] an 8-week clinical trial, nortriptyline (serum level 50–150 ng/mL) proved more effective than placebo in reducing depressive symptoms for 14 patients each with type 1 and type 2 diabetes, but it had no effect on HbA1C levels and may have impaired glycemic control as measured by serum glucose. Fluoxetine (≤40 mg/day) was also superior to placebo for depressive symptoms in an 8-week trial of 60 patients with type 1 or type 2 diabetes.[39] Effective treatment of depression was not accompanied by improvement in HbA1C, but fluoxetine, unlike nortriptyline, did not increase serum glucose. In the largest controlled trial to date, Katon and colleagues randomly assigned 329 patients with diabetes and major depression or dysthymia, who were enrolled in a large health maintenance organization, to usual outpatient primary care or enhanced depression treatment consisting of case management, medication adherence interventions, and problem-solving therapy.[40] Patients in the enhanced treatment group demonstrated better adherence to treatment at 6 and 12 months, greater reductions in depressive symptoms, and larger improvements in quality of life. However, glycemic control as measured by HbA1C did not improve. In this study, patients in both groups were exposed to the HMO's diabetes management program and baseline HbA1C levels were only mildly elevated at 8%, both of which could have reduced the ability of the treatment intervention to demonstrate improvements in glycemic control. Williams and colleagues studied 293 patients over age 60 with diabetes identified from a larger trial of enhanced treatment of depression in primary care.[41] Interventions were similar to the Katon study.[40] Depression was significantly improved at 6 and 12 months. Glycemic control did not change, though patients generally had good control at baseline (mean HbA1C = 7.3%).

Only one controlled trial has investigated the effectiveness of a full course of psychotherapy.[38] Lustman and colleagues randomly assigned 51 patients with type 2 diabetes to a 10-week course of cognitive behavioral therapy (CBT) for depression plus a diabetes education program or the education program alone. CBT was more effective for depressive symptoms and it reduced HbA1C by 0.7% compared to the education program alone, a statistically and clinically significant result. This difference was recorded 6 months after treatment, but was not seen at the 12-month follow-up assessment. In summary, controlled studies of antidepressant interventions published to date have demonstrated that depression can be treated successfully in patients with diabetes. However, effective treatment of depression did not result in sustained reductions in HbA1C. It is not known if other elements of the total burden of illness (e.g., functional impairment, frequency of doctor visits, and so on) improved with the reduction in depressive symptoms.

Uncontrolled trials of antidepressant medications and psychosocial interventions have demonstrated more direct effects on glycemic parameters in patients without clinically significant depressive symptoms. In obese, nondepressed, patients with type 2 diabetes, two studies showed that 4 weeks of treatment with fluoxetine, 60 mg/day, improved insulin sensitivity. Patients did not lose weight or show a reduction in their HbA1C levels.[74,75] In two other trials of fluoxetine treatment (60 mg/day) in nondepressed patients with type 2 diabetes, HbA1C and weight dropped at 6 months,[100,101] but this effect was lost at 12 months.[101] A group stress management program that did not involve depressed patients also demonstrated improvement in glycemic control.[102] That investigation compared 5 weeks of group stress management training plus diabetes education to diabetes education alone. No differences were noted until the 1-year follow-up assessment, when the stress management patients showed a 0.5% reduction in HbA1C levels.

Considerations in Choosing Antidepressant Therapies

Pending the completion of additional controlled trials of antidepressant treatment in patients with diabetes, the results of uncontrolled studies can be used to guide treatment choices.

Medication Options

Since the introduction of antidepressant medications in the 1960s, they have been known to affect plasma glucose concentrations. The hydrazine monoamine oxidase inhibitors (MAOIs), phenelzine and isocarboxazid, have been shown to slightly reduce plasma glucose levels.[60,69] However, their dietary restrictions may complicate patients' dietary control of diabetes and their potential to cause orthostatic hypotension may worsen orthostatic intolerance in patients with diabetic peripheral neuropathy.[103] Tricyclic antidepressants (TCAs), at low dose, have long been used to treat diabetic peripheral neuropathy. Placebo-controlled, clinical trials found the TCAs, desipramine, and amitriptyline, to be more effective than the SSRI, fluoxetine, for treating this condition.[104,105] At these low doses, potential TCA side effects such as weight gain, hyperglycemia, orthostatic hypotension, and quinidine-like effects on cardiac conduction may not be problematic.[37,103] However, they may present greater difficulties when used at the higher doses needed for effective antidepressant activity.

SSRIs and the other new generation antidepressant compounds, venlafaxine, duloxetine, bupropion, mirtazapine, and nefazodone appear to offer improved tolerability and safety advantages for depressed patients with diabetes. They lack the troublesome anticholinergic, antiadrenergic, and cardiac conduction effects of the TCAs and the orthostasis, dietary restrictions, and drug-drug interaction of the MAOIs.[96] In an 8-week trial of depressed patients without diabetes, 19 patients treated with fluoxetine 20–40 mg/day dropped their mean fasting blood glucose from 88 to 80 mg/dL, whereas a similar number of patients treated with imipramine 75–200 mg/day had their mean fasting glucose increase from 87 to 97 mg/day.[106]

This would make SSRIs seem like the medications of choice for depressed patients with diabetes. However, several of these newer agents have the potential for drug-drug interactions because of their ability to inhibit one or more hepatic, cytochrome (CYP) P450 isoenzymes. Nefazodone, fluoxetine, and fluvoxamine inhibit CYP 3A4, and therefore, may inhibit the metabolism of pioglitazone (Actos), repaglinide (Prandin), and nateglinide (Starlix), causing unexpected bouts of hypoglycemia. Fluoxetine, fluvoxamine, and high-dose sertraline inhibit CYP 2C9, which metabolizes the sulfonylureas, tolbutamide (Orinase), and glimepride (Amaryl). However, there have not been any clinical reports of significant interactions with SSRIs and these drugs.[107] In healthy volunteers, high-dose sertraline (200 mg/day) decreased tolbutamide clearance by only 16%.[108]

Several psychotropic medications that may be used in patients with depression have a significant potential for weight gain. Among the antidepressants, mirtazapine is most likely to cause this adverse effect.[109,110] New generation (atypical) antipsychotic drugs and anticonvulsants may be used as adjuncts in the treatment of depression. A few of these agents have a significant potential for weight gain (e.g., valproate, olanzapine, quetiapine). Furthermore, the FDA recently required manufacturers of all atypical antipsychotics to label their products with warnings about the potential for new-onset diabetes, worsening diabetes control, and increased lipids. At the present time, there is considerable debate about which of these drugs have the fewest metabolic side effects. Until this matter is resolved, closer metabolic screening may be needed when patients with diabetes require these agents.[111–113]

Psychosocial Interventions

In addition to the controlled trial of psychotherapy discussed above,[37] several other studies of psychologic interventions for patients with diabetes have been reported using techniques such as biofeedback,[114] computerized self-monitoring of depressive symptoms,[115] and stress management training.[116] These investigations included patients without depression or only low levels of depressive symptoms. Therefore, they have limited value in guiding decisions about the psychosocial treatment of depression in patients with diabetes. When depressive symptoms were present, they responded well to treatment, but persistent improvements in glycemic control were not attained.

Combination Treatment— Antidepressant Medications and Psychotherapy

There are no data on the use of traditional combinations of antidepressant medications and psychotherapy for depression in patients with diabetes. However, this approach is recommended in practice guidelines for treating depression[117] and it was found to be significantly more efficacious than single modality treatments in medically healthy subjects.[118]

► CONCLUSIONS

The prevalence of major depressive disorder and clinically significant depressive symptoms is twice as high in patients with diabetes as it is in the general population. Emerging data suggest that depression may be a risk factor for new-onset diabetes and more significant diabetic complications as well as a secondary complication of the medical illness, itself. Biologic factors including altered insulin and glucagon dynamics, and HPA axis and immune system activation may underlie the relationship between diabetes and depression. Psychosocial factors such as depravation and poor motivation for health-promoting behaviors appear to play a role as well. There are few well-controlled intervention studies to guide treatment of patients with diabetes and depression. Available data suggest that standard antidepressant medications and psychotherapies are effective in reducing depressive symptoms, but consistent improvement in glycemic control has not been demonstrated as yet. Other potential benefits of effective treatment for depression, such as reduced disability, better patient satisfaction, improved pain control, and lower general medical costs have received little attention in studies to date.

REFERENCES

1. Finkelstein EA, Bray JW, Chen H, et al. Prevalence and costs of major depression among elderly claimants with diabetes. *Diabetes Care* 2003;26:415.
2. Goetzel RZ, Hawkins K, Ozminkowski RJ, et al. The health and productivity cost burden of the "top 10" physical and mental health conditions affecting six large U.S. employers in 1999. *J Occup Environ Med* 2003;45:5.
3. Egede LE. Diabetes, major depression, and functional disability among U.S. adults. *Diabetes Care* 2004;27:421.
4. Gilmer TP, O'connor PJ, Rush WA, et al. Predictors of health care costs in adults with diabetes. *Diabetes Care* 2005;28:59.
5. Gavard JA, Lustman PJ, Clouse RE. Prevalence of depression in adults with diabetes. An epidemiological evaluation. *Diabetes Care* 1993;16:1167.
6. Anderson RJ, Freedland KE, Clouse RE, et al. The prevalence of comorbid depression in adults with diabetes: A meta-analysis. *Diab Care* 2001;24:1069.
7. Wild S, Roglic G, Green A, et al. Global prevalence of diabetes: Estimates for the year 2000 and projections for 2030. *Diabetes Care* 2004;27:1047.
8. Centers for Disease Control and Prevention: Serious psychological distress among persons with diabetes—New York City, 2003. *MMWR Morb Mortal Wkly Rep* 2004;53:1089.
9. Amsterdam JD, Schweizer E, Winokur A. Multiple hormonal responses to insulin-induced hypoglycemia in depressed and normal volunteers. *Am J Psychiatry* 1987;144:170.
10. Winokur A, Maislin G, Phillips JL, et al. Insulin resistance after oral glucose tolerance testing in patients with major depression. *Am J Psychiatry* 1988;145:325.
11. Amsterdam JD, Maislin G. Hormonal responses during insulin-induced hypoglycemia in manic-depressed, unipolar depressed and healthy control subjects. *J Clin End Metab* 1991;73:541.
12. Fried SK, Bunkin DA, Greenburg AS. Omental and subcutaneous adipose tissue of obese subjects release interleukin-6: Depot difference and regulation by glucocorticoid. *J Clin End Metab* 1998;83:847.
13. Fernandez-Real JM, Vayred M, Richart C, et al. Circulating interleukin 6 levels, blood pressure, and insulin insensitivity in apparently healthy men and women. *J Clin Endo Metab* 86:1154, 2001.
14. Paolisso G, Rizzo MR, Mazziotti G, et al. Advancing age and insulin resistance: Role of plasma tumor necrosis factor-alpha. *Am J Physiol* 1998;275(2 pt 1):E294.
15. Hotamisligil GS, Peraldi P, Budavari A, et al. IRS-1-mediated inhibition of insulin receptor tyrosine kinase activity in TNF-alpha- and obesity-induced insulin resistance. *Science* 1994;271:665.
16. Hotamisligil GS, Spiegelman BM. Tumor necrosis factor a: A key component of the obesity-diabetes link. *Diabetes* 1994;43:1271.
17. Kern PA, Saghizadeh M, Ong JM, et al. The expression of tumor necrosis factor in human adipose tissue. Regulation by obesity, weight loss, and relationship to lipoprotein lipase. *J Clin Invest* 1995;95:2111.
18. Saghizadeh M, Ong JM, Garvey WT, et al. The expression of TNFa by human muscle. Relationship to insulin resistance. *J Clin Invest* 1996;97:1111.
19. Kent S, Bluthe RM, Kelley KW, et al. Sickness behavior as a new target for drug development. *Trends Pharmacol Sci* 1992;13:24.
20. Yirmiya R. Endotoxin produces a depressive-like episode in rats. *Brain Res* 1996;711:163.
21. Maes M, Delange J, Ranjan R, et al. Acute phase proteins in schizophrenia, mania and major depression: Modulation by psychotropic drugs. *Psychiatr Res* 1996;66:1.
22. Berk M, Wadee AA, Kuschke RH, et al. Acute phase proteins in major depression. *J Psychosom Res* 1997;43:529.
23. Frommberger UH, Bauer J, Haselbauer P, et al. Interleukin-6-(IL-6) plasma levels in depression and schizophrenia: Comparison between the acute state and after remission. *Eur Arch Psychiatr Clin Neurosci* 1997;247:228.

24. Musselman DL, Miller AH, Porter MR, et al. Higher than normal plasma interleukin-6 concentrations in cancer patients with depression. *Am J Psychiatry* 2001;158:1252.

25. Miller GE, Stetler CA, Carney RM, et al. Clinical depression and inflamatory risk markers for coronary heart disease. *Am J Cardiol* 2002;90:1279.

26. Lloyd CE, Matthews KA, Wing RR, et al. Psychosocial factors and complications of IDDM: The Pittsburgh Epidemiology of Diabetes Complications Study. *Diabetes Care* 1992;15:166.

27. Kumari M, Head J, Marmot M. Prospective study of social and other risk factors for incidence of type 2 diabetes in the Whitehall II study. *Arch Intern Med* 2004;164:1873.

28. Lustman PJ, Anderson RJ, Freedland KE, et al. Depression and poor glycemic control: A meta-analytic review of the literature. *Diabetes* 2000;23:934.

29. de Groot M, Anderson R, Freedland KE, et al. Association of depression and diabetes complications: A meta-analysis. *Psychosom Med* 2001;63:619.

30. Peyrot M, Rubin RR. Levels and risks of depression and anxiety symptomatology among diabetic adults. *Diabetes Care* 1997;20:585.

31. Vinnamaki H, Niskanen L, Uusitupa M. Mental well-being in people with non-insulin dependent diabetes. *Acta Psychiatr Scand* 1995;92:392.

32. Ziemer DC, Ferguson SY, Royal-Fletcher L, et al. Depression: A major barrier to diabetes management. *Diabetes* 1999;48(Suppl 1):A320.

33. Xu L, Ren J, Cheng M, et al. Depressive symptoms and risk factors in Chinese persons with type 2 diabetes. *Arch Med Res* 2004;35:301.

34. Ludman EJ, Katon W, Russo J, et al. Depression and diabetes symptom burden. *Gen Hosp Psychiatry* 2004;26:430.

35. Goldney RD, Phillips PJ, Fisher LJ, et al. Diabetes, depression, and quality of life: A population study. *Diabetes Care* 2004;27:1066.

36. Musselman DL, Betan E, Larsen H, et al. Relationship of depression to diabetes types 1 and 2: Epidemiology, biology, and treatment. *Biol Psychiatry* 2003;54:317.

37. Lustman PJ, Griffith LS, Clouse RE, et al. Effects of nortriptyline on depression and glucose regulation in diabetes: Results of a double-blind, placebo-controlled trial. *Psychosom Med* 1997;59:241.

38. Lustman PJ, Griffith LS, Freedland KE, et al. Cognitive behavior therapy for depression in type 2 diabetes mellitus: A randomized, controlled trial. *Ann Intern Med* 1998;129:613.

39. Lustman PJ, Freedland KE, Griffith LS, et al. Fluoxetine for depression in diabetes: A randomized, double-blind, placebo-controlled trial. *Diabetes Care* 2000;23:618.

40. Katon WJ, Von Korff M, Lin EH, et al. The Pathways Study: A randomized trial of collaborative care in patients with diabetes and depression. *Arch Gen Psychiatry* 2004;61:1042.

41. Williams Jr JW, Katon W, Lin EH, et al. The effectiveness of depression care management on diabetes-related outcomes in older patients. *Ann Intern Med* 2004;140:1015.

42. Yach D, Hawkes C, Gould CL, et al. The global burden of chronic diseases: Overcoming impediments to prevention and control. *JAMA* 2004;291:2616.

43. Fox CS, Coady S, Sorlie PD, et al. Trends in cardiovascular complications of diabetes. *JAMA* 2004;292:2495.

44. Beem SE, Machala M, Holman C, et al. Aiming at "de feet" and diabetes: A rural model to increase annual foot examinations. *Am J Public Health* 2004;94:1664.

45. Moreland ME, Kilbourne AM, Engelhardt JB, et al. Diabetes preventive care and non-traumatic lower extremity amputation rates. *J Healthc Qual* 2004;26:12.

46. Gregg EW, Sorlie P, Paulose-Ram R, et al. Prevalence of lower-extremity disease in the US adult population >=40 years of age with and without diabetes: 1999-2000 national health and nutrition examination survey. *Diabetes Care* 2004;27:1591.

47. Cusick M, Chew EY, Hoogwerf B, et al. Risk factors for renal replacement therapy in the Early Treatment Diabetic Retinopathy Study (ETDRS), Early Treatment Diabetic Retinopathy Study Report No. 26. *Kidney Int* 2004;66:1173.

48. Centers for Disease Control and Prevention (CDC): Prevalence of visual impairment and selected eye diseases among persons aged >/=50 years with and without diabetes—United States, 2002. *MMWR Morb Mortal Wkly Rep* 2004;53:1069.

49. Evans DL, Charney DS. Mood disorders and medical illness: A major public health problem. *Biol Psychiatry* 2003;54:177.

50. Skaer TL, Robison LM, Sclar DA, et al. Use of antidepressant pharmacotherapy within the first year after diagnosis of diabetes mellitus: A study of a Medicaid population. *Curr Ther Res Clin Exp* 1999;60:415.

51. Katon WJ, Simon G, Russo J, et al. Quality of depression care in a population-based sample of patients with diabetes and major depression. *Med Care* 2004;42:1222.

52. Testa MA, Simonson DC. Health economic benefits and quality of life during improved glycemic control in patients with type 2 diabetes mellitus. *JAMA* 1998;280:1490.

53. Bisschop MI, Kriegsman DM, Deeg DJ, et al. The longitudinal relation between chronic diseases and depression in older persons in the community: The Longitudinal Aging Study Amsterdam. *J Clin Epidemiol* 2004;57:187.

54. Husaini BA, Hull PC, Sherkat DE, et al. Diabetes, depression, and healthcare utilization among African Americans in primary care. *J Natl Med Assoc* 2004;96:476.

55. Fisher L, Chesla CA, Mullan JT, et al. Contributors to depression in Latino and European-American patients with type 2 diabetes. *Diabetes Care* 2001;24:1751.

56. Lustman PJ, Griffith LS, Clouse RE. Depression in adults with diabetes. Results of 5-yr follow-up study. *Diabetes Care* 1988;11:605.

57. McCowan PK, Quastel JH. Blood sugar studies in abnormal mental states. *J Mental Sci* 1931;77:525.

58. Freeman H. Resistance to insulin in mentally disturbed soldiers. *Arch Neurol Psychiatry* 1946;56:74.

59. Pryce IG. The relationship between glucose tolerance, body weight, and clinical state. *J Mental Sci* 1958;104:1079.

60. Van Praag HM, Leijnse B. Depression, glucose tolerance, peripheral glucose uptake and their alterations under the influence of anti-depressive drugs of the hydrazine type. *Psychopharmacologia (Berlin)* 1965;8:65.

61. Mueller PS, Heninger GR, McDonald RK. Intravenous glucose tolerance test in depression. *Arch Gen Psychiatry* 1968;21:470.

62. Sachar EJ, Finkelstein J, Hellman L. Growth hormone responses in depressive illness, 1: Response to insulin tolerance test. *Arch Gen Psychiatry* 1971;25:263.

63. Casper RC, Davis JM, Pandey G, et al. Neuroendocrine and amine studies in affective illness. *Psychoneuroendocrinology* 1977;2:105.

64. Wright JH, Jacisin JJ, Radin NS, et al. Glucose metabolism in unipolar depression. *Br J Psychiatry* 1978;132:386.

65. Crammer J, Gillies C. Psychiatric aspects of diabetes mellitus: Diabetes and depression. (Letter to editor) *Br J Psychiatry* 1981;139:171.

66. Kronfol Z, Greden J, Carroll B. Psychiatric aspects of diabetes mellitus: Diabetes and depression. (Letter to editor) *Br J Psychiatry* 1981;139:172.

67. Finestone DH, Weinwe RD. Effects of ECT on diabetes mellitus. *Acta Psychiatr Scand* 1984;70:321.

68. Yudofsky SC, Rosenthal NE. ECT in a depressed patient with adult onset diabetes mellitus. *Am J Psychiatry* 1980;137:100.

69. Goodnick PJ, Kumar A, Henry JH, et al. Sertraline in coexisting major depression and diabetes mellitus. *Psychopharmacol Bull* 1997;33:261.

70. Amsterdam JD, Maislin G, Winokur A, et al. The assessment of abnormalities in hormonal responsiveness at multiple levels of the hypothalamic-pituitary-adrenocortical axis in depressive illness. *Psychoneuroendocrinol* 1989;14:43.

71. Goodnick PJ, Henry JH, Buki VMV. Treatment of depression in patients with diabetes mellitus. *J Clin Psychiatry* 1995;56:128.

72. Erenmemisoglu A, Ozdogan UK, Saraymen R, et al. Effect of some antidepressants on glycaemia and insulin levels of normoglycaemic and alloxan-induced hyperglycaemic mice. *J Pharm Pharmacol* 1999;51:741.

73. Gray DS, Fujioka K, Devine W, et al. Fluoxetine treatment of the obese diabetic. *Int J Obesity* 1992;16:193.

74. Potter van Loon BJ, Radder JK, Frolich M, et al. Fluoxetine increases insulin action in obese non-diabetic and in obese non-insulin-dependent diabetic individuals. *Int J Obesity* 1992;16:79.

75. Mahuex P, Ducros F, Bourque J, et al. Fluoxetine improves insulin sensitivity in obese patients with non-insulin-dependent diabetes mellitus independently of weight loss. *Int J Obesity* 1997;21:97.

76. Hayward C. Psychiatric illness and cardiovascular disease risk. *Epidemiol Rev* 1995;17:129.

77. Eaton WW, Armenian H, Gallo J, et al. Depression and risk for onset of type II diabetes: A prospective population-based study. *Diabetes Care* 1996;22:109.

78. Kawakami N, Tkatsuka N, Shimuza H, et al. Depressive symptoms and occurrence of type 2 diabetes among Japanese men. *Diabetes Care* 1999;22.

79. Arroyo C, Hu FB, Ryan LM, et al. Depressive symptoms and risk of type 2 diabetes in women. *Diabetes Care* 2004;27:129.

80. Everson-Rose SA, Meyer PM, Powell LH, et al. Depressive symptoms, insulin resistance, and risk of diabetes in women at midlife. *Diabetes Care* 2004;27:2856.

81. Golden SH, Williams JE, Ford DE, et al. Depressive symptoms and the risk of type 2 diabetes: The Atherosclerosis Risk in Communities study. *Diabetes Care* 2004;27:429.

82. Palinkas LA, Lee PP, Barrett-Connor E. A prospective study of Type 2 diabetes and depressive symptoms in the elderly: The Rancho Bernardo Study. *Diabetes Med* 2004;21:1185.

83. van den Akker M, Schuurman A, Metsemakers J, et al. Is depression related to subsequent diabetes mellitus? *Acta Psychiatr Scand* 2004; 110:178.

84. Kessing LV, Nilsson FM, Siersma V, et al. Increased risk of developing diabetes in depressive and bipolar disorders? *J Psychiatr Res* 2004;38:395.

85. Saydah SH, Brancati FL, Golden SH, et al. Depressive symptoms and the risk of type 2 diabetes mellitus in a US sample. *Diabetes Metab Res Rev* 2003;19:202.

86. Carnethon MR, Kinder LS, Fair JM, et al. Symptoms of depression as a risk factor for incident diabetes: Findings from the National Health and Nutrition Examination Epidemiologic Follow-up Study, 1971-1992. *Am J Epidemiol* 2003;158:416.

87. Ciechanowski PS, Katon WJ, Russo JE. Depression and diabetes: Impact of depressive symptoms on adherence, function, and costs. *Arch Int Med* 2000;1160:3278.

88. Lin EH, Katon W, Von Korff M, et al. Relationship of depression and diabetes self-care, medication adherence, and preventive care. *Diabetes Care* 2004;27:2154.

89. McKellar JD, Humphreys K, Piette JD, et al. Depression increases diabetes symptoms by complicating patients' self-care adherence. *Diabetes Educ* 2004;30:485.

90. Park H, Hong Y, Lee H, et al. Individuals with type 2 diabetes and depressive symptoms exhibited lower adherence with self-care. *J Clin Epidemiol* 2004;57:978.

91. Katon WJ, Von Korff M, Lin E, et al. Population-based care of depression: Effective disease management strategies to decrease prevalence. *Gen Hosp Psychiatry* 1997;19:169.

92. Black SA, Markides KS, Ray LA. Depression predicts increased incidence of adverse health outcomes in older Mexican Americans with type 2 diabetes. *Diabetes Care* 2003;26:2822.

93. Whittemore R, Kanner S, Singleton S, et al. Correlates of depressive symptoms in adolescents with type 1 diabetes. *Pediatr Diabetes* 2002;3:135.

94. Katon WJ, Lin EH, Russo J, et al. Cardiac risk factors in patients with diabetes mellitus and major depression. *J Gen Intern Med* 2004;19:1192.

95. Marcus MD, Wing RR, Guare J, et al. Lifetime prevalence of major depression and its effect on treatment outcome in obese type II diabetic patients. *Diabetes Care* 1992;15:253.

96. Evans DL, Staab JP, Petitto JM, et al. Depression in the medical setting: Biopsychological interactions and treatment considerations. *J Clin Psychiatry* 1999;60(Suppl 4):40.

97. Staab JP, Datto, CJ, Weinrieb RM, et al. Detection and diagnosis of psychiatric disorders in primary medical care settings. *Med Clin North Am* 2001; 85:579.

98. Lustman PJ, Freedland KE, Carney RM, et al. Similarity of depression in diabetic and psychiatric patients. *Psychosom Med* 1992;54:602.

99. Lustman PJ, Griffith LS, Clouse RE, et al. Depression in adults with diabetes. Results of 5-yr follow-up study. *Diabetes Care* 1988;11:605.

100. O'Kane M, Wiles PG, Wales JK. Fluoxetine in the treatment of obese type 2 diabetic patients. *Diabetes Med* 1994;11:105.

101. Bruem L, Bjerre U, Bak JF, et al. Long-term effects of fluoxetine on glycemic control in obese patients with non-insuline-dependent diabetes mellitus or glucose intolerance: Influence on muscle glycogen synthase and insulin receptor kinase activity. *Metab Clin Exp* 1995;44:1570.

102. Surwit RS, Williams RB, Siegler IC, et al. Hostility, race, and glucose metabolism in nondiabetic individuals. *Diabetes Care* 2002;25:835.

103. Rabkin J, Quitkin F, Harrison W, et al. Adverse reactions to monoamine oxidase inhibitors, I: A comparative study. *J Clin Psychopharmacol* 1984;4:270.

104. Max MB, Kishore-Kumar R, Schafer SC, et al. Efficacy of desipramine in painful diabetic neuropathy: A placebo-controlled trial. *Pain* 1991;45:3.

105. Max MB, Lynch SA, Muir J, et al. Effects of desipramine, amitriptyline, and fluoxetine in diabetic neuropathy. *N Engl J Med* 1992;326:1250.

106. Ghaeli P, Shahsavand E, Mesbahi M, et al. Comparing the effects of 8-week treatment with

fluoxetine and imipramine on fasting blood glucose of patients with major depressive disorder. *J Clin Psychopharmacol* 2004;24:386.

107. DeVane CL, Markowitz JS. Psychoactive drug interactions with pharmacotherapy for diabetes. *Psychopharmacol Bull* 2002;36:40.

108. Tremaine LM, Wilner KD, Preskorn SH. A study of the potential effect of sertraline on the pharmacokinetics and protein binding of tolbutamide. *Clin Pharmacokinet* 1992;32(Suppl 1):31.

109. Sussman N, Ginsberg DL, Bikoff J. Effects of nefazodone on body weight: A pooled analysis of selective serotonin reuptake inhibitor-and imipramine-controlled trials. *J Clin Psychiatry* 2001;62:256.

110. Fava M. Weight gain and antidepressants. *J Clin Psychiatry* 2002;61(Suppl 11):37.

111. Dunlop BW, Sternberg M, Phillips LS, et al. Disturbed glucose metabolism among patients taking olanzapine and typical antipsychotics. *Psychopharmacol Bull* 2003;37:99.

112. Serynak MJ, Leslie DL, Alarcon RD, et al. Association of diabetes mellitus with use of atypical neuroleptics in the treatment of schizophrenia. *Am J Psychiatry* 2002;159:561.

113. American Diabetes Association, American Psychiatric Association, American Association of Clinical Endocrinologists, et al. Consensus development conference on antipsychotic drugs and obesity and diabetes. *Diabetes Care* 2004;27:596.

114. Lane JD, McCaskill CC, Williams PG, et al. Personality correlates of glycemic control in type 2 diabetes. *Diabetes Care* 2000;23:1321.

115. Pouwer F, Snoek FJ, van der Ploeg HM, et al. Monitoring of psychological well-being in outpatients with diabetes: Effects on mood, HbA(1c), and the patient's evaluation of the quality of diabetes care: A randomized controlled trial. *Diabetes Care* 2001;24:1929.

116. Spiess K, Sachs G, Pietschmann P, et al. A program to reduce onset distress in unselected type I diabetic patients: Effects on psychological variables and metabolic control. *Eur J Endocrinol* 1995;132:580.

117. American Psychiatric Association: Major depressive disorder (second edition), in American Psychiatric Association Practice Guidelines for the Treatment of Psychiatric Disorders. Washington, DC: American Psychiatric Publishing, 2004.

118. Keller MB, McCullough JP, Klein DN, et al. A comparison of nefazodone, the cognitive behavioral-analysis system of psychotherapy, and their combination for the treatment of chronic depression. *N Engl J Med* 2000;342:1462.

CHAPTER 7

Depression and Obesity

ALBERT STUNKARD, MYLES S. FAITH, AND KELLY C. ALLISON

▶ DIAGNOSIS

Obesity is a condition characterized by excessive accumulation of fat in the body.[1] In clinical practice, overweight (i.e., weight corrected for height) is used as a surrogate for body fat. Since body weight and fat are highly correlated, especially at greater degrees of overweight, this practice seems reasonable. Overweight has been defined in terms of the body mass index (BMI = weight in kilograms divided by height in meters squared).[1] Overweight is classified as a BMI of 25–30 and obesity as a BMI greater than 30.[2] These values have been arbitrarily defined and there is no physiologically defined cutoff point for overweight or obesity. For most practical purposes, the eyeball test is adequate: if a person *looks* fat the person *is* fat.

Obesity is a common disorder which is becoming ever more common. At the present time, 30.5% of the population in the United States is obese with another 34% overweight.[3] Prevalence varies by age, race, socioeconomic status (SES), and other variables.

▶ PATHOGENESIS

What causes obesity? In one sense, the answer is simple: consuming more calories than are expended as energy. The causes of obesity are to be found in the regulation of body weight (which is primarily the regulation of body fat). We still have only an imperfect understanding of how this regulation is achieved. We do know, however, that weight is regulated with great precision. During a lifetime, the average person consumes at least 60 million kcals. A gain or loss of 20 lb, representing 72,000 kcal, constitutes an error of no more than 0.001%.[4] The determinants of obesity can be divided into genetic, environmental, and regulatory factors.

Classic twin studies have estimated high levels of heritability of body weight, the percent of variance accounted for is about 80%.[5] Even a study of identical twins separated at birth, a method that avoids the bias in classic twin studies, estimated heritability at nearly this level.[6] Environmental factors clearly influence the development of obesity, as shown by the powerful influence of social class[7] and, strikingly, by the rapid, epidemic increase in obesity in recent years. These influences include the consumption of calorically dense, highly palatable foods and a deficit in physical activity.

▶ RELATIONSHIP OF OBESITY TO DEPRESSION

Overweight and obesity combined afflict almost 65% of Americans.[3] Since the prevalence of depression has been estimated at 10%[8] there is a strong probability that the two disorders will occur together by chance and for years it was assumed that any relationship of depression to obesity in the general population was largely coincidental. Research in the recent past, however, has uncovered a large number of moderating and mediating variables that relate depression and obesity. Depression influences obesity under some circumstances and obesity influences depression under others.

The influence of moderating and mediating variables is attracting increasing attention in psychiatry.[9] Moderators specify for whom and under what conditions agents exert their effects; mediators identify why and how they exert their effect. Moderators precede what they moderate which, in turn, precedes the outcome; mediators always come between what they mediate and the outcome. In this review, moderators are defined as variables on which the obesity-depression covariation is conditional, whereas mediators are causal agents between obesity and depression.

Identifying moderators such as gender, ethnicity, or age would pinpoint those obese persons among whom depression is more likely to occur and who may be the most appropriate candidates for psychiatric treatment. Similarly, identification of mediators (physiologic or behavioral) would lead to better pharmacologic and lifestyle interventions as causal pathways are delineated.

▶ MODERATORS AND MEDIATORS

Table 7-1 shows a list of potential moderators and mediators.

Potential Moderating Variables

Severity of Depression

The first variable that may moderate the relationship between depression and obesity is severity of the depression. At least one prospective study has shown that the presence of *clinical* depression predicts the development of obesity. Pine et al.[10] found that major depression among 6–19 year olds

▶ **TABLE 7-1** POTENTIAL MODERATORS AND MEDIATORS OF DEPRESSION AND OBESITY

Moderators	Mediators
Severity of depression	Eating and
Severity of obesity	physical activity
Gender	Teasing
Socioeconomic status	Disordered eating
Gene-environment	Stress
interactions	
Adverse childhood	
experience	

predicted a greater BMI in adult life than that of persons who had not been depressed (BMI of 26.1 vs. 24.2). Other studies have not detected an association between *subclinical* depression levels and obesity.[11] Results of these studies suggest that severity of depression may moderate the relationship with obesity.

Severity and Nature of Obesity

Just as severity of depression moderates the relationship with obesity, so may the severity of obesity moderate the relationship with depression. An example is illustrated in Fig. 7-1, from National Health and Nutrition Examination Survey (NHANES)-III data, which shows the relationship between severity of obesity and the prevalence of major depression (Martin and Moore, personal communication, April 24, 2002). Among the leanest adolescents, aged 15–19, depression was uncommon and, in fact, not present among the leanest boys. Among the most obese subjects, in the 95–100th percentile, on the other hand, the prevalence of major depression was highly significant (20% for boys and 30% for girls).

In a study of the predictors of weight change occurring during unipolar depression, Stunkard et al.[6] assessed 53 unmedicated outpatients across two distinct episodes of severe depression. There were at least two notable findings from this study. First, there was a high correspondence in the direction of weight change across the two episodes. Thus, patients who had gained weight

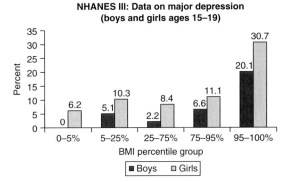

Figure 7-1. Relationship of BMI to major depression among boys and girls aged 15–19. There is little difference in the prevalence of major depression as a function of BMI until the 95th percentile is reached. Here, however, the prevalence of major depression (20% for boys, 30% for girls) is unusually high for adolescents.

Source: Reproduced from Martin and Moore. Personal communication, April 24, 2002. Data are used by permission from Shapeup America. (www.shapeup.org)

▶ **TABLE 7-2** ADJUSTED ODDS RATIOS* FOR THE CATEGORICAL AND CONTINUOUS WEIGHT-BY-SEX INTERACTIONS

	Major Depression, OR (95% CI)
Continuous weight (BMI)†	
Men	0.55 (0.48, 0.63)
Women	1.22 (1.06, 1.40)
Obese vs. average weight	
Men	0.63 (0.60, 0.67)
Women	1.37 (1.09, 1.65)

Abbreviations: OR = odds ratio; 95% CI = 95% confidence interval.

All ORs are adjusted for race, age, education, past year income, self-reported disease history, and the race-by-weight interaction term.

†*Odds ratios are presented for a 10-unit change in body mass index (BMI).*

Source: Table reproduced in part from Carpenter et al., 2000, p. 256.

during the first episodes tended to gain weight during the second episode, whereas patients who had lost weight during the first episode also tended to lose weight again during the second episode. Second, BMI was positively associated with weight change during depressive episodes, such that heavier individuals tended to gain more weight ($r = 0.30$, $P < 0.05$), thereby suggesting that the association between obesity and depression may depend on patients' initial weight status.

A recent finding suggests that the distribution of body fat may mediate the relationship between obesity and depression.[12] Depressive mood was positively associated with visceral adipose tissue ($P = 0.007$) even after controlling other confounding factors. It was not, however, related to subcutaneous fat. The relationship seems specific to depression, for BMI and waist circumference were positively related to both visceral and subcutaneous adipose tissue.

Gender
Several studies report that the relationship between obesity and depression differs for men and women.

Istvan et al.,[13] for example, showed a positive relationship between depression and obesity among women but not among men. Similarly, Faith et al.[14] found a positive relationship between neuroticism and BMI in women but not in men. A striking example of the different relationship between depression and obesity among men and women is shown in Table 7-2 from Carpenter et al.[15] Obesity in women was associated with a 37% *increase* in major depression whereas among men obesity was associated with a 37% *decrease* in major depression.

Socioeconomic Status
The relationship between depression and obesity appears to differ across SES levels.[16] Figure 7-2, adapted from data of the Midtown Manhattan Study,[17] shows that the difference in percent depressed between obese and normal weight men was not related to their SES. Among women, however, SES predicted the nature of the relationship between depression and obesity. Being obese was associated with greater depression among women of high SES but with reduced depression among women of low SES. Carpenter

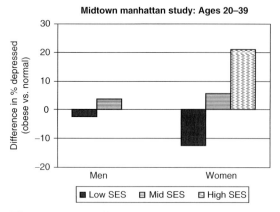

Midtown manhattan study: Ages 20–39

Figure 7-2.   Difference in depression prevalence as a function of gender and socioeconomic status in the Midtown Manhattan Study (adapted from Moore et al., 1962). Among high SES men, the difference in depression prevalence was approximately zero and so the corresponding bar is not visible in the figure.

et al.[15] found similar relationships among both White and Black women.

Age

DiPietro et al.[18] tested the prospective association between depressive symptoms, measured by the Center for Epidemologic Studies Depression Scale (CED-S), and weight change in a population-based sample. Participants were enrolled in the NHANES in 1971–1975, and were subsequently tracked in the National Health Epidemiologic Follow-up Study in 1982–1984. Results indicated distinct patterns for participants who were younger than, versus older than, 55 years of age (i.e., *younger* and *older* participants, respectively). Among younger males, those who were depressed at baseline gained nearly 3 kg more at follow-up than those who were not depressed at baseline. This effect was further moderated by education, such that young males who were depressed and had <12 years of education at baseline gained more weight over time than young males who were depressed but had ≥12 years of education at baseline (6.2 kg vs. 1.2 kg, respectively). By contrast,

young women who were depressed at baseline gained slightly less weight over time than those who were not depressed at baseline. Education also moderated this association in young women, such that those with <12 years of education gained more weight over time than those with ≥12 years of education at baseline (−3.2 kg vs. 0.6 kg, respectively). Among older participants, however, being depressed at baseline was associated with greater weight loss over time in both males and females.

Adverse Childhood Experiences

An association between obesity and depression may result from exposure to adverse childhood experiences. Exposure to childhood adversities is clearly associated with an increase in obesity. Although these studies did not examine obesity-depression comorbidity per se, these life experiences may promote both disorders. Let us begin with obesity. A prospective study in Copenhagen by Lissau and Sorensen,[19] found a striking relationship between childhood neglect and adult obesity. Children (*n* = 756) selected by their teachers as being "neglected" at age 10 had a risk ratio of 7.1, i.e., 7.1 times more likely to be obese at age 20 (*P* < 0.0001) than those not selected, while those identified by teachers being as "dirty and neglected" had a risk ratio for adult obesity of 9.8 (*P* < 0.0001). Felitti and colleagues[20–23] also proposed that childhood abuse (sexual, verbal, physical, and fear of physical abuse) was associated with adult obesity in a study of 13,177 members of a health maintenance organization. Exposure to all four types of abuse at the greatest level of severity resulted in a relative risk for a BMI ≥30 and ≥40 of 1.46 (1.16–1.85) and 2.54 (1.21–3.35). Regarding treatment, King et al.[24] have reported that 22 obese women who had been sexually abused in childhood or adolescence lost significantly less weight (15.3 ± 10.1 kg) than 22 nonsexually abused women in the same weight reduction program (23.5 ± 8.8 kg; *P* < 0.01).

Turning to the effects of physical abuse in childhood on depression, Harris (2001) implicated early childhood adversities in the development of depression in later life. He speaks to the detrimental effects of powerlessness, loss, and humiliation as contributing pathways to depression. For example, girls who were exposed to physical or sexual abuse were significantly more likely to experience depressive symptoms compared to girls who were not exposed in a national sample.[25] Felitti et al.[21] found that a high level of childhood abuse was associated with a relative risk of 4.6 (3.8, 5.6) for clinical depression. Furthermore, a history of childhood abuse predicted adenosie corticotropin hormone (ACTH) response during a laboratory test among a sample of adult women.[26]

Gene-Environment Interactions

A theoretical possibility is that the relationship of depression and obesity may be moderated by gene-environment interactions. This possibility is depicted in Fig. 7-3 in which BMI-depression covariation might be attributable to a common set of underlying genes and common environmental

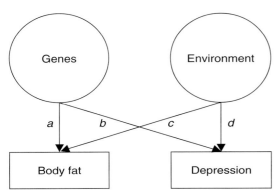

Figure 7-3. Pictorial representation of "genetic correlation" and "environmental correlation" between depression and obesity. Pathways a and b refer to a common set of genes that influence both body fat and depression, respectively, and can be used to estimate a genetic correlation between body fat and depression. Pathways c and d refer to a common set of environmental experiences that influence both body fat and depression, respectively, and can be used to estimate an environmental correlation between body fat and depression.

factors. Such a model has been developed by Kendler et al.[27] for studies of genetic epidemiology. Evidence for a genetic correlation can be estimated from path coefficients a and b. Evidence for an "environmental correlation" can be estimated from path coefficients c and d. Using these models, Kendler and colleagues found that a common set of genes underlies major depression and alcoholism, while a different set of genes underlies phobia, generalized anxiety disorder, panic disorder, and bulimia nervosa.[27] Evidence for a comparable genetic correlation between depression and body weight has also been reported in the literature.[28]

Potential Mediating Variables

Eating and Physical Activity

Among the most important determinants of obesity are eating and physical activity, and both may play an important part in linking depression with obesity. Although the DSM-IV finds both overeating, with weight gain (and undereating, with weight loss) among the diagnostic criteria for major depression,[29] the study of eating and physical activity as potential mediators of a link between depression and obesity has been limited. There is reason to expect such a relationship. Thus, physical inactivity not only characterizes many depressed persons,[30,31] but also predicts weight gain. Furthermore, physical activity has been used with modest success in the treatment of depression.[32]

Teasing

Everyone has observed the effects of teasing upon confidence and self-esteem, and many of us have experienced this problem in our own lives. Obese persons, from childhood on, are subject to such verbal abuse and its effects have been documented in the significantly greater rate of depression experienced by obese persons.[33] A recent study has shown that the stigma of obesity, already severe in 1960, has increased measurably in the past 43 years.[34] An instructive 3-year prospective study of adolescents demonstrated how teasing mediated the relationship between obesity and later levels of depression.[35] The obesity status of these adolescents elicited teasing which, in turn, elicited depression through their increased dissatisfaction with their appearance. Jackson et al.[36] also reported that those obese women with binge eating disorder (BED) who experienced teasing about their appearance developed body dissatisfaction and depression.

Disordered Eating

Disordered eating may mediate the relationship between depression and obesity. The experience of binge eating (and its associated feelings of uncontrollable eating) may promote depression. From the first descriptions, BED has been strongly associated with depression.[37–39] Among persons suffering from BED, 54% had a history of major depressive disorder compared to 14% of nonbinge eating obese persons.[39] Sherwood et al.[40] showed that improvements in binge eating status predicted greater weight loss in treatment through a pathway that involved a decrease in depression. The night eating syndrome (NES) (morning anorexia, evening hyperphagia, insomnia, and nighttime awakenings to eat)[41] may place persons at increased risk for depression. In one study, 44% of night eaters had a history of major depressive disorder compared to 18% of noneating disordered obese persons (Allison et al., unpublished observations). Obese patients with the NES show levels of depression that are consistently higher than they are among control patients matched for weight and age[42] (Allison et al., unpublished observations). A particularly interesting characteristic of the depression exhibited by many night eaters is its distinctive circadian quality. Thus, among these patients depressive mood is minimal in the morning, rises during the afternoon and evening, and reaches its peak late at night in conjunction with the most intense hyperphagia.[41]

Stress

Depressed individuals may experience increased stress that, in turn, may promote obesity. The influence of stress upon obesity is exerted via both psychologic and physiologic mechanisms. Attention to a healthy diet and adequate physical activity are key elements in preventing obesity and in controlling it once it has begun. One of the primary influences of stress is to disrupt these habits and these concerns, fostering the development of obesity. Similarly, stress leads to depression via *psychologic routes*, as shown in the stunning impact of bereavement, marital separation, and job loss.

Stress may impact both depression and obesity via its action on the hypothalamic-pituitary-adrenal (HPA) axis. Elevated levels of cortisol, indicating HPA activation, are not uncommon among obese persons and are believed to give rise to so-called abdominal obesity—fat primarily within the abdominal wall. This fat distribution is notable for its malign association with many bodily functions. Activation of the HPA axis in depression appears to be responsible for the small but statistically significant associations between depression and abdominal body fat.[43,44] Rosmond and Bjorntorp[45] identified a group of subjects whom they termed "anxio-depressive" who scored high on measures of *psychologic disturbance*. These authors found that nonresponse to the dexamethasone suppresion test, indicative of elevated HPA axis activity, was significantly associated with BMI ($P = 0.03$), waist-to-hip ratio ($P = 0.008$), and sagittal diameter ($P = 0.05$).

A similar finding was noted in obese persons suffering from the NES. In controlled metabolic studies, serum cortisol was significantly higher among persons suffering from this disorder than among matched control subjects.[41]

▶ TREATMENT OF OBESE PATIENTS WITH DEPRESSION

There is a fascinating relationship between the treatment of depression in the presence of obesity and vice versa. Treatment of obesity often leads to a decrease in depression. A dramatic example is the striking improvement in mood that accompanies the large weight losses achieved by gastric bypass surgery.[46,47] Moderate weight losses also lead to reduction in depression, but only modestly.[48] Just as severe obesity, but not modest obesity, is associated with depression, large, but not modest, weight losses lead to large decreases in depression.

In contrast to the favorable results of the treatment of obesity on depression, the treatment of depression can have a negative effect on obesity. The treatment of depression has rarely had a stronger impact upon another disorder than it does on obesity. Table 7-3 shows the effects of pharmacotherapeutic agents for depression on body weight. Traditional tricyclic antidepressants have long been known to produce weight gain. The advent of the selective serotonin reuptake inhibitors (SSRIs) has had a salutary effect on this problem; initial studies suggested that most SSRIs induce less weight gain compared to tricyclic antidepressants and monoamine oxidase inhibitors (MAOIs). However, this evidence came primarily from short-term treatment outcome studies. More recent and long-term studies suggest that weight gain may occur after several months of treatment.[49] There is also evidence that the weight gain associated with paroxetine might be greater than that associated with fluoxetine or sertraline; in one study, the number of patients whose weight increased >7% from baseline was significantly greater among paroxetine-treated patients compared to patients treated by either of the other drugs.[50] The dual reuptake inhibitor duloxetine initially shows minimal weight loss, but over the course of a year shows weight increases that are statistically but not necessarily clinically significant.[51] Similarly, there was no significant weight gain associated with venlafaxine, a serotonin-norepinepherine reuptake inhibitor, in a randomized clinical trial.[52] Finally, it should be noted that cognitive-behavioral therapies for depression are effective for many persons. In one study of 65 outpatients with early-onset chronic depression, its efficacy was similar to that of interpersonal therapy and imipramine.[53] Improvements in depression did not differ significantly among the three groups. There are no published data addressing weight changes associated with these treatments for depression.

The problem of weight gain with pharmacotherapy for bipolar disorder is another matter, and a serious one (Table 7-4). Some of the newer agents for the treatment of bipolar disorder produce weight gains so large as to seriously compromise treatment of the mood disorder, not to mention serious weight gain. There can hardly be a more urgent need in all of pharmacotherapy than for the development of agents for bipolar disorder that do not cause large weight gains.

Although very little research has examined the relationship between "atypical depression"

► **TABLE 7-3** EFFECTS OF PHARMACOTHERAPY FOR DEPRESSION ON WEIGHT

Medication	Effect on Weight
Tricyclics	Most produce weight gain
SSRIs:	
Citalopram, fluoxetine, fluvoxamine, and sertraline	Neutral (short-term); potential gain (longer-term)
Paroxetine	Gain
Duloxetine	Limited/not clinically significant gain
Bupropion	Loss
Mirtazapine	Gain
Venlafaxine	Neutral

Source: Table compiled from Sifton,[55] Fuller and Sajatovic,[56] Aronne et al.,[57] Raskin et al.,[58] Khan et al.,[59] and Schatzberg.[60]

▶ **TABLE 7-4** EFFECTS OF PHARMACO-
THERAPY FOR BIPOLAR DISORDER ON
WEIGHT

Medication	Effect on Weight
Lithium	Gain
Valproate	Gain
Olanzapine	Gain
Carbamazepine	Neutral
Lamotrigine	Neutral
Topiramate	Loss
Aripriprizole	Neutral or gain
Ziprasidone	Neutral or gain
Risperidone	Gain
Quetiapine	Gain

*Source: Table compiled Sifton,[55] Fuller and Sajatovic,[56]
and American Diabetes Association/American
Psychiatric Association.[61]*

and obesity, this may be an important direction
for future research. Atypical depression is associated with hyperphagia in some research.[54]

▶ **CONCLUSION**

Obesity and depression traditionally have been
conceptualized as distinct and nonoverlapping
disorders with respect to etiology and treatment.
The data reviewed in this article challenge this
viewpoint and suggest the need to better understand why these disorders cooccur in certain
individuals and how to develop more efficacious
pharmacologic and behavioral interventions.

REFERENCES

1. Heymsfield SB, Wang Z, Baumgartner RN, et al.
   Human body composition: Advances in models
   and methods. *Ann Rev Nutr* 1998;17:527–558.
2. National Heart, Lung and Blood Institute. *Clinical
   Guidelines for the Identification, Evaluation, and
   Treatment of Overweight and Obesity in Adults:
   The Evidence Report.* Bethesda, MD: National Heart,
   Lung and Blood Institute, 1998.
3. Flegal KM, Carroll MD, Ogden CL, et al. Prevalence and trends in obesity among US adults.
   JAMA 2002;288:1723–1727.
4. Stunkard AJ, Wadden TA. Obesity. In: Kelley WN
   (ed.), *Textbook of Internal Medicine*, 3rd ed.
   Philadelphia, PA: Lippincott-Raven, pp. 192–198,
   1997.
5. Allison DB, Kaprio J, Korkeila M, et al. The heritability of body mass index among an international sample of monozygotic twins reared apart.
   Int J Obes Relat Metab Disord 1996;20(6):
   501–506.
6. Stunkard AJ, Harris JK, Pedersen NL, et al. The
   body mass index of twins who have been reared
   apart. *N Engl J Med* 1990;322:1483–1487.
7. Sobal J, Stunkard AJ. Socioeconomic status and
   obesity. A review of the literature. *Psych Bull*
   1989;18:260–275.
8. Kessler RC, McGonagle KA, Zhao S, et al. Lifetime and 12-month prevalence of DSM-III-R psychiatric disorders in the United States: Results
   from the National Comorbidity Survey. *Arch Gen
   Psychiatry* 1994;51:8–19.
9. Kraemer HC, Wilson GT, Fairburn CG, et al. Mediators and moderators of treatment effects in randomized clinical trials. *Arch Gen Psychiatry*
   2002;59:877–883.
10. Pine DS, Goldstein RB, Wolk S, et al. The associa-
    tion between childhood depression and adulthood
    body mass index. *Pediatrics* 2001;107:1049–1056.
11. Friedman MA, Brownell KD. Psychological corre-
    lates of obesity: Moving to the next research gen-
    eration. *Psych Bull* 1995;117:3–20.
12. Woo OS, Sook LE, Sangyeoup L, et al. Depressive
    mood and abdominal fat distribution in pre-
    menopausal overweight women. *Int J Obes* 2004;
    28:S54.
13. Istvan J, Zavela K, Weidner G, et al. Body weight
    and psychological distress in NHANES I. *Int J
    Obes* 1992;16:999–1003.
14. Faith MS, Berman N, Heo M, et al. Effects of con-
    tingent-TV on physical activity and TV-viewing
    in obese children. *Pediatrics* 2001;107:1043–
    1048.
15. Carpenter KM, Hasin DS, Allison DB, et al. Rela-
    tionships between obesity and DSM-IV major
    depressive disorder, suicide ideation, and suicide
    attempts: Results from a general population study.
    Am J Public Health 2000;90(2):251–257.
16. Faith MS, Matz PE, Jorge MA. Obesity-depression
    associations in the population. *J Psychosom Res*
    2002;53:935–942.
17. Moore ME, Stunkard A, Srole L. Obesity, social
    class, and mental illness. *JAMA* 1962;181:962–966.

18. DiPietro L, Anda RF, Williamson DF, et al. Depressive symptoms and weight change in a national cohort of adults. *Int J Obes* 1992;16:745–753.

19. Lissau I, Sorensen TIA. Parental neglect during childhood and increased risk of obesity in young adulthood. *Lancet* 1994;343:324–327.

20. Felitti VJ. Childhood sexual abuse, depression, and family dysfunction in adult obese patients. *South Med J* 1993;86:732–735.

21. Felitti VJ, Anda RF, Nordenberg D, et al. Relationship of childhood abuse and household dysfunction to many of the leading causes of death in adults. The Adverse Childhood Experiences (ACE) Study. *Am J Prevent Med* 1998;14:245–258.

22. Felitti VJ. Long-term medical consequences of incest, rape and molestation. *South Med J* 1991;84: 328–331.

23. Williamson DF, Thompson TJ, Anda RF, et al. Body weight and obesity in adults and self-reported abuse in childhood. *Int J Obes* 2002;26:1075–1082.

24. King TK, Clark MM, Pera V. History of sexual abuse and obesity treatment outcome. *Addict Behav* 1996;21:283–290.

25. Diaz A, Simantov E, Rickert VI. Effect of abuse on health: Results of a national survey. *Arch Pediatr Adolesc Med* 2002;156(8):811–817.

26. Heim C, Newport DJ, Wagner D, et al. The role of early adverse experience and adulthood stress in the prediction of neuroendocrine stress reactivity in women: A multiple regression analysis. *Depress Anxiety* 2002;15(3):117–125.

27. Kendler KS, Walters EE, Neale MC, et al. The structure of the genetic and environmental risk factors for six major psychiatric disorders in women: Phobia, generalized anxiety disorder, panic disorder, bulimia, major depression, and alcoholism. *Arch Gen Psychiatry* 1995;52:374–383.

28. Maes HH, Neale MC, Eaves LJ. Genetic and environmental factors for body mass index and depression in the Virginia 30,000. *Behav Genet* 1999;29:363.

29. American Psychiatric Association. *Diagnostic and Statistical Manual of Mental Disorders*, 4th ed., Text Revision. Washington, DC: American Psychiatric Association, 2000.

30. Posternak MA, Zimmerman M. Symptoms of atypical depression. *Psychiatry Res* 2001;104(2):175–181.

31. Camacho TC, Roberts RE, Lazarus NB, et al. Physical activity and depression: Evidence from the Alameda County Study. *Am J Epidemiol* 1991;134: 220–231.

32. Babyak M, Blumenthal JA, Herman S, et al. Exercise treatment for major depression: Maintenance of therapeutic benefit at 10 months. *Psychosom Med* 2000;62:633–638.

33. Thompson JK, Heinberg LJ, Altabe M, et al. *Exacting Beauty: Theory, Assessment, and Treatment of Body Image Disturbance*. Washington, DC: American Psychological Association.

34. Latner JD, Stunkard AJ. Getting worse: Stigmatization of obese children. *Obes Res* 2003;11:452–456.

35. Thompson JK, Coovert M, Richards KJ, et al. Development of body image and eating disturbance in young females: Covariance structure modeling and longitudinal analyses. *Int J Eat Disord* 1995;18:221–236.

36. Jackson TD, Grilo CM, Masheb RM. Teasing history, onset of obesity, current eating disorder psychopathology, body dissatisfaction, and psychological functioning in binge eating disorder. *Obes Res* 2000;8:451–458.

37. Marcus MD, Wing RR, Ewing L, et al. Psychiatric disorders among obese binge eaters. *Int J Eat Disord* 1996;9:69–77.

38. Mitchell JE, Mussell MP. Comorbidity and being eating disorder. *Addict Behav* 1995;20:725–732.

39. Yanovski SZ. Binge eating disorder: Current knowledge. *Obes Res* 1993;1:306–324.

40. Sherwood NE, Jeffery RW, Wing RR. Binge status as a predictor of weight loss treatment outcome. *Int J Psychiatry* 1999;23:485–493.

41. Birketvedt GS, Florholmen J, Sundsfjord J, et al. Behavioral and neuroendocrine characteristics of the night-eating syndrome. *JAMA* 1999;282: 657–663.

42. Gluck ME, Geliebter A, Satov T. Night eating syndrome is associated with depression, low self-esteem, reduced daytime hunger, and less weight loss in obese out patients. *Obes Res* 2001;9:264–267.

43. Bjorntorp P, Rosmond R. Obesity and cortisol. *Nutrition* 2000;16:924–936.

44. Larsson B, Seidell J, Svardsudd K, et al. Obesity, adipose tissue distribution and health in men–the study of men born in 1913. *Appetite* 1989;13:37–44.

45. Rosmond R, Bjorntorp P. Endocrine and metabolic aberrations in men with abdominal obesity in relation to anxio-depressive infirmity. *Metab Clin Exp* 1998;47:1187–1193.

46. Waters GS, Pories WJ, Swanson MS, et al. Long-term studies of mental health after the Greenville gastric bypass operation for morbid obesity. *Am J Surg* 1991;161:154–158.

47. Dymek MP, le Grange D, Neven K, et al. Quality of life and psychosocial adjustment in patients after Roux-en-Y gastric bypass: A brief report. *Obes Surg* 2001;11:32–39.

48. Gladis MM, Wadden TA, Vogt R, et al. Behavioral treatment of obese binge eaters: Do they need different care? *J Psychosom Res* 1998;44: 375–384.

49. Aronne LJ. *A Practical Guide to Drug-Induced Weight Gain*. New York: McGraw-Hill, 2002.

50. Fava M, Judge R, Hoog SL, et al. Fluoxetine versus sertraline and paroxetine in major depressive disorder: Changes in weight with long-term treatment. *J Clin Psychiatry* 2000;61:863–867.

51. Raskin J, Goldstein DJ, Mallinckrodt CH, et al. Duloxetine in the long-term treatment of major depressive disorder. *J Clin Psychiatry* 2003;64: 1237–1244.

52. Kahn A, Upton GV, Rudolph RL, et al. The use of venlafaxine in the treatment of major depression and major depression associated with anxiety: A dose-response study. *J Clin Psychopharmacol* 1998;18:19–25.

53. Agosti V, Ocepek-Welikson K. The efficacy of imipramine and psychotherapy in early-onset chronic depression: A reanalysis of the National Institute of Mental health Treatment of Depression Collaborative Research Program. *J Affect Disord* 1997;43(3):181–186.

54. Posternak MA, Zimmerman M. Partial validation of the atypical features subtype of major depressive disorder. *Arch Gen Psychiatry* 2001;59:70–76.

55. Sifton DW (ed.). *PDR Drug Guide for Mental Health Professionals*. Montvale, NJ: Thompson Medical Economics, 2002.

56. Fuller MA, Sajatovic M. *Psychotropic Drug Information Handbook*, 4th ed. Hudson, OH: Lexi-Comp, American Pharmaceutical Association, 2003.

57. Aronne LJ, Allison DB, Rozen TD, et al. *A Pratical Guide to Drug-Induced Weight Gain*. New York: McGraw-Hill, 2002.

58. Raskin J, Goldstein DJ, Mallinckrodt CH, et al. Duloxetine in the long-term treatment of major depressive disorder. *J Clin Psychiatry* 2003; 64(10):1237–1244.

59. Khan A, Upton GV, Rudolph RL, et al. The use of venlafaxine in the treatment of major depression and major depression associated with anxiety: A dose-response study. *J Clin Psychopharmacol* 1998;18:19–25.

60. Schatzberg AF. Efficacy and Tolerability of duloxetine. A novel dual reuptake inhibitor, in the treatment of major depressive disorder. *J Clin Psychiatry* 2003:64(Suppl 13):30–37.

61. American Diabetes Association/American Psychiatric Association. Consensus Development Conference on Antipsychotic Drugs and Obesity and Diabetes. *Diabetes Care* 2004;27:596–601.

CHAPTER 8

Major Depression and Osteoporosis Risk

GIOVANNI CIZZA

▶ INTRODUCTION

This presentation summarizes the knowledge on the relationship between depression and osteoporosis. Existing studies have been quite heterogeneous in their design and usage of diagnostic instruments to assess the clinical severity of depression, which may have contributed to the different results on the comorbidity of these two conditions. Nevertheless, these studies reveal a strong association between depression and osteoporosis. The endocrine and immune factors such as increased levels of cytokines, depression-induced hypersecretion of corticotropin releasing hormone (CRH), and hypercortisolism may play a critical role in the bone loss observed in subjects suffering from major depressive disorder (MDD).

Depression is a common disorder affecting 5–9% of women and 1–2% of men.[1] This disorder carries a considerable risk of morbidity and is associated with a two- to threefold increase in all-cause, non-suicide-related mortality, especially in men.[2] Hypercortisolism, a frequent finding in depressed patients,[3] may possibly contribute to some of the somatic consequences of depression, including bone loss, possibly periodontitis, and alterations in body composition.[4–7]

Osteoporosis is a condition characterized by bone fragility and increased risk of bone fracture.[8] Prevention of this common disorder should be reserved for subjects at risk; however, there is debate regarding which risk factors warrant further evaluation by measurements of bone mineral density (BMD). Evidence suggests that the diagnosis of osteoporosis should be considered when one or more of the accepted risk factors are present (i.e., personal history or family history of prior fracture, thinness, or current smoking). The identification of unrecognized risk factors for osteoporosis is therefore central in the diagnosis of osteoporosis and not only has scientific interest, but also has considerable clinical consequences.

As recently reviewed, decreased BMD is more frequently seen in depressed subjects than in the general population[9]; since this review was published the number of studies on this topic has doubled. As low BMD is one of the most important risk factors for having an osteoporotic fracture,[10] these studies suggest that depression may be a significant, but ignored risk factor for osteoporosis. The purpose of this chapter is to summarize the most recent evidence of depression as a risk factor for osteoporosis and to balance this relevance of depression against currently established risk factors for osteoporosis. To accomplish this, we reviewed the published studies on the association between depression and osteoporosis. The endocrine and immune factors potentially responsible for the bone loss observed in subjects with depression such as, hypercortisolism, hypogonadism, and growth hormone (GH) deficiency are discussed in further detail.

▶ DEPRESSION AND OSTEOPOROSIS

Depression, BMD, and Fractures

A database search was conducted on osteoporosis and depression. The most important studies which were found on this relationship are summarized in Table 8-1.

In the first study, trabecular bone density, assessed by a single-energy quantitative computed tomography (CT) scan at the lumbar spine, was approximately 15% lower in 80 depressed men and women older than 40 years, as compared with 57 nondepressed men and women.[11] Important factors with the potential to influence bone loss such as, smoking, lifetime history of excessive or inadequate physical exercise, or a history of estrogen treatment did not affect the regression model, suggesting indirectly that depression supposedly had an effect on bone mass. However, age of onset and total duration of depression did not reveal a significant influence on bone mass. As pointed out in a subsequent letter,[12] both female and male comparison subjects had a similar lumbar BMD values, which raises the question of just how representative the comparison group was to the general population.

A follow-up study conducted in 18 depressed men and women with 21 comparison subjects from the original cohort indicated that the bone loss over a period of at least 24 months was 10–15% greater in the depressed subjects than in the comparison subjects.[13] Interestingly, the bone loss was also about 6% greater in depressed men than in depressed women. The small number of subjects included in the follow-up study limited the statistical power of the study and this made the matching of controls by gender, age, and body mass index (BMI) uncertain.

In the third study, BMD was measured by dual-energy x-ray absorptiometry (DEXA) at the spine, hip, and radius in 22 pre- and 2 postmenopausal women with previous or current MDD.[14] The 24 controls were matched by age, menopausal status, race, and BMI. BMD was 6–14% lower at the spine and hip in the depressed women as compared with the controls. In 10 of the depressed premenopausal women, the BMD was at least 2 standard deviations (SD) below the young normal mean value, which corresponds to having severe osteopenia.[8] Contrastingly, no premenopausal woman in the control group had a deficit of any similar magnitude. As the risk of fracture increased by a factor of 1.5–3 for each SD reduction in BMD,[15] a substantial lifetime risk of osteoporotic fractures related to depression was already established before menopause. Markers of bone turnover, serum osteocalcin (OC), urinary deoxypyridinoline (DPD) crosslinks, and urinary N-telopeptide (NTX) crosslinks of type I collagen were about 15–30% lower in depressed women as compared with the controls, which indicates a reduced bone turnover in depressed patients. Although still within the normal range in many of the patients, the urinary-free cortisol excretion was about 40% higher in depressed women than in controls.

In a multicenter, prospective, cohort study of 7414 elderly women, the association among depression, BMD, falls and the risk of fracture was examined.[16] The study employed the Geriatric Depression Score, which is a 15-item validated checklist of symptoms designed to detect depression in the elderly. BMD was measured by DEXA at the spine and the hip. Incident vertebral fractures were documented by follow-up spine x-rays, and all self-reported falls were ascertained at follow-up visits. The prevalence of depression was found to be 6%, a consistent

► **TABLE 8-1** SUMMARY OF REPORTS ON DEPRESSION AND OSTEOPOROSIS

Authors	Subjects (Mean age)	Bone and other Measurements	Study Design/ Setting	Evaluation Of Depression	Findings
Amsterdam and Hooper (1998)	6 depressed (3 men, 3 women) (41 years old), 5 healthy controls 38 years old)	Spine BMD by DEXA 24 h UFC	Cross-sectional	DSM-3R Hamilton Depression Score greater than 20	No differences in BMD
Coelho et al. (1999)	102 women, randomly selected (58 years)	BMD at the spine- and hip by DEXA	Cross-sectional population-based	Beck Depression Inventory Hopkins Symptom Checklist-90	25–35% higher scores of depressive symptoms and depression in women with osteoporosis
Forsén et al. (1999)	18,612 Norwegian women (50–101 years; mean 66 years)	Hip fractures	Prospective (3 years of follow-up), population-based study of association between mental distress and hip fractures	Mental distress index. No specific evaluation for depression.	Women in the highest (10%) mental distress category have a twofold increase in hip fractures (CI 1.15; 3.29)after adjusting for use of medications, smoking, BMI, physical activity, and other factors
Greendale et al. (1999)	684 men and women fracture-free at baseline (70–79 years). Part of the MacArthur Study of Successful Aging	Self-reported fractures 12 h UFC at baseline	Prospective study 7 years of follow-up	Depressive symptoms, Hopkins Symptoms Checklist	70 fractures seen in 7 years with 684 participants. Subjects in the highest quartile of the higher baseline UFC are predictive of increased risk of fractures, more so in men (OR: women 2.08; men: 5.19)
Herran et al. (2000)	19 antidepressant-free women (45 years) with a single depressive episode 19 controls, matched by age, BMI, and post-menopausal state	Osteocalcin, bone-specific alkaline phosphatase, telopeptide, type I collagen propeptide serum cortisol	Cross-sectional	Hamilton Depression Scale (mean score 21)	Higher cortisol and increased bone turnover as indicated by increased bone formation (osteocalcin), Increased bone resorption (telopeptide and cross-laps) in depressed women
Halbreich et al. (1995)	33 women (44 years), 35 men (36 years) with various mental disorders; 21 depressed subjects	BMD by DPA at the spine and hip testosterone (in men), estradiol (in women), prolactin, cortisol	Observational study of hospitalized patients	DSM-III R	Low BMD in depressed subjects, especially in depressed men. Inverse correlation between plasma cortisol and BMD

(Continued)

Authors	Subjects (Mean age)	Bone and other Measurements	Study Design/ Setting	Evaluation Of Depression	Findings
Kavuncu et al. (2002)	42 depressed women (35 years), 42 healthy controls matched by age	BMD by DEXA biochemical markers of bone turnover	Cross-sectional	DSM-IV plus a Hamilton Depression Score greater than 14	No difference in BMD between depressed women and control women. Increased bone resorption in women with depression
Michelson et al. (1996)	24 depressed women (41 years), 24 control women (41 years)	BMD by DEXA at the spine, hip, and radius. Biochemical markers of bone turnover cortisol, PTH, vitamin D, IGF-I	Cross-sectional	DSM-III R	6–14% lower BMD in depressed women at the spine and hip
Reginster (1999)	121 healthy post-menopausal women (63 years)	BMD at the spine and hip by DEXA	Cross-sectional, study of screened patients at a clinic for osteoporosis	General health questionnaire	No association between depressive symptoms and BMD
Robbins et al. (2001)	Random sampling of 1566 (65 years or older) enrolled in the Cardiovascular Health Study	BMD of the total hip by DEXA	Cross-sectional evaluation of a large cohort of elderly	Center for Epidemiological Studies Depression Scale (CES-Dm)	16% of subjects were depressed (CES-Dm > than 10) 25% of men and 13% of women were osteoporotic (T score lower than 2.5 SD). Depression negatively associated with total hip BMD (stronger association in women than men). Depression scores predictive of bone loss 2 years later. Hip BMD 5% lower in subjects with depression
Schweiger et al. (1994)	27 depressed men (58 years), 53 depressed women (62 years), 30 nondepressed men (63 years), 58 nondepressed women (58 years)	Spine BMD by single-energy CT scan	Cross-sectional	DSM-III R	15% lower spine BMD in depressed subjects

Study	Subjects	Measurements	Design	Diagnosis	Results
Schweiger et al. (2000)	10 depressed men (57 years), 8 depressed women (61 years), 14 nondepressed men (65 years), 7 nondepressed women (63 years)	Same as study 1 (Schweiger et al., 1994)	Longitudinal, at least 24 months follow-up on study 1	Same as study 1	10–15% greater bone loss over at least 24 months in depressed subjects, 6% greater bone loss in depressed men as compared to depressed women
Yazici et al. (2003)	25 premenopausal women with depression (31 years; duration of illness 6 months; Hamilton score 23), 15 control women matched by age, BMI, calcium intake, physical activity, and SES	BMD by DEXA at the spine and hip sites bone chemical markers: alkaline phosphatase, osteocalcin, and urinary deoxypyridinoline	Cross-sectional	DSM-IV	11–12% lower BMD at the total femur and spine in depressed women, 50% increase in bone resorption. No differences in plasma cortisol or bone formation. Bone loss was not related to clinical indices of depression
Vrkljan et al. (2001)	31 depressed subjects (19 men, 12 women) (37 years), 17 healthy male controls (39 years)	BMD (skeletal site not specified) plasma cortisol, 24 h UFC, and 1 mg dexamethasone suppression test	Cross-sectional	Unspecified	Negative correlation between T score and years of antidepressant therapy
Whooley et al. (1999)	467 depressed women (75 years), 6949 controls (73 years)	BMD by DEXA at the spine and hip falls fractures	Prospective cohort over 3.7 years	Geriatric depression scale	Greater incidence of falls (OR 1.6) and fractures (OR 2.3), but no difference in BMD between depressed and nondepressed women

value reported by others.[1] Depressed women were more likely to fall (70% vs. 59%), and had a greater incidence of vertebral (11% vs. 5%) and nonvertebral (28% vs. 21%) fractures as compared with the controls. In the tertile of women with the highest BMI (above 27.6 kg/m^2), the depressed women showed a 3–5% lower BMD in the spine and hip. However, there were no differences shown in BMD in the depressed and nondepressed women in the any other BMI tertiles, nor in the cohort as a whole. Correction for a greater propensity to fall in depressed women partly explained the increased risk of fracture in this group. Adjustment for the use of antidepressants, sedatives, and hypnotics did not influence the association between depression and fractures. The authors proposed that the falls in depressed women may be related to nonspecific factors, such as poor adjustment to old age, suggesting that the association between depression and low BMD might therefore be limited to younger women and/or to women with more severe, long-lasting depression. Degenerative bone changes are known to make BMD measurements less reliable in the elderly,[17] which may in part explain the vague association between BMD and fracture in this population. Nevertheless, this study underscores the importance of depression as a risk factor for osteoporotic fractures.

In a study of 35 men and 33 women consecutively hospitalized for mental disorders, BMD was measured by dual-photon densitometry at the spine and hip.[18] The patients suffered from depression, schizophrenia, mania, schizoaffective disorder, or from adjustment disorders. Patients with depression or schizophrenia had significantly lower BMD than age- and gender-matched controls, and in general the bone loss was more severe in depressed men than in depressed women. A negative association between serum cortisol levels and BMD was observed in depressed subjects of both genders. In men there was a positive correlation between BMD and testosterone levels, whereas in women estradiol levels were not correlated with BMD.

The relationship between osteoporosis and indices of well-being or psychopathology was evaluated in a community sample of 105 ambulatory middle-age women.[19] Depressive symptoms were evaluated by the Beck Depression Inventory and BMD was measured by DEXA at the spine and hip. The prevalence of osteoporosis in this sample was 47%, which corresponds to reports from epidemiologic studies.[20] Depression was significantly more common in women with osteoporosis than in women without it (77% vs. 54%), corresponding to an odds ratio (OR) of depression in women with osteoporosis of 2.9 (95% CI: 1.0–7.6); women with osteoporosis had about 25–35% higher depressive scores than women with normal bone mass. The association between depression and osteoporosis was independent of other risk factors for osteoporosis, such as age or BMI. No differences were found in the general well-being scores, suggesting that depression was not a consequence of pain or physical distress in these asymptomatic women with a diagnosis of osteoporosis based on BMD determination.

Depressive symptomatology was assessed by the general health questionnaire (GHQ) in 121 postmenopausal women that spontaneously attended a screening visit for osteoporosis.[21] BMD was measured by DEXA at the spine and hip. Importantly, this study did not find any association between depressive symptoms nor a depressive trait and low BMD, suggesting that only fully developed depression is a risk factor for osteoporosis.

Three small, cross-sectional studies recently conducted in Europe all reported that lower spine and hip BMD were associated with increased bone resorption in subjects with depression, in addition, there was a negative correlation between T scores and years of antidepressant usage.[22,23] We are currently conducting at the National Institutes of Health Clinical Center (NIH CC) the P.O.W.E.R. (premenopausal, osteoporosis, women, alendronate, depression) Study, a prospective study of premenopausal women with major depression and matched controls. This study has enrolled more than 90 patients and 40 controls who have been followed for up to 24 months.

Most recently primary hyperparathyroidism, a secondary cause of osteoporosis, has been associated with depression.[24] In a consecutive series of 360 subjects who underwent surgery for primary hyperparathyroidism, 35 subjects met criteria for major depression. Postoperatively, 90% of these subjects stated that depression no longer impacted their ability to work or to do daily activities and many had stopped antidepressant medications. The mechanisms leading to depression in subjects with primary hyperparathyroidism are unclear but may possibly involve the effects of hypercalcemia on the central nervous system (CNS).

Not only is there a correlation with major depression and osteoporosis, but "stress" per se is also associated with osteoporosis and fractures. In a large, population-based, prospective study conducted in Norway, women with the highest level of stress, defined by a composite index that included life satisfaction, nervousness, loneliness, and sleep disorders, were 50% more likely to suffer from hip fractures, after correcting for many factors including the use of medications.[25] Specifically, the 10% of women with the highest mental distress had a twofold increased risk of hip fracture as compared with the 10% of women with the lowest mental distress category. Therefore, the mental problems that led to the use of psychotropic medications may have had a direct effect on fracture risk, independent of the medication. The potential causes were not explored in this study; however, in another large study conducted in elderly subjects one of the potential causes for bone loss was thought to be an increase in cortisol level.[26] In 684 elderly subjects that were part of the MacArthur Study of Successful Aging, higher urinary cortisol at baseline was predictive of the possibility of increased fractures. Interestingly, the predictive value was stronger for men than for women.

If depression is a cause for osteoporosis, one would expect in principle some kind of dose-relationship between these two factors with more severe depression being associated with greater bone loss. The existence of such a link should be apparent in large, prospective studies of long duration. The Cardiovascular Health Study is a population-based prospective study of more than 5000 subjects. In a random subset of 1566 elderly subjects, depression was negatively associated with hip BMD, and the clinical severity of depression was predictive of future bone loss 2 years later.[27]

For completeness, it should be noted that although the preponderance of reports on BMD in women with major depression found an association between these two conditions, however this was not universally the case. In a well-conducted cross-sectional study of 42 premenopausal women suffering from MDD and 42 closely matched controls, there were no differences in BMD between the groups; however, bone resorption was increased in women with major depression.[28] In another small study with 6 depressed and 5 controls subjects, there were no differences in BMD observed.[29]

In summary, the existence of an association between depression and osteoporosis has been reported in different settings and populations, and should, therefore, be considered real.

Psychotropic Medications for Falls and Fractures

The use of antidepressants, sedatives, and hypnotics is associated with a greater incidence of falls and fractures, especially in the elderly.[30] These medications can increase the risk of falling by various mechanisms, such as inducing orthostatic hypotension and syncope, dizziness, vertigo, blurred vision, ataxia, or somnolence. The association between hip fractures, falls, and the usage of two commonly prescribed classes of antidepressants, tricyclic antidepressants (TCA) and selective serotonin-reuptake inhibitors (SSRIs), was investigated in a case-control study.[31] Each of the 8239 elderly men and women treated in a hospital setting for hip fractures (cases) within a 12-month period was matched by age and gender to five controls. Hospital records determined comorbidity and risk of falls during the 3 years preceding the hip fracture. Most of the cases were women (78%), and a large proportion of these women were older than 85 years (40%). Depression was approximately threefold more common in patients with hip fracture compared with controls (14.9% vs. 5.7%). Of the patients with hip fracture, 6.6% had been exposed to SSRI, 2.6% to secondary TCA, and 9.0% to tertiary TCA. After adjusting for confounding variables, the OR for hip fracture was 1.5 in patients exposed to tertiary TCA and 2.4 in patients exposed to SSRI. Consistently, current users of antidepressants were at higher risk than former users were, and there was no relationship between dose of antidepressants and the risk of hip fracture. Because BMD was not measured in this study, it was not possible to establish whether the increased risk of fracture observed in depressed subjects reflected an underlying association between low BMD and depression. In addition, the study design did not allow for conclusions on cause-relationship, resulting in the remaining possibility that depression was in part the result of a debilitating fracture.

In another case-control study of elderly residents of a long-term facility, the incidence of falls was correlated to the general health of the residents and their use of medications.[32] Falls and use of medications were significantly related, and in general this association was more related to the prescribed drug than to the underlying condition which initially required the prescription. In addition, the use of three or more drugs increased the risk of falling. Only depression and osteoarthritis were consistently associated with an increase risk of falling across the 12 therapeutic classes of drugs, which suggests an independent effect of these two medical conditions.

In addition to potentially impairing arousal and balance and hereby increasing the risk of falls, many of the drugs prescribed for depression have an effect on calcium metabolism and possibly on BMD. It is, however, unclear if this effect contributes to the fractures resulting from drug-related falls. Lithium carbonate, a drug primarily used for bi- and unipolar affective disorders, potentiates the calcium-induced inhibition of parathyroid hormone (PTH) secretion.[33] Use of this drug has been associated with secondary hyperparathyroidism.[34,35] In a small cross-sectional study, BMD at the hip and spine, plasma calcium, and PTH levels were all found to be normal in 23 patients (5 men and 18 women), all of whom were treated with lithium for various affective disorders over a period of 0.6–9.9 years.[36] Thyroid stimulating hormone (TSH)-suppressive doses of thyroxine treatment have been found to have a negative effect on BMD.[37] Both thyroxine and triiodothyronine are sometimes used in doses sufficient to suppress TSH as adjunct treatment to antidepressive therapy in patients with major depression or rapid-cycling bipolar disorders; however, little is known about the effects of this treatment on BMD. A small cross-sectional study evaluated the BMD in 10 (9 pre- and 1 postmenopausal) women with bipolar disorder treated with thyroxine for at least 18 months.[38] In this small series of patients, the use of thyroxine was not associated with a decrease in BMD at any site. A similar study conducted in 26 women with affective disorders followed for a period of 12 months or longer reached similar conclusions.[39]

Carbamazepine, phenytoin, and other anticonvulsivants are sometimes used in certain forms of severe and psychotic depression, especially in elderly subjects. A large prospective study of elderly, community-dwelling women reported a greater rate of decline at the calcaneus and hip levels in continuous phenytoin users. Such a decline would increase the risk of hip fractures by 29% over 5 years among women 65 years and older.[40]

In summary, various class of psychotropic medications have been shown to increase the fractures rate, mainly by increasing the risk of falling, although some other class of medications, such as the anticonvulsivants, may also have a direct effect on bone turnover. Fracture risk is especially high in elderly subjects taking psychotropic medications: in addition to limit drug exposure as medically indicated, various interventions aimed at modifying the living environment to decrease the risk of falling (i.e., adequate light, eliminating physical barriers, walking aids, proper shoes) should be implemented.

Glucocorticoid-Induced Osteoporosis

Osteoporosis is a known consequence of chronic steroid usage. The mechanism of bone loss in glucocorticoid-induced osteoporosis is similar to that observed in endogenous Cushing syndrome, and it has relevance to depression-related osteoporosis since hypercortisolism is commonly observed in depressed subjects.[9]

Bone Loss in Endogenous Cushing Syndrome

Bone loss induced by hypercortisolism seems to be primarily caused by decreased bone formation,[41] whereas the relative contribution of increased bone resorption is unknown. Bone loss is more pronounced in trabecular than in cortical bone, and it more frequently leads to fractures.[42] The degree of bone loss correlates with the severity and the duration rather than the underlying cause of the condition.[41] This includes the factitious and drug-related form.[43] Bone mass is only partially regained once the disease is cured, and this process may take many years.[41]

In a series of 20 consecutive patients with Cushing syndrome, the majority had a bone loss at the spine and femoral neck of similar magnitude.[42] Most patients did not fully regain BMD for up to 60 months after the correction of hypercortisolism. About 3 months after curative surgery, the level of OC and DPD increased, thus suggesting a reactivation of both osteoblastic and osteoclastic activity. Interestingly, depressed women experienced a more pronounced bone loss at the hip than observed in subjects with Cushing syndrome. This suggests that other biologic factors in addition to hypercortisolism may contribute to bone loss in depressed subjects.[9]

Endogenous hypercortisolism is particularly deleterious to bone during growth. This was demonstrated in a longitudinal study of two identical twin girls, one of whom was diagnosed at 14 years of age with an adrenocorticotropic hormone (ACTH)-secreting pituitary adenoma.[44] The affected twin had a spine BMD of minus 3.2 SD as compared with her age-matched control's mean value, and a decrease in OC and DPD levels. Surgical cure led to increased bone formation, as indicated by OC levels. However, more than 2 years after surgery, the BMD had only improved to a level of minus 1.9 SD. Additionally, the affected twin was 21 cm shorter, had a delayed puberty with suppressed gonadotropin and estradiol secretion, and exhibited a decrease in lean mass with an increase in fat mass.

Bone loss in Cushing syndrome can be restored by specific antiosteoporotic treatments. Bisphosphonates inhibit osteoclast-related resorption of bone.[45] In a prospective, open-label study, treatment with the bisphosphonate alendronate increased BMD at the hip and spine in patients with Cushing syndrome.[46] Thirty nine consecutive patients with Cushing disease (18 women and 21 men, all 29–51 years of age) underwent selective adenomectomy. Cured patients ($n = 21$) were randomly allocated for either treatment with alendronate (10 mg daily) or for no treatment. Noncured patients ($n = 18$) were randomly assigned to either treatment with ketoconazole (200–600 mg/day [$n = 8$]), which is an inhibitor of adrenal steroidogenesis, or to treatment with ketoconazole plus alendronate (10 mg/day [$n = 10$]). BMD was lower at the hip and spine in all patients with Cushing syndrome, as compared with their healthy control subjects matched for age and BMI. Nine patients with Cushing syndrome had osteoporosis and 20 patients had osteopenia. Treatment with alendronate for 12 months increased BMD both in the cured patients and in the patients with active disease by 1.7–2.4% at the spine and by 1.2–1.8% at the hip. No improvements in BMD were observed in patients with the active disease who received only ketoconazole.

Bone loss is common in patients who receive long-term glucocorticoid therapy.[41] A 48-week, randomized, double-blind, placebo-controlled study of alendronate in 477 men and women

(17–83 years of age), all whom received glucocorticoid therapy for various diseases was recently published.[47] Patients requiring long-term therapy (at least 1 year), with a daily dose of at least 7.5 mg prednisolone or its equivalent, were followed for 48 weeks after randomization for daily placebo or alendronate treatment. All patients also received a daily supplement of 800–1000 mg calcium and a 250–500 IU of vitamin D. At baseline, 32% of the patients had osteoporosis and 16% had asymptomatic vertebral fractures. After 48 weeks of treatment with daily 10 mg alendronate, the BMD of these patients had increased by 2.9% at the spine, whereas the placebo group experienced a decrease of 0.4%. Similar results were obtained in a study of 141 subjects with glucocorticoid-induced osteoporosis who were treated with bisphosponate etidronate.[48]

Hypercortisolism may affect the calcium metabolism by various mechanisms: decreased calcium absorption, increased calcium excretion, or transient hypocalcemia; all of which may trigger secondary hyperparathyroidism.[48] The conversion of vitamin D to its active metabolites is also affected by hypercortisolemia, resulting in further impairment of intestinal calcium absorption.[49] Treatment with calcium and vitamin D are effective preventive treatments of glucocorticoid-induced osteoporosis.[50] A total of 103 patients starting corticosteroid therapy were randomly assigned to receive 1000 mg calcium per day and either oral calcitriol (0.5–1 g/day) plus intranasal salmon calcitonin (400 IU/day), calcitriol plus a placebo nasal spray, or a double placebo for 1 year.[50] Treatment with calcitriol with or without calcitonin prevented spinal bone loss more effectively than calcium did alone. However, bone loss at the femoral neck and distal radius was not significantly affected by any of the treatments.

Potential Mechanisms of Bone Loss in Depression

One of the mechanisms by which depression may induce bone loss is hypercortisolism.

Osteoporosis is in fact one known consequence of hypercortisolism, usually seen in the form of endogenous Cushing syndrome or in chronic steroidal use. Bone loss in Cushing syndrome seems to be primarily caused by decreased bone formation,[41] whereas the relative contribution of increased bone resorption is unknown. Bone loss is more pronounced in trabecular rather than in cortical bone, and it frequently leads to fractures.[42] The degree of bone loss correlates with the severity and the duration of this condition rather than with the underlying cause.[41] This includes the factitious and drug-related forms.[43] Bone mass is only partially regained once the disease is cured, and this process may take many years.[41] Depression does seem to be associated, in any case, with increased bone turnover which is indicated by a small cross-sectional study in 19 women, all of whom suffered from a moderate single depressive episode with reportedly both increased markers of bone formation and turnover.[51]

Hypercortisolism, a well-known biologic correlate of depression, may be the consequence of a dysregulation of the CRH system and the hypothalamic-pituitary-adrenocortical (HPA) axis[5] (Fig. 8-1). CRH hypersecretion and hypercortisolism in turn lead to inhibition of the reproductive axis and hypogonadism. The latter is an established risk factor for bone loss in both genders.[52] In addition, CRH hypersecretion and hypercortisolism tend to decrease the activity of the GH/IGF-1 axis, an important enhancer of bone formation.[53] In depression, a dysregulation of several inflammatory mediators, including interleukin-6 (IL-6), has been reported.[54] This cytokine may also be implicated in some of the other medical consequences of major depression, such as cardiovascular disease and insulin resistance.[55,56] IL-6, a major mediator of bone resorption, is elevated in depressed subjects, especially at an older age.[57] Increased sympathetic activity, often observed in depressed subjects,[58] also tends to increase IL-6 secretion. As recently reviewed,[59] the reproductive axis is altered in women with major depression; however, no clear hormonal abnormalities have

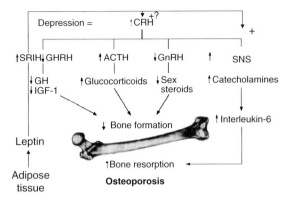

Figure 8-1. *Schematic representation of the proposed endocrine mechanisms contributing to bone loss in subjects suffering from depression.*

Major depression is associated with increased secretion of CRH and glucocorticoids along the HPA axis. CRH, in turn, inhibits the gonadal axis affecting the hypothalamic release of GnRH, and inhibits the GH axis via stimulation of somatostatin and inhibition of GHRH. Increased secretion of cortisol, decreased secretion of GH and insulin-like growth factor 1 (IGF-1), and decreased secretion of sex steroids result in decreased bone formation and increased bone resorption. High levels of catecholamines stimulate the production of IL-6, a potent bone resorption factor. Most recently, leptin, an adipocyte-producing hormone, has been shown to exert, at least in experimental animals, an inhibitory effect on bone formation which is centrally mediated. The concurrent effect of increased bone formation and decreased bone resorption lead to a net bone loss in subjects with depression.

been documented in this axis in women with major depression. More studies are needed to evaluate the influence of depression on the age at menarche, menopause, the actual levels of circulating hormones, and on the proper rhythmicity of these hormones in women. When this reliable information on both the clinical characteristics and the length of the menstrual cycle in women with major depression is prospectively collected, it will serve to be very useful.

Recently it has been reported that leptin, a hormone secreted by the white adipose tissue,

inhibits bone formation through a central mechanism involving a hypothalamic relay.[60,61] Intracerebroventricular administration of leptin to leptin-deficient (ob/ob) mice, a strain characterized by abnormally elevated bone mass, not only caused a markedly decrease in food intake, an increase in energy expenditure, and a decrease weight loss, but it also induced bone loss. This effect is centrally mediated at the level of the hypothalamus, and does not involve any direct effect of circulating leptin on the bone cells, for no leptin receptors are present on any osteoblasts or on any other bone cells. As the secretion of leptin is increased at night in depressed subjects,[62] we hypothesize that an additional potential mechanism of bone loss in major depression may include central inhibition of bone formation by leptin. We have recently also speculated that seasonal changes in leptin levels may also be implicated in preserving bone mass during the winter in hibernating animals.[63] Interestingly, the phenotype of the ob/ob mice also includes hypercortisolism and hypogonadism, two features also commonly seen in depressed subjects. Finally, both major depression and osteoporosis are likely to be associated with multiple genes, perhaps involved in the regulation of phospholipids.[64] Whether or not depression and osteoporosis share a common genetic predisposition, or whether both are mediated by a common genetic set-up still remains to be determined.

The nature of the relationship between depression and osteoporosis has therefore been discussed based upon the novel perspective that depression may induce bone loss via all the potential biologic mechanisms discussed above. Osteoporosis may be a silent disease and as such, may go undiagnosed for quite a long time; that is, until pathologic fractures ensue. Several of the studies reviewed have reported subjects suffering from major depression, in all of whom bone loss had gone asymptomatic and undiagnosed. It would be very difficult to sustain the notion that osteoporosis, a largely asymptomatic condition which the subject is not aware of having, could induce depressive symptoms.

However, bone loss does eventually cause fractures and if these fractures are present at the hip site, they could cause a very serious and disabling condition. For example, the quality of life is profoundly threatened by falls and hip fractures among elderly women.[65] In this scenario, it is conceivable that clinical osteoporosis, especially if causing pain and physical disability, may induce reactive depressive symptoms. Whether such depressive symptoms are in turn followed by changes in cortisol and other hormones remains to be determined. In summary, the relationship between depression and osteoporosis, similarly to other clinical situations such as stroke, rheumatoid arthritis, and any other debilitating conditions in which depression coexists with a medical condition, should be seen as a bidirectional one, with the two conditions influencing each other leading to a vicious circle.

► CONCLUSIONS

The studies outlined found a consistent association between depression and osteoporosis, thus suggesting that depression is a substantial, yet previously unrecognized risk factor for osteoporosis, being similar to other well-established risk factors such as low BMI,[66] smoking, or a family history of osteoporosis.[67] Despite the evidence presented, the nature of the relationship between these two conditions is so far only partly elucidated. It is therefore important to note some of the limitations of the literature reviewed. To begin with, most studies were cross-sectional and were, by design, only able to indicate associations, not causal links. Furthermore, different diagnostic systems were used to diagnose and estimate the severity of depression. These differences may have contributed to the wide range of the prevalence of depression reported in subjects affected by osteoporosis. In several studies of bone loss, actively depressed subjects were pooled with subjects who only carried a historic diagnosis of depression. It is problematic to not know whether the impact of bone loss in those with current depression is equivalent to those who had a past history of depression. Retrospective evaluation of depression certainly has limited reliability, since it is solely based upon subject recollection. In addition, many of these studies were small with heterogeneous patients. It is also important to note that those studies which used the diagnosis of major depression as the "threshold" for severity of depression, a far more severe condition than depressive symptomatology, found a clear association between depression and osteoporosis.

Finally, it should be noted that any review of the literature of this kind may have an inherent selective publication bias, due to the fact that studies which fail to prove the original hypothesis, either because of lack of statistical power or because the hypothesis proved to be untrue, are three or more times less likely not to be published than positive studies, a phenomenon known as the "file drawer problem."[68] Therefore, it is possible that there may be unpublished studies of which we are unaware, which may have failed to find an association between depression and osteoporosis, or which may have proven that there is no association between these two terms. To reduce the possibility of such bias, some researchers are now advocating that their institution use a registry listing of all the clinical studies which were started on a given research topic.

Within these limitations, all of the studies discussed raise questions that should be addressed in the future. The existence of a causal link between depression and osteoporosis as well as whether bone loss only occurs when a patient is actively depressed should be determined. Additionally, it should be established whether or not successful treatments of depression and/or use of antidepressants have any important impact on bone turnover. The prevalence of osteoporosis in depressed subjects should be further investigated as well as whether there exists a particular subgroup of these depressed subjects that are more at risk of becoming osteoporotic, for many may be candidates for treatment.

Moreover, additional research is needed to understand the putative role of depression in male osteoporosis, as this condition is poorly understood, and until recently this condition has been relatively neglected, being labeled as "idiopathic" in approximately one-third of the subjects.[69,70] At a mechanistic level, it is crucial to understand the specific roles of the endocrine and paracrine factors responsible for the bone loss in depression, and their relative contribution to the bone loss of decreased bone formation and of increased bone resorption.

Only prospective, long-term studies with sufficient statistical power will be able to answer these questions and allow the needed insight into the pathogenesis of bone loss in depression. In conclusion, the clinical evaluation of subjects with idiopathic bone loss, especially in premenopausal women and in young/middle-aged men, should also include an assessment of depression. Conversely, a history of nontraumatic fractures in a depressed subject should alert the physician to the possibility of undiagnosed osteoporosis. From a practical perspective, patients with current or past history of major depression or depressive symptoms should be evaluated for osteoporosis by DEXA measurement of spine or femoral BMD, or, whenever bone densitometry measurements were not feasible, by blood measurement of biochemical markers of bone turnover. This would be especially indicated for depressed subjects that have lost height, have poor nutrition and calcium intake, are smokers, show clinical evidence of hypogonadism, or have a strong family history for osteoporosis.

REFERENCES

1. Robins LN, Helzer JE, Weissman MM, et al. Lifetime prevalence of specific psychiatry disorders in three sites. *Arch Gen Psychiatry* 1984;41:949–958.
2. Zheng D, Ferguson JE, Macera CA, et al. Major depression and all-cause mortality among white adults in the United States. *Ann Epidemiol* 1997;7: 213–218.
3. Steckler T, Holsboer F, Reul JM. Glucocorticoids and depression. *Baillieres Best Pract Res Clin Endocrinol Metab* 1999;4:597–614.
4. Bjorntorp P, Rosmond R. The metabolic syndrome-a neuroendocrine disorder? *Br J Nutr* 2000; 83(Suppl 1):S49–S57.
5. Chrousos GP, Gold PW. A healthy body in a healthy mind—and vice versa—the damaging power of "uncontrollable" stress. *J Clin Endocrinol Metab* 1998;83:1842–1845.
6. Genco RJ, Ho AW, Grossi SG, et al. Relationship of stress, distress and inadequate coping behaviors to periodontal disease. *J Periodontol* 1999;70: 711–723.
7. Rosmond R, Bjorntorp P. Endocrine and metabolic aberrations in men with abdominal obesity in relation to anxio-depressive infirmity. *Metabolism* 1998;10:187–193.
8. Consensus Development Conference Diagnosis: Prophylaxis and treatment of osteoporosis. *Am J Med* 1993;94:636–638.
9. Cizza G, Ravn P, Chrousos GP, et al. Depression: A major, unrecognized risk factor for osteoporosis? *Trends Endocrinol Metab* 2001;12:198–203.
10. Ross PD, Davis JW, Vogel JM, et al. A critical review of bone mass and the risk of fractures in osteoporosis. *Calcif Tissue Int* 1990;46:149–161.
11. Schweiger U, Deuschle M, Korner A. Low lumbar bone mineral density in patients with major depression. *Am J Psychiatry* 1994;151:1691–1693.
12. Hay P. Treatable risk factor for osteoporosis? *Am J Psychiatry* 1996;153:140.
13. Schweiger U, Weber B, Deuschle M, et al. Lumbar bone mineral density in patients with major depression: Evidence of increased bone loss at follow-up. *Am J Psychiatry* 2000;157:118–120.
14. Michelson D, Stratakis C, Hill L, et al. Bone mineral density in women with depression. *N Engl J Med* 1996;335:1176–1181.
15. Schuit SC, van der Klift M, Weel AE, et al. Fracture incidence and association with bone mineral density in elderly men and women: The Rotterdam Study. *Bone* 2004;34:195–202.
16. Whooley MA, Kip KE, Cauley JA, et al. Depression, falls and risk of fracture in older women Study of Osteoporotic Fractures Research Group. *Arch Intern Med* 1999;159:484–490.
17. Drinka PJ, DeSmet AA, Bauens SF, Rogot A. The effect of overlying calcification on lumbar bone densitometry. *Calcif Tissue Int* 1992;50(6): 507–510.
18. Halbreich U, Rojansky N, Palter S, et al. Decreased bone mineral density in medicated psychiatric patients. *Psychosom Med* 1995;57:485–491.

19. Coelho R, Silva C, Maia A, et al. Bone mineral density and depression: A community study in women. *J Psychosom Res* 1999;46:29–35.

20. Melton LJ 3rd, Chrischilles EA, Cooper C, et al. Perspective: How many women have osteoporosis? *J Bone Miner Res* 1992;7:1005–1010.

21. Reginster JY, Deroisy R, Paul I, et al. Depressive vulnerability is not an independent risk factor for osteoporosis in postmenopausal women. *Maturitas* 1999;33:133–137.

22. Vrkljan M, Thaller V, Lovricevic I, et al. Depressive disorder as possible risk factor of osteoporosis. *Coll Antropol* 2001;25:485–492.

23. Yazici KM, Akinci A, Sutcu A, et al. Bone mineral density in premenopausal women with major depressive disorder. *Psychiatry Res* 2003;117: 271–275.

24. Wilhelm SM, Lee J, Prinz RA. Major depression due to primary hyperparathyroidism: A frequent and correctable disorder. *Am Surg* 2004;70:175–180.

25. ForsÇn L, Meyer HE, Sogaard AJ, et al. Mental distress and risk of hip fracture. Do broken hearts lead to broken bones? *J Epidemiol Community Health* 1999;53:343–347.

26. Greendale GA, Unger JB, Rowe JW, et al. The relation between cortisol excretion and fractures in healthy older people: Results from the MacArthur studies-Mac. *J Am Geriatr Soc* 1999;47:799–803.

27. Robbins J, Hirsch C, Whitmer R, et al. The association of bone mineral density and depression in an older population. *J Am Geriatr Soc* 2001;49: 732–736.

28. Kavuncu V, Kuloglu M, Kaya A, et al. Bone metabolism and bone mineral density in premenopausal women with mild depression. *Yonsei Med J* 2002; 43:101–108.

29. Amsterdam JD, Hooper MB. Bone density measurement in major depression. *Prog Neuropsychopharmacol Biol Psychiatry* 1998;22:267–277

30. Leipzig RM, Cumming RG, Tinetti ME. Drugs and falls in older people: A systematic review and meta-analysis: I. Psychotropic drugs. *J Am Geriatr Soc* 1999;47:30–39.

31. Liu B, Anderson G, Mittmann N, et al. Use of selective serotonin-reuptake inhibitors or tricyclic antidepressants and risk of hip fractures in elderly people. *Lancet* 1998;351:1303–1307.

32. Brown EM. Lithium induces abnormal calcium-regulated PTH release in dispersed bovine parathyroid cells. *J Clin Endocrinol Metab* 1981; 52:1046–1048.

33. Granek E, Baker SP, Abbey H, et al. Medications and diagnoses in relation to falls in a long-term care facility. *J Am Geriatr Soc* 1987;35:503–511.

34. Bendz H, Sjodin I, Toss G, et al. Hyperparathyroidism and long-term lithium therapy: A cross-sectional study and the effect of lithium withdrawal. *J Intern Med* 1996;240:357–365.

35. Mak TW, Shek CC, Chow CC, et al. Effects of lithium therapy on bone mineral metabolism: A two-year prospective longitudinal study. *J Clin Endocrinol Metab* 1998;83:3857–3859.

36. Cohen O, Rais T, Lepkifker E, et al. Lithium carbonate therapy is not a risk factor for osteoporosis. *Horm Metab Res* 1998;30:594–597.

37. Greenspan SL, Greenspan FS. The effect of thyroid hormone on skeletal integrity. *Ann Intern Med* 1999;130:750–758.

38. Gyulai L, Jaggi J, Bauer MS, et al. Bone mineral density and L-thyroxine treatment in rapidly cycling bipolar disorder. *Biol Psychiatry* 1997;41: 503–506.

39. Gyulai L, Bauer M, Garcia-Espana F, et al. Bone mineral density in pre-and post-menopausal women with affective disorder treated with long-term L-thyroxine augmentation. *J Affect Disord* 2001;66:185–191.

40. Ensrud KE, Walczak TS, Blackwell T, et al. Antiepileptic drug use increases rates of bone loss in older women: A prospective study. *Neurology* 2004;62:2051–2057.

41. Ziegler R, Kasperk C. Glucocorticoid-induced osteoporosis: Prevention and treatment. *Steroids* 1998;63:344–348.

42. Hermus AR, Smals AG, Swinkels LM, et al. Bone mineral density and bone turnover before and after surgical cure of Cushing's syndrome. *J Clin Endocrinol Metab* 1995;80:2859–2865.

43. Cizza G, Nieman LK, Doppman JL, et al. Factitious Cushing syndrome. *J Clin Endocrinol Metab* 1996;81:3573–3577.

44. Leong GM, Mercado-Asis LB, Reynolds JC, et al. The effect of Cushing's syndrome on bone mineral density, body composition, growth, and puberty: A report of an identical adolescent twin pair. *J Clin Endocrinol Metab* 1996;81:1905–1911.

45. Fleisch H. Bisphosphonates: Mechanism of action. *Endocr Rev* 1998;19:80–100.

46. Di Somma C, Colao A, Pivonello R, et al. Effectiveness of chronic treatment with alendronate in the osteoporosis of Cushing's disease. *Clin Endocrinol (Oxf)* 1998;48:655–662.

47. Saag KG, Emkey R, Schnitzer TJ, et al. Alendronate for the prevention and treatment of glucocorticoid-induced osteoporosis. Glucocorticoid-Induced Osteoporosis Intervention Study Group. *N Engl J Med* 1998;339:292–299.

48. Adachi JD, Bell MJ, Bensen WG, et al. Intermittent etidronate therapy to prevent corticosteroid-induced osteoporosis. *N Engl J Med* 1997;337:382–387.

49. Chan SD, Chiu DK, Atkins D. Mechanism of the regulation of the 1 alpha, 25-dihydroxyvitamin D3 receptor in the rat jejunum by glucocorticoids. *J Endocrinol* 1984;103:295–300.

50. Sambrook P, Birmingham J, Kelly P, et al. Prevention of corticosteroid osteoporosis. A comparison of calcium, calcitriol, and calcitonin. *N Engl J Med* 1993;328:1747–1752.

51. Herran A, Amado JA, Garcia-Unzueta MT, et al. Increased bone remodeling in first-episode major depressive disorder. *Psychosom Med* 2000;62:779–782.

52. Harper KD, Weber TJ. Secondary osteoporosis. Diagnostic considerations. *Endocrinol Metab Clin North Am* 1998;27:325–348.

53. Chrousos GP, Gold PW. The concepts of stress and stress system disorders: Overview of physical and behavioral homeostasis. *JAMA* 1992;267:1244–1252.

54. Cizza G, Mistry S, Eskandari F, et al. A group of 21 to 45-year old women with major depression exhibits greater plasma proinflammatory and lower anti-inflammatory cytokines: Potential implications for depression-induced osteoporosis and other medical consequences of depression. Paper presented at the annual meeting of the Endocrine Society, New Orleans, LA, 2004.

55. Papanicolaou DA, Wilder RL, Manolagas SC, et al. The pathophysiologic roles of interleukin-6 in human disease. *Ann Intern Med* 1998;128: 127–137.

56. Licinio J, Wong ML. The role of inflammatory mediators in the biology of major depression: central nervous system cytokines modulate the biological substrate of depressive symptoms, regulate stress-responsive systems, and contribute to neurotoxicity and neuroprotection. *Mol Psychiatry* 1999;4:317–327.

57. Dentino AN, Pieper CF, Rao MK, et al. Association of interleukin-6 and other biological variables with depression in older people living in the community. *J Am Geriatr Soc* 1999;47:6–11.

58. Wong ML, Kling MA, Munson PJ, et al. Pronounced and sustained central hypernoradrenergic function in major depression with melancholic features: Relation to hypercortisolism and corticotropin-releasing hormone. *Proc Natl Acad Sci USA* 2000;97:325–330.

59. Young EA, Korszun A. The hypothalamic-pituitary-gonadal axis in mood disorders. *Endocrinol Metab Clin North Am* 2002;31:63–78.

60. Ducy P, Amling M, Takeda S, et al. Leptin inhibits bone formation through a hypothalamic relay: A central control of bone mass. *Cell* 2000;100: 197–207.

61. Takeda S, Elefteriou F, Levasseur R, et al. Leptin regulates bone formation via the sympathetic nervous system. *Cell* 2002;111:305–317.

62. Antonijevic IA, Murck H, Friebos RM, et al. Elevated nocturnal profiles of serum leptin in patients with depression. *J Psychiatr Res* 1998;32: 403–410.

63. Cizza G, Mistry S, Phillips T. Serum markers of bone metabolism show bone loss in hibernating bears. *Clin Orthop* 2004;422:281–283.

64. Horrobin DF, Bennett CN. Depression and bipolar disorder: Relationships to impaired fatty acid and phospolipids metabolism and to diabetes, cardiovascular disease, immunological abnormalities, cancer ageing, and osteoporosis. Possible candidate genes. *Prostaglandins Leukot Essent Fatty Acids* 1999;60:217–34.

65. Salkeld G, Cameron ID, Cummin RG, et al. Quality of life related to fear of falling and hip fracture in older women: A time trade off study. *Br Med J* 2000;320:241–246.

66. Ravn P, Cizza G, Bjamason NH, et al. Low body mass index is an important risk factor for low bone mass and increased bone loss in early postmenopausal women. Early Postmenopausal Intervention Cohort (EPIC) study group. *J Bone Miner Res* 1999;14:1622–1627.

67. Lindsay R, Meunier P. Osteoporosis: Review of the evidence for prevention, diagnosis and treatment and cost-effectiveness analysis. *Osteoporos Int* 1998;8:11–21.

68. Thornton A, Lee P. Publication bias in meta-analysis: Its causes and consequences. *J Clin Epidemiol* 2000;53:207–216.

69. Orwoll E, Ettinger M, Weiss S, et al. Alendronate for the treatment of osteoporosis in men. *N Engl J Med* 2000;343:604–610.

70. Ebeling PR. Osteoporosis in men: New insights into aetiology, pathogenesis, prevention and management. *Drugs Aging* 1998;13:421–434.

CHAPTER 9

Reproductive Endocrinology and Mood Disorders in Women

Peter J. Schmidt and David R. Rubinow*

▶ INTRODUCTION

The effects of the reproductive system on mood regulation are dramatic, clinically significant, and heuristically invaluable. In this chapter, we will describe the reproductive endocrine system in women, particularly as it changes over the menstrual cycle, during pregnancy and the postpartum, and during the perimenopause and menopause. We then will describe the neurobiologic effects of gonadal steroids and will emphasize those actions that are shared by psychotropic agents and are relevant to current hypotheses regarding the etiopathogenesis of depression. Three reproductive endocrine-related mood disorders will be discussed in detail, following which the interactions of these disorders and changes in reproductive function with classical mood disorders will be presented. The theme throughout is that the reproductive system offers a unique and valuable perspective

*The views expressed in this book do not necessarily represent the views of the National Institutes of Health or the U.S. Govt.

from which to understand and treat affective disorders.

▶ REPRODUCTIVE ENDOCRINE SYSTEM

Hypothalamic-Pituitary-Ovarian Axis and Gonadal Steroids (Fig. 9–1)

Under the control of neural inputs, gonadotropin releasing hormone (GnRH) neurons in the hypothalamus secrete the decapeptide GnRH into the portal hypophyseal blood to regulate the release of follicle stimulating hormone (FSH) and luteinizing hormone (LH) by cells in the anterior pituitary (i.e., gonadotropes). FSH and LH are released into the systemic circulation to act directly on cells in the ovary and stimulate the release of hormones (e.g., estradiol and progesterone) from the ovary. GnRH secretion is in turn regulated by both pituitary and ovarian hormones. Additionally, a variety of other local or peripheral neuromodulators (e.g., beta-endorphin, corticotropin releasing hormone [CRH], and neurosteroid metabolites of progesterone) regulate GnRH secretion.

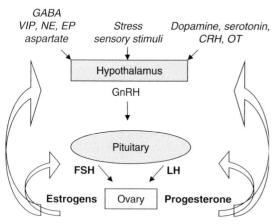

Figure 9-1. The hypothalamic-pituitary-ovarian axis. Secretory products of the axis are in bold type, and modulators of the axis are in italics. Solid arrows indicate stimulation, and hollow arrows indicate inhibition. The ovarian products display feedback effects at both the pituitary level and the hypothalamic level.

Dynamics of the Menstrual Cycle, Pregnancy, Postpartum, Menopause

Menstrual cycle: The first day of menstruation is, by convention, the first day of the menstrual cycle, when estrogen and progesterone levels are low. GnRH is secreted in a pulsatile fashion from the hypothalamus and stimulates the secretion of FSH from the pituitary. FSH stimulates the secretion of estrogen from the ovarian follicles, resulting in the proliferation of the uterine lining. Estrogen and another ovarian hormone, inhibin, exert negative feedback on FSH release from the pituitary. At the end of the first menstrual cycle week, one follicle is selected and becomes the predominant follicle. That follicle undergoes maturation and secretes increasing amounts of estrogen.

The amplitude and particularly the frequency of GnRH pulses increase during the second menstrual cycle week, with the increasingly frequent GnRH pulses giving rise to a surge of LH secretion, the trigger for the expulsion of the egg from the follicle (ovulation) between 35 and 44 hours

after the onset of the LH surge. Before the LH surge the rising estrogen levels through undetermined mechanisms suddenly exert a positive, rather than a negative, feedback on gonadotropin secretion and are responsible for the changes in GnRH secretion that result in the LH surge. Ovulation marks the end of the follicular phase.

After ovulation and under the influence of LH stimulation, the remains of the ovarian follicle, the corpus luteum, secretes large amounts of progesterone and, to a smaller extent, estradiol. During this phase of the menstrual cycle, the luteal phase, the amplitude of the GnRH pulses increases, and the frequency greatly decreases under the influence of brain opiates. If fertilization and implantation of the egg do not take place, the corpus luteum atrophies. Progesterone levels precipitously decline, and that decline initiates the shedding of the uterine lining, menstruation, within approximately 12–16 days of ovulation. During the last few days of the luteal phase, declining estradiol levels remove the negative feedback on FSH secretion, thereby initiating the rise in FSH levels that will give rise to the next menstrual cycle.

Pregnancy and the postpartum: The successful implantation of the developing embryo initiates a series of physiologic events within the lining of the uterus, including the formation of the decidua, the development of the maternal-feto-placental vascular system, the stimulation of local growth factors, and the secretion of human chorionic gonadotrophin (hCG).[1] In turn, hCG stimulates the maternal ovary and corpus luteum to produce increasing quantities of sex steroids (e.g., progesterone, 17-alpha-hydroxyprogesterone, estradiol, and estrone) as well as other hormones (e.g., relaxin). The high levels of the mother's ovarian hormones maintain pregnancy until the placenta is developed and able to produce these hormones independent of corpus luteal activity. This transition from the corpus luteum to the placenta occurs usually in the eighth or ninth week of pregnancy, and the corpus luteum can be safely removed without causing an abortion after the ninth week.[2]

Hormone production by the fetal-placental-maternal unit is responsible for normal growth and development as well as the onset of parturition. Compared to the adult ovary, however, neither the placenta nor the fetal cortex have complete sets of synthetic enzymes, and, therefore, the adrenal cortex, placenta, as well as the maternal system combine to produce the profile of steroid hormones that characterize pregnancy.

In the fetus, three tissues are the principle sites of steroid hormone production. First, the hypothalamic pituitary system is developed by about 16–17 weeks of gestation, and the majority of hypothalamic hormones (e.g., CRH) present in the adult are detectable in the fetus by 14–18 weeks of pregnancy and the pituitary hormones by 16 weeks of pregnancy. Second, the fetal adrenal cortex is a critical regulator of fetal development, including intrauterine homeostasis, growth and maturation of the organ systems, and possibly the timing of delivery. In primates, the fetal zone of the adrenal gland is active by 10–12 weeks of gestation and accounts for the majority of the adrenal hormones produced by the fetus. Cortisol secretion is present by the 16th week of gestation. The fetal zone is regulated by fetal pituitary adrenocorticotropic hormone (ACTH) as well as by paracrine and autocrine effects of local growth factors. The steroids synthesized by the fetal adrenal zone are limited by a reflection of the type of synthetic enzymes present in the tissue. Specifically, the fetal zone is characterized by high levels of both 17-alpha-hydroxylase and sulfotransferase as well as the relative absence of 3-beta-hydroxy steroid dehydrogenase (the latter hormone is present in the outer adrenal cortex but never appears in the fetal zone). Thus, the steroid precursor pregnenolone is shunted to the delta five pathway (Fig. 9-2), converted to dehydroepiandrosterone (DHEA), which is then promptly sulfated to form DHEA-S. The DHEA-S is not a substrate for 3-beta-hydroxy steroid dehydrogenase; therefore, DHEA-S leaves the adrenal and circulates in the fetal vasculature. The production of DHEA-S by the fetus is approximately 200 mg/day by term.[1,3] Some DHEA-S reaches the placenta where it is desulfated by placental sulfatase

enzymes and converted through the actions of placental 3-beta- and 17-beta-hydroxy steroid dehydrogenases into testosterone and in turn, by the actions of placental aromatase, into estradiol. However, the majority of circulating DHEA-S passes into the liver, the fetus's third major synthetic tissue. The fetal liver is characterized by high 16-alpha-hydroxylase activity, and DHEA-S is metabolized into 16-alpha-hydroxy DHEA-S (i.e., a second hydroxyl group is added). Thus, large quantities of this latter compound pass through the fetal-placental unit where it is converted to estriol (by the same pathway as DHEA-S described above), an estrogenic steroid with a structure similar to that of estradiol. By the 12th week of gestation, estriol concentrations in the maternal circulation rapidly increase by approximately a 100-fold coinciding with the enlargement of the fetal zone of the adrenal cortex. The development of the fetal ovary results in peak germ cell production at 16–20 weeks of gestation with approximately six million primordial follicles that are reduced to two million at term. By 12 weeks the ovarian interstitial cells have the enzymatic capacity to synthesize steroids; however, there is no evidence that fetal ovaries are active during pregnancy, in contrast to the fetal testes, which are actively producing and secreting androgens from the Leydig cells by about 8 weeks with a peak around 15–18 weeks of gestation.

In addition to metabolizing the massive amounts of fetal-source DHEA-S into estriol, the placenta also serves a vital role in the production of progesterone. The placenta produces progesterone largely from the maternal source of LDL cholesterol, which is converted to pregnenolone and shunted into the delta four pathways in which it is made into progesterone (placenta has 3-beta-hydroxy steroid dehydrogenase). By term, progesterone is produced in quantities of approximately 250 mg/day, resulting in maternal plasma levels of progesterone of approximately 130 ng/mL (approximately 10 times plasma levels observed in the mid luteal phase of the normal menstrual cycle). Progesterone

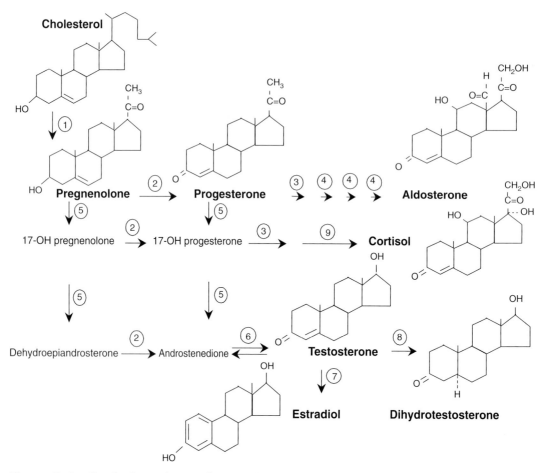

Figure 9-2. Synthetic pathways for steroid hormones. Circled numbers identify synthetic enzymes: 1 = cytochrome P450 (CYP) 11A (cholesterol desmolase); 2 = 3β-hydroxysteroid dehydrogenase; 3 = CYP21 (21-hydroxylase); 4 = CYP11B2 (11β-hydroxylase, 18-hydroxylase, 18-oxidase); 5 = CYP17 (17α-hydroxylase, 17,20-lyase); 6 = 17β-hydroxysteroid dehydrogenase (or oxidoreductase); 7 = aromatase; 8 = 5α-reductase; 9 = CYP11B1 (11β-hydroxylase).

plays a critical role in maintaining pregnancy, as reflected by miscarriages induced by the administration of progesterone receptor antagonists. In addition to its actions to inhibit uterine contractility, progesterone is thought to reduce cellular immune responsivity and contribute to the longevity of pregnancy. In contrast, the role of estrogens in pregnancy has been questioned.[3] As described above, 90% of the estrogens produced by the fetal-placental unit is in the form

of estriol. Estriol has a potency of approximately 0.01 times that of estradiol in all functions with the exception of its ability to increase utero-placental blood flow, in which it is equipotent with estradiol. Thus, if there is a role of estrogen in pregnancy it would be to generate the high vascular flow needed to maintain normal growth and development of the fetus.

Both the fetal hypothalamus as well as placenta produce identical forms of CRH, and there is a 20-fold increase in placental CRH mRNA in the last 5 weeks of pregnancy. In contrast to hypothalamic CRH, placental CRH is regulated by a positive feedback effect of cortisol. Thus, as cortisol increases during the last trimester there is an increase in CRH production causing a progressive increase in both ACTH and cortisol secretion. Additionally, there is a progressive decrease in CRH binding protein during the last 4 weeks of pregnancy, which results in an increase in free CRH. Indeed, enhanced CRH activity may be a critical facilitator to the onset of parturition.[1,4]

In addition to the placenta's production of estriol, progesterone, and CRH, the decidua and surrounding fetal membranes become important producers of both prolactin and relaxin; as well, these tissues are capable of vitamin D metabolism. Thus, placental hormones contribute to the regulation of both uterine contractility (prolactin and relaxin) and calcium homeostasis and bone development in the fetus.

Pregnancy is accompanied by a sustained elevation in the secretion of several steroid and peptide hormones, followed by a sudden drop in hormone levels over the first few days after delivery. During the third trimester of pregnancy, plasma progesterone levels in the mother are approximately 130 ng/mL and estradiol reaches plasma levels of approximately 10–15 ng/mL, levels that are increased 10- and 50-fold, respectively, beyond maximum menstrual cycle levels.[5] After parturition, progesterone and estradiol levels drop to early follicular phase levels within days,[6] and the puerperium is characterized by relative hypogonadism.

During the postpartum period the secretion of estradiol and progesterone as well as ovulation are sufficiently compromised so as to result in relative hypogonadism and the absence of follicular development. The absence of ovarian activity during the postpartum is a reflection of reduced gonadotropin secretion. Normal LH pulsatility reappears after 6–8 weeks; however, lactation may enhance the restraint on hypothalamic GnRH secretion and LH pulsatility. The exact mechanism mediating the suppression of pulsatile hypothalamic GnRH secretion during the postpartum and lactation remains to be fully clarified.[7] There is substantial individual variability in the duration of postpartum hypogonadism and amenorrhea prior to the resumption of normal follicular development and cyclic ovarian steroid production.

Peri- and postmenopause: The menopause has been defined as the permanent cessation of menstruation resulting from loss of ovarian activity and is characterized endocrinologically by tonically elevated gonadotropin (FSH, LH) secretion, persistently low levels of ovarian steroids (estradiol, progesterone), and relatively low (50% decrease compared to younger age groups) androgen secretion (Fig. 9-3).[8] The perimenopause has been defined as the transitional period from reproductive to nonreproductive life.[9] As the perimenopause progresses, ovarian follicular depletion occurs, the ovary becomes less sensitive to gonadotropin stimulation, and a state of relative hypoestrogenism occurs; gonadotropin secretion is elevated across the menstrual cycle; ovulatory cycles are fewer; and menstrual cycle irregularity ensues. However, in contrast to the postmenopause, episodic (not tonic) gonadotropin secretion is present, and both ovulation and normal (or at times increased) estradiol secretion may occur.[9,10] The late perimenopause is characterized endocrinologically by tonic elevations of plasma FSH, sustained menstrual cycle irregularity with periods of amenorrhea, and hypoestrogenism. The levels of several other hormones that may also impact on mood and behavior decrease with aging concomitant with changes in reproductive function: androgens (testosterone and androstenedione),[8,10] which begin to decline in the 20s and reach peak decline during the late 40s and 50s; DHEA; and insulin-like growth factors and binding proteins.

Gonadal Steroid Hormones

Gonadal steroids, like all steroid hormones, are derivatives of cholesterol. Steroidogenic acute regulatory protein (STAR) is the critical regulator

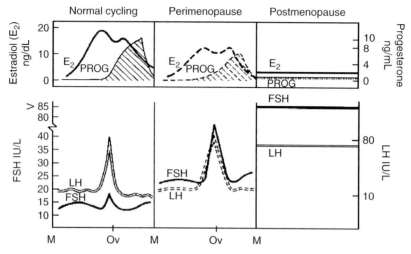

Figure 9-3. Levels of the ovarian steroids estradiol (E_2) and progesterone (PROG) (top) and the pituitary gonadotropic hormones follicle-stimulating hormone (FSH) and luteinizing hormone (LH) at three phases of reproductive life. Ov, ovulation; M, menses. The illustrated hormonal patterns for the climacteric do not reflect intra- and interindividual variability in frequency of ovulation and length of menstrual cycle during this phase.

of cholesterol's availability within the mitochondria, where it is converted by the enzyme cholesterol desmolase to pregnenolone.[3,11] Pregnenolone then serves as the precursor of the family of steroid hormones, individual members of which are generated through the actions of a relatively small number of enzymes with multiple sites of action (see Fig. 9-2). The tissue in which metabolism occurs and the enzymes present in that tissue determine the resulting end products of this cascade. For example, testosterone may be the end product and act directly at the androgen receptor, or it may be reduced to a form with greater affinity for the androgen receptor (dihydrotestosterone), converted to a form with less affinity for the androgen receptor (androsterone), or aromatized to estradiol and act through the estrogen receptor.

The classic action of steroid hormones occurs after the steroid binds (activates) its intracellular receptor, which, after undergoing phosphorylation and release from heat shock proteins, binds (usually as a dimer) to a hormone response element on a gene and directs or modifies transcription of that gene. Once the ligand-receptor complex binds to the hormone response element (which is located on or near the promoter of the gene), the result can be either the initiation or repression of transcription of messages coding for an array of proteins, including synthetic and metabolic enzymes for neurotransmitters, neuropeptides, receptor proteins, transporters, and second messengers.

Several factors may influence the actions of gonadal steroids and account for their widespread and variable effects. First, isoforms of both the androgen and progesterone receptors exist, which have different transcriptional effects, and two separate estrogen receptors, alpha and beta, have been identified, coded for by genes on the 6th and 14th chromosomes, respectively. These estrogen receptors have different distributions in the brain, different transcriptional actions, and even possess additional isoforms (e.g., insertional and deletional variants of ER alpha and beta). Second, the activated steroid receptor regulates transcription by binding protein intermediaries called coregulators (both stimulatory and inhibitory). Coregulators are expressed in a tissue-specific fashion, and their differential localization may contribute to opposite effects of the same hormone in different tissues despite the presence of similar concentrations of hormone receptor. Third, activated hormone receptors can influence the transcription of genes that do not possess hormone response elements through interactions with other cellular proteins called cointegrators, which translate hormone signals to a variety of genes lacking hormone response elements. Fourth, hormones display acute nongenomic actions; i.e., they can, in a receptor isoform-specific fashion, modify the activity of neurotransmitter gated ion channels, can directly bind and regulate ion channels, and can initiate signal transduction through membrane rather than cytoplasmic or nuclear receptors. In the CNS, these membrane-related steroid receptors are thought to be present in caveoli-like domains within the cell membrane.[12] Fifth, steroid hormone receptors can be activated by a variety of neurotransmitters (e.g., dopamine through D_1 receptor) and growth factors, even in the absence of steroid hormones. In this fashion environmental events (e.g., stressors) can impact the response to a steroid hormone signal. Finally, hormones may influence each other's activity by competing for cofactors or by producing opposing regulatory effects on genes through integrator proteins.

▶ REPRODUCTIVE ENDOCRINE SYSTEMS AND THE PATHOPHYSIOLOGY OF MOOD DISORDERS

Recent advances in cell biology, pharmacology, and neuroimaging techniques have contributed greatly to hypotheses about the causes of mood disorders and potential treatments. Our knowledge of the intricacies of cellular signaling, transcriptional regulation, and the processes of cellular resilience, neuroplasticity, and apoptosis in the CNS have increased the number of

potential candidate pathophysiologic processes that could mediate mood disorders. As well, both brain imaging and neuropathologic studies have permitted the mapping of many brain regions involved in the regulation of affect and cognition, abnormalities of which may underlie disturbances in mood. In this section, those systems currently implicated in the pathophysiology of mood disorders will be reviewed, followed by a presentation of the effects of reproductive endocrine events (or specific gonadal steroids) on the regulation of these same systems.

Neurotransmitters

Affective disorders have traditionally been considered to reflect an underlying dysregulation of one or more of the classic neurotransmitter systems. Thus, preclinical studies as well as those in humans suggested that mood disorders arose from either deficiencies or excesses within the synapse of serotonin, dopamine, noradrenaline, acetylcholine, or gamma-aminobutyric acid (GABA) in brain regions that subserve the regulation of mood and behavior. Indeed, the treatments of depression were reported to influence these same systems as an integral part of their therapeutic actions. Reports of abnormal levels of these neurotransmitters and their metabolites in the cerebrospinal fluid (CSF), urine, plasma, or in peripheral cells in depression supported this concept.[13] Moreover, pharmacologic challenge studies employing agents that targeted these neurotransmitter systems demonstrated differences between depressed subjects and controls in several outcomes including neuroendocrine, behavioral, and temperature measures. For example, the acute depletion of either serotonin or noradrenaline/dopamine in humans induced depression in antidepressant-treated subjects[14] as well as changes in the pattern of activation in the prefrontal cortex.[15,16] More recently, postmortem and in vivo radioligand imaging studies have identified abnormalities in neurotransmitter receptor levels or function that distinguish depressed patients from controls, including decreased serotonin 1A receptors (postmortem and in vivo) and alpha-2- and beta-adrenergic receptors (postmortem).[17]

Cell Signaling Pathways

Although the mood stabilizers, lithium, valproate, and carbamazepine do not act like antidepressants on monoamine activity, they do influence several of the signal transduction pathways regulated by traditional neurotransmitters and antidepressants. For example, in vitro studies have reported that mood stabilizers (lithium, valproate) and antidepressants alter the levels of many components and targets of these systems: cAMP levels and cAMP response element-binding protein (CREB) (increased), Brain-derived neurotrophic factor (BDNF) (increased), Entracellular signal-regulated kinase/mitogen-activated protein kinase (ERK-MAP) kinase activity (increased), bcl-2 (increased), Wnt cascade—glycogen synthesis kinase-3-beta (GSK-3-beta) (decreased) and beta-catenin (increased).[17] The roles of these small molecules in cellular resilience, neurogenesis, and cell death became apparent and were integrated into hypotheses about the pathophysiology of depression. Moreover, interest was renewed in some neurotransmitter systems not previously considered of major importance in mood regulation (e.g., glutamatergic) because of their roles in neuroplasticity.[17]

Brain Regional Morphologic Changes

Abnormalities in brain regional activity also supported the concept that neurogenesis could be an integral part of both the pathophysiology and treatment of affective disorders. For example, brain-imaging studies in depressed subjects have identified abnormalities (both increased and decreased) in the function (e.g., blood flow) of the following brain regions: amygdala (increased); dorsomedial and dorsoanterolateral prefrontal cortex (decreased); and subgenual and pregenual areas of the cingulate gyrus (increased), although the subgenual changes were initially reported as a decrease due to the failure to correct for the lower cortical volume in this region in depression. Structural imaging studies have confirmed abnormalities in similar brain regions, and postmortem studies have identified both glial and neuronal cell loss in some of these same brain regions in patients with affective disorders compared to controls. Moreover, the functional abnormalities in some but not all of these brain regions reverse with successful antidepressant treatment.[18,19] Finally, human and animal brain mapping studies have shown that many of these brain regions are involved in the regulation of emotion, including the integration of the emotional, cognitive, and physiologic responses to stress, the ability to experience pleasure, the identification of internal cues and vegetative state, the response to reward, as well as decision making.

The Hypothalamic-Pituitary-Adrenal Axis

Stress is considered to be a central component in the pathophysiology of mood disorders. Some of the most consistent neuroendocrine abnormalities in depression have been hypercortisolemia, enhanced CRH secretion, blunted feedback inhibition, a blunted ACTH response to CRH administration, as well as several other abnormalities in the regulation of the hypothalamic-pituitary-adrenal axis.

Under normal conditions, information about specific stressors is transmitted from higher cortical centers to the mediobasal hypothalamus, where CRH along with several other factors are released into the hypophysial-portal circulation. CRH acts through at least two CRH receptors on the corticotropes in the anterior pituitary gland.[20] Additionally, hormones such as arginine vasopressin (AVP) modulate the stimulatory effects of CRH on ACTH secretion. ACTH circulates in the blood and when in contact with the adrenal cortex stimulates production of both glucocorticoids and the adrenal androgen DHEA. Glucocorticoid production is regulated by feedback systems at the levels of the pituitary and the hypothalamus mediated through both the type 1 and type 2 corticosteroid receptors, also present in other areas of the CNS. After glucocorticoids bind to their receptor, the ligand-receptor complex undergoes a series of events and ultimately binds glucocorticoid response elements in the genome. However, as with other members of the steroid family of receptors, glucocorticoids also may act through nongenomic or membrane-related mechanisms. In addition to their roles in metabolism, the stress response, immunity and the inflammatory response, glucocorticoids may play an important role in cellular resilience and neuroplasticity in brain regions including the adult hippocampus.[21]

The enhanced CRH secretion and hypercortisolemia in depression may contribute to many of the long-term sequela of depression, including decreased neuronal cells in the hippocampus (mediated by the neurotoxic effects of hypercortisolemia), decreased bone density, and the metabolic syndrome.[22] However, recent evidence suggests that some of the effects on the CNS presumed to be due to hypercortisolemia may instead be inherited, including, for example, the size of the hippocampi.[23] Thus, smaller hippocampi may increase the vulnerability to the effects of stress and, possibly, the development of mood disorders rather than be caused by stress.

Role of Gonadal Steroids in Modulating the Systems Involved in Mood Disorders

Results from animal studies demonstrate that gonadal steroids influence several of the neuroregulatory systems thought to be involved in both the pathophysiology of affective disorders and the efficacy of antidepressant therapies.[24–26]

Preclinical studies have documented the myriad effects of gonadal steroids on neurotransmitter system activities, including regulation of synthetic and metabolic enzyme production as well as receptor and transporter protein activity. The modulatory effects of ovarian steroids on the serotonin system have been extensively studied, reflecting in part interest in the higher prevalence of depression in women and the efficacy of selective serotonin reuptake inhibitors (SSRIs) in some reproductive endocrine-related mood disorders. In some, but not all (reviewed in[27]), experimental paradigms, estradiol, like antidepressants, has been observed to inhibit serotonin transporter (SERT) mRNA,[28] decrease activity of 5-HT_{1A} receptors (down regulation and uncoupling from its G-protein),[29,30] increase 5-HT_{2A}[31] binding and mRNA,[32] and facilitate imipramine-induced down regulation of 5-HT_2 receptors in the rat frontal cortex, an action seen to accompany antidepressant administration.[33] 5-HT_{1A} receptor binding, which is decreased in depression, is modulated by both estradiol[34–39] and progesterone.[40–43] Similarly, SERT message, protein and binding have been reported to be changed by ovarian steroids in preclinical studies.[27,28,43–46]

In animals, gonadal steroids determine several observed sexual dimorphisms in serotonergic function including the following: female rats have increased serotonin and serotonin metabolites in the brain,[47,48] increased susceptibility to the serotonin behavioral syndrome,[49] increased serotonin synthesis,[50] and increased response to application of the serotonin 1A agonist 8-OH-DPAT in some (cortisol)[51] but not all (hyperphagia)[52,53] measures. Estrus cycle phase-dependent changes in serotonergic function also have been observed, including a reduced response to 8-OH-DPAT during proestrus.[42,54] Finally, progesterone receptors are colocalized with serotonin neurons in the dorsal and medial raphe nuclei of the rat, and progesterone regulates prolactin secretion through its action on the central serotonergic system.[55,56]

In humans, there are patterns of effects of gender and gonadal steroids on the serotonin system similar to those observed in animals. First, sexual dimorphisms have been reported in the following measures: whole brain serotonin synthesis (decreased in women),[57] 5-HT_2 receptor binding capacity (decreased in women),[58] behavioral response to tryptophan depletion (increased in women),[59–61] and the prolactin responses to d-fenfluramine and to m-chlorophenylpiperazine (m-CPP) (increased in women).[62–64] Second, menstrual cycle phase effects on the products of serotonergic stimulation include an increased prolactin secretion during the luteal phase after m-CPP[65] and buspirone[66] administration compared to the early follicular phase, and a decreased prolactin response following L-tryptophan[67] or d-fenfluramine[68] compared to midcycle. Third, hormone replacement in menopausal women is associated with increased urinary 5-hydroxyindole acetic acid (5-HIAA),[69,70] increased[71] (or unchanged)[72] platelet imipramine binding sites, and increased m-CPP-stimulated cortisol and prolactin.[73] Fourth, prolactin secretion is increased after progesterone administration in women with GnRH agonist-induced hypogonadism.[74] Finally, although the effect of estrogen on 5-HT$_{1A}$ receptor binding has not been examined in humans, one uncontrolled study reported an increase in 5-HT$_{2A}$ binding (F18 altanserin) in the anterior cingulate, dorsolateral prefrontal cortex, and lateral orbital frontal cortex during combined estrogen and progestin replacement (but not after estradiol alone).[75]

As noted above, several nonclassical neural signaling systems have been identified as potential mediators of the therapeutic actions of antidepressants and Electro convalsive therapy (ECT) (e.g., CREB and BDNF[76]), based on observations that these systems are modulated by a range of therapies effective in depression (e.g., serotonergic and noradrenergic agents and ECT) and exhibit a pattern of change consistent with the latency to therapeutic efficacy for most antidepressants.[77] For example, antidepressants increase the expression and activity of CREB in certain brain regions (e.g., hippocampus)[78] and regulate (in a brain region-specific manner) activity of genes with a cAMP response element.[77] Genes for BDNF and its receptor trkB have been proposed as potential targets for antidepressant-related changes in CREB activity.[77] Similarly, estradiol has been reported to influence many of these same neuroregulatory processes. Specifically, ovariectomy has been reported to decrease, and estradiol increase, BDNF levels in the forebrain and hippocampus.[79] Estrogen also increases CREB activity,[80] trkA,[81] and decreases GSK-3-beta activity (Wnt pathway)[82] in the rat

brain in a direction similar to that of mood stabilizer drugs. In contrast, an estradiol-induced decrease in BDNF has been reported to mediate estradiol's regulation of dendritic spine formation in hippocampal neurons.[83] Thus, the therapeutic potential of gonadal steroids in depression is suggested not only by their widespread actions on neurotransmitter systems but also by certain neuroregulatory actions shared by both ovarian steroids and traditional therapies for depression (i.e., antidepressants, ECT).

Modulation of neural and glial survival during aging provides yet another means by which reproductive steroids may influence the susceptibility to neuropsychiatric illness, given the putative role of neurodegeneration in depression.[84–86] Indeed, both reproductive steroids and mood regulating therapies regulate cell death and survival through effects on cell survival proteins (e.g., Bcl-2, BAX), signal transduction (e.g., MAPK, Wnt, Akt), and free radical species generation.[87–91]

Several studies have employed neuroimaging techniques (i.e., positron emmission tomography [PET] or functional magnetic resonance imaging [fMRI]) to examine the effects of ovarian steroids on regional cerebral blood flow under conditions of cognitive activation. First, Berman et al.[92] employed the Wisconsin Card Sort Test, a measure of executive function and cognitive set shifting, and observed that GnRH agonist-induced hypogonadism was associated with a loss of the characteristic pattern of cortical activation in brain regions including the dorsolateral prefrontal cortex, the inferior parietal lobule, and the posterior inferior temporal cortex. No differences were observed in those brain regions involved with the motor or the visual components of this task, and the changes in regional cerebral blood flow were, therefore, relatively specific to cognitive performance. Moreover, the normal pattern of cognitive activation was restored with the replacement of physiologic levels of either estradiol or progesterone after 2–3 weeks each. Finally, Berman et al. noted that hippocampal activation was increased on estradiol and decreased on progesterone compared to hypogonadism.[92] Changes in cortical activation could not be attributed to performance differences, since performance did not change across hormonal conditions. Thus, both estradiol and progesterone (as well as the hypogonadal state) regulated cortical activity in brain regions (prefrontal cortex, parietal and temporal cortex, and hippocampus) also reported to be involved in the regulation of mood. Second, Shaywitz et al.[93] reported in a randomized, double-blind, placebo-controlled crossover trial that postmenopausal women did not perform differently on estrogen therapy (ET) compared with placebo, but functional MRI during ET showed significantly increased activation in the inferior parietal lobule and right superior frontal gyrus during verbal encoding, with significant decreases in the inferior parietal lobule during nonverbal coding. Third, in a cross-sectional observational study, Resnick observed that hormone replacement therapy (HRT) users had enhanced regional cerebral blood flow (PET imaging) in the right parahippocampal gyrus, right precuneous, and right frontal regions during verbal memory processing, and in the right parahippocampal and inferior parietal regions during figural memory processing.[94] Additionally, performance was enhanced in those taking HRT compared with those not taking HRT.[94] Finally, Maki and Resnick employed PET and extended their initial cross-sectional findings (employing both verbal and figural memory tasks) by performing repeated measures after a 2-year period on or off HRT. The only consistent difference observed across the sampling period between ET users and nonusers was limited to the right inferior frontal cortex during the verbal memory task.[95] Additionally, when they combined activation patterns at rest and after both verbal and visual tasks and compared results after 2 years with baseline, ET users and nonusers showed different activation patterns. The relevance of the differential pattern of region-specific increases with time in brain activation in the ET users and nonusers remains to be clarified, as no differences in performance in the activation tasks were observed over the 2-year period but several other aspects of cognitive function improved. Thus, although the brain regions potentially regulated by estrogen are somewhat ill defined, the activities in the frontal cortex and hippocampus, areas subserving memory and the regulation of affect, appear to be regulated by ovarian steroids.

Extensive studies in animals demonstrate that both gender and reproductive steroids regulate basal and stimulated HPA axis function. In general, low-dose, short-term administration of estradiol inhibits HPA axis responses in ovariectomized animals,[96–99] while higher doses and longer treatment regimens enhance HPA axis reactivity to stressors.[100–102] The regulatory effects of changes in reproductive steroids or menstrual cycle phase on the HPA axis in women are less well studied. Although some studies using psychologic stressors identified increased stimulated cortisol in the luteal phase,[103,104] others using psychologic[105,106] or physiologic (e.g., insulin-induced hypoglycemia, exercise)[107,108] stressors failed to find a luteal phase increase in HPA axis activity.

Altemus et al.[109] recently demonstrated that exercise-stimulated HPA responses were increased in the midluteal compared with the follicular phase. However, in contrast to a large animal literature documenting the ability of estradiol to increase HPA axis secretion, Roca et al.[110] found that progesterone, but not estradiol, significantly increased exercise-stimulated AVP, ACTH, and cortisol secretion compared with a leuprolide-induced hypogonadal condition or estradiol replacement. The mechanism by which progesterone augments stimulated HPA axis activity is currently unknown but could include the following: modulation of cortisol feedback restraint of the axis[96,111–114]; neurosteroid-related down regulation of GABA receptors[115]; up regulation of AVP (consistent with luteal phase reductions in the threshold for AVP release).[116] Alternatively, Aguilera et al. (Ochedalski, Wynn, and Aguilera, unpublished manuscript) suggest that progesterone enhances oxytocin-induced CRH.

Pregnancy is also associated with marked changes in adrenocortical function. Plasma levels of cortisol, desoxycorticosterone, aldosterone, and corticosteroid-binding globulin all increase considerably during gestation. Cortisol levels, for example, rise to three or four times normal, peak during delivery, and return to normal levels quickly after delivery,[117] although a high rate of dexamethasone suppression test (DST) nonsuppression persists in the postpartum.[118] Additionally, CRH is produced by the placenta in large amounts, particularly in the third trimester. One study in normal pregnant women showed increases in CRH from 50 pg/mL at 28 weeks' gestation to over 1400 pg/mL at 40 weeks.[119]

As stated earlier, stress-induced elevations of glucocorticoids may have negative effects on cellular resilience and be neurotoxic. Indeed, several neuroprotective factors including BDNF are reduced by stress, further diminishing cellular viability. In contrast, some antidepressants and reproductive steroids (e.g., DHEA) will not only stimulate neuroprotective cascades such as BDNF, but may have direct actions to protect cells from glucocorticoid-induced damage.[120–122]

▶ REPRODUCTIVE ENDOCRINE-RELATED MOOD DISORDERS

Premenstrual Dysphoria

Prevalence

Premenstrual dysphoria (PMD), a severe form of premenstrual syndrome, is a prevalent and serious disorder that affects approximately 5% of women of reproductive age. Community-based studies have observed rates of severe PMD ranging from 1 to 11% in women of reproductive age, with larger proportions (up to 18%) reporting PMD symptoms associated with functional impairment (but without meeting full syndromal criteria).[123–128] In a community-based study, Angst observed that 8% of women reported distressing perimenstrual symptoms (presumed severe and hence a proxy for PMD), whereas menses-related symptom changes were reported by 44% (irritability) and 29% (depressed mood) of the women studied.[129]

In a large multicenter trial, it was found that during the luteal phase women with this disorder experience substantially impaired social adjustment, equivalent to that experienced by women

with dysthymia on all seven factors of the Social Adjustment Scale (except for the parental factor, which is significantly more impaired in women with PMD). In the social/leisure and parental scales, the impairment is not different from that experienced by women with chronic major depression or recurrent major depression, with impairment on the marital factor greater in women with PMD.[128]

The degree of impairment is even more striking when expressed in terms of the "burden" of PMD, calculated according to the burden of disease model of the World Health Organization.[130] This model determines the Disability Adjusted Life Years, the years of life lost to premature death or years lived with a disability of specific severity and duration. The severity weight of PMD during the luteal phase is between 0.36 and 0.5 (with one being death), with that for unipolar depression ranging from 0.5 to 0.7.[128] Given the prevalence of PMD and the years at risk, the average woman would be expected to experience 459 cycles with an average of 6.1 days of severe symptoms, a total of 2800 days or 7.67 years of symptoms. This translates into 1400 days or 3.84 years of disability for each woman (given a severity weight of 0.5). As there are at least 3.8 million women who meet criteria for PMD, the total Disability Adjusted Life Years in the United States would be approximately 14.5 million, a burden of considerable and obvious consequence.[128] Increased rates and odds ratios of suicide attempts are reported for PMD, consonant with the not uncommon marked suicidal ideation reported by these women, but the data are inadequate to determine the risk.

In our clinic, the severity of symptoms of several patients was such that they elected to have surgical removal of their ovaries following determination in our studies of a clear link between their symptoms and reproductive function. Clearly, the public health implications of developing effective treatments for this disorder are substantial.

Diagnosis and Presenting Symptoms

Unlike other diagnoses in medicine, PMD is a time-oriented and not a symptom-oriented diagnosis. The symptoms are relatively nonspecific; rather it is their exclusive appearance during the luteal phase that defines the disorder. As such the diagnosis cannot be made on the basis of history but instead requires a prospective demonstration that symptoms are confined to the luteal phase, disappearing at or soon after the onset of menses. While many variations on this theme potentially exist, use of a more restrictive definition has been necessary in order to assure the homogeneity of samples across studies necessary for comparison and generalization of results obtained. Employment of the two existing sets of diagnostic guidelines[131,132] has confirmed the existence of PMD and resolved many (but not all) controversies in the literature regarding the neurobiologic basis of PMD.

Pathophysiology

Given the coincidence of symptoms with the luteal phase in women with PMD, early investigators sought, as an etiology, a disturbance in reproductive endocrine function. Comparisons of basal plasma hormone levels in women with PMD and controls have revealed no consistent diagnosis-related differences. Specifically, no diagnosis-related differences in the plasma levels, areas under the curve, or patterns of hormone secretion have been observed for estradiol, progesterone, FSH, or LH.[133–136] Results for studies of androgen levels have been inconsistent, demonstrating both normal and decreased testosterone levels[137–139] and elevated and decreased free testosterone levels.[138,139] Additionally, two of four studies failed to find any diagnosis-related differences in the pattern of LH pulsatility or in the gonadotropin response to GnRH[140] (Smith et al., in press).[136,141] Finally, studies of a variety of other hormonal factors have been similarly unrevealing.[139,142–150] Several studies do, however, suggest that levels of estrogen, progesterone, or "neurosteroids" (e.g., pregnenolone sulfate) may be correlated with symptom severity in women with PMD.[151–153]

Recent speculations about the etiology of PMD have focused on putative abnormal neurosteroid levels. Observations central to these speculations include the following: (1) the GABA receptor (the presumed mediator of anxiolysis) is positively modulated by the 5-alpha- and beta-reduced metabolites of progesterone (allopregnanolone and pregnanolone, respectively)[154]; (2) withdrawal of progesterone in rats produces anxiety and insensitivity to benzodiazepines due to withdrawal of allopregnanolone, with consequent induction of $GABA_A$ alpha-4 subunit levels and inhibition of GABA currents[115,155]; (3) decreased plasma allopregnanolone levels are seen in major depressive disorder and in depression associated with alcohol withdrawal, with an increase in levels seen in plasma and CSF following successful antidepressant treatment[156–159]; (4) allopregnanolone displays anxiolytic effects in several animal anxiety models[160–162] and may be involved in the stress response[163]; (5) antidepressants may promote the reductive activity of one of the synthetic enzymes (3-alpha-hydroxysteroid oxidoreductase), thus favoring the formation of allopregnanolone[164,165]; (6) PMD patients show differences from controls in pregnanolone-modulated saccadic eye velocity (SEV) and sedation in the luteal phase[166] (although the reported differences seem attributable to an SEV response to vehicle in those with PMD and a blunted sedation response in the follicular phase in controls); high severity PMD patients show blunted SEV and sedation responses to $GABA_A$ receptor agonists—pregnanolone[166] or midazolam[167]—compared with low severity PMD patients. While several investigators observed decreased serum allopregnanolone levels in women with PMD compared to controls on menstrual cycle day 26,[168] during the luteal phase only,[169] or during the follicular phase only,[170] PMD patients in the last two studies had lower progesterone levels, which may explain the observed decreased allopregnanolone levels. This explanation is supported by the observation of Girdler et al.[171] that women with PMD had both higher progesterone and allopregnanolone levels during the luteal phase compared with controls. Further, other studies showed no diagnosis-related differences in allopregnanolone or pregnanolone[172,173] nor any difference in allopregnanolone levels in women with PMD before and after successful treatment with citalopram.[174] Wang et al.[173] did find that if two cycles differed in the area under the curve (AUC) of one of the hormones measured by more than 10%, the cycle with the lower levels of allopregnanolone and higher levels of estradiol, pregnanolone, and pregnanolone sulfate was accompanied by higher levels of symptom severity.

In general, no differences have been observed in basal plasma cortisol levels, urinary free cortisol, the circadian pattern of plasma cortisol secretion, or basal plasma ACTH levels.[175] (Both decreased ACTH levels in PMD patients across the menstrual cycle and no differences from controls have been reported).[139,176–178] In contrast, the cortisol responses to the serotonin$_{2C}$ (5-HT$_{2C}$) agonist/5-HT$_{2A}$ antagonist m-CPP,[65] a psychologic stressor,[171] and CRH[178] or naloxone[179] were blunted in patients with PMD during the luteal phase. Finally, in a study of CSF, Eriksson et al.[180] observed no differences in CSF monoamine metabolites in PMD patients compared with controls, nor were there menstrual cycle-related differences in either group. Similarly, Parry et al.[181] found no cycle-related differences (midcycle vs. premenstrual) in CSF ACTH, beta-endorphin, GABA, 5-HIAA, homovanillic acid (HVA), or norepinephrine; a slight but significant premenstrual increase in CSF 3-methoxy-4-hydroxyphenyl glycol (MHPG) was noted.

Recently, Roca et al.[110] reported that women with PMD also fail to show the luteal phase enhancement of exercise-stimulated HPA axis activity seen in normal control women. The differential HPA axis response to exercise stimulation in women with PMD provides strong additional evidence for the dysregulation of stress response physiology in this disorder. PMD patients failed to show the luteal phase increase in AVP, ACTH, and cortisol seen in controls; indeed, stimulated hormone levels in women with PMD were higher (albeit insignificantly) in the follicular phase. Differences seen were not attributable to differences in the level of stress achieved, as similar stimulated levels of lactate were obtained in both menstrual cycle phases in patients and controls. In addition to the abnormal response to menstrual cycle phase, women with PMD showed (at a trend level) reduced adrenal response to ACTH in both cycle phases. The failure of prior studies to demonstrate these significant differences in HPA axis function may reflect the nature of the stimulation paradigms employed: graded exercise stimulation is a more robust activator of the axis than most others used (e.g., CRH, m-CPP) and additionally permits a similar degree of stress across individuals by indexing the stimulus parameters to those required to elicit 90% of the individual's maximal aerobic capacity.

In conclusion, there are no consistently demonstrated endocrine or other biologic abnormalities in PMD. Further, for the overwhelming majority of biologic factors for which diagnostic group-related differences have been suggested or demonstrated, the difference is not confined to the luteal phase but rather appears in both follicular and luteal phases.[65,67,138,139,177,178,182–188] Even if these differences are confirmed, their persistence across the menstrual cycle would appear to argue against their direct role in the expression of a disorder confined to the luteal phase. Presently, then, there is no clearly demonstrated luteal phase-specific physiologic abnormality in PMD.

PMD does not, therefore, appear to reflect an abnormality of the reproductive endocrine axis. Indeed, we administered a progesterone receptor blocker, mifepristone, with or without human chorionic gonadotropin (hCG) to women with PMD during the early to mid luteal phase and demonstrated that hormonal events and gonadal steroid levels of the mid to late luteal phase were irrelevant to PMD, as they could be eliminated without altering subsequent symptom appearance.[189] It, nonetheless, remained possible that the follicular phase or early luteal phase gonadal steroids might be critical to the appearance of PMD, a speculation supported by reports of the therapeutic efficacy in PMD of ovarian suppression through either medical (GnRH agonist; danocrine)[190–199] or surgical (oophorectomy)[200,201] means. Consequently, we evaluated the effect of elimination of ovarian steroid secretion on PMD symptoms as well as the effect of ovarian steroid replacement in those whose symptoms were responsive to ovarian steroid suppression. We confirmed the therapeutic efficacy of GnRH agonist-induced ovarian suppression[202] and, consistent with data from Mortola and Muse,[195,203] demonstrated that either estrogen or progesterone could precipitate the return of typical symptoms in women with PMD.[202] In contrast, a group of control women lacking PMD showed no perturbation of mood during GnRH agonist-induced hypogonadism nor during hormone addback with either progesterone or estradiol, despite achieving hormone levels comparable to those seen in the women with PMD. Women with PMD, therefore, are differentially sensitive to gonadal steroids such that they experience mood destabilization with levels or changes in gonadal steroids that are without effect on mood in women without a history of PMD. Gonadal steroids, then, are necessary but not sufficient for PMD: They can trigger PMD, but only in women who are otherwise vulnerable to experience mood state destabilization. Thus, PMD could represent a disorder of mood state that is triggered by hormone-related events occurring prior to the mid to late luteal phase of the menstrual cycle. Nonetheless, the system(s) that underlies the vulnerability to gonadal steroid-induced mood disturbances in PMD remains to be identified. One potential candidate system that may mediate the differential behavioral sensitivity is the central serotonergic system.

Several observations have suggested the importance of interactions between the serotonin system and gonadal steroids in the pathophysiology of PMD. First, in a potential animal model of menstrual cycle-related irritability (resident intruder model),[204] female rat aggression is ovarian steroid dependent and is prevented by serotonin reuptake inhibitors (as is PMD).[205] Second, serotonin has a role in behaviors (e.g., appetite, impulsivity, mood, sleep, sexual interest) that vary with the menstrual cycle in PMD. Third, women with PMD have altered imipramine

binding and platelet 5-HT uptake compared to controls[145,146,206–209] as well as altered platelet paroxetine binding (which normalize with successful treatment with GnRH agonist[210]). Fourth, pharmacologic challenge studies, although limited by the absence of selective agonists/antagonists of the 5-HT system, suggest that 5-HT regulation differs between women with and without PMD. For example, blunted endocrine responses to serotonergic agonists (e.g., L-tryptophan, *m*-CPP) have been described in PMD (although not confined to the luteal phase).[65,67,205] Additionally, the 5-HT$_{1A}$ system, implicated in one study as disturbed in PMD,[211] is involved in the regulation of GABA activity,[39,212–216] abnormalities of which have been described or inferred in PMD.[115,153,155,166–169,172,174,217–220] Finally, serotonin reuptake inhibitors, but not nonserotonergic antidepressants, are efficacious in the treatment of PMD (suggesting increased SERT activity in PMD),[221] and the therapeutic efficacy of serotonin agonists can be reversed by tryptophan depletion[222] or serotonin receptor blockade.[223] While alterations in serotonin function are clearly relevant to the successful treatment of PMD symptoms, it remains unclear whether alterations in serotonin function underlie the differential mood response to ovarian steroids in PMD.

Management

Until recently, the ability of medical professionals to help women with PMD was limited and for the most part confined to unproved therapies (e.g., progesterone) or to lifestyle and dietary manipulations. Some nutritional, behavioral, and cognitive approaches, such as the initiation of regular exercising, restriction of caffeine consumption, and education regarding sleep hygiene, may benefit some women. However, these strategies are not usually effective in women with clinically significant symptoms.

Our approach to treatment is founded on the principle that the cornerstone of effective treatment is a careful evaluation. A complete medical and psychiatric history and review of systems is required to rule out medical disorders (e.g., hypothyroidism) that may manifest as a recurrent mood disorder as well as psychiatric disorders, the symptoms of which may or may not vary in a menstrual cycle phase-specific fashion. The patient is then told that, for both purposes of evaluation and to establish a baseline against which the efficacy of treatment can be measured, it will be necessary for her to rate the intensity of her symptoms on a daily basis for the next few cycles. Either 100 mm line scales or 6-point severity scales can be used to track the appearance and intensity of commonly experienced symptoms or those symptoms that the patient identifies as most characteristic of her syndrome. For practical purposes, the Daily Rating Form[224] permits the patient and physician to determine at a glance the relationship between symptom appearance and menstrual cycle phase. These daily ratings serve several functions. First, they establish whether symptoms appear during and are confined to the luteal phase, or whether they occur chronically with premenstrual exacerbation, or whether they lack menstrual cycle-related variation (e.g., depression or recurrent brief depression). Second, they provide considerable information about the life and symptom determinants of the patient, irrespective of the diagnosis. Third, they provide considerable therapeutic benefit: the patient not only develops self-observational skills that can assist her treatment but additionally may experience relief in response to the validation, predictability, and control that are conferred by the rating process.

For most women with PMD, manipulations of lifestyle are not sufficient, and usually some form of medication is prescribed. A multitude of vitamins and minerals, such as pyridoxine (vitamin B_6), vitamin E, vitamin A, and magnesium, have been studied as treatment modalities for PMD. All of these agents have shown inconsistent results and have not been proved to be superior to placebo. Other agents such as diuretics, beta-blockers, prostaglandin inhibitors, and prolactin inhibitors may have some beneficial effects for specific symptoms but are not, overall, effective treatments for PMD.[225–228] Thys-Jacobs demonstrated symptomatic relief following calcium administration, but these findings require replication.[229] The two options that at this time are associated with replicable efficacy are the SSRIs[227,228,230–233] and ovarian suppression.[190–195, 197, 234] As such, a trial of an SSRI is indicated in someone with PMD, with either continuous therapy or the intermittent administration of medication from (approximately) ovulation until the onset of menses. SSRIs are effective in only 50–60% of patients with PMD, with predictors of efficacy currently undetermined.[205] In most studies the effective dose of SSRI in PMD is lower than that required for the treatment of major depression and may additionally require adjustment of dose (up or down) or time of administration (a.m. or p.m.) to maximize efficacy or manage side effects (particularly sleep disturbance). For those who are unresponsive or for whom side effects (e.g., sexual dysfunction) may be treatment limiting, any of the other putative therapeutic agents may be employed, albeit with even less of a guarantee of success. Use of ovarian suppression should be reserved for those women with severe PMD and for whom oophorectomy would be a potential option (i.e., women who will not wish to have additional children). While requiring application of both the art and science of medicine, menstrual cycle-related mood disorders are treatable conditions.

Prognosis

Premenstrual dysphoria is a chronic disorder that continues until the onset of the menopause in most women. Two recent studies[235,236] have documented that the diagnosis of PMD in most instances is stable over time and does not develop into another psychiatric or medical condition. Moreover, Bloch et al. demonstrated that over the short term the symptom profile of PMD displays considerable stability from month to month.[237] Finally, the increased lifetime prevalence of mood disorders in women with PMD documented in several studies suggests that these women have an increased risk for the development of major or minor depressive episodes independent of the luteal phase.[238–240]

Postpartum Psychiatric Disorders

Prevalence

Affective syndromes that occur during the post-partum period have traditionally been divided into three categories: (1) postpartum "blues," (2) postpartum depression (PPD), and (3) puerperal psychosis. PPD is associated with more persistent symptoms and a higher rate of morbidity than the blues but is less severe (depressions of minor to moderate severity) than postpartum psychotic depressions. The 2–3-month prevalence rates of PPD in studies using conventional diagnostic criteria (e.g., research diagnostic criteria (RDC), diagnostic and statistical manual of mental disorders-version 3 (DSM-III) have been reported to be in the range of 8.2–14.9%.[241–244] Some studies[242,245,246] have reported that the incidence of depression is increased significantly during the first 3 months after birth as compared to during prepregnancy, pregnancy, or the period after the first postpartum year. Others have disputed this association, arguing that the prevalence of depression during the postpartum period is no greater than that in comparably aged nonpuerperal women.[247–251] In fact, recent epidemiologic studies[248,249] observed that the last trimester of pregnancy was associated with a prevalence of depression comparable to the postpartum, but neither were significantly increased relative to the non-puerperal women. Thus, the peripartum (last trimester and early postpartum) is not associated with an increased prevalence of major or minor depression. Nonetheless, it is not the increased prevalence of depression but the linkage of the onset of depression to a specific phase of reproductive change that distinguishes this condition.

Diagnosis and Presenting Symptoms

The DSM-IV includes the postpartum as a course modifier for major depression. Thus, subjects who meet criteria for major depression and in whom the onset of depression is within 4 weeks of delivery fulfill DSM criteria for PPD.[131] Although not formally acknowledged in DSM-IV, a similar temporal criterion would be employed to characterize the 50% or more of PPDs that are minor

depressions. Several studies have extended the 4-week window within which depressions must occur to 3 and 6 months from delivery.[252] As suggested by DSM-IV, the main symptoms of PPD are not distinct from those present in other forms of depression and include sleep disturbance, excessive fatigue, as well as sadness and anhedonia, excessive guilt, psychomotor and cognitive disturbances. Clinically women with PPD may present with severe ruminations (again not unlike depressions at other times in a woman's life)[253] and obsessional-like behaviors and thought disorders.

Pathophysiology

A number of studies have attempted to determine the relationship between postpartum mood symptoms and gonadal steroid level changes by examining basal levels, or changes in levels, during pregnancy and the postpartum period. O'Hara et al. showed that women with PPD (diagnosed at 9 weeks postpartum by self-administered Beck Depression Inventories) were not distinguished from controls by basal plasma estradiol or progesterone levels (with the exception of lower plasma estradiol levels during week 36 of gestation and day 2 postpartum),[247] nor by differences in the rate of change of either estradiol or progesterone during the peripartum. Similarly, Harris et al.[254] observed no associations between salivary progesterone levels and PPD during the peripartum. In contrast, another study showed higher progesterone, but not estradiol, levels at day 7 postpartum in women who went on to develop PPD at 6–10 weeks after delivery compared with control mothers who did not develop PPD.[255]

In addition to levels of estradiol and progesterone, studies have focused on measures that may predict a woman's vulnerability to develop gonadal steroid-induced depression. Examples of such measures include apomorphine-induced growth hormone response and alterations in neurosteroid levels in postpartum psychiatric illness. Wieck et al.[256] demonstrated that an increased growth hormone response to apomorphine on postpartum day 4 (before the usual onset of illness) was associated with an increased risk of a recurrent episode of depression. The authors speculated that these findings reflected increased sensitivity of central dopamine receptors, which may be triggered by the sharp fall in circulating estrogen concentrations after delivery (i.e., estradiol uncouples D_2 receptors,[257] with an acute upregulation in D_2 receptors possibly resulting in psychiatric disturbance following the sudden postpartum drop in estradiol levels). As described above, neurosteroid metabolites of gonadal steroids are known to have acute, nongenomic modulatory effects at GABA and glutamate receptors. Levels of one such potent progesterone metabolite, allopregnanolone, rise progressively during pregnancy[258] and drop abruptly after parturition (as levels are closely correlated with plasma progesterone levels[172]). Preliminary data (Daly, unpublished data) suggest that women with a history of PPD show a significant correlation between decreasing levels of this anxiolytic neurosteroid and mood symptoms. Pearson-Murphy also has suggested a role for alterations in progesterone metabolites in PPD, with higher levels of 5α dihydroprogesterone observed in depressed patients compared to controls during the last trimester of pregnancy.[259]

Finally, in a scaled-down model of pregnancy and the postpartum, Bloch et al.[260] demonstrated that women with a past history of PPD, but not those without such a history, experienced a recurrence of depressive symptoms after the blinded withdrawal of supraphysiologic levels of estradiol and progesterone. Although the maximal change in mood occurred after withdrawal in some women with PPD, mood symptoms began prior to withdrawal while still on supraphysiologic levels of gonadal steroids (similar to observations, of the onset of PPD symptoms prior to parturition).[248,249] Thus, Bloch et al. suggested that, as with PMD, symptoms of PPD may reflect a differential sensitivity to the mood destabilizing effects of changes in gonadal steroids, in this case substantial increases or withdrawal of estradiol and progesterone.

To summarize the above data, no consistent differences in gonadal steroid levels have been demonstrated, either in pregnancy or the postpartum, between women with and those without PPD, suggesting that the condition does not represent a simple gonadal steroid excess or deficiency state. Our data would, nonetheless, suggest that alterations in the levels of gonadal steroids are implicated in the development of the condition, either during the period of elevated levels or during withdrawal from such levels.

Higher cortisol levels at the end of pregnancy have been reported in association with more severe blues, and cortisol levels have been shown to correlate with postpartum mood in breastfeeding mothers during the first week postpartum.[261] Most studies, however, have failed to show any association of blues or PPD with plasma or salivary cortisol or with urinary metabolites.[255,262–265]

Abnormalities of CRH-stimulated ACTH (but not cortisol) have been reported in mixed samples of PPD and blues.[266] Magikou et al.[267] showed that women with the blues or PPD had a more severe and longer lasting suppression of hypothalamic CRH secretion in the postpartum period than euthymic mothers. Additionally, Bloch et al. (JCEM, in press) observed greater CRH-stimulated cortisol in euthymic women with a history of PPD compared with controls during a hormone addback state simulating pregnancy. These dynamic abnormalities of the HPA axis suggest that adaptive response to stress may be compromised in women who experience or are susceptible to PPD.

Finally, no clear relationship between thyroid dysfunction and PPD exists, and although thyroid dysfunction may contribute to postpartum mood disorders, other factors would appear to play more defining roles in the development of the condition.

In summary, gonadal steroids appear to play a key role in the development of PPD, but the exact nature of this role has yet to be fully determined. Only a subgroup of women appear to have an underlying biologic\sensitivity that ultimately manifests as PPD.

Management

The treatment of a PPD involves both the careful monitoring of women at risk as well as the careful evaluation of any persistent mood symptoms occurring during the third trimester and the peripartum. Thus, treatments are aimed at prophylaxis for those women at increased risk and prompt evaluation and care if symptoms develop in any woman. Women with a past history of PPD should be counseled prior to future pregnancies about their increased risk for depression, and a plan should be instituted to communicate any evidence of mood symptoms to the treatment team. Particular attention should be paid to strategies designed to protect the sleep of the patient. The presence of psychotic symptoms, suicidal ideas, or statements suggesting the risk of infanticide should be treated as a medical emergency, and care should be provided immediately along with efforts to maintain the safety of both the mother and child. There have been few randomized-controlled trials of therapies in PPD. In fact with the exception of a trial demonstrating the efficacy of interpersonal therapy compared to placebo,[268] there has been no double-blind, placebo-controlled trial of any psychotropic monotherapy in the treatment or prophylaxis of PPD. Nonetheless, a non-placebo controlled trial of an SSRI showed efficacy compared to a psychotherapeutic intervention,[269] and estradiol was demonstrated under double-blind conditions to have a superior effect compared to placebo in women with PPD, the majority of whom were on some form of antidepressant.[270] Indeed, several studies[271,272] have shown that open-label treatment of PPD with estradiol results in a rapid (2–3 weeks) onset of antidepressant action in PPD, similar to the time course observed in perimenopause-related depression.[273] Finally, one open study showed that the perinatal administration of estradiol in women at high risk for developing a PPD reduced the rate of onset of depression significantly compared to high-risk women not taking estrogen prophylactically.[274] A similar reduction in the rate of PPD was observed in women receiving postpartum sertraline (started on postpartum day 1–2) compared with those on placebo.[275] In addition to potential prophylactic effects of estrogen and sertraline in PPD, studies have examined the effects of nonpharmacologic interventions. A recent meta-analysis showed that contact with a midwife, counseling, and brief psychotherapy

provide a measurable level of primary prevention in this condition.[276] Finally, some studies, but not all, have suggested that lithium prophylaxis is effective in women at risk for relapse of their bipolar illness during the postpartum,[277] whereas a recent study could not demonstrate that sodium valproate (taken within 48 hours after birth) reduced the rate of recurrence during the postpartum period in women with a history of bipolar disorder.[278]

The decision to use any medication during the postpartum obviously must be made in the context of the woman's preference to nurse her child. Most currently available antidepressants including SSRIs have been reported to pass into the breast milk[279] and, therefore, may exert effects on the infant's developing brain. This possibility is strenghthened by the observation that the infants of women who use SSRIs during pregnancy show disruptions in several neurobehavioral meaasures.[280] While the safety of SSRIs during nursing remains to be established, considerable evidence suggests the adverse effects on child developement of untreated PPD. Consequently, treatment with SSRIs is still clinically justified. An SSRI combined with interpersonal therapy would be predicted to yield the best therapeutic effect given results of the few trials in PPD and the much larger literature in non-PPDs. Support is critical, and the use of patient-oriented support groups are anecdotally reported to be of value. Finally, if a woman has had PPD for the first time she should be counseled about the risks discussed below for developing subsequent depressions either related to the postpartum period and subsequent pregnancies or independent of any change in reproductive function.

Prognosis

Several studies have suggested that a past history of PPD predisposes women to develop episodes of PPD during subsequent pregnancies. In longitudinal prospective studies,[281–283] women with a past history of PPD had a significantly higher rate of PPD during a subsequent pregnancy than women without a history of PPD, specifically, 28–40% compared with 10%. These findings are corroborated by preliminary results from a longitudinal prospective study conducted at the Massachusetts General Hospital suggesting a higher relative risk of PPD during subsequent pregnancies in women with a prior episode of PPD (Lee Cohen, personal communication). Additionally, studies have identified potential negative effects of PPD on the developing infant.[284] Mediators of these effects are unknown but could include environmental (impaired mother), physiologic (increased cortisol), or pharmacologic (psychotropic medications) factors.

Perimenopausal Depression

Prevalence

Although the postmenopause has not been associated with an increased risk for developing depression in women,[285–287] depressive symptoms have been observed more frequently in perimenopausal women compared to postmenopausal women in some longitudinal, community-based studies.[288,289] Similarly, depressive-like symptoms have been evaluated in perimenopausal women attending gynecology clinics,[290–292] with one study observing that up to 45% of the sample had high scores (consistent with clinically significant depression) on standardized rating scales for depression.[292] In two additional studies from gynecology clinics, perimenopausal women reported significantly more symptoms than postmenopausal women.[290,291] Thus, both clinic-based surveys and epidemiologic studies suggest the relevance of the perimenopause in disturbances of mood in a substantial number of women.

Community-based surveys of the prevalence of affective syndromes (conditions meeting standardized diagnostic criteria, such as major or minor depression) have identified patterns of morbidity consistent with those reported in the surveys examining mood symptoms. Several epidemiologic studies examining gender and age-related differences in the 6 months to 1 year prevalence of major depression reported no increased prevalence of major depression in women at midlife

(age range approximately 45–55 years).[293,294] Nonetheless, several more recent studies that characterized the reproductive status of subjects demonstrated increased depressive syndromes during the perimenopause. The Study of Women's Health Across the Nation (SWAN)[295] employed a measure of "psychologic distress" as a proxy for the syndrome of depression by requiring that core depressive symptoms (sadness, anxiety, and irritability) persist for at least 2 weeks. Similar to the studies of depressive symptoms, SWAN's initial cross-sectional survey observed that perimenopausal women reported significantly more psychologic distress than either pre- or postmenopausal women (defined by self-reported menstrual cycle status).[295] Moreover, the increased psychologic distress appeared independent of the presence of vasomotor symptoms.[296] Two recent studies have found results similar to the SWAN data. First, Freeman et al.[297] identified an increased risk for significant depression (defined by elevated CES-D scale scores and the Primary Care Evaluation of Mental Disorders [PRIME MD][298]) during the perimenopause compared to the pre- or postmenopause. Moreover, this association remained after adjusting for several variables including past history of depression, severe premenstrual syndrome, poor sleep, and hot flushes. Levels of depression were increased relative to those found in the postmenopausal women; however, only 3% of the sample (approximately 10 women) were followed through to the postmenopausal phase. We (Schmidt et al., AJP, in press) followed 29 asymptomatic, premenopausal women until 6–12 months after their last menstrual period and demonstrated that the late perimenopause was associated with a 14-fold increase in the risk for developing major and minor depressions compared to a 31-year time period antecedent to the perimenopause. These data, therefore, provide additional evidence supporting the role of the perimenopause (the time when ovarian hormones change), but not the postmenopause, in the development of mood disorders in some women.

Episodes of both major and minor depression occur during the perimenopause (as well as the postpartum). Major depressions are well-established medical conditions; however, even within the psychiatric community some have questioned the clinical relevance of minor depressions. Minor depressions, by definition, have fewer and less severe symptoms than major depressions.[299,300] Nonetheless, they are associated with disability comparable to that of major depression.[301–303] In fact, major depressions of moderate severity are not distinguished from minor depressions by family history,[304,305] course (i.e., both major and minor depressions occur in the same subjects over their lifetime),[299,304] or biologic characteristics.[306,307] Finally, depressive symptoms as a comorbid condition (regardless of minor or major depression) may worsen the prognosis of several medical illnesses including heart disease.[308,309] Indeed, depressive symptoms increased the risk of death from cardiovascular disease by 50% after adjustment for an extensive list of other risk factors.

Diagnosis and Presenting Symptoms

Perimenopausal depression is a condition defined by the onset of depression at middle age in association with the onset of menstrual cycle irregularity or amenorrhea. Perimenopausal reproductive status is confirmed by the presence of menstrual cycle irregularity (or amenorrhea of less than 1 year in duration) and hormonal evidence of ovarian dysfunction. This latter criterion has been operationalized to include either a single elevated plasma FSH level or more persistent elevations of plasma FSH levels (e.g., three out of four $\geq$ 2 standard deviations above average FSH levels for women of reproductive age).[310] A recent workshop proposed detailed criteria for defining different stages of reproductive aging (Fig. 9-4) to more precisely characterize the perimenopausal transition.[311] DSM-IV[132] includes neither perimenopausal depression as a distinct mood disorder nor the perimenopause as a course specifier (as it does

Stages:	–5	–4	–3	–2	–1	0	+1	+2
						Final menstrual period (FMP) ▼		
Terminology:	Reproductive			Menopausal transition			Postmenopause	
	Early	Peak	Late	Early	Late*		Early*	Late
				Perimenopause				
Duration of stage:	Variable			Variable		(a) 1 yr	(b) 4 years	Until demise
Menstrual cycles:	Variable to regular	Regular		Variable cycle length (>7 days different from normal)	≥2 skipped cycles and an interval of amenorrhea (≥60 days)	Amen x 12 mos	None	
Endocrine:	Normal FSH		↑FSH	↑FSH			↑FSH	

*Stages most likely to be characterized by vasomotor symptoms   ↑ = Elevated

Figure 9-4.   Stages of Reproductive Aging Workshop (STRAW) criteria. (Source: Soules et al., Executive summary: stages of reproductive aging workshop (STRAW). *Fertility and Sterility*, 2001;76:874–878, with permission from American Society for Reproductive Medicine.

the postpartum). Perimenopausal depressions are not distinguished from major or minor depressive disorder on the basis of phenomenology, course, or family or personal history of mood disorder. As mentioned above, however, their distinction at present lies in the linkage of onset of depression to a period of reproductive endocrine change.

Pathophysiology

There have been no consistent abnormalities of reproductive or adrenal hormones identified in women with perimenopausal depression compared to controls. Nonetheless, the relevance of changes in pituitary-ovarian function to depression during the perimenopause is suggested by evidence that mood symptoms may change concordantly with FSH levels[312] and that estradiol therapy has acute mood enhancing effects in perimenopausal women with depression.[274,313]

Several additional reports indirectly support a role for reproductive hormones during the perimenopause in depression: hormone replacement beneficially affects both hot flushes and mood in hypogonadal women,[314–318] and lower gonadotropin levels are observed in postmenopausal depressed women compared to asymptomatic comparison groups.[319–322] The observed improvement in depressive symptoms after hormone replacement suggests the contribution of hypoestrogenism to mood disturbances, permitting the speculation that depressed perimenopausal women are relatively more estrogen deficient than nondepressed perimenopausal women. Perimenopausal women with depressive symptoms have been reported to have lower plasma estrone (E_1) levels[323] than nondepressed perimenopausal women, and an association has been described between increased plasma FSH levels and depression[324] (contradicting studies cited above). In contrast, three studies of perimenopausal and postmenopausal women observed either no diagnosis-related differences in plasma estradiol (E_2) and FSH[325] or no correlation between plasma levels of estrogens or androgens and severity of depressive symptoms.[326,327]

In a study of 21 women with their first episode of depression occurring during the perimenopause and 21 asymptomatic perimenopausal controls,[328] we were unable to confirm previous reports of lower basal plasma levels of LH[319–322] or E_1[323] in perimenopausal and postmenopausal women with depression compared to matched controls. Additionally, we observed no diagnosis-related differences in basal plasma levels of FSH, E_2, testosterone (T) or free T. Our data are consistent with those of Barrett-Connor et al.[326] and of Cawood et al.,[327] who found no correlation between mood symptoms and plasma levels of E_1, E_2, or T. Notwithstanding the limitations of basal hormonal measures, data suggest that depressed perimenopausal women are not distinguished from nondepressed perimenopausal women by being "more" estrogen deficient.

Age-related differences in the function of several physiologic systems have been observed in both animals and humans. Some of these differences may occur coincident with the perimenopause and, therefore, may potentially contribute to mood dysregulation at this time. Although, postmenopausal women have been reported to exhibit increased stress-induced plasma norepinephrine levels compared to premenopausal women,[288] only one previous study[323] reported elevated urinary cortisol levels in perimenopausal women reporting depressive symptoms compared to asymptomatic controls. Unfortunately, to date no systematic study has been performed of HPA axis function in perimenopausal women with a depressive syndrome.

A role for the adrenal androgen DHEA and its sulfated metabolite (DHEA-S) in the regulation of mood state has been suggested by both its effects on neural physiology[329–331] and its potential synthesis within the central nervous system.[332,333] Moreover, in clinical trials, DHEA administration has been reported to improve mood in some,[334–337] but not all, studies.[338] Finally, abnormalities of DHEA secretion have been observed in depressive disorders, with both increased and decreased levels observed relative to nondepressed controls.[339–342] DHEA's potential role in the onset of depression may be particularly relevant at midlife given the declining levels of DHEA production with aging and the accelerated decrease in DHEA levels reported in women, but not men, during midlife.[343,344] Plasma levels of DHEA and DHEA-S decline progressively from the third decade at a rate of about 2–3% per year,[345] reaching about 50% of peak levels during the fifth to sixth decades.[346–348] It is possible, therefore, that declining secretion (or abnormally low secretion) of DHEA may interact with perimenopause-related changes in ovarian function to trigger the onset of depression in some women. In fact, in perimenopausal and postmenopausal women, mood is correlated with DHEA(S) levels, with lower DHEA levels associated with more depression and higher levels associated with greater well-being.[326,327] We measured morning plasma levels of DHEA, DHEA-S, and cortisol in a separate sample of women with their first onset of depression during the perimenopause and in nondepressed women matched for age and reproductive status. Depressed perimenopausal women had significantly lower levels of both plasma DHEA and DHEA-S but not cortisol compared to controls.[328] Thus, DHEA, but not adrenal glucocorticoid secretion, differed in depressed and nondepressed perimenopausal women.

Finally, despite the antidepressant efficacy of estradiol and linkage of perimenopausal depression to a time of estrogen withdrawal, we still do not know by what mechanisms either declining estradiol levels or acute estradiol withdrawal induce changes in CNS function that increase a woman's vulnerability to develop depression.

Management

The therapeutic efficacy of estradiol in perimenopausal depression has been demonstrated in two randomized-controlled trials employing similar methodologies to define both depression and the perimenopause. We examined the efficacy of estradiol therapy (ET) in 34 women (approximately half of whom had no prior history of depression) with perimenopausal depression under double-blind, placebo-controlled conditions.[274] A full or partial therapeutic response was seen in 80% of subjects on estradiol and in 22% of those on placebo, consistent with the observed effect size for ET in a meta-analysis of studies examining estrogen's effects on mood[349] as well as with subsequent reports of estradiol's efficacy in perimenopausal[314,350] but not postmenopausal[351] depression. Neither baseline nor posttreatment estradiol levels predicted therapeutic response. Further, antidepressant efficacy was observed in women without hot flushes (suggesting that estrogen's effect on depression is not solely a product of its ability to reduce the distress of hot flushes). Additionally, the findings emphasize that the stage of reproductive senescence may predict response to estrogen, as originally reported by Appleby et al.[352] Thus, perimenopausal women who are undergoing changes in reproductive function may be more responsive to estrogen than postmenopausal women whose hormonal changes have long since stabilized.

The differential diagnosis of perimenopause-related depression includes the following: dysphoria secondary to hot flush-induced dysomnia; depression secondary to adverse or stressful life events; and medical illness presenting as depression. As such, from both research and clinical perspectives, the assessment of perimenopause-related depression should include a careful history focused on several phenomena: (1) the presence of somatic symptoms such as hot flushes or vaginal dryness, (2) the prominence of affective and behavioral symptoms relative to somatic symptoms such as hot flushes or vaginal dryness; (3) the presence of any past history of depression or hypomania, in order to compare the similarity of current symptoms to those of previous episodes; (4) possible comorbid or preexisting conditions; (5) the temporal relationship between the severity of mood symptoms and possible changes in menstrual cycle function (regular to irregular); (6) the current social and vocational context; (7) potential risk factors for osteoporosis, which may suggest the potential benefits of ET; and (8) the presence of contraindications to ET, such as a personal or family history of breast cancer. Reproductive status may be characterized by serial plasma FSH or estradiol levels to confirm the presence of the perimenopause and to track improvements in mood if they occur in relation to changes in pituitary-ovarian hormone secretion.

In addition to the possible antidepressant efficacy of estrogen in perimenopausal depression, some but not all,[353] studies have suggested that the response of peri-menopausal (Soares et al., personal communication) and post-menopausal women[354,355] to some antidepressants (i.e., SSRIs) may be enhanced by the use of estrogen replacement. Consequently, if not otherwise contraindicated, estrogen augmentation may be of value in the treatment of peri-menopausal-depressed women who ostensibly are antidepressant nonresponders.[356]

The decision to prescribe estradiol for perimenopausal depression must further be informed by associated risks and the availability of alternative treatments. The potential risks for cardiovascular morbidity, breast cancer, clotting abnormalities, and dementia after prolonged ET appear to offset the benefits of ET as a first-line treatment for depression.[357–361] Additionally, several adequate treatments for depression exist, and, therefore, the first-line medication for perimenopausal women presenting with depression is a traditional antidepressant such as a, SSRI. Nonetheless, treatment of depression with estradiol may be considered under the following circumstances: (1) as an alternative for the 50% or so of ambulatory depressed patients who fail to respond to a conventional, first-line intervention[361]; (2) women who refuse to take psychotropic agents or who otherwise prefer treatment with estradiol; (3) women who will undertake treatment with estradiol for other acute symptoms (e.g., hot flushes) and who, therefore, could delay treatment with antidepressants until determining whether estradiol treatment was sufficient. While estradiol treatment may no longer be appropriate for prophylaxis, it still is reasonably prescribed for acute symptoms and syndromes, including depression.[363,364] Finally, progestin may induce a dysphoric state in some women receiving ET; however, progestin-induced

dysphorias are not uniformly experienced in all women, nor are predictors of the dysphoric response known. Thus, progestins are not contraindicated in the presence of an antidepressant response to estradiol in a depressed perimenopausal woman.

Prognosis

The long-term courses of perimenopause-related major and minor depressions have not been described. However, two epidemiologic studies[294,365] have documented a poorer outcome and a more chronic course compared to male depressives in women with the onset of depression during mid to later life (greater than 45 years).

▶ COMORBIDITY AND COURSE MODIFICATION

Reproductive Endocrine-Related Mood Disorders

Few studies have systematically investigated the cooccurrence of PMD, PPD, and perimenopause-related depression. Nonetheless, several observations have suggested that these disorders cooccur with greater than expected frequency. First, clinic-based studies have reported that women with perimenopausal depressions or PPDs report higher rates of PMD than expected from the reported community prevalence rates for PMD.[366–368] Second, longitudinal studies have suggested that PMD is a risk factor for the development of both PPD and perimenopause-related depression.[369–371] Finally, several authors have hypothesized that these conditions share a common pathophysiology, due to some reports of the efficacy of estradiol therapy in all three conditions.[372–374] Nevertheless, problems interpreting these studies make it premature to infer that these are in fact variable expressions of the same disorder. For example, the definition of both PMD and PPD in these studies was often based upon a retrospective self-report, which has been demonstrated to be subject to considerable recall bias. Moreover, the definition of perimenopause-related depression in many of these studies included neither hormonal evidence of perimenopausal reproductive status nor a standardized definition for depression and, therefore, might overstate the association between these conditions (vs. primary affective disorders). For example, in a recent study (Richards et al., in press) we employed prospective daily ratings to define significant PMD and found that women developing a depression during the perimenopause were not distinguished from asymptomatic perimenopausal women by a higher rate of prospectively confirmed PMD.

The clustering of reproductive endocrine-related mood disorders in a subgroup of women could reflect the presence of an extreme sensitivity to the potential mood destabilizing effects of changes in gonadal steroids. Nevertheless, the comorbidity of reproductive endocrine-related mood disorders is not a uniformly experienced phenomenon, and many women will experience one condition without another. Thus, the presence of one disorder does not predictably increase the risk of the other conditions. Additionally, until more is learned about the relative comorbidities of these conditions in women with other non-reproductive-related depression, a general reproductive endocrine-related mood disorder phenotype is only speculation. The coprevalence of these conditions may simply reflect the high rate of comorbidity with primary (nonreproductive endocrine-related) depression.

Reproductive Endocrine-Related Mood Disorders and Primary Mood Disorders

Several studies have documented an increased prevalence of comorbid mood and anxiety disorders in women with reproductive endocrine-related mood disorders. Additionally, similarities in symptom profile, family histories, heritability, and treatment response characteristics have suggested that reproductive endocrine-related mood disorders represent variants of primary affective disorder.[375–376] Comorbidity among primary psychiatric disorders is not uncommon. In fact, the National Comorbidity Survey reported that more than 56% of the respondents who had at least one lifetime disorder had two or more disorders. Additionally, comorbidity is associated with a more serious course of illness and a greater utilization of health care services.[379]

PMD is a stable diagnosis and only rarely represents the prodrome of a primary affective disorder[236]; however, studies have identified that between 30 and 60% of women with PMD have another nonreproductive endocrine-related depression over the course of their lifetime (with elevated rates of comorbid anxiety and somatoform disorders).[241,380] Similarly, PPD is associated with an increased risk of developing a depression during both subsequent postpartum periods as well as nonpuerperal phases of life.[282,381,382] Studies also have identified a substantial association between the heritability of bipolar disorder and PPD.[383] The risk of a severe form of PPD, puerperal psychosis, is significantly greater in parous women with bipolar disorder who had a family history of puerperal psychosis in a first-degree relative compared to those parous women with bipolar disorder with no such family history (74% vs. 30%).[383] Thus, in addition to bipolar disorder itself, the puerperal trigger for an episode of bipolar disorder is an inherited phenomenon.

Studies systematically examining the presence of reproductive endocrine-related mood disorders in women with primary affective disorders suggest considerable overlap. The presence of concurrent symptoms makes it difficult to establish the presence of the reproductive endocrine-related mood disorder independent of the primary psychiatric disorder. Nonetheless, in one study[384] the prevalence of PMD in women with seasonal affective disorder (who experience a remission of their seasonal affective disorder (SAD) during the summer as part of their condition) was 46%, well above published community prevalence figures for PMD (5–11%). The increased prevalence rate of PMD in seasonal affective disorder is consistent with the possibility that the presence of a primary mood disorder conveys an increased vulnerability for developing episodes of depression during periods of reproductive endocrine change. As mentioned earlier, a history of recurrent unipolar and bipolar disorder increases risk of PPD, and several studies have suggested that a past history of depression may increase the risk as well for developing depression during the perimenopause. Nonetheless, recent longitudinal studies show that a past history of depression does not uniformly predict the onset of depression during the perimenopause, and in many women, the depression during the perimenopause is the first onset.[297,385]

Reproductive Endocrinology as a Course Modifier of Primary Affective Disorders

A series of observations have suggested that alterations in reproductive function may influence or alter the expression of the symptoms of primary psychiatric disorders. First, menstrual cycle phase-related symptom exacerbation has been noted, with several reports of psychiatric patients (manic or schizophrenic patients) whose symptoms increased in severity prior to menses and improved after menses.[386] For example, Malikian et al.[386] described the premenstrual worsening of the symptoms of depression in a sample of women with chronic depressive illness. Similarly, the potential influence of the menstrual cycle on the expression of the symptoms of psychiatric illness has been inferred from numerous reports of the disproportionate occurrence of suicide attempts and/or psychiatric admissions during the premenstrual phase.[388–391] However, a postmortem study employing endometrial biopsies as a method of dating menstrual cycle phase found no increased proportion of suicides occurring during the premenstruum.[392]

Altered reproductive function may influence the appearance (as opposed to the severity) of symptoms of a concurrent psychiatric disorder. The episodic symptoms of certain psychiatric disorders (e.g., panic disorder) are observed to be reduced during pregnancy and increased during the postpartum[393] and postmenopause.[394] On the other hand, prospective studies have failed to identify a menstrual cycle phase-related exacerbation or clustering of the symptoms of panic or anxiety in patients with panic disorder.[395–397]

There are several ways in which pregnancy could influence the course of a mood disorder. For example, many women stop medications during the first trimester, and the risk of recurrence of a mood disorder in the 6 months after antidepressant treatment is discontinued is estimated to be as high as 50%.[398–400] Although the effect of discontinuing antidepressant medication during or before pregnancy remains controversial, a recent prospective study reported relapse rates of 75% (most during the first trimester) after antidepressants were discontinued close to the time of conception.[401] Similarly, whether pregnancy reduces or increases the risk of relapse in bipolar illness in those women choosing to withdraw from mood stabilizers remains unclear, and case reports have described both outcomes.[402] Nevertheless, studies have documented the negative impact of withdrawing mood stabilizers in nonpregnant bipolar patients, suggesting that withdrawal from mood stabilizing treatment during pregnancy will increase the likelihood of relapse.[403,404] Clearly, women with bipolar illness have an increased risk of relapse during the postpartum period, with relapse rates ranging from 33 to 50%.[253,405] Finally, Altschuler et al.[405] also have emphasized the effects of pregnancy on plasma volume, hepatic microsomal enzyme activity, and/or renal clearance, which may impact on antidepressant levels; the clinical implications vis-à-vis likelihood of depressive relapse during pregnancy are unknown.

The second, midlife peak in the onset of bipolar disorder originally described by Angst (present in women but not men) was recently found to occur in both genders and, therefore, is unlikely related to specific effects of ovarian decline in the perimenopause.[407,408] Nonetheless, Kukopulos described the perimenopause and midlife in women as associated with an increased risk for the development of rapid cycling bipolar illness, a condition that is more prominent in women.[409] Finally, Freeman et al. suggest that women with bipolar illness who are not taking menopausal hormone therapy have an increased risk of developing a relapse of their symptoms during the perimenopause.[410]

► CONCLUSIONS

Familiarity with the role of the reproductive system in the regulation and dysregulation of mood is important for a variety of reasons. Substantial percentages of women suffer or will suffer from affective disorders triggered by reproductive events. These disorders, which are attended by disability and suffering, are frequently overlooked or misdiagnosed. Reproductive hormonal therapies are efficacious in these disorders and thus provide important additions to the psychotherapeutic armamentarium, either as primary or augmenting agents. As reproductive steroids are able to precipitate affective disturbances in some women, they provide a neurobiologic probe or tracer that can help elucidate the neurocircuitry and molecular physiology of affective state regulation; i.e., in contrast to classical affective disorders, the biologic trigger is known. Finally, reproductive endocrine-related mood disorders represent the convergent effects of a reproductive trigger and a susceptibility to experience affective dysregulation, since the same biologic trigger is without effect on mood in women lacking this susceptibility. As such, these disorders provide an unparalleled opportunity to uncover the biologic and environmental underpinnings of vulnerability to affective dysregulation.

REFERENCES

1. Yen SSC, Jaffe RB, Barbieri RL. *Reproductive Endocrinology: Physiology, Pathophysiology, and Clinical Management*. Philadelphia, PA: W.B. Saunders, 1999.
2. Csapo AI, Pulkkinen MO, Wiest WG. Effects of luteectomy and progesterone replacement therapy in early pregnant patients. *Am J Obstet Gynecol* 1973;115:759–765.
3. Miller WL. Steroid hormone biosynthesis and actions in the materno-feto-placental unit. *Clin Perinatol* 1998;25:799–817.
4. Weiss G. Endocrinology of parturition. *J Clin Endocrinol Metab* 2000;85:4421–4425.
5. Tulchinsky D, Hobel CJ, Yeager EM. Plasma estrone, estradiol, estriol, progesterone and 17-hydroxyprogesterone in human pregnancy. *Am J Obstet Gynecol* 1972;112:1095–1100.
6. Speroff L, Glass RH, Kase NG. *Clinical Gynecologic Endocrinology and Infertility*. Baltimore, MD: Williams & Wilkins, 1983.
7. McNeilly AS. Lactational endocrinology: The biology of lam. *Adv Exp Med Biol* 2002;503:199–205.
8. Couzinet B, Meduri G, Lecce MG, et al. The postmenopausal ovary is not a major androgen-producing gland. *J Clin Endocrinol Metab* 2001;86:5060–5066.
9. Santoro N, Brown JR, Adel T, et al. Characterization of reproductive hormonal dynamics in the perimenopause. *J Clin Endocrinol Metab* 1996;81:1495–1501.
10. Burger HG, Dudley EC, Hopper JL, et al. The endocrinology of the menopausal transition: A cross-sectional study of a population-based sample. *J Clin Endocrinol Metab* 1995;80:3537–3545.
11. Miller WL. Androgen biosynthesis from cholesterol to DHEA. *Mol Cell Endocrinol* 2002;198:7–14.
12. Huang C, Zhou J, Feng AK, et al. Nerve growth factor signaling in caveolae-like domains at the plasma membrane. *J Biol Chem* 1999;274:36707–36714.
13. Potter WZ, Manji HK. Catecholamines in depression: An update. *Clin Chem* 1994;40:279–287.
14. Booij L, Van der Does AJW, Riedel WJ. Monoamine depletion in psychiatric and healthy populations: Review. *Mol Psychiatry* 2003;8:951–973.
15. Neumeister A, Nugent AC, Waldeck T, et al. Neural and behavioral responses to tryptophan depletion in unmedicated patients with remitted major depressive disorder and controls. *Arch Gen Psychiatry* 2004;61:765–773.
16. Bremner JD, Vythilingam M, Ng CK, et al. Regional brain metabolic correlates of a-methylparatyrosine-induced depressive symptoms: Implications for the neural circuitry of depression. *J Am Med Assoc* 2003;289:3125–3134.
17. Manji HK, Drevets WC, Charney DS. The cellular neurobiology of depression. *Nat Med* 2001;7:541–547.

18. Drevets WC. Neuroimaging studies of mood disorders. *Biol Psychiatry* 2000;48:813–829.

19. Drevets WC. Neuroimaging and neuropathological studies of depression: Implications for the cognitive-emotional features of mood disorders. *Curr Opin Neurobiol* 2001;11:240–249.

20. Plotsky PM, Owens MJ, Nemeroff CB. Psychoneuroendocrinology of depression: Hypothalamic-pituitary-adrenal axis. *Psychoneuroendocrinology* 1998;21:293–307.

21. Gallagher M, Landfield PW, McEwen B, et al. Hippocampal neurodegeneration in aging. *Science* 1996;274:484–485.

22. Brown ES, Varghese FP, McEwen BS. Association of depression with medical illness: Does cortisol play a role? *Biol Psychiatry* 2004;55:1–9.

23. Gilbertson MW, Shenton ME, Ciszewski A, et al. Smaller hippocampal volume predicts pathologic vulnerability to psychological trauma. *Na Neurosci* 2002;5:1242–1247.

24. Woolley CS, Schwartzkroin PA. Hormonal effects on the brain. *Epilepsia* 1998;39:S2–S8.

25. McEwen BS, Alves SE, Bulloch K, et al. Ovarian steroids and the brain: Implications for cognition and aging. *Neurology* 1997;48(Suppl 7):S8–S15.

26. Rachman IM, Unnerstall JR, Pfaff DW, et al. Estrogen alters behavior and forebrain c-fos expression in ovariectomized rats subjected to the forced swim test. *Proc Natl Acad Sci USA* 1998;95:13941–13946.

27. Rubinow DR, Schmidt PJ, Roca CA. Estrogen-serotonin interactions: Implications for affective regulation. *Biol Psychiatry* 1998;44:839–850.

28. Pecins-Thompson M, Brown NA, Bethea CL. Regulation of serotonin re-uptake transporter mRNA expression by ovarian steroids in rhesus macaques. *MolBrain Res* 1998;53:120–129.

29. Clarke WP, Maayani S. Estrogen effects on 5-HT$_{1A}$ receptors in hippocampal membranes from ovariectomized rats: Functional and binding studies. *Brain Res* 1990;518:287–291.

30. Thomas ML, Bland DA, Clarke CH, et al. Estrogen regulation of serotonin (5-HT) transporter and 5-HT$_{1A}$ receptor mRNA in female rat brain. *Abstr Soc Neurosci* 1997;23:1501.

31. Sumner BEH, Fink G. Estrogen increases the density of 5-hydroxytryptamine$_{2A}$ receptors in cerebral cortex and nucleus accumbens in the female rat. *J Steroid Biochem Molec Biol* 1995;54:15–20.

32. Sumner BEH, Fink G. Effects of acute estradiol on 5-hydroxytryptamine and dopamine receptor subtype mRNA expression in female rat brain. *Mol Cell Neurosci* 1993;4:83–92.

33. Kendall DA, Stancel GM, Enna SJ. Imipramine: Effect of ovarian steroids on modifications in serotonin receptor binding. *Science* 1981;211:1183–1185.

34. Wissink S, van der Burg B, Katzenellenbogen BS, et al. Synergistic activation of the serotonin-1A receptor by nuclear factor-$_{KB}$ and estrogen. *Molecular Endocrinol* 2001;15:543–552.

35. Bethea CL, Mirkes SJ, Su A, et al. Effects of oral estrogen, raloxifene and arzoxifene on gene expression in serotonin neurons of macaques. *Psychoneuroendocrinology* 2002;27:431–445.

36. Gundlah C, Pecins-Thompson M, Schutzer WE, et al. Ovarian steroid effects on serotonin 1A, 2A and 2C receptor mRNA in macqaque hypothalamus. *Mol Brain Res* 1999;63:325–339.

37. McEwen BS, Alves SE. Estrogen actions in the central nervous system. *Endocr Rev* 1999;20:279–307.

38. Osterlund MK, Halldin C, Hurd YL. Effects of chronic 17β-estradiol treatment on the serotonin 5-HT$_{1A}$ receptor mRNA and binding levels in the rat brain. *Synapse* 2000;35:39–44.

39. Krezel W, Dupont S, Krust A, et al. Increased anxiety and synaptic plasticity in estrogen receptor β-deficient mice. *Proc Natl Acad Sci USA* 2001;98:12278–12282.

40. Lu NZ, Bethea CL. Ovarian steroid regulation of 5-HT$_{1A}$ receptor binding and G protein activation in female monkeys. *Neuropsychopharmacology* 2002;27:12–24.

41. Hery M, Becquet D, Francois-Bellan AM, et al. Stimulatory effects of 5HT1A receptor agonists on luteinizing hormone-releasing hormone release from cultured fetal rat hypothalamic cells: Interactions with progesterone. *Neuroendocrinology* 1995;61:11–18.

42. Maswood S, Stewart G, Uphouse L. Gender and estrous cycle effects of the 5-HT$_{1A}$ agonist, 8-OH-DPAT, on hypothalamic serotonin. *Pharmacol Biochem Behav* 1995;51:807–813.

43. Bethea CL, Lu NZ, Gundlah C, et al. Diverse actions of ovarian steroids in the serotonin neural system. *Front Neuroendocrinol* 2002;23:41–100.

44. Sumner BEH, Grant KE, Rosie R, et al. Effects of tamoxifen on serotonin transporter and 5-hydroxytryptamine$_{2A}$ receptor binding sites and mRNA levels in the brain of ovariectomized rats with or without acute estradiol replacement. *Mol Brain Res* 1999;73:119–128.

45. Fink G, Sumner BEH. Oestrogen and mental state. *Nature* 1996;383:306.

46. McQueen JK, Wilson H, Dow RC, et al. Oestradiol-17β increases serotonin transporter (SERT) binding sites and SERT mRNA expression in discrete regions of female rat brain. *J Physiol* 1996;495.P:114P.

47. Carlsson M, Svensson K, Ericksson E, et al. Rat brain serotonin: Biochemical and functional evidence for a sex difference. *J Neural Transm* 1985;63:297–313.

48. Carlsson M, Carlsson A. A regional study of sex differences in rat brain serotonin. *Prog Neuropsychopharmacol Biol Psychiatry* 1988;12:53–61.

49. Fischette CT, Biegon A, McEwen BS. Sex steroid modulation of the serotonin behavioral syndrome. *Life Sci* 1984;35:1197–1206.

50. Haleem DJ, Kennett GA, Curzon G. Hippocampal 5-hydroxytryptamine synthesis is greater in female rats than in males and more decreased by 5-HT$_{1A}$ agonist 8-OH-DPAT. *J Neural Transm* 1990;79:93–101.

51. Haleem DJ, Kennett GA, Whitton PS, et al. 8-OH-DPAT increases corticosterone but not other 5-HT$_{1A}$ receptor-dependent responses more in females. *Eur J Pharmacol* 1989;164:435–443.

52. Ebenezer IS, Tite R. Sex difference in the feeding responses of non-deprived rats to the 5-HT$_{1A}$ agonists 8-OH-DPAT and gepirone. *Methods Find Exp Clin Pharmacol* 1997;16:91–96.

53. Salamanca S, Uphouse L. Estradiol modulation of the hyperphagia induced by the 5-HT$_{1A}$ agonist, 8-OH-DPAT. *Pharmacol Biochem Behav* 1992;43:953–955.

54. Uphouse L, Salamanca S, Caldarola-Pastuszka M. Gender and estrous cycle differences in the response to the 5-HT$_{1A}$ agonist 8-OH-DPAT. *Pharmacol Biochem Behav* 1991;40:901–906.

55. Bethea CL. Colocalization of progestin receptors with serotonin in raphe neurons of macaque. *Neuroendocrinology* 1993;57:1–6.

56. Bethea CL. Regulation of progestin receptors in raphe neurons of steroid-treated monkeys. *Neuroendocrinology* 1994;60:50–61.

57. Nishizawa S, Benkelfat C, Young SN, et al. Differences between males and females in rates of serotonin synthesis in human brain. *Proc Natl Acad Sci USA* 1997;94:5308–5313.

58. Biver F, Lotstra F, Monclus M, et al. Sex difference in 5HT$_2$ receptor in the living human brain. *Neurosci Lett* 1996;204:25–28.

59. Ellenbogen MA, Young SN, Dean P, et al. Mood response to acute tryptophan depletion in healthy volunteers: Sex differences and temporal stability. *Neuropsychopharmacology* 1996;15:465–474.

60. Anderson IM, Parry-Billings M, Newsholme EA, et al. Dieting reduces plasma tryptophan and alters brain 5-HT function in women. *Psychol Med* 1990;20:785–791.

61. Walsh AES, Oldman AD, Franklin M, et al. Dieting decreases plasma tryptophan and increases the prolactin response to d-fenfluramine in women but not men. *J Affect Disord* 1995;33:89–97.

62. Goodwin GM, Murray CL, Bancroft J. Oral d-fenfluramine and neuroendocrine challenge: Problems with the 30 mg dose in men. *J Affect Disord* 1994;30:117–122.

63. Charney DS, Woods SW, Goodman WK, et al. Serotonin function in anxiety: II. Effects of the serotonin agonist MCPP in panic disorder patients and healthy subjects. *Psychopharmacology* 1987;92:14–24.

64. Murphy DL, Mueller EW, Hill JL, et al. Comparative anxiogenic, neuroendocrine, and other physiologic effects of m-chlorophenylpiperazine given intravenously or orally to healthy volunteers. *Psychopharmacology* 1989;98:275–282.

65. Su T-P, Schmidt PJ, Danaceau M, et al. Effect of menstrual cycle phase on neuroendocrine and behavioral responses to the serotonin agonist m-chlorophenylpiperazine in women with premenstrual syndrome and controls. *J Clin Endocrinol Metab* 1997;82:1220–1228.

66. Dinan TG, Barry S, Yatham LN, et al. The reproducibility of the prolactin response to buspirone: Relationship to the menstrual cycle. *Int Clin Psychopharmacol* 1990;5:119–123.

67. Bancroft J, Cook A, Davidson D, et al. Blunting of neuroendocrine responses to infusion of L-tryptophan in women with perimenstrual mood change. *Psychol Med* 1991;21:305–312.

68. O'Keane V, O'Hanlon M, Webb M, et al. d-Fenfluramine/prolactin response throughout the menstrual cycle: Evidence for an oestrogen-induced alteration. *Clin Endocrinol* 1991;34:289–292.

69. Lippert TH, Filshie M, Möck AO, et al. Serotonin metabolite excretion after postmenopausal estradiol therapy. *Maturitas* 1996;24:37–41.

70. Mueck AO, Seeger H, Kabpohl-Butz S, et al. Influence of norethisterone acetate and estradiol on the serotonin metabolism of postmenopausal women. *Horm Metab Res* 1997;29:80–83.

71. Sherwin BB, Suranyi-Cadotte BE. Up-regulatory effect of estrogen on platelet 3H-imipramine binding sites in surgically menopausal women. *Biol Psychiatry* 1990;28:339–348.

72. Best NR, Barlow DH, Rees MP, et al. Lack of effect of oestradiol implant on platelet imipramine and 5-HT2 receptor binding in menopausal subjects. *Psychopharmacology* 1989;98:561.

73. Halbreich U, Rojansky N, Palter S, et al. Estrogen augments serotonergic activity in postmenopausal women. *Biol Psychiatry* 1995;37: 434–441.

74. Schmidt PJ, Raju J, Danaceau M, et al. The effects of gender and gonadal steroids on the neuroendocrine and temperature response to m-chlorophenylpiperazine in leuprolide-induced hypogonadism in women and men. *Neuropsychopharmacology* 2002;27:900–812.

75. Moses EL, Drevets WC, Smith G, et al. Effects of estradiol and progesterone administration on human serotonin 2A receptor binding: A PET study. *Biol Psychiatry* 2000;48:854–860.

76. Nestler EJ, Terwilliger RZ, Duman RS. Chronic antidepressant administration alters the subcellular distribution of cyclic AMP-dependent protein kinase in rat frontal cortex. *J Neurochem* 1989;53:1644–1647.

77. Duman RS, Heninger GR, Nestler EJ. A molecular and cellular theory of depression. *Arch Gen Psychiatry* 1997;54:597–606.

78. Nibuya M, Nestler EJ, Duman RS. Chronic antidepressant administration increases the expression of cAMP response element-binding protein (CREB) in rat hippocampus. *J Neurosci* 1996;16:2365–2372.

79. Sohbrabji F, Miranda RC, Toran-Allerand CD. Estrogen differentially regulates estrogen and nerve growth factor receptor mRNAs in adult sensory neurons. *J Neurosci* 1994;14:459–471.

80. Zhou Y, Watters JJ, Dorsa DM. Estrogen rapidly induces the phosphorylation of the cAMP response element binding protein in rat brain. *Endocrinology* 1996;137:2163–2166.

81. Sohrabji F, Greene LA, Miranda RC, et al. Reciprocal regulation of estrogen and NGF receptors by their ligands in PC12 cells. *J Neurobiol* 1994;25:974–988.

82. Cardona-Gomez P, Perez M, Avila J, et al. Estradiol inhibits GSK3 and regulates interaction of estrogen receptors, GSK3, and beta-catenin in the hippocampus. *Mol Cell Neurosci* 2004;25:363–373.

83. Murphy DD, Cole NB, Segal M. Brain-derived neurotrophic factor mediates estradiol-induced dendritic spine formation in hippocampal neurons. *Proc Natl Acad Sci USA* 1998;95:11412–11417.

84. Ongur D, Drevets WC, Price JL. Glial reduction in the subgenual prefrontal cortex in mood disorders. *Proc Natl Acad Sci USA* 1998;95: 13290–13295.

85. Rajkowska G, Miguel-Hidalgo JJ, Wei J, et al. Morphometric evidence for neuronal and glial prefrontal cell pathology in major depression. *Biol Psychiatry* 1999;45:1085–1098.

86. Rajkowska G. Postmortem studies in mood disorder indicate altered numbers of neurons and glial cells. *Biol Psychiatry* 2000;48:766–777.

87. Watters JJ, Campbell JS, Cunningham MJ, et al. Rapid membrane effects of steroids in neuroblastoma cells: Effects of estrogen on mitogen activated protein kinase signalling cascade and c-fos immediate early gene transcription. *Endocrinology* 1997;138:4030–4033.

88. Garcia-Segura LM, Cardona-Gomez P, Naftolin F, et al. Estradiol upregulates Bcl-2 expression in adult brain neurons. *Neuroendocrinology* 1998; 9:593–597.

89. Gouras GK, Xu H, Gross RS, et al. Testosterone reduces neuronal secretion of Alzheimer beta-amyloid peptides. *Proc Natl Acad Sci USA* 2000; 97:1202–1205.

90. Zhang L, Li B, Zhao W, et al. Sex-related differences in MAPKs activation in rat astrocytes: Effects of estrogen on cell death. *Mol Brain Res* 2002;103:1–11.

91. Zhang L, Li B, Ma W, et al. Dehydroepiandrosterone (DHEA) and its sulfated derivative (DHEAS) regulate apoptosis during neurogenesis by triggering the Akt signaling pathway in opposing ways. *Mol Brain Res* 2002;98:58–66.

92. Berman KF, Schmidt PJ, Rubinow DR, et al. Modulation of cognition-specific cortical activity by gonadal steroids: A positron-emission tomography study in women. *Proc Natl Acad Sci USA* 1997;94:8836–8841.

93. Shaywitz SE, Shaywitz BA, Pugh KR, et al. Effect of estrogen on brain activation patterns in postmenopausal women during working memory tasks. *J Am Med Assoc* 1999;281:1197–1202.

94. Resnick SM, Maki PM, Golski S, et al. Effects of estrogen replacement therapy on PET cerebral blood flow and neuropsychological performance. *Horm Behav* 1998;34:171–182.

95. Maki PM, Resnick SM. Longitudinal effects of estrogen replacement therapy on PET cerebral

blood flow and cognition. *Neurobiol Aging* 2000; 21:373–383.

96. Redei E, Li L, Halasz I, et al. Fast glucocorticoid feedback inhibition of ACTH secretion in the ovariectomized rat: Effect of chronic estrogen and progesterone. *Neuroendocrinology* 1994;60:113–123.

97. Young EA, Altemus M, Parkinson V, et al. Effects of estrogen antagonists and agonists on the ACTH response to restraint stress in female rats. *Neuropsychopharmacology* 2001;25:881–891.

98. Dayas CV, Xu Y, Buller KM, et al. Effects of chronic oestrogen replacement on stress-induced activation of hypothalamic-pituitary-adrenal axis control pathways. *J Neuroendocrinol* 2000;12:784–794.

99. Komesaroff PA, Esler M, Clarke IJ, et al. Effects of estrogen and estrous cycle on glucocorticoid and catecholamine responses to stress in sheep. *Am J Physiol* 1998;275:E671–E678.

100. Burgess LH, Handa RJ. Chronic estrogen-induced alterations in adrenocorticotropin and corticosterone secretion, and glucocorticoid receptor-mediated functions in female rats. *Endocrinology* 1992;131:1261–1269.

101. Carey MP, Deterd CH, de Koning J, et al. The influence of ovarian steroids on hypothalamic-pituitary-adrenal regulation in the female rat. *J Endocrinol* 1995;144:311–321.

102. Viau V, Meaney MJ. Variations in the hypothalamic-pituitary-adrenal response to stress during the estrous cycle in the rat. *Endocrinology* 1991;129:2503–2511.

103. Marinari KT, Leschner AI, Doyle MP. Menstrual cycle status and adrenocortical reactivity to psychological stress. *Psychoneuroendocrinology* 1976;1:213.

104. Kirschbaum C, Kudielka BM, Gaab J, et al. Impact of gender, menstrual cycle phase, and oral contraceptives on the activity of the hypothalamic-pituitary-adrenal axis. *Psychosom Med* 1999;61:154–162.

105. Collins A, Eneroth P, Landgren B. Psychoneuroendocrine stress responses and mood as related to the menstrual cycle. *Psychosom Med* 1985;47:512–527.

106. Ablanalp JM, Livingston L, Rose RM, et al. Cortisol and growth hormone responses to psychological stress during the menstrual cycle. *Psychosom Med* 1977;39:158–177.

107. Long TD, Ellingrod VL, Kathol RG, et al. Lack of menstrual cycle effects on hypothalamic-pituitary-adrenal axis response to insulin-induced hypoglycaemia. *Clin Endocrinol* (Oxford) 2000; 52:781–787.

108. Galliven EA, Singh A, Michelson D, et al. Hormonal and metabolic responses to exercise across time of day and menstrual cycle phase. *J Appl Physiol* 1997;83:1822–1831.

109. Altemus M, Roca C, Galliven E, et al. Increased vasopressin and adrenocorticotropin responses to stress in the midluteal phase of the menstrual cycle. *J Clin Endocrinol Metab* 2001;86:2525–2530.

110. Roca CA, Schmidt PJ, Altemus M, et al. Differential menstrual cycle regulation of hypothalamic-pituitary-adrenal axis in women with premenstrual syndrome and controls. *J Clin Endocrinol Metab* 2003;88:3057–3063.

111. Keller-Wood M, Silbiger J, Wood CE. Progesterone attenuates the inhibition of adrenocorticotropin responses by cortisol in nonpregnant ewes. *Endocrinology* 1988;123:647–651.

112. Turner BB. Influence of gonadal steroids on brain corticosteriod receptors: A minireview. *Neurochem Res* 1997;22:1375–1385.

113. Patchev VK, Almeida OFX. Gonadal steroids exert facilitating and "buffering" effects on glucocorticoid-mediated transcriptional regulation of corticotropin-releasing hormone and corticosteroid receptor genes in rat brain. *J Neurosci* 1996;16:7077–7084.

114. Young EA. The role of gonadal steroids in hypothalamic-pituitary-adrenal axis regulation. *Crit Rev Neurobiol* 1995;9:371–381.

115. Smith SS, Gong QH, Hsu F-C, et al. GABA$_A$ receptor alpha-4 subunit suppression prevents withdrawal properties of an endogenous steroid. *Nature* 1998;392:926–930.

116. Spruce BA, Baylis PH, Burd J, et al. Variation in osmoregulation of arginine vasopressin during the human menstrual cycle. *Clin Endocrinol* 1985;22:37–42.

117. Smith R, Thomson M. Neuroendocrinology of the hypothalamo-pituitary-adrenal axis in pregnancy and the puerperium. *Baillieres Clin Endocrinol Metab* 1991;5:167–186.

118. Wisner KL, Stowe ZN. Psychobiology of postpartum mood disorders. *Semin Reprod Endocrinol* 1997;15:77–89.

119. Campbell EA, Linton EA, Wolfe CD, et al. Plasma corticotropin-releasing hormone concentrations during pregnancy and parturition. *J Clin Endocrinol Metab* 1987;64:1054–1059.

120. Kalimi M, Shafagoj Y, Loria R, et al. Anti-gluco-corticoid effects of dehydroepiandrosterone (DHEA). *Mol Cell Biochem* 1994;131:99–104.

121. Adams MR, Kaplan JR, Manuck SB, et al. Inhibition of coronary artery atherosclerosis by 17-beta estradiol in ovariectomized monkeys: Lack of an effect of added progesterone. *Arteriosclerosis* 1990;10:1051–1957.

122. Coyle JT, Duman RS. Finding the intracellular signaling pathways affected by mood disorder treatments. *Neuron* 2003;38:157–160.

123. Ramcharan S, Love EJ, Fick GH, et al. The epidemiology of premenstrual symptoms in a population-based sample of 2650 urban women: Attributable risk and risk factors. *J Clin Epidemiol* 1992;45:377–392.

124. Campbell EM, Peterkin D, O'Grady K, et al. Premenstrual symptoms in general practice patients: Prevalence and treatment. *J Reprod Med* 1997;42:637–646.

125. Hylan TR, Sundell K, Judge R. The impact of premenstrual symptomatology on functioning and treatment-seeking behavior: Experience from the United States, United Kingdom, and France. *J Womens Health Gend Based Med* 1999;8:1043–1052.

126. Gehlert S, Hartlage S. A design for studying the DSM-IV research criteria of premenstrual dysphoric disorder. *J Psychosom Obstet Gynaecol* 1997;18:36–44.

127. Deuster PA, Adera T, South-Paul J. Biological, social, and behavioral factors associated with premenstrual syndrome. *Arch Fam Med* 1999;8:122–128.

128. Halbreich U, Borenstein J, Pearlstein T, et al. The prevalence, impairment, impact, and burden of premenstrual dysphoric disorder (PMS/PMDD). *Psychoneuroendocrinology* 2003; 28:1–23.

129. Angst J, Sellaro R, Stolar M, et al. The epidemiology of perimenstrual psychological symptoms. *Acta Psychiatr Scand* 2001;104:110–116.

130. Lopez AD, Murray CCJL. The global burden of disease, 1990–2020. *Nat Med* 1998;4:1241–1243.

131. *Diagnostic and Statistical Manual of Mental Disorders*, 4th ed. Washington, DC: American Psychiatric Association, 1994.

132. *NIMH Premenstrual Syndrome Workshop Guidelines*. Rockville, MD: National Institute of Mental Health, (not published), 1983.

133. Rubinow DR, Hoban MC, Grover GN, et al. Changes in plasma hormones across the men-strual cycle in patients with menstrually related mood disorder and in control subjects. *Am J Obstet Gynecol* 1988;158:5–11.

134. Backstrom T, Sanders D, Leask R, et al. Mood, sexuality, hormones, and the menstrual cycle: II. Hormone levels and their relationship to the premenstrual syndrome. *Psychosom Med* 1983; 45:503–507.

135. Redei E, Freeman EW. Daily plasma estradiol and progesterone levels over the menstrual cycle and their relation to premenstrual symptoms. *Psychoneuroendocrinology* 1995;20:259–267.

136. Facchinetti F, Genazzani AD, Martignoni E, et al. Neuroendocrine changes in luteal function in patients with premenstrual syndrome. *J Clin Endocrinol Metab* 1993;76:1123–1127.

137. Backstrom T, Aakvaag A. Plasma prolactin and testosterone during the luteal phase in women with premenstrual tension syndrome. *Psychoneuroendocrinology* 1981;6:245–251.

138. Eriksson E, Sundblad C, Lisjo P, et al. Serum levels of androgens are higher in women with premenstrual irritability and dysphoria than in controls. *Psychoneuroendocrinology* 1992;17:195–204.

139. Bloch M, Schmidt PJ, Su T-P, et al. Pituitary-adrenal hormones and testosterone across the menstrual cycle in women with premenstrual syndrome and controls. *Biol Psychiatry* 1998;43:897–903.

140. Reame NE, Marshall JC, Kelch RP. Pulsatile LH secretion in women with premenstrual syndrome (PMS): Evidence for normal neuroregulation of the menstrual cycle. *Psychoneuroendocrinology* 1992;17:205–213.

141. Facchinetti F, Genazzani AD, Martignoni E, et al. Neuroendocrine correlates of premenstrual syndrome: Changes in the pulsatile pattern of plasma LH. *Psychoneuroendocrinology* 1990;15: 269–277.

142. Schmidt PJ, Grover GN, Roy-Byrne PP, et al. Thyroid function in women with premenstrual syndrome. *J Clin Endocrinol Metab* 1993;76:671–674.

143. Facchinetti F, Martignoni E, Petraglia F, et al. Premenstrual fall of plasma B-endorphin in patients with premenstrual syndrome. *Fertil Steril* 1987;47:570–573.

144. Chuong CJ, Coulam CB, Kao PC, et al. Neuropeptide levels in premenstrual syndrome. *Fertil Steril* 1985;44:760–765.

145. Taylor DL, Mathew RJ, Ho BT, et al. Serotonin levels and platelet uptake during premenstrual tension. *Neuropsychobiology* 1984;12:16–18.

146. Ashby CR Jr, Carr LA, Cook CL, et al. Alteration of platelet serotonergic mechanisms and monoamine oxidase activity in premenstrual syndrome. *Biol Psychiatry* 1988;24:225–233.

147. Malmgren R, Collins A, Nilsson CG. Patelet serotonin uptake and effects of vitamin B6-treatment in premenstrual tension. *Neuropsychobiology* 1987;18:83–88.

148. Veeninga AT, Westenberg HGM. Serotonergic function and late luteal phase dysphoric disorder. *Psychopharmacology* 1992;108:153–158.

149. Tulenheimo A, Laatikainen T, Salminen K. Plasma β-endorphin immunoreactivity in premenstrual tension. *Br J Obstet Gynaecol* 1987;94:26–29.

150. Hamilton JA, Gallant S. Premenstrual symptom changes and plasma β-endorphin/β-lipotropin throughout the menstrual cycle. *Psychoneuroendocrinology* 1988;13:505–514.

151. Schechter D, Strasser TJ, Endicott J, et al. Role of ovarian steroids in modulating mood in premenstrual syndrome. Abstracts of the Society of Biological Psychiatry 51st Annual Meeting 1996;646.

152. Halbreich U, Endicott J, Goldstein S, et al. Premenstrual changes and changes in gonadal hormones. *Acta Psychiatr Scand* 1986;74:576–586.

153. Wang M, Seippel L, Purdy RH, et al. Relationship between symptom severity and steroid variation in women with premenstrual syndrome: Study on serum pregnenolone, pregnenolone sulfate, 5α-pregnane-3,20-dione and 3α-hydroxy-5α-pregnan-20-one. *J Clin Endocrinol Metab* 1996;81:1076–1082.

154. Majewska MD, Harrison NL, Schwartz RD, et al. Steroid hormone metabolites are barbiturate-like modulators of the GABA receptor. *Science* 1986;232:1004–1007.

155. Smith SS, Gong QH, Li X, et al. Withdrawal from 3α-OH-5α-pregnan-20-one using a pseudopregnancy model alters the kinetics of hippocampal GABA$_A$-gated current and increases the GABA$_A$ receptor α4 subunit in association with increased anxiety. *J Neurosci* 1998;18: 5275–5284.

156. Ströhle A, Romeo E, Hermann B, et al. Concentrations of 3α-reduced neuroactive steroids and their precursors in plasma of patients with major depression and after clinical recovery. *Biol Psychiatry* 1999;45:274–277.

157. Romeo E, Brancati A, de Lorenzo A, et al. Marked decrease of plasma neuroactive steroids during alcohol withdrawal. *Clin Neuropharmacol* 1996; 19:366–369.

158. Romeo E, Strohle A, Spalletta G, et al. Effects of antidepressant treatment on neuroactive steroids in major depression. *Am J Psychiatry* 1998; 155:910–913.

159. Uzunova V, Sheline Y, Davis JM, et al. Increase in the cerebrospinal fluid content of neurosteroids in patients with unipolar major depression who are receiving fluoxetine or fluvoxamine. *Proc Natl Acad Sci USA* 1998; 95:3239–3244.

160. Bitran D, Purdy RH, Kellogg CK. Anxiolytic effect of progesterone is associated with increases in cortical allopregnanolone and GABA$_A$ receptor function. *Pharmacol Biochem Behav* 1993; 45:423–428.

161. Bitran D, Hilvers RJ, Kellogg CK. Anxiolytic effects of 3α-hydroxy-5α[β]-pregnan-20-one: Endogenous metabolites of progesterone that are active at the GABA$_A$ receptor. *Brain Res* 1991;561: 157–161.

162. Wieland S, Lan NC, Mirasedeghi S, et al. Anxiolytic activity of the progesterone metabolite 5α-pregnan-3α-ol-one. *Brain Res* 1991;565: 263–268.

163. Purdy RH, Morrow AL, Moore PH Jr, et al. Stress-induced elevations of gamma-aminobutyric acid type A receptor-active steroids in the rat brain. *Proc Natl Acad Sci USA* 1991;88:4553–4557.

164. Uzunov DP, Cooper TB, Costa E, et al. Fluoxetine-elicited changes in brain neurosteroid content measured by negative ion mass fragmentography. *Proc Natl Acad Sci USA* 1996;93: 12599–13604.

165. Griffin LD, Mellon SH. Selective serotonin reuptake inhibitors directly alter activity of neurosteroidogenic enzymes. *Proc Natl Acad Sci USA* 1999;96:13512–13517.

166. Sundstrom I, Andersson A, Nyberg S, et al. Patients with premenstrual syndrome have a different sensitivity to a neuroactive steroid during the menstrual cycle compared to control subjects. *Neuroendocrinology* 1998;67:126–138.

167. Sundstrom I, Nyberg S, Backstrom T. Patients with premenstrual syndrome have reduced sensitivity to midazolam compared to control subjects. *Neuropsychopharmacology* 1997;17:370–381.

168. Rapkin AJ, Morgan M, Goldman L, et al. Progesterone metabolite allopregnanolone in women with premenstrual syndrome. *Obstet Gynecol* 1997;90:709–714.

169. Monteleone P, Luisi S, Tonetti A, et al. Allopregnanolone concentrations and premenstrual syndrome. *Eur J Endocrinol* 2000;142:269–273.

170. Bicikova M, Dibbelt L, Hill M, et al. Allopregnanolone in women with premenstrual syndrome. *Horm Metab Res* 1998;30:227–230.

171. Girdler SS, Straneva PA, Light KC, et al. Allopregnanolone levels and reactivity to mental stress in premenstrual dysphoric disorder. *Biol Psychiatry* 2001;49:788–797.

172. Schmidt PJ, Purdy RH, Moore PH Jr, et al. Circulating levels of anxiolytic steroids in the luteal phase in women with premenstrual syndrome and in control subjects. *J Clin Endocrinol Metab* 1994;79:1256–1260.

173. Wang G-J, Volkow ND, Overall J, et al. Reproducibility of regional brain metabolic responses to lorazepam. *J Nucl Med* 1996;37:1609–1613.

174. Sundstrom I, Backstrom T. Citalopram increases pregnanolone sensitivity in patients with premenstrual syndrome: An open trial. *Psychoneuroendocrinology* 1998;23:73–88.

175. Rubinow DR, Schmidt PJ. The neuroendocrinology of menstrual cycle mood disorders. *Ann N Y Acad Sci* 1995;771:648–659.

176. Redei E, Freeman EW. Preliminary evidence for plasma adrenocorticotropin levels as biological correlates of premenstrual symptoms. *Acta Endocrinol* 1993;128:536–542.

177. Rosenstein DL, Kalogeras KT, Kalafut M, et al. Peripheral measures of arginine vasopressin, atrial natriuretic peptide and adrenocorticotropic hormone in premenstrual syndrome. *Psychoneuroendocrinology* 1996;21:347–359.

178. Rabin DS, Schmidt PJ, Campbell G, et al. Hypothalamic-pituitary-adrenal function in patients with the premenstrual syndrome. *J Clin Endocrinol Metab* 1990;71:1158–1162.

179. Facchinetti F, Fioroni L, Martignoni E, et al. Changes of opioid modulation of the hypothalamo-pituitary-adrenal axis in patients with severe premenstrual syndrome. *Psychosom Med* 1994; 56:418–422.

180. Eriksson E, Alling C, Andersch B, et al. Cerebrospinal fluid levels of monoamine metabolites: A preliminary study of their relation to menstrual cycle phase, sex steroids, and pituitary hormones in healthy women and in women with premenstrual syndrome. *Neuropsychopharmacology* 1994;11:201–213.

181. Parry BL, Gerner RH, Wilkins JN, et al. CSF and endocrine studies of premenstrual syndrome. *Neuropsychopharmacology* 1991;5:127–137.

182. Roy-Byrne PP, Rubinow DR, Hoban MC, et al. TSH and prolactin responses to TRH in patients with premenstrual syndrome. *Am J Psychiatry* 1987;144:480–484.

183. Lee KA, Shaver JF, Giblin EC, et al. Sleep patterns related to menstrual cycle phase and premenstrual affective symptoms. *Sleep* 1990;13:403–409.

184. Howard R, Mason P, Taghavi E, et al. Brainstem auditory evoked responses (BAERs) during the menstrual cycle in women with and without premenstrual syndrome. *Biol Psychiatry* 1992;32: 682–690.

185. Parry BL, Berga SL, Kripke DF, et al. Altered waveform of plasma nocturnal melatonin secretion in premenstrual syndrome. *Arch Gen Psychiatry* 1990;47:1139–1146.

186. Parry BL, Mendelson WB, Duncan WB, et al. Longitudinal sleep EEG, temperature, and activity measurements across the menstrual cycle in patients with premenstrual depression and in age-matched controls. *Psychiatry Res* 1989;30:285–303.

187. Sherwood RA, Rocks BF, Stewart A, et al. Magnesium and the premenstrual syndrome. *Ann Clin Biochem* 1986;23:667–670.

188. Rosenstein DL, Elin RJ, Hosseini JM, et al. Magnesium measures across the menstrual cycle in premenstrual syndrome. *Biol Psychiatry* 1994; 35:557–561.

189. Schmidt PJ, Nieman LK, Grover GN, et al. Lack of effect of induced menses on symptoms in women with premenstrual syndrome. *N Engl J Med* 1991;324:1174–1179.

190. Muse KN, Cetel NS, Futterman LA, et al. The premenstrual syndrome: Effects of "medical ovariectomy". *N Engl J Med* 1984;311:1345–1349.

191. Hammarback S, Backstrom T. Induced anovulation as a treatment of premenstrual tension syndrome: A double-blind cross-over study with GnRH-agonist versus placebo. *Acta Obstet Gynecol Scand* 1988;67:159–166.

192. Brown CS, Ling FW, Andersen RN, et al. Efficacy of depot leuprolide in premenstrual syndrome: Effect of symptom severity and type in a controlled trial. *Obstet Gynecol* 1994;84:779–786.

193. West CP, Hillier H. Ovarian suppression with the gonadotrophin-releasing hormone agonist goserelin (Zoladex) in management of the premenstrual tension syndrome. *Hum Reprod* 1994;9:1058–1063.

194. Hussain SY, Massil JH, Matta WH, et al. Buserelin in premenstrual syndrome. *Gynecol Endocrinol* 1992;6:57–64.

195. Mortola JF, Girton L, Fischer U. Successful treatment of severe premenstrual syndrome by combined use of gonadotropin-releasing hormone agonist and estrogen/progestin. *J Clin Endocrinol Metab* 1991;71:252A–252F.

196. Bancroft J, Boyle H, Warner P, et al. The use of an LHRH agonist, buserelin, in the long-term management of premenstrual syndromes. *Clin Endocrinol* 1987;27:171–182.

197. Mezrow G, Shoupe D, Spicer D, et al. Depot leuprolide acetate with estrogen and progestin add-back for long-term treatment of premenstrual syndrome. *Fertil Steril* 1994;62:932–937.

198. Sarno AP, Miller EJ Jr, Lundblad EG. Premenstrual syndrome: Beneficial effects of periodic, low-dose danazol. *Obstet Gynecol* 1987;70:33–36.

199. Halbreich U, Rojansky N, Palter S. Elimination of ovulation and menstrual cyclicity (with danazol) improves dysphoric premenstrual syndromes. *Fertil Steril* 1991;56:1066–1069.

200. Casson P, Hahn PM, VanVugt DA, et al. Lasting response to ovariectomy in severe intractable premenstrual syndrome. *Am J Obstet Gynecol* 1990;162:99–105.

201. Casper RF, Hearn MT. The effect of hysterectomy and bilateral oophorectomy in women with severe premenstrual syndrome. *Am J Obstet Gynecol* 1990;162:105–109.

202. Schmidt PJ, Nieman LK, Danaceau MA, et al. Differential behavioral effects of gonadal steroids in women with and in those without premenstrual syndrome. *N Engl J Med* 1998;338:209–216.

203. Muse K. Gonadotropin-releasing hormone agonist-suppressed premenstrual syndrome (PMS): PMS symptom induction by estrogen, progestin, or both. *Abstr Soc Gynecol Investig* 1989;118.

204. Ho HP, Olsson M, Westberg L, et al. The serotonin reuptake inhibitor fluoxetine reduces sex steroid-related aggression in female rats: An animal model of premenstrual irritability? *Neuropsychopharmacology* 2001;24:502–510.

205. Dimmock PW, Wyatt KM, Jones PW, et al. Efficacy of selective serotonin-reuptake inhibitors in premenstrual syndrome: A systematic review. *Lancet* 2000;356:1131–1136.

206. Steege JF, Stout AL, Knight DL, et al. Reduced platelet tritium-labeled imipramine binding sites in women with premenstrual syndrome. *Am J Obstet Gynecol* 1992;167:168–172.

207. Rojansky N, Halbreich U, Zander K, et al. Imipramine receptor binding and serotonin uptake in platelets of women with premenstrual changes. *Gynecol Obstet Invest* 1991;31:146–152.

208. Rapkin AJ, Edelmuth E, Chang LC, et al. Whole-blood serotonin in premenstrual syndrome. *Obstet Gynecol* 1987;70:533–537.

209. Ashby CR Jr, Carr LA, Cook CL, et al. Alteration of 5-HT uptake by plasma fractions in the premenstrual syndrome. *J Neural Transm* 1990;79: 41–50.

210. Bixo M, Allard P, Backstrom T, et al. Binding of [^{3}H]paroxetine to serotonin uptake sites and of [^{3}H]lysergic acid diethylamide to 5-HT$_{2A}$ receptors in platelets from women with premenstrual dysphoric disorder during gonadotropin releasing hormone treatment. *Psychoneuroendocrinology* 2001;26:551–564.

211. Yatham LN. Is 5HT$_{1A}$ receptor subsensitivity a trait marker for late luteal phase dysphoric disorder? A pilot study. *Can J Psychiatry* 1993;38:662–664.

211. Adell A, Celada P, Abellan MT, et al. Origin and functional role of the extracellular serotonin in the midbrain raphe nuclei. *Brain Res Rev* 2002;39: 154–180.

213. Sibille E, Pavlides C, Benke D, et al. Genetic inactivation of the serotonin$_{1A}$ receptor in mice results in downregulation of major GABA$_A$ receptor α subunits, reduction of GABA$_A$ receptor binding and benzodiazepine-resistant anxiety. *J Neurosci* 2000;20:2758–2765.

214. Kishimoto K, Koyama S, Akaike N. Presynaptic modulation of synaptic gamma-aminobutyric acid transmission by tandospirone in rat basolateral amygdala. *Eur J Pharmacol* 2000;407:257–265.

215. Koyama S, Kubo C, Rhee J-S, et al. Presynaptic serotonergic inhibition of GABAergic synaptic transmission in mechanically dissociated rat basolateral amygdala neurons. *J Physiol* 1999; 518(2):525–538.

216. Stutzmann GE, LeDoux JE. GABAergic antagonists block the inhibitory effects of serotonin in the lateral amygdala: A mechanism for modulation of sensory inputs related to fear conditioning. *J Neurosci* 1999;19:RC8 1–RC8 4.

217. Gulinello M, Gong QH, Li X, et al. Short-term exposure to a neuroactive steroid increases α4 GABA$_A$ receptor subunit levels in association with increased anxiety in the female rat. *Brain Res* 2001;910:55–66.

218. Halbreich U, Petty F, Yonkers K, et al. Low plasma gamma-aminobutyric acid levels during the late luteal phase of women with premenstrual dysphoric disorder. *Am J Psychiatry* 1996; 153:718–720.

219. Smith MJ, Adams LF, Schmidt PJ, et al. Effects of ovarian hormone on human cortical excitability. *Ann Neurol* 2002;51:599–603.

220. Sundstrom I, Ashbrook D, Backstrom T. Reduced benzodiazepine sensitivity in patients with premenstrual syndrome: A pilot study. *Psychoneuroendocrinology* 1997;22:25–38.

221. Freeman EW. Premenstrual syndrome: Current perspectives on treatment and etiology. *Curr Opin Obstet Gynecol* 1997;9:147–153.

222. Menkes DB, Coates DC, Fawcett JP. Acute tryptophan depletion aggravates premenstrual syndrome. *J Affect Disord* 1994;32:37–44.

223. Roca CA, Schmidt PJ, Smith MJ, et al. Effects of metergoline on symptoms in women with premenstrual dysphoric disorder. *Am J Psychiatry* 2002;159:1876–1881.

224. Endicott J, Halbreich U. Retrospective report of premenstrual depressive changes: Factors affecting confirmation by daily ratings. *Psychopharmacol Bull* 1982;18:109–112.

225. Altshuler LL, Hendrick V, Parry B. Pharmacological management of premenstrual disorder. *Harv Rev Psychiatry* 1995;2:233–245.

226. Rausch JL, Parry BL. Treatment of premenstrual mood symptoms. *Psychiatr Clin North Am* 1993; 16:829–839.

227. Steiner M, Steinberg S, Stewart D, et al. Fluoxetine in the treatment of premenstrual syndrome. *N Engl J Med* 1995;332:1529–1534.

228. Yonkers KA, Halbreich U, Freeman E, et al. Symptomatic improvement of premenstrual dysphoric disorder with sertraline treatment: A randomized controlled trial. *J Am Med Assoc* 1997; 278:983–988.

229. Thys-Jacobs S, Starkey P, Bernstein D, et al. Calcium carbonate and the premenstrual syndrome: Effects on premenstrual and menstrual symptoms. Premenstrual Syndrome Study Group. *Am J Obstet Gynecol* 1998;179:444–452.

230. Stone AB, Pearlstein TB, Brown WA. Fluoxetine in the treatment of late luteal phase dysphoric disorder. *J Clin Psychiatry* 1991;52:290–293.

231. Su T-P, Schmidt PJ, Danaceau MA, et al. Fluoxetine in the treatment of premenstrual dysphoria. *Neuropsychopharmacology* 1997;16:346–356.

232. Sundblad S, Modigh K, Andersch B, et al. Clomipramine effectively reduces premenstrual irritability and dysphoria: A placebo-controlled trial. *Acta Psychiatr Scand* 1992;85:39–47.

233. Wood SH, Mortola JF, Chan Y-F, et al. Treatment of premenstrual syndrome with fluoxetine: A double-blind, placebo-controlled, crossover study. *Obstet Gynecol* 1992;80:339–344.

234. Freeman EW, Sondheimer SJ, Rickels K, et al. Gonadotropin-releasing hormone agonist in treatment of premenstrual symptoms: With and without comorbidity of depression: A pilot study. *J Clin Psychiatry* 1993;54:192–195.

235. Roca CA, Schmidt PJ, Rubinow DR. A follow-up study of premenstrual syndrome. *J Clin Psychiatry* 1999;60:763–766.

236. Wittchen H-U, Becker E, Lieb R, et al. Prevalence, incidence and stability of premenstrual dysphoric disorder in the community. *Psychol Med* 2002;32:119–132.

237. Bloch M, Schmidt PJ, Rubinow DR. Premenstrual syndrome—evidence for symptom stability across cycles. *Am J Psychiatry* 1997;154:1741–1746.

238. Stout AL, Steege JF, Blazer DG, et al. Comparison of lifetime psychiatric diagnoses in premenstrual syndrome clinic and community samples. *J Nerv Ment Dis* 1986;174:517–522.

239. Hartlage SA, Arduino KE, Gehlert S. Premenstrual dysphoric disorder and risk for major depressive disorder: A preliminary study. *J Clin Psychiatry* 2001;57:1571–1578.

240. DeJong R, Rubinow DR, Roy-Byrne PP, et al. Premenstrual mood disorder and psychiatric illness. *Am J Psychiatry* 1985;142:1359–1361.

241. Cutrona CE. Causal attributions and perinatal depression. *J Abnorm Psychol* 1983;92:161–172.

242. Kumar R, Mordecai Robson K. A prospective study of emotional disorders in childbearing women. *Br J Psychiatry* 1984;144:35–47.

243. O'Hara MW. Social support, life events, and depression during pregnancy and the puerperium. *Arch Gen Psychiatry* 1986;43:569–573.

244. Wisner KL, Parry BL, Piontek CM. Postpartum depression. *N Engl J Med* 2002;347:194–199.

245. Brockington IF, Winokur G, Dean C. Puerperal psychosis. In: Brockington IF, Kumar R (eds.), *Motherhood and Mental Illness*. London: Academic Press, 1982, pp. 37–69.

246. Cox JL, Murray D, Chapman G. A controlled study of the onset, duration and prevalence of postnatal depression. *Br J Psychiatry* 1993;163: 27–31.

247. O'Hara MW, Schlechte JA, Lewis DA, et al. Controlled prospective study of postpartum mood disorders: Psychological, environmental, and hormonal variables. *J Abnorm Psychol* 1991;100: 63–73.

248. Josefsson A, Berg G, Nordin C, et al. Prevalence of depressive symptoms in late pregnancy and postpartum. *Acta Obstet Gynecol Scand* 2001; 80:251–255.

249. Evans J, Heron J, Francomb H, et al. Cohort study of depressed mood during pregnancy and after childbirth. *Br Med J* 2001;323:257–260.

250. Yonkers KA, Ramin SM, Rush AJ, et al. Onset and persistence of postpartum depression in an inner-city maternal health clinic system. *Am J Psychiatry* 2001;158:1856–1863.

251. Halbreich U. Prevalence of mood symptoms and depressions during pregnancy: Implications for clinical practice and research. *CNS Spectr* 2004;9:177–184.

252. Kendell RE, Chalmers JC, Platz C. Epidemiology of puerperal psychoses. *Br J Psychiatry* 1987; 150:662–673.

253. Nolen-Hoeksema S, Grayson C, Larson J. Explaining the gender difference in depressive symptoms. *J Person Soc Psychol* 1999;77:1061–1072.

254. Harris B, Lovett L, Smith J, et al. Cardiff puerperal mood and hormone study. III. Postnatal depression at 5 to 6 weeks postpartum, and its hormonal correlates across the peripartum period. *Br J Psychiatry* 1996;168:739–744.

255. Abou-Saleh MT, Ghubash R, Karim L, et al. Hormonal aspects of postpartum depression. *Psychoneuroendocrinology* 1998;23:465–475.

256. Wieck A, Kumar R, Hirst AD, et al. Increased sensitivity of dopamine receptors and recurrence of affective psychosis after childbirth. *Br Med J* 1991;303:613–616.

257. Maus M, Bertrand P, Drouva S, et al. Differential modulation of D1 and D2 dopamine-sensitive adenylate cyclases by 17β-estradiol in cultured striatal neurons and anterior pituitary cells. *J Neurochem* 1989;52:410–418.

258. Luisi S, Petraglia F, Benedetto C, et al. Serum allopregnanolone levels in pregnant women: Changes during pregnancy, at delivery, and in hypertensive patients. *J Clin Endocrinol Metab* 2000;85:2429–2433.

259. Pearson Murphy BE, Steinberg SI, Hu FY, et al. Neuroactive ring A-reduced metabolites of progesterone in human plasma during pregnancy: Elevated levels of 5α-dihydroprogesterone in depressed patients during the latter half of pregnancy. *J Clin Endocrinol Metab* 2001;86: 5981–5987.

260. Bloch M, Schmidt PJ, Danaceau M, et al. Effects of gonadal steroids in women with a history of postpartum depression. *Am J Psychiatry* 2000; 157:824–930.

261. Bonnin F. Cortisol levels in saliva and mood changes in early puerperium. *J Affect Disord* 1992;26:231–240.

262. O'Hara MW, Schlechte JA, Lewis DA, et al. Prospective study of postpartum blues: Biologic and psychosocial factors. *Arch Gen Psychiatry* 1991;48:801–806.

263. Kuevi V, Causon R, Dixson AF, et al. Plasma amine and hormone changes in "post-partum blues". *Clin Endocrinol* 1983;19:39–46.

264. Harris B, Lovett L, Newcombe RG, et al. Maternity blues and major endocrine changes: Cardiff puerperal mood and hormone study II. *Br Med J* 1994;308:949–953.

265. Feksi A, Harris B, Walker RF, et al. "Maternity blues" and hormone levels in saliva. *J Affect Disord* 1984;6:351–355.

266. Magiakou MA, Mastorakos G, Rabin D, et al. The maternal hypothalamic-pituitary-adrenal axis in the third trimester of human pregnancy. *Clin Endocrinol* 1996;44:419–428.

267. Magiakou MA, Mastorakos G, Rabin D, et al. Hypothalamic cortico-releasing hormone suppression during the postpartum period: Implications for the increase in psychiatric manifestations at this time. *J Clin Endocrinol Metab* 1996;81:1912–1917.

268. O'Hara MW, Stuart S, Gorman LL, et al. Efficacy of interpersonal psychotherapy for postpartum depression. *Arch Gen Psychiatry* 2000;57: 1039–1045.

269. Appleby L, Warner R, Whitton A, et al. A controlled study of fluoxetine and cognitive-behavioural counselling in the treatment of postnatal depression. *Br Med J* 1997;314:932–936.

270. Gregoire AJP, Kumar R, Everitt B, et al. Transdermal oestrogen for treatment of severe postnatal depression. *Lancet* 1996;347:930–933.

271. Ahokas A, Aito A, Rimon R. Positive treatment effect of estradiol in postpartum psychosis: A pilot study. *J Clin Psychiatry* 2000;61:166–169.

272. Ahokas A, Kaukoranta J, Wahlbeck K, et al. Estrogen deficiency in severe postpartum depression: Successful treatment with sublingual physiologic 17β-estradiol: A preliminary study. *J Clin Psychiatry* 2001;62:332–336.

273. Schmidt PJ, Nieman L, Danaceau MA, et al. Estrogen replacement in perimenopause-related depression: A preliminary report. *Am J Obstet Gynecol* 2000;183:414–420.

274. Sichel DA, Cohen LS, Robertson LM, et al. Prophylactic estrogen in recurrent postpartum affective disorder. *Biol Psychiatry* 1995;38:814–818.

275. Wisner KL, Perel JM, Piendl KS, et al. Prevention of postpartum depression: A pilot randomized clinical trial. *Am J Psychiatry* 2004;161:1290–1292.

276. Ogrodniczuk JS, Piper WE. Preventing postnatal depression: A review of research findings. *Harv Rev Psychiatry* 2003;11:291–307.

277. Yonkers KA, Wisner KL, Stowe Z, et al. Management of bipolar disorder during pregnancy and the postpartum period. *Am J Psychiatry* 2004;161:608–620.

278. Wisner KL, Hanusa BH, Peindl KS, et al. Prevention of postpartum episodes in women with bipolar disorder. *Biol Psychiatry* 2004;56: 592–596.

279. Burt VK, Suri R, Altschuler L, et al. The use of psychotropic medications during breast-feeding. *Am J Psychiatry* 2001;158:1001–1009.

280. Zeskind PS, Stephens LE. Maternal selective serotonin reuptake use during pregnancy and new born neurobehavior, *Pediatrics* 2004;113: 368–375.

281. Marks MN, Wieck A, Checkley SA, et al. Contribution of psychological and social factors to psychotic and non-psychotic relapse after childbirth in women with previous histories of affective disorders. *J Affect Disord* 1992;29:253–263.

282. Davidson J, Robertson E. A follow-up study of post partum illness, 1946–1978. *Acta Psychiatr Scand* 1985;71:451–457.

283. Garvey MJ, Tuason VB, Lumry AE, et al. Occurrence of depression in the postpartum state. *J Affect Disord* 1983;5:97–101.

284. Grace SL, Evindar A, Stewart DE. The effect of postpartum depression on child cognitive development and behavior: A review and critical analysis of the literature. *Arch Womens Men Health* 2003;6:263–274.

285. McKinlay JB, McKinlay SM, Brambilla D. The relative contributions of endocrine changes and social circumstances to depression in mid-aged women. *J Health Soc Behav* 1987;28: 345–363.

286. Kaufert PA, Gilbert P, Tate R. The Manitoba project: A re-examination of the link between menopause and depression. *Maturitas* 1992;14:143–155.

287. Avis NE, Brambilla D, McKinlay SM, et al. A longitudinal analysis of the association between menopause and depression: Results from the Massachusetts Women's Health Study. *Ann Epidemiol* 1994;4:214–220.

288. Matthews KA. Myths and realities of the menopause. *Psychosom Med* 1992;54:1–9.

289. Hunter M. The South-East England longitudinal study of the climacteric and postmenopause. *Maturitas* 1992;14:117–126.

290. Stewart DE, Boydell K, Derzko C, et al. Psychologic distress during the menopausal years in women attending a menopause clinic. *Int J Psychiatry Med* 1992;22:213–220.

291. Dennerstein L, Smith AMA, Morse C, et al. Menopausal symptoms in Australian women. *Med J Aust* 1993;159:232–236.

292. Hay AG, Bancroft J, Johnstone EC. Affective symptoms in women attending a menopause clinic. *Br J Psychiatry* 1994;164:513–516.

293. Weissman MM, Leaf PJ, Tischler GL, et al. Affective disorders in five United States communities. *Psychol Med* 1988;18:141–153.

294. Kessler RC, McGonagle KA, Swartz M, et al. Sex and depression in the National Comorbidity Survey I: Lifetime prevalence, chronicity and recurrence. *J Affect Disord* 1993;29:85–96.

295. Bromberger JT, Meyer PM, Kravitz HM, et al. Psychologic distress and natural menopause: A multiethnic community study. *Am J Publ Health* 2001;91:1435–1442.

296. Avis NE, Stellato R, Crawford S, et al. Is there a menopausal syndrome? Menopausal status and symptoms across racial/ethnic groups. *Soc Sci Med* 2001;52:345–356.

297. Freeman EW, Sammel MD, Liu L, et al. Hormones and menopausal status as predictors of depression in women in transition to menopause. *Arch Gen Psychiatry* 2004;61:62–70.

298. Spitzer RL, Williams JBW, Kroenke K, et al. Utility of a new procedure for diagnosing mental disorders in primary care: The PRIME-MD 100 study. *J Am Med Assoc* 1994;272:1749–1756.

299. Judd LL, Rapaport MH, Paulus MP, et al. Subsyndromal symptomatic depression: A new mood disorder? *J Clin Psychiatry* 1994;55: 18–28.

300. Rapaport MH, Judd LL, Schettler PJ, et al. A descriptive analysis of minor depression. *Am J Psychiatry* 2002;159:637–643.

301. Judd LL, Schettler PJ, Akiskal HS. The prevalence, clinical relevance, and public health significance of subthreshold depressions. *Psychiatr Clin North Am* 2002;25:685–698.

302. Broadhead WE, Blazer DG, George LK, et al. Depression, disability days, and days lost from work in a prospective epidemiologic survey. *J Am Med Assoc* 1990;264:2524–2528.

303. Judd LL, Paulus MP, Wells KB, et al. Socioeconomic burden of subsyndromal depressive symptoms and major depression in a sample of the general population. *Am J Psychiatry* 1996; 153:1411–1417.

304. Angst J. Minor and recurrent brief depression. In: Akiskal HS, Cassano GB (eds.), *Dysthymia and the Spectrum of Chronic Depressions*. New York: The Guilford Press, 1997, pp. 183–190.

305. Kendler KS, Gardner CO Jr. Boundaries of major depression: An evaluation of DSM-IV criteria. *Am J Psychiatry* 1998;155:172–177.

306. Akiskal HS, Judd LL, Gillin C, et al. Subthreshold depressions: Clinical and polysomnographic validation of dysthymic, residual and masked forms. *J Affect Disord* 1997;45:53–63.

307. Kumar A, Jin Z, Bilker W, et al. Late-onset minor and major depression: Early evidence for common neuroanatomical substrates detected by using MRI. *Proc Natl Acad Sci USA* 1998;95: 7654–7658.

308. Carney RM, Rich MW, Freedland KE, et al. Major depressive disorder predicts cardiac events in patients with coronary artery disease. *Psychosom Med* 1988;50:627–633.

309. Frasure-Smith N, Lesperance F, Talajic M. Depression following myocardial infarction: Impact on 6-month survival. *J Am Med Assoc* 1993;270:1819–1825.

310. Schmidt PJ, Rubinow DR. Mood and the perimenopause. *Contemp Ob Gyn* 1994;39:68–75.

311. Soules MR, Sherman S, Parrott E, et al. Stages of Reproductive Aging Workshop (STRAW). *J Womens Health Gend Based Med* 2001;10:843–848.

312. Daly RC, Danaceau MA, Rubinow DR, et al. Concordant restoration of ovarian function and mood in perimenopausal depression. *Am J Psychiatry* 2003;160:1842–1846.

313. Soares CD, Almeida OP, Joffe H, et al. Efficacy of estradiol for the treatment of depressive disorders in perimenopausal women: A double-blind, randomized, placebo-controlled trial. *Arch Gen Psychiatry* 2001;58:529–534.

314. Steingold KA, Laufer L, Chetkowski RJ, et al. Treatment of hot flashes with transdermal estradiol administration. *J Clin Endocrinol Metab* 1985;61:627–632.

315. Brincat M, Studd JWW, O'Dowd T, et al. Subcutaneous hormone implants for the control of climacteric symptoms: A prospective study. *Lancet* 1984;1:16–18.

316. Montgomery JC, Brincat M, Tapp A, et al. Effect of oestrogen and testosterone implants on psychological disorders in the climacteric. *Lancet* 1987;1:297–299.

317. Ditkoff EC, Crary WG, Cristo M, et al. Estrogen improves psychological function in asymptomatic postmenopausal women. *Obstet Gynecol* 1991;78:991–995.

318. Sherwin BB, Gelfand MM. Differential symptom response to parenteral estrogen and/or androgen administration in the surgical menopause. *Am J Obstet Gynecol* 1985;151:153–160.

319. Brambilla F, Maggioni M, Ferrari E, et al. Tonic and dynamic gonadotropin secretion in depressive and normothymic phases of affective disorders. *Psychiatry Res* 1990;32:229–239.

320. Amsterdam JD, Winokur A, Lucki I, et al. Neuroendocrine regulation in depressed postmenopausal women and healthy subjects. *Acta Psychiatr Scand* 1983;67:43–49.

321. Altman N, Sachar EJ, Gruen PH, et al. Reduced plasma LH concentration in postmenopausal depressed women. *Psychosom Med* 1975;37: 274–276.

322. Guicheney P, Léger D, Barrat J, et al. Platelet serotonin content and plasma tryptophan in peri- and postmenopausal women: Variations with plasma oestrogen levels and depressive symptoms. *Eur J Clin Investig* 1988;18:297–304.

323. Ballinger S. Stress as a factor in lowered estrogen-levels in the early postmenopause. *Ann N Y Acad Sci* 1990;592:95–113.

324. Huerta R, Mena A, Malacara JM, et al. Symptoms at perimenopausal period: Its association with attitudes toward sexuality, life-style, family function, and FSH levels. *Psychoneuroendocrinology* 1995;20:135–148.

325. Saletu B, Brandstatter N, Metka M, et al. Hormonal, syndromal and EEG mapping studies in menopausal syndrome patients with and without depression as compared with controls. *Maturitas* 1996;23:91–105.

326. Barrett-Connor E, von Muhlen D, Laughlin GA, et al. Endogenous levels of dehydroepiandrosterone sulfate, but not other sex hormones, are associated with depressed mood in older women: The Rancho Bernardo study. *J Am Geriatr Soc* 1999; 47:685–691.

327. Cawood EHH, Bancroft J. Steroid hormones, the menopause, sexuality and well-being of women. *Psychol Med* 1996;26:925–936.

328. Schmidt PJ, Murphy JH, Haq N, et al. Basal plasma hormone levels in depressed peri-menopausal women. *Psychoneuroendocrinology* 2002;27:907–920.

329. Majewska MD, Demirgören S, Spivak CE, et al. The neurosteroid dehydroepiandrosterone sulfate is an allosteric antagonist of the GABA$_A$ receptor. *Brain Res* 1990;526:143–146.

330. Compagnone NA, Mellon SH. Dehydroepiandrosterone: A potential signalling molecule for neocortical organization during development. *Proc Natl Acad Sci USA* 1998;95:4678–4683.

331. Baulieu E-E, Robel P. Dehydroepiandrosterone (DHEA) and dehydroepiandrosterone sulfate (DHEAS) as neuroactive neurosteroids. *Proc Natl Acad Sci USA* 1998;95:4089–4091.

332. Robel P, Baulieu E–E. Neurosteroids, biosynthesis and function. *Trends Endocrinol Metab* 1994; 5:1–8.

333. Zwain IH, Yen SSC. Dehydroepiandrosterone: Biosynthesis and metabolism in the brain. *Endocrinology* 1999;140:880–887.

334. Morales AJ, Nolan JJ, Nelson JC, et al. Effects of replacement dose of dehydroepiandrosterone in men and women of advancing age. *J Clin Endocrinol Metab* 1994;78:1360–1367.

335. Wolkowitz OM, Reus VI, Keebler A, et al. Double-blind treatment of major depression with dehydroepiandrosterone. *Am J Psychiatry* 1999;156:646–649.

336. Wolkowitz OM, Reus VI, Roberts E, et al. Dehydroepiandrosterone (DHEA) treatment of depression. *Biol Psychiatry* 1997;41:311–318.

337. Bloch M, Schmidt PJ, Danaceau MA, et al. Dehydroepiandrosterone treatment of mid-life dysthymia. *Biol Psychiatry* 1999;45:1533–1541.

338. Wolf OT, Neumann O, Hellhammer DH, et al. Effects of a two-week physiological dehydroepiandrosterone substitution on cognitive performance and well-being in healthy elderly women and men. *J Clin Endocrinol Metab* 1997; 82:2363–2367.

339. Goodyer IM, Herbert J, Altham PME, et al. Adrenal secretion during major depression in 8- to 16-year-olds, I. Altered diurnal rhythms in salivary cortisol and dehydroepiandrosterone (DHEA) at presentation. *Psychol Med* 1996;26: 245–256.

340. Goodyer IM, Herbert J, Altham PME. Adrenal steroid secretion and major depression in 8- to 16-year-olds, III. Influence of cortisol/DHEA ratio at presentation on subsequent rates of disappointing life events and persistent major depression. *Psychological Medicine* 1998;28: 265–273.

341. Ferrari E, Locatelli M, Arcaini A, et al. Chronobiological study of some neuroendocrine features of major depression in elderly people. Abstracts of the 79th Annual Meeting of the Endocrine Society, 1997.

342. Heuser I, Deuschle M, Luppa P, et al. Increased diurnal plasma concentrations of dehydroepiandrosterone in depressed patients. *J Clin Endocrinol Metab* 1998;83:3130–3133.

343. Laughlin GA, Barrett-Connor E. Sexual dimorphism in the influence of advanced aging on adrenal hormone levels: The Rancho Bernardo study. *J Clin Endocrinol Metab* 2000;85:3561–3568.

344. Cumming DC, Rebar RW, Hopper BR, et al. Evidence for an influence of the ovary on circulating dehydroepiandrosterone sulfate levels. *J Clin Endocrinol Metab* 1982;54:1069–1071.

345. Gray A, Feldman HA, McKinlay JB, et al. Age, disease and changing sex hormone levels in middle-aged men: Results of the Massachusetts male aging study. *J Clin Endocrinol Metab* 1991; 73:1016–1023.

346. Orentreich N, Brind JL, Rizer RL, et al. Age changes and sex differences in serum dehydroepiandrosterone sulfate concentrations throughout adulthood. *J Clin Endocrinol Metab* 1984;59:551–555.

347. Orentreich N, Brind JL, Vogelman JH, et al. Long-term longitudinal measurements of plasma dehydroepiandrosterone sulfate in normal men. *J Clin Endocrinol Metab* 1992;75:1002–1004.

348. Belanger A, Candas B, Dupont A, et al. Changes in serum concentrations of conjugated and unconjugated steroids in 40- to 80-year-old men. *J Clin Endocrinol Metab* 1994;79:1086–1090.

349. Zweifel JE, O'Brien WH. A meta-analysis of the effect of hormone replacement therapy upon depressed mood. *Psychoneuroendocrinology* 1997;22:189–212.

350. Rasgon NL, Altshuler LL, Fairbanks LA, et al. Estrogen replacement therapy in the treatment of major depressive disorder in perimenopausal women. *J Clin Psychiatry* 2002;63:45–48.

351. Morrison MF, Kallan MJ, Ten Have T, et al. Lack of efficacy of estradiol for depression in

postmenopausal women: A randomized, controlled trial. *Biol Psychiatry* 2004;55:406–412.

352. Appleby L, Montgomery J, Studd J. Oestrogens and affective disorders. In: Studd J (ed.), *Progress in Obstetrics and Gynaecology*. Edinburgh: Churchill Livingstone, 1981, pp. 289–302.

353. Amsterdam J, Garcia-Espana F, Fawcett J, et al. Fluoxetine efficacy in menopausal women with and without estrogen replacement. *J Affect Disord* 1999;55:11–17.

354. Schneider LS, Small GW, Hamilton SH, et al. Estrogen replacement and response to fluoxetine in a multicenter geriatric depression trial. *Am J Geriatr Psychiatry* 1997;5:97–106.

355. Schneider LS, Small GW, Clary CM. Estrogen replacement therapy and antidepressant response to sertraline in older depressed women. *Am J Geriatr Psychiatry* 2001;9:393–399.

356. Cohen LS, Soares CN, Poitras JR, et al. Short-term use of estradiol for depression in perimenopausal and postmenopausal women: A preliminary report. *Am J Psychiatry* 2003;160: 1519–1522.

357. Writing Group for the Women's Health Initiative Investigators: Risks and benefits of estrogen plus progestin in healthy postmenopausal women: Principal results from the Women's Health Initiative randomized controlled trial. *J Am Med Assoc* 2002;288:321–333.

358. Shumaker SA, Legault C, Kuller L, et al. Conjugated equine estrogens and incidence of probable dementia and mild cognitive impairment in postmenopausal women: Women's health initiative memory study. *J Am Med Assoc* 2004;291: 2947–2958.

359. Espeland MA, Rapp SR, Shumaker SA, et al. Conjugated equine estrogens and global cognitive function in postmenopausal women: Women's health initiative memory study. *J Am Med Assoc* 2004;291:2959–2968.

360. Shumaker SA, Legault C, Rapp SR, et al. Estrogen plus progestin and the incidence of dementia and mild cognitive impairment in postmenopausal women: The Women's Health Initiative Memory Study: A randomized controlled trial. *J Am Med Assoc* 2003;289:2651–2662.

361. The Women's Health Initiative Steering Committee: Effects of conjugated equine estrogen in postmenopausal women with hysterectomy. The women's health initiative randomized controlled trial. *J Am Med Assoc* 2004;291:1701–1712.

362. Fava M, Abraham M, Alpert J, et al. Gender differences in Axis I comorbidity among depressed outpatients. *J Affect Disord* 1996;38:129–133.

363. Rubinow DR, Schmidt PJ. Hormone replacement therapy: The last waltz or a new step? *Science SAGE* [Online]. 2004.

364. Naftolin F, Taylor HS, Karas R, et al. The women's health initiative could not have detected cardioprotective effects of starting hormone therapy during the menopausal transition. *Fertil Steril* 2004;81:1498–1501.

365. Sargeant JK, Bruce ML, Florio LP, et al. Factors associated with 1-year outcome of major depression in the community. *Arch Gen Psychiatry* 1990;47:519–526.

366. Stewart DE, Boydell KM. Psychologic distress during menopause: Associations across the reproductive cycle. *Int J Psychiatry Med* 1993;23: 157–162.

367. Collins A, Landgren B-M. Reproductive health, use of estrogen and experience of symptoms in perimenopausal women: A population-based study. *Maturitas* 1995;20:101–111.

368. Soares CD, Almeida OP. Depression during the perimenopause. *Arch Gen Psychiatry* 2001;58: 306.

369. Dennerstein L, Lehert P, Burger H, et al. Mood and the menopausal transition. *J Nerv Ment Dis* 1999;187:685–691.

370. Harlow BL, Cohen LS, Otto MW, et al. Prevalence and predictors of depressive symptoms in older premenopausal women: The Harvard study of mood and cycles. *Arch Gen Psychiatry* 1999;56:418–424.

371. Warner P, Bancroft J, Dixson A, et al. The relationship between perimenstrual depressive mood and depressive illness. *J Affect Disord* 1991;23:9–23.

372. Smith RNJ, Studd JWW, Zamblera D, et al. A randomised comparison over 8 months of 100 μg and 200 μg twice weekly doses of transdermal oestradiol in the treatment of severe premenstrual syndrome. *Br J Obstet Gynecol* 1995;102:475–484.

373. Watson NR, Savvas M, Studd JWW, et al. Treatment of severe premenstrual syndrome with oestradiol patches and cyclical oral norethisterone. *Lancet* 1989;2:730–732.

374. Arpels JC. The female brain hypoestrogenic continuum from the premenstrual syndrome to menopause: A hypothesis and review of supporting data. *J Reprod Med* 1996;41:633–639.

375. Schmidt PJ, Rubinow DR. Parallels between premenstrual syndrome and psychiatric illness. In:

Smith S, Schiff I (eds.), *Modern Management of Premenstrual Syndrome*. New York: W.W. Norton & Company, 1993, pp. 71–81.

376. Endicott J, Amsterdam J, Eriksson E, et al. Is premenstrual dysphoric disorder a distinct clinical entity? *J Womens Health Gend Based Med* 1999; 8:663–679.

377. Endicott J. The menstrual cycle and mood disorders. *J Affect Disord* 1993;29:193–200.

378. Yonkers KA. Anxiety symptoms and anxiety disorders: How are they related to premenstrual disorders? *J Clin Psychiatry* 1997;58(Suppl 3): 62–67.

379. Kessler RC, McGonagle KA, Zhao S, et al. Lifetime and 12-month prevalence of DSM-III-R psychiatric disorders in the United States: Results from the National Comorbidity Survey. *Arch Gen Psychiatry* 1994;51:8–19.

380. Kim DR, Gyulai L, Freeman EW, et al. Premenstrual dysphoric disorder and psychiatric co-morbidity. *Arch Womens Ment Health* 2004;7:37–47.

381. Philipps LHC, O'Hara MW. Prospective study of postpartum depression: 4 1/2-year follow-up of women and children. *J Abnorm Psychol* 1991; 100:151–155.

382. Wisner KL, Perel JM, Peindl KS, et al. Timing of depression recurrence in the first year after birth. *J Affect Disord* 2004;78:249–252.

383. Jones I, Craddock N. Familiality of the puerperal trigger in bipolar disorder: Results of a family study. *Am J Psychiatry* 2001;158:913–917.

384. Praschak-Rieder N, Willeit M, Neumeister A, et al. Prevalence of premenstrual dysphoric disorder in female patients with seasonal affective disorder. *J Affect Disord* 2001;63:239–242.

385. Smith PJ, Haq MA, Rubinow DR. A longitudinal evaluation of the relationship between reproductive status and mood in perimenopausal women. *Am J Psychiatry*, in press.

386. Rubinow DR, Roy-Byrne PP. Premenstrual syndromes: Overview from a methodologic perspective. *Am J Psychiatry* 1984;141:163–172.

387. Malikian JE, Hurt S, Endicott J, et al. Premenstrual dysphoric changes in depressed patients. Abstracts of the American Psychiatric Association 142nd Annual Meeting 1989;128.

388. Dalton K. Comparative trials of new oral progestogenic compounds in treatment of premenstrual syndrome. *Br Med J* 1959;5162:1307–1309.

389. Janowsky DW, Gorney R, Castelnuovo-Tedesco P, et al. Premenstrual-menstrual increases in psychiatric admission rates. *Am J Obstet Gynecol* 1969;103:189–191.

390. Mandell AJ, Mandell MP. Suicide and the menstrual cycle. *J Am Med Assoc* 1967;200:792–793.

391. Tonks CM, Rack PH, Rose MJ. Attempted suicide in the menstrual cycle. *J Psychosom Res* 1968;11: 319–323.

392. Vanezis P. Deaths in women of reproductive age and relationship with menstrual cycle phase. An autopsy study of cases reported to the coroner. *Forensic Sci Int* 1990;47:39–57.

393. Metz A, Sichel DA, Goff DC. Postpartum panic disorder. *J Clin Psychiatry* 1988;49:278–279.

394. Smoller JW, Pollack MH, Wassertheil-Smoller S, et al. Prevalence and correlates of panic attacks in postmenopausal women: Results from an ancillary study to the Women's Health Initiative. *Arch Intern Med* 2003;163:2041–2050.

395. Cameron OG, Kuttesch D, McPhee K, et al. Menstrual fluctuation in the symptoms of panic anxiety. *J Affect Disord* 1988;15:169–174.

396. Cook BL, Noyes R Jr, Garvey MJ, et al. Anxiety and the menstrual cycle in panic disorder. *J Affect Disord* 1990;19:221–226.

397. Stein MB, Schmidt PJ, Rubinow DR, et al. Panic disorder and the menstrual cycle: Panic disorder patients, healthy control subjects, and patients with premenstrual syndrome. *Am J Psychiatry* 1989;146:1299–1303.

398. Kupfer DJ, Frank E, Perel JM, et al. Five-year outcome for maintenance therapies in recurrent depression. *Arch Gen Psychiatry* 1992;49:769–773.

399. Frank E, Kupfer DJ, Perel JM, et al. Three-year outcomes for maintenance therapies in recurrent depression. *Arch Gen Psychiatry* 1990;47: 1093–1099.

400. Prien RF, Kupfer DJ. Continuation drug therapy for major depressive episodes: How long should it be maintained? *Am J Psychiatry* 1986;143:18–23.

401. Cohen LS, Nonacs RM, Bailey JW, et al. Relapse of depression during pregnancy following antidepressant discontinuation: A preliminary prospective study. *Arc Womens Ment Health* 2004;7: 217–221.

402. Grof P, Robbins W, Alda M, et al. Protective effect of pregnancy in women with lithium-responsive bipolar disorder. *J Affect Disord* 2000;61:31–39.

403. Viguera AC, Nonacs R, Cohen LS, et al. Risk of recurrence of bipolar disorder in pregnant and nonpregnant women after discontinuing lithium maintenance. *Am J Psychiatry* 2000;157:179–184.

404. Viguera AC, Cohen LJ, Tondo L, et al. Protective effect of pregnancy in women with lithium-responsive bipolar disorder: Letter to the editor. *J Affect Disord* 2002;72:107–108.

405. Reich T, Winokur G. Postpartum psychoses in patients with manic depressive disease. *J Nerv Ment Dis* 1970;151:60–68.

406. Altshuler LL, Hendrick V, Cohen LS. Course of mood and anxiety disorders during pregnancy and the postpartum period. *J Clin Psychiatry* 1998;59(Suppl 2):29–33.

407. Angst J, Preisig M. Course of a clinical cohort of unipolar, bipolar and schizoaffective patients: results of a prospective study from 1959 to 1985.

Schweizer Archiv Fur Neurologie und Psychiatrie 1995;146:5–16.

408. Angst J. The course of affective disorders. II: Typology of bipolar manic-depressive illness. *Archiv Psychiatrie und Nervenkrankheiten* 1978;226:65–73.

409. Kukopulos A, Reginaldi D, Laddomada P, et al. Course of the manic-depressive cycle and changes caused by treatments. *Pharmako-psychiatr Neuropsychopharmakol* 1980;13:156–167.

410. Freeman MP, Wosnitzer Smith K, Freeman SA, et al. The impact of reproductive events on the course of bipolar disorder in women. *J Clin Psychiatry* 2002;63:284–287.

SECTION III

Cardiovascular and Cerebrovascular Disorders

CHAPTER 10

Cardiovascular Disease and Mood Disorders

KAREN E. JOYNT, K. R. R. KRISHNAN, AND CHRISTOPHER M. O'CONNOR

▶ INTRODUCTION

Depression and cardiovascular disease (CVD) are two of the nation's most prevalent health problems. Depression, affecting 18.8 million American adults annually,[1] accounts for direct and indirect costs totaling over $40 billion per year,[2] and is the leading cause of disability worldwide.[3] CVD, affecting 64.4 million Americans annually, is the leading cause of death and hospitalization in the United States, and was responsible for 931,108 deaths, 6.2 million hospital discharges, and $368.4 billion in spending in 2001.[4]

Depression is more prevalent in individuals with CVD than in the general population, may predispose to the development of CVD, and is independently predictive of poor outcomes in patients suffering from CVD.[5–7] The purpose of this chapter is to provide the clinician with an overview of the epidemiologic connection between CVD and depression, as well as to present the available research that might shed light on the mechanistic underpinnings of this linkage. In addition, this chapter will discuss the complexities of diagnosing depression in patients with CVD, and review studies that have investigated the treatment of depression in patients with CVD. Finally, this chapter will outline some of the areas in which future research

might be concentrated in order to better understand the nature of the connection between these two common and important conditions.

▶ DEMONSTRATING THE LINK BETWEEN CVD AND DEPRESSION

A number of studies have demonstrated that depression is more common in patients with CVD than in the general population. According to the National Institute of Mental Health, 5% of the adult population in a given year suffers from major depressive disorder (MDD).[1] In contrast, studies conducted within the last decade investigating depression in individuals with CVD have reported relatively consistent prevalence rates of 16–30%[8–21] (Table 10-1). Clearly, depression is a common and important problem within the CVD patient population. It should be noted, however, that it is somewhat problematic to compare studies because of methodological differences, including varied patient populations, a lack of information regarding the severity of patients' CVD, and the use of numerous diagnostic instruments. The difference in prevalence rates reported in inpatient populations versus outpatient populations deserves particular

▶ **TABLE 10-1** PREVALENCE OF DEPRESSION IN THE SETTING OF CARDIOVASCULAR DISEASE

Author (year)	N	Patient Population	Diagnostic Instrument	Prevalence of Depression
Barefoot et al. (1996)[8]	1250	Admitted for angiography, CAD present	Zung SDS	25.7% mild, 11.2% mod/sev
Burg et al. (2003)[9]	89	Admitted for nonemergent CABG	BDI	28.1%
Bush et al. (2001)[10]	271	Admitted for acute MI	BDI, interview	19.9% by BDI, 9.5% major by interview
Connerney et al. (2001)[11]	309	Post-CABG	BDI, DIS	20% major by DIS
Frasure-Smith et al. (1993)[12]	222	Admitted for acute MI	DIS	16%
Frasure-Smith et al. (1995)[13]	222	Admitted for acute MI	BDI	16%
Kaufmann et al. (1999)[14]	391	Admitted for acute MI	DIS	27.2%
Lane et al. (2001)[15]	288	Admitted for acute MI	BDI	30.9%
Lane et al. (2002)[16]	288	Admitted for acute MI	BDI	29.9%
Lesperance et al. (2000)[17]	430	Admitted for unstable angina	BDI	41.4%
Lesperance et al. (2002)[18]	896	Admitted for acute MI	BDI	23.5% mild, 8.8% mod/sev
Mayou et al. (2000)[19]	344	Admitted for acute MI	HAD	7.6% probable, 9.9% borderline
Penninx et al. (2001)[20]	2847	Community sample	CES-D, interview	17.8% minor, 2.4% major among those with cardiac disease
Strik et al. (2003)[21]	318	One month after first MI	SCL-90	47.1%

Abbreviations: BDI, Beck Depression Inventory; CABG, coronary artery bypass grafting; CAD, coronary artery disease; CES-D, Center for Epidemiological Studies Depression Scale; DIS, Diagnostic Interview Schedule; HAD, Hospital Anxiety and Depression Scale; MI, myocardial infarction; NS, nonsignificant; SCL-90, 90-item Symptom Check List; SDS, Self-Rating Depression Scale.

mention; while inpatient studies that have reported rates for both major and minor depression have shown major depression rates between 8 and 20%,[8,10,11,18] the single large community study reported a major depression rate of only 2.4%.[20]

Perhaps even more provocative are recent studies suggesting that depression might actually increase an individual's risk for the future development of CVD[20,22–34] (Table 10-2). The study with the longest follow-up enrolled 1190 male medical students and followed them for 37 years; this investigation showed that self-reported depression was associated with a relative risk (RR) of 2.12 for myocardial infarction (MI).[27] In a study by Ferketich et al., enrolling nearly 8000 patients with a mean age of 55, depression

▶ TABLE 10-2 IMPACT OF DEPRESSION ON THE DEVELOPMENT OF CARDIOVASCULAR DISEASE

Author (year)	N	Patient Population	Diagnostic Instrument	Follow-up (Mean or Median)	Primary Outcome	Relative Risk (Adjusted when Available) for Primary Outcome, vs. No Depression, P-values ≤ 0.05 Unless Otherwise Indicated
Anda et al. (1993)[22]	2832	Ages 45–77	GWS	12.4 years	Fatal and nonfatal CAD	1.50
Ariyo et al. (2000)[23]	4493	Age 65 and older	CES-D	6 years	Development of CVD, all-cause mortality	1.15 for CVD, 1.16 for mortality
Aromaa et al. (1994)[24]	5355	Ages 40–64	PSE	6.6 years	Fatal and nonfatal MI	2.62 in men, 1.90 in women
Barefoot and Schroll (1996)[25]	730	Born in 1914	MMPI	Max 27 years	Fatal and nonfatal MI	1.7 for 2-SD difference in depression score
Ferketich et al. (2000)[26]	7893	NHANES I participants, mean age 55	CES-D	8.3 years	CAD incidence and mortality	1.73 in women and 1.71 in men for CAD incidence, NS in women and 2.34 in men for CAD mortality
Ford et al. (1998)[27]	1190	Male only, enrolled at average age of 26	Self-reported depression	37 years	CAD incidence, MI	2.12 for CAD incidence, 2.12 for MI
Mendes de Leon et al. (1998)[28]	2812	Age 65 and older	CES-D	Max 9 years	CAD incidence, CAD mortality	1.03 per unit increase in CES-D score in women for both incidence and mortality, NS in men
Penninx et al. (1998)[29]	3701	Age 70 and older	CES-D	4 years	CVD events, CVD mortality	New depression: 2.07 for CVD events and 1.74 for CVD mortality in men, NS in women; chronic depression: NS
Penninx et al. (2001)[20]	2847	Age 55 and older	CES-D, DIS	4.2 years	CVD mortality	NS for minor depression, 3.9 for major depression
Pratt et al. (1996)[30]	1551	Age 18 and older	DIS	Max 12 years	MI	OR = 4.54
Schwartz et al. (1998)[31]	2960	Age 65 and older	CES-D	3 years	MI	2.23
Sesso et al. (1998)[32]	1305	Male only, ages 40–90	MMPI-2	7 years	Total CAD, total CAD and angina	NS for total CAD, 2.07 for total CAD and angina
Wassertheil-Smoller et al. (1996)[33]	4736	Age 60 and older, hypertensive	CES-D	Max 5 years	MI or stroke	Baseline CES-D NS, 1.2 for 5-unit increase in CES-D in women, NS in men
Whooley and Browner (1998)[34]	7518	Female only, age 67 and older	GDS	6 years	All-cause mortality, CVD mortality	2.14 for all-cause mortality, 1.8 for CVD mortality

Abbreviations: BDI, Beck Depression Inventory; CABG, coronary artery bypass grafting; CAD, coronary artery disease; CES-D, Center for Epidemiological Studies Depression Scale; CVD, cardiovascular disease; DIS, Diagnostic Interview Schedule; GDS, Geriatric Depression Scale; GWS, General Well-being Scale; MI, myocardial infarction; MMPI, Minnesota Multiphasic Personality Inventory; NS, nonsignificant; PSE, Present State Examination.

conferred a RR of about 1.7 for CAD incidence for both men and women, but an increased risk for CAD mortality was only found in men (RR = 2.34).[26] This may be in part due to the fact that women tend to develop CVD at a later age than men; therefore, their morbid events may not have been picked up in the follow-up period. A study by Whooley and Browner of 7518 women over the age of 67 showed a RR of 2.14 for all-cause mortality and 1.8 for CVD mortality among those who were depressed.[34] However, results have been inconsistent; Wasserthiel-Smoller et al. found a significant association in women but not in men,[33] while Penninx et al. showed significant results for men but not women, and for new but not chronic depression.[29] For the most part, these epidemiologic studies used patient self-report instruments to assess depression, and therefore may not be as highly specific as a diagnostic interview. The major advantage of these studies is their large size, increasing the studies' ability to detect an effect. It should also be noted, however, that studies of this type may suffer from publication bias, that is, the preferential reporting of analyses in which associations are found to be significant rather than analyses showing no linkage.

Depression may also confer a poor prognosis on patients with existing CVD[8–21] (Table 10-3). Although many of the studies are limited by a small number of events, authors have reported that depression is associated with a 1.5- to 4-fold increased risk of mortality. The largest inpatient study was done by Barefoot et al. in 1250 patients admitted for angiography; the authors found that mild depression was associated with a RR over more than 10 years of follow-up for cardiac mortality of 1.57, and that major depression was associated with a RR of 1.78.[8] In a group of 271 surgical patients, Bush et al. reported that the presence of any depression carried a RR for all-cause mortality in the 4 months following coronary artery bypass grafting of 3.5.[10] Lesperance et al. reported on 896 patients admitted for acute MI, and demonstrated over 5 years of follow-up that mild depression (RR = 2.35) and moderate to severe depression

(RR = 3.57) were both associated with an increased risk for cardiac mortality.[18] Here, too, however, there have been negative results. Lane et al. reported that depression had no impact on all-cause mortality at 12 months[15] or 3 years[16] in a group of 288 post-MI patients, while Mayou et al. demonstrated that a combined depression and anxiety score was not associated with outcomes over 6 months of follow-up for 344 post-MI patients.[19] As survival continues to improve in the immediate post-MI period, decreasing the number of annual events in the post-MI population, it is likely that larger sample sizes and longer follow-up periods will be needed to give the most accurate and complete data regarding the precise magnitude of the negative prognostic impact of depression in CVD.

In sum, the available evidence suggests that depression is common in patients with CVD, may increase the risk of developing CVD, and is an independent risk factor for poor outcomes in the presence of existing CVD. The logical next question, then, is why this should be the case.

▶ THE MECHANISTIC RELATIONSHIP BETWEEN CVD AND DEPRESSION

Despite the evidence that CVD and depression are epidemiologically linked, the mechanistic correlation between the two is not well understood. However, there are a number of potential mediators of this relationship, which are important to explore as we continue to seek ways to improve prognosis for individuals suffering from depression, CVD, or both. For example, pathophysiologic mediation may play a role; depression is associated with physiologic changes, including nervous system activation, cardiac rhythm disturbances, systemic and localized inflammation, and hypercoagulability, that negatively influence the cardiovascular system. In addition, psychosocial factors such as compliance, social support, and stress may contribute to the connection between these

▶ **TABLE 10-3** PROGNOSTIC VALUE OF DEPRESSION IN THE SETTING OF CARDIOVASCULAR DISEASE

Author (year)	N	Patient Population	Diagnostic Instrument	Follow-up	Primary Outcome	Relative Risk (Adjusted when Available) for Primary Outcome, vs. No Depression, P-values ≤ 0.05 Unless Otherwise Indicated
Barefoot et al. (1996)[8]	1250	Admitted for angiography, CAD present	Zung SDS	>11 years	Cardiac mortality	1.57 mild, 1.78 mod/sev
Burg et al. (2003)[9]	89	Admitted for nonemergent CABG	BDI	2 years	Cardiac mortality	23.16
Bush et al. (2001)[10]	271	Admitted for acute MI	BDI, interview	4 months	All-cause mortality	3.5 for any depression
Connerney et al. (2001)[11]	309	Post-CABG	BDI, DIS	12 months	Cardiac events	2.3
Frasure-Smith et al. (1993)[12]	222	Admitted for acute MI	DIS	6 months	All-cause mortality	4.29
Frasure-Smith et al. (1995)[13]	222	Admitted for acute MI	BDI	18 months	Cardiac mortality	OR = 6.64
Kaufmann et al. (1999)[14]	391	Admitted for acute MI	DIS	12 months	All-cause mortality	4.29 at 6 months, NS at 12 months
Lane et al. (2001)[15]	288	Admitted for acute MI	BDI	12 months	All-cause mortality	NS
Lane et al. (2002)[16]	288	Admitted for acute MI	BDI	3 years	Cardiac mortality, all-cause mortality	NS
Lesperance et al. (2000)[17]	430	Admitted for unstable angina	BDI	12 months	Cardiac death or nonfatal MI	OR = 6.73
Lesperance et al. (2002)[18]	896	Admitted for acute MI	BDI	5 years	Cardiac mortality	2.35 mild, 3.57 mod/sev
Mayou et al. (2000)[19]	344	Admitted for acute MI	HAD	6 months	All-cause mortality	NS for combined depression or anxiety
Penninx et al. (2001)[20]	2847	Community sample	CES-D, interview	4 years	All-cause mortality	1.6 minor, 3.0 major among those with cardiac disease
Strik et al. (2003)[21]	318	One month after first MI	SCL-90	3.4 years	Fatal or nonfatal MI	2.32

Abbreviations: BDI, Beck Depression Inventory; CABG, coronary artery bypass grafting; CAD, coronary artery disease; CES-D, Center for Epidemiological Studies Depression Scale; DIS, Diagnostic Interview Schedule; HAD, Hospital Anxiety and Depression Scale; MI, myocardial infarction; NS, nonsignificant; SCL-90, 90-item Symptom Check List; SDS, Self-Rating Depression Scale.

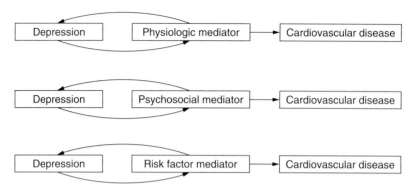

Figure 10-1. Possible mechanistic relationships between depression and CVD. Depression could influence CVD via causation of a physiologic, psychosocial, or risk factor change. Alternately, certain physiologic states, psychosocial influences, or risk factor clusters could cause both depression and CVD.

two conditions. Finally, depression is associated with the presence of cardiovascular risk factors such as smoking and hypertension. This section will explore these three main categories of potential mechanisms underlying the relationship between depression and CVD (Fig. 10-1).

Pathophysiologic Factors

Although depression is classified as a mental disorder, a large body of research suggests that it can have a powerful physical impact as well. Physical manifestations of depression include neurohormonal activation, cardiac rhythm disturbances, systemic and localized inflammation, and hypercoagulability. Each of these disturbances can in turn negatively impact the cardiovascular system, and may therefore play a role in explaining the observed connections between depression and CVD (Table 10-4).

Neurohormonal Activation

Studies have consistently documented hyperactivity of the hypothalamic-pituitary-adrenal (HPA) axis in depressed patients. Depressed patients exhibit hypercortisolemia, elevated corticotropin-releasing factor (CRF) in cerebrospinal fluid, decreased adrenocorticotropic hormone (ACTH) response to CRF challenge, and pituitary and adrenal gland enlargement.[7,35–37] In addition, depressed patients exhibit noncircadian, disorganized patterns of cortisol release,[38] and nonsuppression of cortisol secretion in response to dexamethasone.[35–37] The dexamethasone suppression test is reported to be abnormal in 80% of depressed patients,[39] and the magnitude of nonsuppression may be related to disease severity, particularly in relation to vegetative symptoms.[40]

HPA hyperactivity in turn augments sympathetic hyperactivity via central regulatory pathways. Sympathetic hyperactivity is manifest by elevated plasma norepinephrine (NE) and urinary catecholamine metabolites as well as a hypersecretory catecholamine response to orthostatic challenge, and has been demonstrated in patients suffering from depression.[41,42] For example, Wong et al. showed that depressed patients had significantly higher plasma NE than controls (137.46 pg/mL vs. 102.36 pg/mL, respectively, $P < 0.02$) and significantly higher plasma cortisol than controls (11.6 Êg/dL vs. 8.7 Êg/dL, $P < 0.02$), and that NE and cortisol levels were correlated.[43] Further, these patients exhibited inappropriately high levels of ACTH for their elevated cortisol levels, suggesting a dysregulation of the normal feedback loops of the HPA

▶ **TABLE 10-4** PHYSIOLOGIC PARAMETERS LINKING DEPRESSION AND CARDIOVASCULAR DISEASE

Physiologic Parameter Associated with Depression	Nature of Physiologic Change	Impact on Cardiovascular System or Outcomes
Neurohormonal activation	Hypercortisolemia Nonsuppression with dexamethasone challenge Elevated plasma norepinephrine	Acceleration of atherosclerosis Hypertension Elevated heart rate
Cardiac rhythm disturbances	Decreased HRV Decreased baroreflex cardiac control Increased QT dispersion Increased frequency of ventricular tachycardia	Susceptibility to arrhythmias Increased risk of sudden cardiac death
Inflammation	Elevated plasma concentration of inflammatory molecules (IL-1, IL-6, TNF) Elevated plasma concentration of acute-phase reactants (CRP)	Acceleration of atherosclerosis Instability of atherosclerotic plaques Increased risk of MI and stroke
Hypercoagulability	Increased platelet activation and aggregability Elevated plasma concentration of coagulation factors	Microvascular and/or macrovascular clotting Increased risk of MI and stroke

Abbreviations: CRP, C-reactive protein; IL-1, interleukin-1; IL-6, interleukin-6; MI, myocardial infarction; TNF, tumor necrosis factor.

axis. Veith et al. reported that depressed patients demonstrated elevated appearance but similar clearance of NE when compared with controls.[44] However, not all studies have found this association; a report by Carney et al. suggested no relationship between NE levels and depression in a study of 89 patients with CAD (NE levels for depressed vs. nondepressed patients: 280 pg/mL vs. 323 pg/mL, values log_{10} transformed, $P = 0.36$).[45]

Neurohormonal activation has been shown to speed the development of CVD. Elevated cortisol promotes the development of atherosclerosis and hypertension, and accelerates injury of vascular endothelial cells.[46,47] Elevations in plasma catecholamines lead to vasoconstriction, platelet activation, and elevated heart rate, all of which are damaging to the cardiovascular system.[48] Matthews et al. showed that the magnitude of stress-induced pulse pressure change predicted the appearance of carotid atherosclerosis in 254 initially healthy women, further evidence that sympathetic hyperresponsiveness might impact the development and progression of CVD.[49]

Whether or not the treatment of depression alters neurohormonal parameters is uncertain. Veith et al. reported that the administration of desipramine was associated with a decreased plasma NE appearance rate as well as an increased clearance rate in a group of 17 depressed patients.[44] In a small crossover study of healthy volunteers, Shores et al. found that short-term treatment with the selective serotonin reuptake inhibitor (SSRI) sertraline also led to a decreased plasma NE appearance rate.[50]

Therefore, we can conclude that depression is associated with augmentation of the HPA axis and sympathetic nervous activity, which in turn can damage the cardiovascular system, and may in part explain why depression is associated with the development of CVD and poor outcomes in established CVD. However, further research into the relationship between nervous system activation and outcomes, as well as research regarding the impact of pharmacologic and behavioral treatment of depression on neurohormonal parameters, is needed.

Rhythm Disturbances

Depression is a condition associated with autonomic dysregulation, as discussed above. Measures of heart rate variability (HRV) such as the standard deviation of normal-to-normal RR intervals (SDNN) can quantify the balance between sympathetic and parasympathetic influence on the heart; reduced HRV suggests proportionally reduced vagal modulation of the heart and therefore less parasympathetic protection from arrhythmias.[48,51] The combination of reduced parasympathetic protection and elevated sympathetic activity increases patients' susceptibility to arrhythmias triggered by inadequately opposed sympathetic stimulation.[52]

Depressed patients demonstrate significant disturbances in cardiac rhythm, suggesting dysregulation of the balance between parasympathetic cardioprotection and sympathetic stimulation.[53] Depressed patients have been found to have lower HRV on both linear and nonlinear measures[53,54]; further, some investigators have noted a dose-response effect, i.e., patients with more severe depression have lower HRV.[55] Carney et al., in a study of 674 post-MI subjects, demonstrated that depressed patients had significantly decreased HRV on four HRV indices as compared to nondepressed patients,[56] while Stein et al. showed that CAD patients who were moderately or severely depressed had a mean SDNN of 99 ms, whereas patients without depression had a mean SDNN of 119 ms.[57] Guinjoan et al. found that depression was associated with significantly lower high-frequency HRV, specifi-

cally indicative of impaired parasympathetic influence on the heart, in a group of older patients with acute coronary syndromes.[58]

Additional rhythm abnormalities have been noted in depressed patients as well; Watkins et al. showed that depressive symptoms were associated with a 30% reduction in baroreflex cardiac control, a measure of the body's ability to vary heart rate in response to blood pressure change.[59] Similarly, Yeragani et al. showed that depressed patients had higher QT variability (which may be a particularly poor prognostic sign in patients with concurrent reduction in HRV) than controls.[60] Nahshoni et al. demonstrated increased rate-corrected QT dispersion in a small sample of elderly patients with depression compared to elderly controls (81 ms vs. 43 ms, $P = 0.001$)[61]; QT dispersion is usually between 20 and 50 ms in normal individuals and between 60 and 80 ms in cardiac patients.[61] Dunbar et al., in a study of 176 patients with recent internal cardioverter defibrillator (ICD) implantation, found that mood disturbance was a significant predictor of arrhythmic events at 3 and 6 months even after controlling for left ventricular ejection fraction (LVEF), arrhythmia history, and medication use,[62] and Carney et al. showed that CAD patients with depression were significantly more likely to exhibit episodes of ventricular tachycardia during ambulatory monitoring than those without depression (RR = 8.2, 95% CI 2.14, 31.70).[63]

Rhythm disturbances are associated with a poor prognosis in patients with CVD. Sudden cardiac death accounts for 50% of deaths in patients with CVD,[64–66] and a majority of sudden deaths in patients with CVD result from ventricular arrhythmias.[67,68] Decreased HRV is a known risk factor for sudden death and ventricular arrhythmias in patients with CVD.[51,52]. For example, Kleiger et al. found that CVD patients with low HRV, defined as SDNN less than 50 ms, were 5.3 times as likely to die in 31 months of follow-up as the group with normal HR variability (SDNN > 100 ms)[69] and La Rovere et al. found that SDNN < 70 ms carried a RR of cardiac mortality of 3.2 in a group of 1284 post-MI patients.[70] Additionally, La Rovere et al. showed that low baroreflex sensitivity (<3.0 ms/mmHg) was associated with a RR of cardiac mortality of 2.8.[70] QT dispersion is also a negative prognostic sign; de Bruyne et al. followed a group of 5812 elderly patients and found that those in the highest tertile of QT dispersion had a twofold risk for cardiac death (RR = 2.5, $P < 0.05$) and sudden cardiac death (RR = 1.9, $P < 0.05$) when compared with those in the lowest tertile.[71] Similar findings have been noted in patients with known CVD,[72] although not all studies have supported this finding.[73]

Rhythm disturbances might have a major impact on mortality for patients with both depression and CVD; Frasure-Smith et al., following over 200 patients after MI, found that, while depressed patients had an odds ratio for mortality of 6.64 compared with nondepressed patients, depressed patients with a high frequency of premature ventricular contractions had an odds ratio for mortality of 29.1.[13] Much of the increased risk of mortality was a result of sudden death; the authors hypothesized that this increase might be a result of decreased HRV in the depressed patients in their sample.[13]

Evidence for the effect of treatment of depression on rhythm parameters is somewhat equivocal. The tricyclic antidepressants (TCAs) are known to have cardiac effects, including decreased HRV, and are contraindicated for patients with QT prolongation, heart block, or acute MI.[74,75] However, studies have suggested that the SSRIs have either a neutral[76,77] or even a beneficial effect[78] on rhythm, including increasing HRV. Roose et al., in a study of patients with CAD and depression, found that the TCA nortriptyline caused an increase in heart rate as well as a decrease in HRV, while the SSRI paroxetine had no effect on these measures.[76] McFarlane et al. found that 12 depressed post-MI patients demonstrated a recovery in HRV when treated with the SSRI sertraline that was similar to a nondepressed post-MI group, while 15 depressed post-MI patients who received placebo demonstrated continuing decline in HRV over the study period; there was no correlation between improvement of depressive symptoms and improvement in HRV measures.[78] In contrast, a recent study of sertraline in 369 depressed post-MI patients demonstrated no significant effect on ventricular arrhythmias, QT interval, or HRV; the treatment group had fewer cardiovascular events than the control group (14.5% vs. 22.4%), although the difference did not reach statistical significance.[77] Agelink et al. reported that nefazodone treatment was associated with decreases in mean resting heart rate and blood pressure, but had no impact on HRV.[79] Interestingly, Khaykin et al. showed that responders to treatment (i.e., those whose depressive symptoms improved) with either the TCA doxepin or the SSRI fluoxetine demonstrated increased HRV, while nonresponders showed a small decrease in HRV[80]; this finding raises the question of whether symptom remission rather than pharmacologic effects might be the mechanism underlying the effect of antidepressants on HRV. Supporting this hypothesis, Carney et al. showed that 16 sessions of cognitive behavioral therapy led to a decrease in heart rate as well as a significant increase in short-term HRV in severely depressed patients with stable CAD.[81]

Taken together, these findings suggest that depression is associated with rhythm disturbances that could predispose to arrhythmias, and may in part account for the deleterious effect of depression on prognosis in CVD. Additional research is needed to link alterations in rhythm to outcomes in studies of depressed patients with CVD, as well as to examine the impact of treatment of depression on mortality related to arrhythmic events.

Inflammation

Elevated plasma levels of proinflammatory cytokines are characteristic of depression.[82–86] These cytokines, such as interleukin (IL)-1, IL-6, and tissue necrosis factor-alpha (TNF-α), reflect the body's response to acute or chronic, localized or general stress, and may be signaled via a beta-adrenergic receptor mechanism.[84,87] The increased levels of inflammatory molecules seen in depressed patients may therefore represent a response to acute or chronic psychologic distress.[88] Maes et al., in a study of 115 patients, showed that plasma concentrations of IL-6 were more than twice as high in the depressed group as in controls (5.52 pg/mL vs. 2.50 pg/mL, $P =$ 0.00002)[89]; Sluzewska et al. replicated these findings in a study of 64 subjects (4.28 pg/mL vs. 1.24 pg/mL, $P < 0.0001$),[82] and Miller et al. in patients with CAD and depression versus patients with CAD alone (3.0 pg/mL vs. 1.9 pg/mL, $P =$ 0.007).[90] Interestingly, a recent report investigating a group of 53 healthy men without a diagnosis of major depression showed that the presence of even mild to moderate depressive symptoms was correlated with elevated inflammatory markers, suggesting that depression may have a harmful physiologic impact well before it becomes clinically apparent.[91] Musselman et al. showed that depressed cancer patients had IL-6 levels that were significantly higher than nondepressed healthy controls and nondepressed controls with cancer, but comparable to depressed healthy controls.[92] Appels et al. found that depression was associated with elevated IL-1 in angioplasty patients,[86] while Owen et al. similarly found elevated IL-1 in both major and postviral depression compared with both healthy and postviral controls.[93] Increased serum TNF concentrations in depressed patients were reported by Mikova et al.,[94] and increased interferon gamma by Seidel et al.[95] However, these studies have shown no association between severity of depression and degree of cytokine elevation, raising the possibility that elevated proinflammatory cytokines are a trait marker for depression rather than a state marker for current depression.[89,92,93]

Conversely, ILs and other cytokines might actually cause depression.[88] Patients undergoing immunotherapy with IL-1, IL-2, TNF, or interferon alpha for cancer or chronic viral infection tend to develop symptoms such as depressed mood, anxiety, anorexia, and fatigue that are independent of the primary illness.[84,96] Mood and cognitive facets of this syndrome have been shown to be responsive to SSRI treatment, while anorexia and fatigue are not, suggesting that

cytokines may mediate distinct components of depression via distinct mechanisms.[96]

It is also possible that ILs and other cytokines might affect the onset and progression of depression via local endothelial damage and ischemia rather than by systemic effects. Inflammatory hyperresponsiveness has been postulated to play a role in endothelial damage of the cerebral vasculature, and thus contribute to the development of a specific subtype of depression known as "vascular depression." Vascular depression is characterized by apathy, psychomotor changes, and cognitive impairment; it is more common in the elderly and less often associated with a family history of depression.[97–99] In both population studies and focused studies of depressed individuals, vascular changes, defined by lesions visualized on MRI, are associated with worse depressive symptoms.[98,99] Further, these vascular changes correlate with the degree of atherosclerosis present, supporting the likelihood of a common underlying process.[97] Steffens et al. recently conducted a prospective study, showing that cerebrovascular disease at baseline predicted the worsening of symptoms of depression over time.[99] Taylor et al. demonstrated that the degree of worsening of MRI-visualized lesions was correlated with patients' likelihood of having poor outcomes in depression, that is, in failing to reach and sustain remission of symptoms.[100] Thomas et al. showed that expression of intercellular adhesion molecule-1, a marker of ischemia-induced inflammation, is higher in the dorsolateral prefrontal cortex in depressed patients.[101] Taylor et al. found that MRI-visualized lesions were seen in the frontal cortices of depressed patients more often in their nondepressed counterparts.[102] These findings suggest that cerebrovascular disease, and resulting ischemia, can lead to inflammatory damage in brain areas implicated in depression.[101] Currently, there is no evidence to suggest that vascular depression is more common in patients with CVD than without; a correlation would lend further support to the idea that inflammation-accelerated atherosclerosis is the common underlying pathology in depression and CVD that could explain their association.

Proinflammatory cytokines have been implicated in the pathogenesis of atherosclerosis and consequent CVD.[103–105] Damage to the endothelium of coronary vessels leads to the release of proinflammatory cytokines including IL-1, IL-6, and TNF-α. These cytokines induce leukocyte chemoattraction, while exposure of adhesion molecules causes inflammatory cells to adhere to the endothelium.[106] Macrophages and T-cells then invade the vascular wall and further activate cytokine cascades and growth factor release. In response, intimal smooth muscle cells proliferate and atherosclerosis accelerates. Continued degradation of the plaque matrix by macrophages can cause plaques to become unstable, promoting thrombus formation and consequent vascular occlusion.[103,104]

Proinflammatory cytokines increase hepatic production of acute-phase reactants, including C-reactive protein (CRP), fibrinogen, haptoglobin, and alpha-1-acid glycoprotein (AGP). Depression is also associated with this acute-phase response; Kop et al. found that the presence of depression was associated with small elevations in CRP and fibrinogen in a sample of 4268 individuals without CVD,[85] while Maes et al. found depressed subjects to have elevated haptoglobin, fibrinogen, and AGP compared to controls and independent of disease severity.[107] Seidel et al. noted increased CRP in individuals with major depression compared to controls (0.45 mg/dL vs. 0.31 mg/dL, $P < 0.05$),[95] and and Lanquillon et al. reported similar findings (5.45 mg/L vs. 1.95 mg/L, $P < 0.001$).[108] Sluzewska et al. showed that AGP was significantly elevated in depressed patients as well as directly correlated with IL-6 levels, supporting the role of IL-6 in triggering the release of acute-phase reactants.[82]

The magnitude of this proinflammatory acute-phase response to endothelial damage may predict progression and prognosis of coronary disease. Elevated plasma CRP, a surrogate action marker for IL-6,[87] have been reported in patients with acute ischemia and/or MI, and

predict recurrent ischemia and MI among patients with unstable angina.[106,109,110] Ridker et al. showed that initially healthy men who had elevated baseline levels of CRP were at greater risk for MI and stroke than those with normal levels; men in the highest CRP quartile had three times the risk of MI of those in the lowest quartile over 8 years of follow-up.[110] Further, aspirin, an anti-inflammatory drug, had its greatest effects in reducing the risk of MI in men with the highest levels of CRP.[110] These data suggest that the degree of baseline inflammation for any individual may impact the body's response to the initiation of the atherosclerotic process.

Evidence for the effect of the treatment of depression on inflammation is mixed. Antidepressants from a variety of classes may exert anti-inflammatory effects via reestablishment of feedback control in the HPA axis, normalization of sympathetic hyperactivity, or direct inhibition of the release of proinflammatory cytokines from monocytes.[88] However, Maes et al. reported that chronic treatment with SSRIs had no effect on acute-phase or inflammatory molecules, further supporting the idea that these are a trait rather than state marker of depression.[89] Mikova et al. reported that responders to pharmacologic treatment (defined by reduction in depressive symptoms) demonstrated decreased inflammation whereas nonresponders showed no change,[94] and Lanquillon et al. similarly noted a decrease in TNF-α only among treatment responders following treatment with amitriptyline.[108] A lack of data regarding changes in inflammation from stress reduction or cognitive-behavioral therapy make it difficult to determine whether it is symptom remission or pharmacology that may impact inflammation. Further, no studies have been undertaken that combine measures of CVD, depression, and inflammation, and no data exist to suggest that an antidepressant-induced decrease in inflammation leads to any improvement in outcomes for either depressed patients or patients with heart disease.

Evidence suggests, therefore, that depression is associated with increased serum levels of inflammatory mediators and inflammatory markers, including acute-phase reactants. The heightened inflammation seen in depressed patients may contribute to the development of CVD in susceptible patients or the progression of CVD in established disease. However, correlational data do not allow us to determine whether the inflammation seen in depressed patients is a trait marker of depression, or whether inflammation contributes to the pathogenesis of depression. Additional research is needed to prospectively examine these processes.

Hypercoagulability

Studies have consistently shown that untreated depressed patients have a variety of abnormalities in platelet function that lead to increased platelet aggregation.[111–113] Platelet reactivity up to 40% greater than controls, as measured by β-TG, platelet factor 4 (PF4), and anti-ligand-induced binding site (LIBS) antibody plasma levels, has been demonstrated in studies of depressed patients[114–116]; the degree of activation is similar to that seen in patients with large-vessel atherosclerotic disease.[117,118] However, studies of depressed patients' platelet aggregation in response to thrombin, adenosine diphosphate, and collagen have shown mixed results.[118,119]

Depression has been found to be associated with an increased density of platelet serotonin 5-HT$_{2A}$ receptors[120–122]; these findings are of particular interest given the implication of serotonin abnormalities in the pathophysiology of depression.[123] The impact of this increase in receptor density is unclear; many studies have reported that depressed patients demonstrate decreased platelet aggregation in response to serotonin,[124] although Shimbo et al. recently reported that platelet reactivity to serotonin was significantly increased in depressed patients, while reactivity to adenosine diphosphate was identical between depressed patients and matched controls.[125] Whyte et al. showed that depressed patients with the serotonin-transporter-linked promoter region *l/l* genotype (associated with a greater number of serotonin transporters) had increased platelet activation

relative to both nondepressed controls and depressed patients without the l/l genotype, suggesting that genetic differences may influence the effect of depression-related serotonin dysregulation on platelet activation.[126]

Treatment studies provide additional insight into the relationship between depression and platelet function. An in vitro study of the SSRI sertraline and its metabolite N-desmethylsertraline found both to inhibit platelets in a dose-dependent and significant fashion.[127] Serebruany, in a study of 126 CAD patients presenting for revascularization, found that patients with antecedent SSRI therapy had significantly lower baseline platelet activation by a broad range of measures than those not using SSRIs.[128] Pollock demonstrated that the administration of the SSRI paroxetine to depressed patients with ischemic heart disease and elevated PF4/β-TG caused a significant reduction in PF4 and β-TG, while nortriptyline failed to impact platelet measures[129]; Musselman et al. similarly found that platelet activation was reduced to levels comparable to controls after 6 weeks of paroxetine treatment.[130] Serebruany et al. found that sertraline administration significantly decreased platelet activation compared to placebo even with concomitant administration of aspirin and clopidogrel.[131] However, it is still unknown whether the normalization of platelet function after SSRI treatment is the result of a decrease in depressive symptoms or a direct effect on platelets.[130]

Studies investigating plasma procoagulant factors in depression have found limited evidence of hypercoagulability in depressed individuals.[132] The Coronary Artery Risk Development in Young Adults (CARDIA) Study suggested that fibrinogen levels were positively associated with the presence of depressive symptoms, although the degree of increase was small.[133] Kop et al., in a study including 4268 subjects free of CAD, found that depressed individuals exhibited elevated fibrinogen and factor VIIc even after controlling for demographic and clinical variables, but these associations became nonsignificant when physical factors such as grip strength and activity level were added to the model.[85] The relationship of procoagulant factors to depression may be mediated by HPA or sympathetic hyperactivity, as both have been shown to stimulate blood coagulation; hypercortisolism is associated with increases in factor VIII and von Willebrand Factor as well as a decrease in fibrinolytic activity, while elevated NE is associated with concurrent increases in coagulation and fibrinolysis.[132]

Platelet activation also clearly plays a role in CVD. Thaulow et al. conducted a prospective study of 487 apparently healthy men, and found that over nearly 14 years of follow-up, baseline platelet concentration and aggregability was predictive of future coronary events.[134] A recent investigation by Heeschen et al. in a group of patients with unstable CAD demonstrated that elevation of soluble CD40 ligand levels was associated with an increased risk of cardiovascular events (RR = 2.71, $P < 0.001$), and that antiplatelet therapy significantly reduced this risk.[135] In addition, the potent ability of antiplatelet therapies such as aspirin and glycoprotein IIb/IIIa inhibitors to improve long-term survival in patients with evolving MI or unstable angina supports the centrality of platelets in cardiovascular outcomes.[136]

In addition to platelet activity, plasma coagulation factors and fibrinolysis are also crucial in the development and prognosis of CVD.[137] When these components are dysregulated, a hypercoagulable state can result; the consequent promotion of fibrin deposition in the vasculature augments progression of CVD. Increased plasma levels of coagulation-promoting entities (including fibrinogen, factor VII activity, factor VIII activity, von Willebrand Factor antigen, tissue-type plasminogen activator antigen, type 1 tissue-type plasminogen activator inhibitor antigen, D-dimer, and plasmin-#2 antiplasmin complex) have been shown to predict coronary syndromes, such as unstable angina, MI, and sudden cardiac death, in patients with CVD as well as healthy individuals.[138] The importance of hypercoagulability in prognosis for CVD patients is further supported by the therapeutic benefits of anticoagulant and fibrinolytic therapy in treating patients with both acute and chronic coronary syndromes.[139,140]

Taken as a whole, the available evidence suggests that depression is associated with abnormalities in coagulation; these abnormalities may negatively influence the microvasculature in susceptible individuals as well as in CVD patients. Prospective research concurrently measuring depressive symptoms, coagulation parameters, and cardiovascular outcomes is needed.

Psychosocial Factors

Psychosocial factors, including compliance, social support, and stress, may also mediate the relationship between cardiovascular disease and depression (Table 10-5).

Compliance

Compliance with medical recommendations includes taking medication correctly, following a diet when prescribed, engaging in exercise when prescribed, attending appointments, and making healthy lifestyle choices.[141] Depressed patients with a range of medical illnesses, including end-stage renal disease, cancer, and rheumatoid arthritis, have an odds ratio of 3.03 (95% CI 1.96, 4.89) when compared with non-depressed patients with similar illnesses for non-compliance with medical recommendations, according to a 2000 meta-analysis by DiMatteo et al.[141] In addition, a recent study of 496 patients being treated for hypertension found depression to be the only variable independently associated with higher odds of noncompliance,[142] and investigations have shown that patients who are depressed are less likely to adhere to cardiac rehabilitation programs after MI.[143,144] One study looking at psychosocial variables and compliance in heart failure patients found that higher mental health was predictive of overall compliance behavior.[145] Therefore, depressed patients may be at a higher risk of nonadherence to both pharmacologic and behavioral recommendations.

▶ **TABLE 10-5** PSYCHOSOCIAL PARAMETERS LINKING DEPRESSION AND CARDIOVASCULAR DISEASE

Psychosocial Parameter Associated with Depression	Nature of Change	Impact on Cardiovascular System or Outcomes
Compliance	Decreased compliance with medications and rehabilitation programs	Less use of evidence-based therapies Independent poor outcomes associated with noncompliance
Social support	Decreased social support	Increased cardiovascular mortality
Stress	Mental stress-induced myocardial ischemia Nervous system hyperactivity Inflammation	Increased ambulatory myocardial ischemia

Treatment of CVD often involves complicated medication regimens as well as significant lifestyle modifications. A large number of randomized, placebo-controlled trials in the post-MI population have been conducted, and meta-analyses suggest a 20–25% RR reduction in mortality with aspirin, a 20–30% RR reduction with beta-blockers, a 20–25% RR reduction with angiotensin converting enzyme (ACE) inhibitors, and a 25–40% RR reduction with HMG-CoA reductase inhibitors (statins).[139] These four classes of medication, when taken by individuals with CAD, are estimated to cumulatively confer a 70–75% RR reduction of recurrent cardiac events.[146] However, patients who are nonadherent with their medications or lifestyle recommendations will not experience the proven benefits of these interventions. Evidence suggests that many of these medications are in fact underutilized; Butler et al. reported that among 846 post-MI patients, less than half of the study population was discharged on beta-blockers; of those discharged on beta-blockers, 85% had filled a prescription by 30 days postdischarge, but only 63 and 61% were still taking the medication at 6 months and 1 year, respectively.[147] A population-based study of more than 100,000 older adults in Canada showed that 2-year adherence rates to statin therapy for patients

with an initial prescription were only 40.1% for patients with recent acute coronary syndrome and 36.1% for patients with chronic CAD.[148]

Interestingly, noncompliance itself may also be detrimental to prognosis. The Coronary Drug Project Research Group found a relative mortality risk for subjects nonadherent with clofibrate and placebo of 1.7 and 1.9, respectively, when compared to patients adherent with each ($P < 0.001$ for each),[149] while the beta-blocker heart attack trial showed that nonadherers to either propanolol or placebo had an odds ratio for mortality of 2.6 ($P = 0.03$).[150] While not all studies have found this association, a meta-analysis by McDermott suggests that noncompliance to either placebo or active medication is associated with a higher risk of both rehospitalization and mortality.[151]

Only a small number of studies examining the impact of pharmacologic or behavioral interventions for depression on adherence have been published to date. Two small studies in depressed patients with diabetes, one using nortriptyline[152] and one using cognitive-behavioral therapy,[153] succeeded in decreasing depression and improving glucose control, but there was no improvement in adherence to glucose monitoring. Rich et al. showed that a multidisciplinary intervention was successful in improving compliance in heart failure patients, but no morbidity or mortality data were available in this study.[154] Although these reports suggest that behavioral interventions might improve compliance and consequently decrease hospitalization and mortality, no direct evidence is available and conclusions therefore must be drawn with caution.

It seems likely that compliance plays a role in the interaction between depression and CVD, but the current evidence does not allow firm conclusions to be drawn. In order to determine the true nature of this link, prospective research incorporating careful measures of depressive symptoms, compliance, and outcomes is needed.

Social Support

Social support may significantly impact depression. The presence of social support was shown to correlate with a lower risk for depression in a study of 2810 older patients with chronic disease.[155] Cross-sectional twin-twin studies suggest that a lack of social support is correlated with depression, although twin-twin longitudinal data did not find a lack of social support to be a prospective risk factor for the development of depression.[156] Social support may impact the course of depression; a study of 166 elderly patients found that subjective social support was associated with an OR of 1.21 (95% CI 1.09, 1.35) for nonremission of depression,[157] and the presence of social support has been shown to buffer the functional decline associated with depression in elderly patients.[158]

Lack of social support has been correlated with poor outcomes in a number of conditions, including stroke[159,160] and cardiac disease.[161–165] For example, Berkman et al. demonstrated that a pre-MI lack of emotional support predicted a nearly threefold increased risk of death in the 6 months following an MI (OR 2.9, $P < 0.05$).[161] A study of nearly 2000 patients with CAD showed that a lack of emotional resources (patients who lacked a confidant and were unmarried) was associated with a RR of 5-year mortality of 3.34 ($P < 0.0001$).[163] Similarly, among 1234 patients studied by Case et al., living alone was associated with a RR of 1.54 for a recurrent cardiac event

over the subsequent 2 years.[164] In an initially healthy group of 32,624 men, Kawachi et al. demonstrated that social isolation carried a RR of 1.90 for cardiovascular mortality ($P < 0.05$) over more than 120,000 patient-years of follow-up.[165] In addition, social support may have a positive impact on patient compliance,[145] another potential mechanism via which social support could affect outcomes.

Few studies in CVD patients with depression have attempted to specifically boost social support; Krumholz et al. reported that an education and support intervention for heart failure patients was successful in decreasing hospitalizations and mortality (RR = 0.69, 95% CI 0.52, 0.92, $P = 0.01$), but the mechanism via which this occurred, be it increased compliance, patient empowerment, or both, was not specifically evaluated.[166] Multidisciplinary interventions for depressed CAD patients, incorporating support from nurses, nutritionists, counselors, and others, have shown mixed results in their ability to impact morbidity and mortality,[167] and will be discussed in more detail in a later section of this chapter.

The available evidence suggests that a lack of social support may have a deleterious influence on the course of both CVD and depression. Although this observation does not explain the high prevalence of depression in CVD, it may contribute to the negative impact of depression on prognosis in established CVD.

Stress

The biologic definition of stress suggests that it is "a state of threatened homeostasis provoked by a psychologic, environmental, or physiologic stressor."[168] The definition of "stress" is somewhat less strict when moving from controlled laboratory experiments to real-life observations, and many studies use self-reported "stress," a much less precise measure, to evaluate the effect of stress on depression. That caveat noted, evidence suggests that stress in daily life might influence the onset and course of depression.[169–171] In community and clinic samples, stressful life experiences have been shown to correlate with the onset and course of depressive disorders.[172–175] A longitudinal study of 680 pairs of twins investigating genetic, life event, and temperament variables found that a stressful event in the preceding year was the most powerful risk factor for depression.[176] Stressful work environment has been shown to correlate with depressive symptoms[177] as well as to predict a longitudinal increase in depressive symptoms.[178] Bosworth et al. evaluated 335 inpatients with coronary artery disease, and found that self-reported "negative life events" were predictive of depression (OR = 4.30, 95% CI 1.39, 13.27, $P < 0.05$) even after controlling for demographic factors.[179] However, much of the data driving the literature in this area are observational, making conclusions somewhat difficult to draw.[171]

Stress has also been implicated in the development and prognosis of CVD. For example, a prospective study of 73,424 men and women in Japan found that women with self-reported "high stress" had a RR of 2.58 (95% CI 1.21, 5.47, $P < 0.05$) for MI, and 2.28 (95% CI 1.17, 4.43, $P < 0.05$) for coronary artery disease even after adjusting for demographic, medical, and psychologic factors; the associations for men were not significant.[180] A study of 7000 men in Sweden suggested a RR of 1.5 for CVD among men reporting high stress, but found no association between stress and CVD in a smaller subsequent sample.[181] A prospective study, by Tennant et al., of post-MI patients suggested that acute and chronic stress were associated with RR of reinfarction of 2.5 and 2.3, repectively,[182] while two other studies have found no relationship between life-stress level and mortality after MI.[183,184]

There are many ways in which stress may affect cardiovascular health. For example, mental stress can induce myocardial ischemia in individuals with CAD, potentially contributing to worsening cardiac status.[168,185–187] Mental arithmetic under stressful conditions has been shown to cause paradoxical coronary artery constriction in patients with atherosclerotic disease, whereas healthy controls respond with dilation.[188] Blumenthal et al.[189] and Jiang et al.[190]

performed 48-hour ambulatory Holter monitoring on a sample of 132 subjects with documented CVD, and subsequently performed radionuclide ventriculography during mentally stressful tasks (public speaking, mathematical calculations, mirror tracing) and exercise testing.[189] Five-year follow-up suggested that patients who had tested "positive" for mental stress-induced ischemia (new wall motion abnormality or reduction in ejection fraction > 5%) were more likely to experience a cardiac event (death, MI, or revascularization), even after adjusting for age, history of MI, and baseline ejection fraction (OR = 2.8, 95% CI 1.0, 7.7); transforming reduction in ejection fraction into a continuous variable yielded a standardized risk ratio for cardiac events of 2.4.[190] Sheps et al. assessed response to mental stress (a public speaking task) using radionuclide ventriculography in 196 patients with known CVD, and found that the presence of new wall motion abnormalities during mental stress testing was associated with a RR of 2.95 for mortality over 5 years of follow-up.[191] However, patients who demonstrated ischemia during ambulatory Holter monitoring were not at increased risk for events in either study, suggesting that the presence of stress-induced ischemia might be a marker for poor outcomes not because of chronic ischemia but rather via a different mechanism, such as autonomic hyperresponsiveness, an augmented neurohormonal response, or changes in other biologic correlates of psychologic stress that would impact cardiac outcomes.[190]

It is also worth noting that autonomic function and inflammation, two systems discussed previously, may also account for the effect of stress on the cardiovascular system. The stress response is regulated by the HPA axis and the sympathetic nervous system, suggesting that many of the deleterious effects that hyperactivity of these systems can have on the cardiovascular system might be triggered or augmented by stress.[168,192] Similarly, several studies have proposed that inflammation is the intermediary factor; mental stress has been shown to induce cytokine production,[193,194] and cytokine production may have a negative impact on cardiovascular health.

A small number of studies have tested interventions specifically designed to address stress-induced ischemia. Both atenolol and nifedipine were shown to be effective in attenuating the development of wall motion abnormalities in response to mental stress in a small group of individuals with stable angina.[195] A recent study of 121 men with stress-induced ischemia randomized patients to a stress management program, exercise, or usual care and found that the stress management program was associated with a reduction in cardiac events over a 5-year follow-up period ($P = 0.037$).[196] General stress-reduction interventions will be discussed in more detail in a later section of this chapter.

Stress, though difficult to define and even more difficult to quantify, may play a role in the pathogenesis of both depression and CVD. Additional studies are needed in order to further clarify the directionality of this relationship, as well as the potential impact of the reduction of stress-induced ischemia on prognosis in CVD.

Risk Factor Clustering

A number of factors increase an individual's risk for CVD, including smoking, hypertension, diabetes, hypercholesterolemia, and obesity.[197,198] In addition, "novel" risk factors such as homocysteine have been identified.[199] Depressed individuals may be more likely than nondepressed individuals to have one or more of these risk factors, and therefore the link between depression and CVD may be in part due to risk factor clustering (Table 10-6). Although most studies examining this link have controlled for risk factors, the sum of the parts may be greater than the whole; that is, the presence of multiple risk factors may be inadequately controlled for because of the robustness of its effect.

Smoking

Cigarette smoking is associated with an increased risk of CVD; the RR of CVD mortality associated with each additional pack of cigarettes smoked per day is approximately 1.39.[200] In the United States, 49% of individuals with depression smoke,

▶ **TABLE 10-6** CARDIOVASCULAR RISK FACTORS LINKING DEPRESSION AND CARDIOVASCULAR DISEASE

Risk Factor for CVD	Association with Depression	Impact on Cardiovascular System or Outcomes
Smoking	Increased risk of depression Increased risk of smoking if depressed Less likely to quit successfully if depressed	Risk of cardiovascular mortality 1.39 per pack smoked per day
Hypertension	Higher risk of developing hypertension over many years if depressed	Dose-related increased risk of cardiovascular disease with elevated blood pressure
Diabetes	Increased risk of depression	Increased cardiovascular mortality
Hypercholesterolemia	Depression is associated with low cholesterol	Potentially positive
Obesity	Obese women are more likely to be depressed No relationship between obesity and depression in men	Risk of cardiovascular disease increased 64%
Homocysteine	Higher levels in depressed patients	High levels associated with increased cardiovascular risk

whereas only 20–30% of the general population does so.[201] A 1996 study suggested that a history of major depression conferred a threefold increased risk of becoming a smoker.[202] The reverse may also be true; lifetime prevalence rates of depression among smokers are 30–45%, significantly higher than the 5–10% seen in the general population.[203,204] Depressed smokers have repeatedly been shown to be less likely to successfully quit, and more likely to experience withdrawal symptoms during their efforts at abstinence.[201,203,204] These factors combine to make smoking more prevalent within the depressed population than the nondepressed population.

Hypertension

Patients with hypertension are significantly more likely to develop CVD; a prolonged increase of 10 mmHg above normal in diastolic pressure is associated with a 37% increased risk of CVD.[198] A number of studies have investigated the relationship of depression and blood pressure, theorizing that the autonomic hyperactivity seen in patients with anxiety or depression (see later) has a pressor effect on the cardiovascular system, but prospective studies have yielded mixed results. Shinn et al., following 508 adults for 4 years, found no association between either anxiety or depression and blood pressure.[205] However, Jonas et al. followed 3310 initially normotensive patients in the National Health and Nutrition Examination Study (NHANES) I study, and found that symptoms of depression and anxiety at baseline were associated with a higher risk of developing hypertension over 20 years of follow-up (RR [White women] = 1.73, RR [Black women] = 3.12, RR [all men] = 1.56), controlling for demographic and behavioral risk factors for hypertension such as age, smoking status, and body mass index (BMI).[206] Davidson et al. followed 3340 individuals in the CARDIA Study, and found that those with CES-D scores ≥16 were significantly more likely to develop hypertension during 5 years of follow-up, again controlling for demographic and behavioral factors. The effect was particularly robust in Black study subjects (OR = 2.70, 95% CI 1.49, 4.92).[207]

Diabetes

Diabetes is associated with a three- to fourfold increased risk of CVD and cardiovascular mortality.[208] Depression is more prevalent in individuals with diabetes than in the general population; a recent meta-analysis examining 39 studies of depression and diabetes found a composite odds ratio for depression of 2.0 (95% CI 1.8, 2.2).[209] Data from the Epidemiologic Catchment Area study suggested a RR of 2.23 for development of diabetes over a 13-year follow-up for otherwise healthy individuals with depression compared with controls, but the data were found to be statistically nonsignificant ($P = 0.11$, 95% CI 0.90, 5.55).[210] Depression has been shown to negatively influence glycemic control in diabetic patients,[211] as well as to increase the risk of complications including nephropathy, neuropathy, and retinopathy.[212]

Hypercholesterolemia

Hypercholesterolemia is also an established risk factor for CVD. CVD mortality increases 9% for each 10 mg/dL increase in plasma cholesterol,[213] and individuals in the highest quartile of plasma cholesterol levels are three times more likely to die of CVD than those in the lowest quartile.[200] However, a link has been noted not between high cholesterol levels and depression but rather between low cholesterol levels and depression,[214–217] and cholesterol-lowering agents have been reported to cause depressive symptoms.[218] A recent study by Steegmans et al. replicated previous smaller trials, and found that men with chronically low cholesterol levels were more likely to experience depressive symptoms than controls, even after adjusting for potential confounders including age, alcohol use, and chronic disease (RR = 7.0, 95% CI 1.7, 29.5).[217] Olusi et al. showed that clinical recovery from depression was associated with an increase in serum cholesterol to normal levels.[215] One possible explanation for these findings is an alteration of serotonin metabolism: fatty acids compete with tryptophan, a serotonin precursor, for binding to albumin; fewer free fatty acids in the blood leaves more albumin available to bind to tryptophan, thereby decreasing the amount of free tryptophan available for conversion to serotonin in the brain.[216] Supporting this hypothesis, decreased plasma serotonin was associated with low cholesterol levels in a study of 100 individuals.[216] Interestingly, data from the Framingham study suggested that falling cholesterol levels over the first 14 years of observation, found in 14% of men and 20% of women, were associated with an increased risk of CVD death over the subsequent 18 years, although no data on depression are available from this study.[213]

Obesity

Obesity is another known risk factor for CVD. A recent examination of Framingham data showed that overweight (BMI 25.0–29.9) and obesity (BMI ≥ 30) were associated with RR of CVD of 1.2 and 1.64, respectively, in comparison to normal weight subjects (BMI 18.5–24.9).[219] There may be gender differences in the relationship between depression and obesity; a study of 2853 NHANES I subjects showed that obesity was associated with an increased risk of depression among women (OR = 1.38, 95% CI 1.07, 1.69), but not among men.[220] More than 42,000 subjects were included in a 2000 study by Carpenter et al., who demonstrated that obesity was associated with an increased risk of depression among women (OR = 1.37, 95% CI 1.09, 1.73) but a reduced risk of depression among men (OR = 0.63, 95% CI 0.60, 0.67).[221]

Homocysteine

Elevated plasma homocysteine is a novel cardiovascular risk factor; a recent meta-analysis found that a 25% lower homocysteine level was associated with an 11% lower risk of CVD,[222] and reduction of homocysteine levels with B-vitamin supplementation has been shown to reduce vascular event rates after percutaneous coronary intervention.[223] A genetic polymorphism causing elevations in plasma homocysteine was also recently shown to be linked to CVD.[224] Homocysteine levels are higher in depressed patients than in healthy controls, with 20–50% of depressed patients

exhibiting homocysteine levels that would, based on studies of CVD patients, confer an increased risk of CVD mortality.[199] Further, folate supplementation, known to lower plasma homocysteine levels, may augment the antidepressant effects of fluoxetine in women,[225] and folate alone was found to have antidepressant properties in a small trial of elderly patients.[226]

▶ DIAGNOSIS OF DEPRESSION IN PATIENTS WITH CVD

It is clearly important to address the presence of depression in patients with CVD, as its prevalence is high and its negative impact on prognosis is considerable. However, significant limitations stand in the way of clinical efforts to do so.

The first limitation is a lack of attention to depression in the medical community at large. Perhaps in part because of the misconceptions surrounding what constitutes depression, the disorder commonly goes undiagnosed; it has been suggested that 30–50% of cases of depression in the general population are never detected by a medical professional.[227–229] Physicians may not address depression because they have not been adequately trained to recognize both typical and atypical depressive symptoms, because of time constraints in high-volume clinical settings, or because they do not know how to best treat the condition.[230] Patients may be unwilling to disclose emotional distress to their physicians for fear of being stigmatized with a label of mental illness, because they believe their feelings are part of their medical illness, or because they do not want a psychiatric diagnosis recorded in their medical record.[230,231] Data from the recent National Comorbidity Survey Replication, a study that conducted face-to-face interviews with 9090 individuals, suggested that only 57.3% of persons who met criteria for depression had received treatment for depression in the 12 months preceding their interview, and that only 64.3% of these individuals received treatment that met criteria for even minimal adequacy.[232]

Although public health programs to increase awareness of depression are ongoing, and the proportion of Americans who receive treatment for depression is increasing,[233] underdiagnosis remains a considerable problem.[234] It is crucial that both clinicians and patients realize that the presence of major depression is not a standard part of living with CVD. While feeling upset from time to time about having a serious disease may be nearly universal, true major depression is not a normal reaction to illness and should be recognized as the disabling, chronic, and treatable condition that it is.[231]

The second limitation is the difficulty inherent in diagnosing depression in the context of medical illness, particularly in the older population.[235,236] It is hard to diagnose depression in the setting of a disease with symptoms that mimic depression. Depression is characterized by low mood, loss of interest in usual activities, weight loss or gain, difficulty sleeping, low energy, feelings of worthlessness, and decreased ability to concentrate,[229,237] while CVD, particularly when complicated by heart failure, is often associated with fatigue, malaise, and insomnia.[238] Further, effects of pharmacotherapy may mimic or increase depressive symptoms. It has been reported, for example, that the use of beta-blockers is associated with an increased risk of depression.[239,240] A recent meta-analysis,[241] as well as a number of focused reports,[242,243] have not found this to be the case, but both clinicians and patients may attribute depressive symptoms to a medication regimen rather than an underlying mood disorder.

The variability of case-finding instruments for depression also complicates its diagnosis; Koenig et al. showed that the prevalence of major depression in a population of 460 medically ill older inpatients varied by a factor of 2—from 10 to 21%—depending on which diagnostic scheme was utilized.[244] This difficulty is compounded when symptoms of medical illness overlap symptoms of depression, as most depression inventories do not take such overlap into account.[245] For research purposes, it is important to recognize and quantify depression as precisely as possible. To this end, the Depression Interview and Structured Hamilton (DISH) was specifically developed to diagnose and assess the severity of depression via interview in the setting of medical illness; it was utilized in the Enhancing Recovery in Coronary Heart Disease (ENRICHD) trial and was found to be valid as well as efficient to administer.[193] Researchers should consider utilizing the DISH, or other instruments that have been designed specifically for the diagnosis of depression in the medically ill, for future studies of depression in HF.

In contrast, in the clinical setting, the identification of depression is more important than a precise quantification of depressive symptoms. Screening for depression is currently recommended by the U.S. Preventive Services Task Force as part of routine medical care, but often does not take place due to time constraints or a lack of familiarity with available instruments.[246] However, a study testing seven depression questionnaires in a population of 590 patients at an urgent care clinic found that a two-question case-finding instrument for depression had 96% sensitivity and 57% specificity for depression, similar to the other six, much longer, instruments.[237] The two questions were "During the past month, have you often been bothered by feeling down, depressed, or hopeless?" and "During the past month, have you often been bothered by little interest or pleasure in doing things?"[237] Utilization of even this simple instrument, particularly practical in busy clinical settings with significant time constraints, could help to identify cases of depression that are currently going unrecognized in patients with CVD.

▶ TREATMENT OF DEPRESSION IN PATIENTS WITH CVD

As the relationship between depression and CVD has become increasingly recognized and accepted in the medical community, a number of trials have begun to examine the impact of pharmacologic and nonpharmacologic interventions on depression in patients with heart disease. In theory, if depression has a damaging influence on the cardiovascular system, then treatment of depression should decrease its negative prognostic impact. However, the trials addressing this theory that have been conducted thus far have shown mixed results.[77,167,247,248] Consequently, concern has arisen in the behavioral medicine community regarding the impact that these inconsistent findings might have on future clinical trials.[249] A very important aspect of continued therapeutic advances in this field will be the ability to show a convincing connection between the treatment of depression in patients with heart disease and a reduction in morbidity and mortality associated with the cooccurrence of these conditions.

The purpose of this section is to review the major pharmacologic and nonpharmacologic treatment trials in the field of depression and CVD, and discuss what we can learn from these trials. In addition, this section will outline methodologic complexities commonly enountered in the study of depression and CVD, and suggest ways in which future trials might help shed light on the relationship between depression and cardiovascular morbidity and mortality.

Pharmacologic Treatment of Depression

SADHART

The first trial to investigate the safety and efficacy of sertraline treatment of MDD in patients with CVD, a patient population not previously included in trials of pharmacologic treatment for depression, was the Sertraline Anti-Depressant Heart Attack Trial (SADHART). SADHART investigators enrolled 369 patients with MDD and either acute myocardial infarction or unstable angina in a randomized, double-blind, placebo-controlled trial. After a 2-week single-blind placebo run-in, patients were randomly assigned to receive sertraline in flexible doses of 50–200 mg or placebo for 24 weeks.[77]

From a safety standpoint, SADHART achieved its objectives; no changes were seen in mean LVEF, prolonged QTc interval, or other cardiac measures.[77] In comparison with TCAs, which are known to have potentially harmful cardiac effects

and are generally contraindicated in patients with known cardiac pathology,[74] the trial demonstrated that sertraline can safely be used in patients with ischemic heart disease.

From an efficacy standpoint, however, findings were mixed. Unexpectedly, sertraline was not extremely effective for the treatment of depression in this population. Among all patients, sertraline was statistically superior to placebo on the clinical global impression improvement (CGI-I) scale (measured over 24 weeks, 2.57 vs. 2.75, $P = 0.049$) but not on Hamilton depression (HAM-D) change score (measured over 16 weeks, 8.4 vs. 7.6, $P = 0.14$). However, in predefined subgroup analysis examining patients with recurrent or severe depression, sertraline was shown to be more efficacious than placebo on both CGI-I and HAM-D measurements.[77] Sertraline was associated with significantly improved quality of life and functioning in this group as well.[250] One possible confounder for the overall sample was the placebo response rate of 53%, considerably higher than the rates of 25–35% typically seen in antidepressant trials.[251]

Possibly the most provocative finding from the SADHART investigations was that the incidence of severe cardiac events (death, myocardial infarction, congestive heart failure, stroke, and recurrent angina) was numerically lower among patients receiving sertraline than those receiving placebo (14.5% vs. 22.4%, RR 0.77, 95% CI 0.51–1.16), although this result did not reach statistical significance.[77] In a SADHART substudy, investigators determined that sertraline was associated with decreased platelet and endothelial activation markers, suggesting one mechanism via which sertraline might confer a morbidity and mortality advantage.[252] Although small, this substudy is important because it combines psychologic, cardiovascular, and pharmacologic data into a single database, allowing researchers better insight into the mechanisms that might mediate the outcomes seen in the larger trial. Because SADHART was not powered to detect a difference in morbidity and mortality in this relatively small sample of patients, the impact of sertraline treatment of major depression on hard outcomes in the patient with ischemic heart disease remains unclear. However, SADHART's major contribution was to prove the safety of such treatment, thus opening the door for future investigations adequately powered to more closely examine morbidity and mortality endpoints. The Myocardial INfarction and Depression-Intervention Trial (MIND-IT), currently underway in The Netherlands, will examine mirtazapine, citalopram, and placebo in depressed post-MI patients, and may contribute to our knowledge in this area.[253]

Nonpharmacologic Treatment of Depression

Although a good deal of literature exists to support the efficacy of nonpharmacologic therapy as a treatment for depression,[254,255] little research in this field has been conducted specifically on patients with CVD. Therefore, we can only extrapolate by examining the impact of broader psychosocial interventions on a broader group of patients: multidisciplinary programs for CVD patients, incorporating support from nurses, nutritionists, counselors, and others.

These interventions, however, have shown mixed results in their ability to impact morbidity and mortality, have not reported on physiologic or psychosocial intermediates, and have not assessed patients for depression.[7] For example, Frasure-Smith and Prince found that 229 post-MI patients receiving stress-reducing interventions had a 50% decrease in cardiac mortality (4.5% vs. 9%), although no change was found in readmission rates.[167] Blumenthal et al. showed that 40 post-MI patients in a stress management program had a RR for cardiac events of 0.26 compared to 33 controls.[256] The Montreal Heart Attack Readjustment Trial (M-HART), on the other hand, found that 684 women receiving nonpharmacologic anxiety-reducing intervention after MI were actually more likely to die (RR = 1.39) when compared with 692 controls, with the increased mortality primarily related to sudden death caused by arrhythmias.[248] A 1996 meta-analysis suggested that the addition of

psychosocial interventions to standard care for patients with CAD is associated with an overall improvement in disease recurrence and mortality rates; however, many of the studies that were included in the analysis were limited by sample size and length of follow-up.[257] Interestingly, the three largest trials of psychosocial interventions in patients with CVD that have been conducted to date [248,258,259] have failed to demonstrate a difference in psychosocial or cardiovascular outcomes between intervention and control groups. It is worth noting, however, that the vast majority of these interventions were undertaken on heterogeneous mixes of patients rather than groups of patients explicitly selected because they were suffering from depression.

ENRICHD

A trial specifically focusing on nonpharmacologic treatment of depression in patients with CVD had not been performed until ENRICHD. The first trial in behavioral medicine to be funded by the National Heart, Lung, and Blood Institute (NHLBI), ENRICHD enrolled 2481 patients with myocardial infarction as well as depression and/or low perceived social support.[247] The intervention tested was an individually tailored CBT-based intervention, initiated 2–3 weeks after myocardial infarction and continued for a median of 11 sessions over 6 months. In addition, patients scoring higher than 24 on the Hamilton Rating Scale for Depression (HRSD) or demonstrating a less than 50% reduction in Beck Depression Inventory (BDI) scores after 5 weeks were eligible to receive a SSRI.[247]

Results of the ENRICHD trial were mixed. Psychologic outcomes were better at the 6-month evaluation for patients receiving the intervention in comparison with the control group, with mean BDI score 9.1 in the intervention group versus 12.2 in the control group ($P < 0.001$), but these effects did not persist to the 30-month evaluation. There was no difference in event-free survival between the two groups (75.9% vs. 75.8%, P = ns).[247] In a follow-up analysis attempting to clarify these results, investigators showed that depression was in fact an independent risk factor for death after MI (HR 2.4, 95% CI 1.2–4.7),[260] despite the fact that successful treatment of depression was not associated with a decrease in this risk. One possible confounding factor in this trial was the concomitant use of antidepressant medication, which reached a prevalence of 20.6% in the control group and 28% in the intervention group by the end of follow-up; interestingly, antidepressant medication use was associated with a significant decrease in risk of death or nonfatal MI (adjusted HR, 0.57; 95% CI, 0.38–0.85).[247]

Methodologic Complexity of Trials in Depression and CVD

Treating depression in patients with heart disease is extremely important. Successful treatment of depression can lead to a significant improvement in quality of life for patients who suffer from this debilitating and often chronic disorder.[250,261,262] SADHART showed that the use of sertraline to achieve remission in severe or recurrent depression is safe and effective for patients with ischemic heart disease. ENRICHD proved that the use of nonpharmacologic treatment strategies could also positively impact depressive symptoms in patients after myocardial infarction. However, demonstrating that a relationship exists between the treatment of depression and a subsequent improvement in morbidity and mortality has not yet been convincingly accomplished. Why is this the case?

First, it should be recognized that depression is a complex variable, the definition and measurement of which are inherently difficult. Not all depressed patients are the same; many will remit spontaneously, while many others will go on to develop a lifetime of chronic depression.[263–265] Many patients with CVD will experience mild depression that is not easy to differentiate from a normal grief response to the diagnosis of a significant illness, while many others will experience moderate to severe depression.[8,266] As discussed previously, the diagnosis of depression in the context of CVD and other medical illnesses is also difficult.

Further, the conduct of trials examining treatments for depression is complex. Because of the large standard deviation in psychosocial assessments, sample sizes for trials in depression must often be prohibitively large to be adequately powered to show a connection between changes in psychosocial parameters and hard outcomes. Despite the high prevalence of depression and CVD, finding eligible patients can be daunting; SADHART investigators, for example, screened 11,456 patients to come up with their final sample size of 269, an incredible amount of time and effort to put into a trial with a relatively straightforward design.[77] ENRICHD investigators had the added complexity of a behavioral intervention to contend with, including efforts to standardize treatment across eight clinical centers.[247] Both groups of trial personnel coordinated researchers in at least two clinical departments (psychiatry and cardiology), often a daunting task in today's huge academic centers. Ethical issues often arise as well; some challenge the use of a placebo arm in depression trials because of the availability of known efficacious treatments for the condition,[267] while others argue that placebo-controlled trials are essential for rigorous scientific methodology, and can be conducted while keeping patient safety paramount.[252,268] Crossover represents another significant confounder; patients allocated to the placebo group may initiate antidepressant treatment in consultation with their primary care physician, or may request pharmacologic treatment from their study physician. Failing to include this likelihood in pretrial power calculations can lead to significant underestimation of the sample size needed to show a particular correlation.

Interpreting the results of even the most well designed trials in the field of depression and CVD can also be difficult. Because placebo response rates are quite high in most antidepressant efficacy trials,[251] it can be difficult to sort out the precise impact of a particular intervention on depressive symptoms. Quantifying a dose-response relationship is not straightforward in biobehavioral research; in the case of cognitive-behavioral therapy, for example, use of one-on-one therapy versus group therapy must somehow be entered into a calculation with therapy frequency and duration to determine the appropriate "dose" to achieve a particular outcome.

Adding outcomes such as morbidity and mortality into the mix further complicates research methodology, particularly when examining the relationship between depression and cardiovascular outcomes. Even if symptomatic improvement in depression can be demonstrated, an improvement in morbidity and mortality might not necessarily follow. If the treatment being tested does not address the underlying pathophysiology explaining the increased morbidity and mortality associated with depression in patients with CVD, then an improvement in depression would not have any correlation with these outcomes. For example, if hypercoagulability were the mechanism by which depressed patients were made susceptible to CVD, cognitive-behavioral therapy would hardly be likely to prevent a blood clot. On the other hand, aspirin or clopidogrel might show benefits in depressed CVD patients beyond what is seen in a nondepressed patient with CVD. Because we do not yet fully understand the link between depression and CVD on a pathophysiologic level, it is impossible for us to predict which treatments that are effective for depression might impact hard outcomes like morbidity and mortality. Combined with the complex and variable cardiovascular physiology that many patients with CVD possess, it comes as little surprise that correlating changes in depression with changes in cardiovascular outcomes can be extremely difficult.

▶ CONCLUSIONS

Depression is common in patients with CVD, may contribute to the development of CVD in susceptible populations, and is independently predictive of poor outcomes including hospital readmission and mortality. This effect may be mediated via pathophysiologic pathways shared between CVD and depression, including neurohormonal activation, rhythm disturbances, inflammation, and hypercoagulability. The influence of depression on noncompliance with medical recommendations, the correlation between depression and lack of social support, or the deleterious impact of stress on both mental and physical health may also contribute. Each of these thematic areas of interconnection represents a potential therapeutic target to improve outcomes in CVD. The impact of behavioral and pharmacologic treatment of depression in patients suffering from CVD remains inadequately studied. Understanding the links between depression and CVD will likely require large-scale investigations, with simultaneous collection of both physiologic and outcomes data. The poor outcomes associated with depression demand that clinicians be vigilant in the detection of depression in the setting of CVD, as attention to this powerful prognosticator may improve quality of life, decrease hospitalizations, and decrease mortality for CVD patients suffering from depression.

REFERENCES

1. National Institute of Mental Health. *The Numbers Count: Mental Disorders in America*. NIH Publication 01-4584. Bethesda, MD: National Institutes of Health, 2001.
2. American Psychiatric Association. *Let's Talk Facts About Depression*. Washington, DC: American Psychiatric Association, 1998.
3. Murray CJL, Lopez AD (eds.), *The Global Burden of Disease and Injury Series, Volume 1: A Comprehensive Assessment of Mortality and Disability from Diseases, Injuries, and Risk Factors in 1990 and Projected to 2020*. Cambridge, MA: Harvard School of Public Health on behalf of the World Health Organization and the World Bank, Harvard University Press, 1996.
4. American Heart Association. *Heart Disease and Stroke Statistics—2004 Update*. Dallas, TX: American Heart Association, 2003.
5. Joynt KE, Whellan DJ, O'Connor CM. Depression and cardiovascular disease: Mechanisms of interaction. *Biol Psychiatry* 2003;54:248–261.
6. Musselman DL, Evans DL, Nemeroff CB. The relationship of depression to cardiovascular

disease: Epidemiology, biology, and treatment. *Arch Gen Psychiatry* 1998;55:580–592.

7. Rozanski A, Blumenthal JA, Kaplan J. Impact of psychological factors on the pathogenesis of cardiovascular disease and implications for therapy. *Circulation* 1999;99:2192–2217.

8. Barefoot JC, Helms MJ, Mark DB, et al. Depression and long-term mortality risk in patients with coronary artery disease. *Am J Cardiol* 1996;78: 613–617.

9. Burg MM, Benedetto MC, Soufer R. Depressive symptoms and mortality two years after coronary artery bypass graft surgery (CABG) in men. *Psychosom Med* 2003;65:508–510.

10. Bush DE, Ziegelstein RC, Tayback M, et al. Even minimal symptoms of depression increase mortality risk after acute myocardial infarction. *Am J Cardiol* 2001;88:337–341.

11. Connerney I, Shapiro PA, McLaughlin JS, et al. Relation between depression after coronary artery bypass surgery and 12-month outcome: A prospective study. *Lancet* 2001;358:1766–1771.

12. Frasure-Smith N, Lesperance F, Talajic M. Depression following myocardial infarction. Impact on 6-month survival. *JAMA* 1993;270:1819–1825.

13. Frasure-Smith N, Lesperance F, Talajic M. Depression and 18-month prognosis after myocardial infarction. *Circulation* 1995;91:999–1005.

14. Kaufmann MW, Fitzgibbons JP, Sussman EJ, et al. Relation between myocardial infarction, depression, hostility, and death. *Am Heart J* 1999;138:549–554.

15. Lane D, Carroll D, Ring C, et al. Mortality and quality of life 12 months after myocardial infarction: Effects of depression and anxiety. *Psychosom Med* 2001;63:221–230.

16. Lane D, Carroll D, Ring C, et al. In-hospital symptoms of depression do not predict mortality 3 years after myocardial infarction. *Int J Epidemiol* 2002; 31:1179–1182.

17. Lesperance F, Frasure-Smith N, Juneau M, et al. Depression and 1-year prognosis in unstable angina. *Arch Intern Med* 2000;160:1354–1360.

18. Lesperance F, Frasure-Smith N, Talajic M, et al. Five-year risk of cardiac mortality in relation to initial severity and one-year changes in depression symptoms after myocardial infarction. *Circulation* 2002;105:1049–1053.

19. Mayou RA, Gill D, Thompson DR, et al. Depression and anxiety as predictors of outcome after myocardial infarction. *Psychosom Med* 2000;62: 212–219.

20. Penninx BW, Beekman AT, Honig A, et al. Depression and cardiac mortality: Results from a community-based longitudinal study. *Arch Gen Psychiatry* 2001;58:221–227.

21. Strik JJ, Denollet J, Lousberg R, et al. Comparing symptoms of depression and anxiety as predictors of cardiac events and increased health care consumption after myocardial infarction. *J Am Coll Cardiol* 2003;42:1801–1807.

22. Anda R, Williamson D, Jones D, et al. Depressed affect, hopelessness, and the risk of ischemic heart disease in a cohort of U.S. adults. *Epidemiology* 1993;4:285–294.

23. Ariyo AA, Haan M, Tangen CM, et al. Depressive symptoms and risks of coronary heart disease and mortality in elderly Americans. Cardiovascular Health Study Collaborative Research Group. *Circulation* 2000;102:1773–1779.

24. Aromaa A, Raitasalo R, Reunanen A, et al. Depression and cardiovascular diseases. *Acta Psychiatr Scand Suppl* 1994;377:77–82.

25. Barefoot JC, Schroll M. Symptoms of depression, acute myocardial infarction, and total mortality in a community sample. *Circulation* 1996;93: 1976–1980.

26. Ferketich AK, Schwartzbaum JA, Frid DJ, et al. Depression as an antecedent to heart disease among women and men in the NHANES I study. National Health and Nutrition Examination Survey. *Arch Intern Med* 2000;160:1261–1268.

27. Ford DE, Mead LA, Chang PP, et al. Depression is a risk factor for coronary artery disease in men: The precursors study. *Arch Intern Med* 1998;158:1422–1426.

28. Mendes de Leon CF, Krumholz HM, Seeman TS, et al. Depression and risk of coronary heart disease in elderly men and women: New Haven EPESE, 1982–1991. Established Populations for the Epidemiologic Studies of the Elderly. *Arch Intern Med* 1998;158:2341–2348.

29. Penninx BW, Guralnik JM, Mendes de Leon CF, et al. Cardiovascular events and mortality in newly and chronically depressed persons > 70 years of age. *Am J Cardiol* 1998;81:988–994.

30. Pratt LA, Ford DE, Crum RM, et al. Depression, psychotropic medication, and risk of myocardial infarction. Prospective data from the Baltimore ECA follow-up. *Circulation* 1996;94:3123–3129.

31. Schwartz SW, Cornoni-Huntley J, Cole SR, et al. Are sleep complaints an independent risk factor for myocardial infarction? *Ann Epidemiol* 1998;8: 384–392.

32. Sesso HD, Kawachi I, Vokonas PS, et al. Depression and the risk of coronary heart disease in the Normative Aging Study. *Am J Cardiol* 1998;82:851–856.

33. Wassertheil-Smoller S, Applegate WB, Berge K, et al. Change in depression as a precursor of cardiovascular events. SHEP Cooperative Research Group (Systoloc Hypertension in the elderly). *Arch Intern Med* 1996;156:553–561.

34. Whooley MA, Browner WS. Association between depressive symptoms and mortality in older women. Study of Osteoporotic Fractures Research Group. *Arch Intern Med* 1998;158:2129–2135.

35. Arborelius L, Owens MJ, Plotsky PM, et al. The role of corticotropin-releasing factor in depression and anxiety disorders. *J Endocrinol* 1999;160:1–12.

36. Ehlert U, Gaab J, Heinrichs M. Psychoneuroendocrinological contributions to the etiology of depression, posttraumatic stress disorder, and stress-related bodily disorders: The role of the hypothalamus-pituitary-adrenal axis. *Biol Psychol* 2001;57:141–152.

37. Plotsky PM, Owens MJ, Nemeroff CB. Psychoneuroendocrinology of depression. Hypothalamic-pituitary-adrenal axis. *Psychiatr Clin North Am* 1998;21:293–307.

38. Yehuda R, Teicher MH, Trestman RL, et al. Cortisol regulation in posttraumatic stress disorder and major depression: A chronobiological analysis. *Biol Psychiatry* 1996;40:79–88.

39. Heuser I, Yassouridis A, Holsboer F. The combined dexamethasone/CRH test: A refined laboratory test for psychiatric disorders. *J Psychiatr Res* 1994;28:341–356.

40. Kunzel HE, Binder EB, Nickel T, et al. Pharmacological and nonpharmacological factors influencing hypothalamic-pituitary-adrenocortical axis reactivity in acutely depressed psychiatric in-patients, measured by the Dex-CRH test. *Neuropsychopharmacology* 2003;28:2169–2178.

41. Gold PW, Gabry KE, Yasuda MR, et al. Divergent endocrine abnormalities in melancholic and atypical depression: Clinical and pathophysiologic implications. *Endocrinol Metab Clin North Am* 2000;31:37–62.

42. Maas JW, Katz MM, Koslow SH, et al. Adrenomedullary function in depressed patients. *J Psychiatr Res* 1994;28:357–367.

43. Wong ML, Kling MA, Munson PJ, et al. Pronounced and sustained central hypernoradrenergic function in major depression with melancholic features: Relation to hypercortisolism and corticotropin-releasing hormone. *Proc Natl Acad Sci USA* 2000;97:325–330.

44. Veith RCM, Catecholamines, depressive disorder. Sympathetic nervous system activity in major depression: Basal and desipramine-induced alterations in plasma norepinephrine kinetics.[Article]. *Arch Gen Psychiatry* 1994;51:411–422.

45. Carney RM, Freedland KE, Veith RC, et al. Major depression, heart rate, and plasma norepinephrine in patients with coronary heart disease. *Biol Psychiatry* 1999;45:458–463.

46. Colao A, Pivonello R, Spiezia S, et al. Persistence of increased cardiovascular risk in patients with Cushing's disease after five years of successful cure. *J Clin Endocrinol Metab* 1999;84:2664–2672.

47. Troxler RG, Sprague EA, Albanese RA, et al. The association of elevated plasma cortisol and early atherosclerosis as demonstrated by coronary angiography. *Atherosclerosis* 1977;26:151–162.

48. Remme WJ. The sympathetic nervous system and ischaemic heart disease. *Eur Heart J* 1998;19(Suppl F):F62–F71.

49. Matthews KA, Owens JF, Kuller LH, et al. Stress-induced pulse pressure change predicts women's carotid atherosclerosis. *Stroke* 1998;29:1525–1530.

50. Shores MM, Pascualy M, Lewis NL, et al. Short-term sertraline treatment suppresses sympathetic nervous system activity in healthy human subjects. *Psychoneuroendocrinology* 2001;26:433–439.

51. Huikuri HV, Makikallio TH. Heart rate variability in ischemic heart disease. *Auton Neurosci* 2001;90:95–101.

52. Curtis BM, O'Keefe JH Jr. Autonomic tone as a cardiovascular risk factor: The dangers of chronic fight or flight. *Mayo Clin Proc* 2002;77:45–54.

53. Gorman JM, Sloan RP. Heart rate variability in depressive and anxiety disorders. *Am Heart J* 2000;140:77–83.

54. Yeragani VK, Rao KA, Smitha MR, et al. Diminished chaos of heart rate time series in patients with major depression. *Biol Psychiatry* 2002;51:733–744.

55. Agelink MW, Boz C, Ullrich H, et al. Relationship between major depression and heart rate variability. Clinical consequences and implications for antidepressive treatment. *Psychiatry Res* 2002;113:139–149.

56. Carney RM, Blumenthal JA, Stein PK, et al. Depression, heart rate variability, and acute myocardial infarction. *Circulation* 2001;104: 2024–2028.

57. Stein PK, Carney RM, Freedland KE, et al. Severe depression is associated with markedly reduced

heart rate variability in patients with stable coronary heart disease. *J Psychosom Res* 2000;48:493–500.

58. Guinjoan SM, de Guevara MS, Correa C, et al. Cardiac parasympathetic dysfunction related to depression in older adults with acute coronary syndromes. *J Psychosom Res* 2004;56:83–88.

59. Watkins LL, Grossman P. Association of depressive symptoms with reduced baroreflex cardiac control in coronary artery disease. *Am Heart J* 1999;137:453–457.

60. Yeragani VK, Pohl R, Jampala VC, et al. Increased QT variability in patients with panic disorder and depression. *Psychiatry Res* 2000;93:225–235.

61. Nahshoni E, Aizenberg D, Strasberg B, et al. QT dispersion in the surface electrocardiogram in elderly patients with major depression. *J Affect Disord* 2000;60:197–200.

62. Dunbar SB, Kimble LP, Jenkins LS, et al. Association of mood disturbance and arrhythmia events in patients after cardioverter defibrillator implantation. *Depress Anxiety* 1999;9:163–168.

63. Carney RM, Freedland KE, Rich MW, et al. Ventricular tachycardia and psychiatric depression in patients with coronary artery disease. *Am J Med* 1993;95:23–28.

64. Buxton AE, Lee KL, Hafley GE, et al. Relation of ejection fraction and inducible ventricular tachycardia to mode of death in patients with coronary artery disease: An analysis of patients enrolled in the multicenter unsustained tachycardia trial. *Circulation* 2002;106:2466–2472.

65. Goldstein S, Friedman L, Hutchinson R, et al. Timing, mechanism and clinical setting of witnessed deaths in postmyocardial infarction patients. *J Am Coll Cardiol* 1984;3:1111–1117.

66. Rouleau JL, Talajic M, Sussex B, et al. Myocardial infarction patients in the 1990s—their risk factors, stratification and survival in Canada: The Canadian Assessment of Myocardial Infarction (CAMI) Study. *J Am Coll Cardiol* 1996;27:1119–1127.

67. Bayes dL, Coumel P, Leclercq JF. Ambulatory sudden cardiac death: Mechanisms of production of fatal arrhythmia on the basis of data from 157 cases. *Am Heart J* 1989;117:151–159.

68. Pires LA, Lehmann MH, Steinman RT, et al. Sudden death in implantable cardioverter-defibrillator recipients: Clinical context, arrhythmic events and device responses. *J Am Coll Cardiol* 1999;33:24–32.

69. Kleiger RE, Miller JP, Bigger JT Jr, et al. Decreased heart rate variability and its association with increased mortality after acute myocardial infarction. *Am J Cardiol* 1987;59:256–262.

70. La Rovere MT, Bigger JT Jr, Marcus FI, et al. Baroreflex sensitivity and heart-rate variability in prediction of total cardiac mortality after myocardial infarction. ATRAMI (Autonomic Tone and Reflexes After Myocardial Infarction) Investigators. *Lancet* 1998;351:478–484.

71. de Bruyne MC, Hoes AW, Kors JA, et al. QTc dispersion predicts cardiac mortality in the elderly: The Rotterdam Study. *Circulation* 1998;97:467–472.

72. Dabrowski A, Kramarz E, Piotrowicz R, et al. Predictive power of increased QT dispersion in ventricular extrasystoles and in sinus beats for risk stratification after myocardial infarction. *Circulation* 2000;101:1693–1697.

73. Zabel M, Klingenheben T, Franz MR, et al. Assessment of QT dispersion for prediction of mortality or arrhythmic events after myocardial infarction: Results of a prospective, long-term follow-up study. *Circulation* 1998;97:2543–2550.

74. Glassman AH, Bigger JT Jr. Cardiovascular effects of therapeutic doses of tricyclic antidepressants. A review. *Arch Gen Psychiatry* 1981;38:815–820.

75. Tulen JHM. Cardiovascular variability in major depressive disorder and effects of imipramine or mirtazapine (Org 3770). *J Clin Psychopharmacol* 1996;16:135–145.

76. Roose SP, Laghrissi-Thode F, Kennedy JS, et al. Comparison of paroxetine and nortriptyline in depressed patients with ischemic heart disease. *JAMA* 1998;279:287–291.

77. Glassman AH, O'Connor CM, Califf RM, et al. Sertraline treatment of major depression in patients with acute MI or unstable angina. Sertraline Antidepressant Heart Attack Randomized Trial. *JAMA* 2002;288:701–709.

78. McFarlane AM. Effect of sertraline on the recovery rate of cardiac autonomic function in depressed patients after acute myocardial infarction. *Am Heart J* 2001;142:617–623.

79. Agelink MW, Majewski T, Wurthmann C, et al. Autonomic neurocardiac function in patients with major depression and effects of antidepressive treatment with nefazodone. *J Affect Disord* 2001;62:187–198.

80. Khaykin Y, Dorian P, Baker B, et al. Autonomic correlates of antidepressant treatment using heart-rate variability analysis. *Can J Psychiatry* 1998;43:183–186.

81. Carney RM, Freedland KE, Stein PK, et al. Change in heart rate and heart rate variability during treatment for depression in patients with coronary heart disease. *Psychosom Med* 2000;62:639–647.

82. Sluzewska A, Rybakowski J, Bosmans E, et al. Indicators of immune activation in major depression. *Psychiatry Res* 1996;64:161–167.

83. Anisman H, Merali Z. Cytokines, stress, and depressive illness. *Brain Behav Immun* 2002;16: 513–524.

84. Maes M, Bosmans E, Meltzer HY, et al. Interleukin-1 beta: A putative mediator of HPA axis hyperactivity in major depression? *Am J Psychiatry* 1993;150:1189–1193.

85. Kop WJ, Gottdiener JS, Tangen CM, et al. Inflammation and coagulation factors in persons > 65 years of age with symptoms of depression but without evidence of myocardial ischemia. *Am J Cardiol* 2002;89:419–424.

86. Appels A, Bar FW, Bar J, et al. Inflammation, depressive symptomtology, and coronary artery disease. *Psychosom Med* 2000;62:601–605.

87. Papanicolaou DA, Wilder RL, Manolagas SC, et al. The pathophysiologic roles of interleukin-6 in human disease. *Ann Intern Med* 1998;128: 127–137.

88. Leonard BE. The immune system, depression and the action of antidepressants. *Prog Neuropsychopharmacol Biol Psychiatry* 2001;25: 767–780.

89. Maes M, Meltzer HY, Bosmans E, et al. Increased plasma concentrations of interleukin-6, soluble interleukin-6, soluble interleukin-2 and transferrin receptor in major depression. *J Affect Disord* 1995;34:301–309.

90. Miller GE, Stetler CA, Carney RM, et al. Clinical depression and inflammatory risk markers for coronary heart disease. *Am J Cardiol* 2002;90: 1279–1283.

91. Suarez EC, Krishnan RR, Lewis JG. The relation of severity of depressive symptoms to monocyte-associated proinflammatory cytokines and chemokines in apparently healthy men. *Psychosom Med* 2003;65:362–368.

92. Musselman DL, Miller AH, Porter MR, et al. Higher than normal plasma interleukin-6 concentrations in cancer patients with depression: Preliminary findings. *Am J Psychiatry* 2001;158: 1252–1257.

93. Owen BM, Eccleston D, Ferrier IN, et al. Raised levels of plasma interleukin-1beta in major and postviral depression. *Acta Psychiatr Scand* 2001; 103: 226–228.

94. Mikova O, Yakimova R, Bosmans E, et al. Increased serum tumor necrosis factor alpha concentrations in major depression and multiple sclerosis. *Eur Neuropsychopharmacol* 2001;11:203–208.

95. Seidel A, Arolt V, Hunstiger M, et al. Cytokine production and serum proteins in depression. *Scand J Immunol* 1995;41:534–538.

96. Capuron L, Gumnick JF, Musselman DL, et al. Neurobehavioral effects of interferon-alpha in cancer patients: Phenomenology and paroxetine responsiveness of symptom dimensions. *Neuropsychopharmacology* 2002;26:643–652.

97. Manolio TA, Kronmal RA, Burke GL, et al. Magnetic resonance abnormalities and cardiovascular disease in older adults. The Cardiovascular Health Study. *Stroke* 1994;25:318–327.

98. Krishnan KR, Hays JC, Blazer DG. MRI-defined vascular depression. *Am J Psychiatry* 1997;154: 497–501.

99. Steffens DC, Krishnan KR, Crump C, et al. Cerebrovascular disease and evolution of depressive symptoms in the cardiovascular health study. *Stroke* 2002;33:1636–1644.

100. Taylor WD, Steffens DC, MacFall JR, et al. White matter hyperintensity progression and late-life depression outcomes. *Arch Gen Psychiatry* 2003; 60:1090–1096.

101. Thomas AJ, Ferrier IN, Kalaria RN, et al. Elevation in late-life depression of intercellular adhesion molecule-1 expression in the dorsolateral prefrontal cortex. *Am J Psychiatry* 2000;157: 1682–1684.

102. Taylor WD, MacFall JR, Steffens DC, et al. Localization of age-associated white matter hyperintensities in late-life depression. *Prog Neuropsychopharmacol Biol Psychiatry* 2003;27:539–544.

103. Koenig W. Inflammation and coronary heart disease: An overview. *Cardiol Rev* 2001;9:31–35.

104. Mulvihill NT, Foley JB. Inflammation in acute coronary syndromes. *Heart* 2002;87:201–204.

105. Robbins M, Topol EJ. Inflammation in acute coronary syndromes. *Cleve Clin J Med* 2002; 69(Suppl 2):SII130–SII142.

106. Thompson SG, Kienast J, Pyke SD, et al. Hemostatic factors and the risk of myocardial infarction or sudden death in patients with angina pectoris. European Concerted Action on Thrombosis and Disabilities Angina Pectoris Study Group. *N Engl J Med* 1995;332:635–641.

107. Maes M, Delange J, Ranjan R, et al. Acute phase proteins in schizophrenia, mania and major depression: Modulation by psychotropic drugs. *Psychiatry Res* 1997;66:1–11.

108. Lanquillon S, Krieg JC, Bening-Abu-Shach U, et al. Cytokine production and treatment response in major depressive disorder. *Neuropsychopharmacology* 2000;22:370–379.

109. Liuzzo G, Biasucci LM, Gallimore JR, et al. The prognostic value of C-reactive protein and serum amyloid a protein in severe unstable angina.[comment]. *N Engl J Med* 1994;331:417–424.

110. Ridker PM, Cushman M, Stampfer MJ, et al. Inflammation, aspirin, and the risk of cardiovascular disease in apparently healthy men. *N Engl J Med* 1997;336:973–979.

111. Markovitz JH, Matthews KA. Platelets and coronary heart disease: Potential psychophysiologic mechanisms. *Psychosom Med* 1991;53:643–668.

112. Nair GV, Gurbel PA, O'Connor CM, et al. Depression, coronary events, platelet inhibition, and serotonin reuptake inhibitors. *Am J Cardiol* 1999;84:321–323.

113. Nemeroff CB, Musselman DL. Are platelets the link between depression and ischemic heart disease? *Am Heart J* 2000;140:S57–S62.

114. Kuijpers PM, Hamulyak K, Strik JJ, et al. Beta-thromboglobulin and platelet factor 4 levels in post-myocardial infarction patients with major depression. *Psychiatry Res* 2002;109:207–210.

115. Laghrissi-Thode F, Wagner WR, Pollock BG, et al. Elevated platelet factor 4 and beta-thromboglobulin plasma levels in depressed patients with ischemic heart disease. *Biol Psychiatry* 1997;42:290–295.

116. Musselman DL, Tomer A, Manatunga AK, et al. Exaggerated platelet reactivity in major depression. *Am J Psychiatry* 1996;153:1313–1317.

117. Musselman DL, Marzec U, Davidoff M, et al. Platelet activation and secretion in patients with major depression, thoracic aortic atherosclerosis, or renal dialysis treatment. *Depress Anxiety* 2002;15:91–101.

118. Lederbogen F, Gilles M, Maras A, et al. Increased platelet aggregability in major depression? *Psychiatry Res* 2001;102:255–261.

119. Maes M, Van der Planken M, Van Gastel A, et al. Blood coagulation and platelet aggregation in major depression. *J Affect Disord* 1996;40:35–40.

120. Hrdina PD, Bakish D, Chudzik J, et al. Serotonergic markers in platelets of patients with major depression: Upregulation of 5-HT2 receptors. *J Psychiatry Neurosci* 1995;20:11–19.

121. Neuger J, El Khoury A, Kjellman BF, et al. Platelet serotonin functions in untreated major depression. *Psychiatry Res* 1999;85:189–198.

122. Sheline YI, Bardgett ME, Jackson JL, et al. Platelet serotonin markers and depressive symptomatology. *Biol Psychiatry* 1995;37:442–447.

123. Leonard BE. Evidence for a biochemical lesion in depression. *J Clin Psychiatry* 2000;61(Suppl 6):12–17.

124. Mendelson SD. The current status of the platelet 5-HT(2A) receptor in depression. *J Affect Disord* 2000;57:13–24.

125. Shimbo D, Child J, Davidson K, et al. Exaggerated serotonin-mediated platelet reactivity as a possible link in depression and acute coronary syndromes. *Am J Cardiol* 2002;89:331–333.

126. Whyte EM, Pollock BG, Wagner WR, et al. Influence of serotonin-transporter-linked promoter region polymorphism on platelet activation in geriatric depression. *Am J Psychiatry* 2001;158:2074–2076.

127. Serebruany VL, Gurbel PA, O'Connor CM. Platelet inhibition by sertraline and N-desmethylsertraline: A possible missing link between depression, coronary events, and mortality benefits of selective serotonin reuptake inhibitors. *Pharmacol Res* 2001;43:453–462.

128. Serebruany VL, O'Connor CM, Gurbel PA. Effect of selective serotonin reuptake inhibitors on platelets in patients with coronary artery disease. *Am J Cardiol* 2001;87:1398–1400.

129. Pollock BG, Laghrissi-Thode F, Wagner WR. Evaluation of platelet activation in depressed patients with ischemic heart disease after paroxetine or nortriptyline treatment. *J Clin Psychopharmacol* 2000;20:137–140.

130. Musselman DL, Marzec UM, Manatunga A, et al. Platelet reactivity in depressed patients treated with paroxetine: Preliminary findings. *Arch Gen Psychiatry* 2000;57:875–882.

131. Serebruany VL, Glassman AH, Malinin AI, et al. Platelet/endothelial function in depressed patients treated with a selective serotonin reuptake inhibitor after acute coronary events: The Sertaline AntiDepressant Heart Attack Randomized Trial (SADHART) platelet substudy. *Circulation* 2003;108(8):939–944.

132. von Kanel R, Mills PJ, Fainman C, et al. Effects of psychological stress and psychiatric disorders on blood coagulation and fibrinolysis: A biobehavioral pathway to coronary artery disease? *Psychosom Med* 2001;63:531–544.

133. Folsom AR, Qamhieh HT, Flack JM, et al. Plasma fibrinogen: Levels and correlates in young adults. The Coronary Artery Risk Development in Young Adults (CARDIA) Study. *Am J Epidemiol* 1993; 138:1023–1036.

134. Thaulow E, Erikssen J, Sandvik L, et al. Blood platelet count and function are related to total and cardiovascular death in apparently healthy men. *Circulation* 1991;84:613–617.

135. Heeschen C, Dimmeler S, Hamm CW, et al. Soluble CD40 ligand in acute coronary syndromes. *N Engl J Med* 2003;348:1104–1111.

136. Antithrombotic Trialists' Collaboration: Collaborative meta-analysis of randomised trials of antiplatelet therapy for prevention of death, myocardial infarction, and stroke in high risk patients. *Br Med J* 2002;324:71–86.

137. Fuster V, Badimon L, Badimon JJ, et al. The pathogenesis of coronary artery disease and the acute coronary syndromes (1). *N Engl J Med* 1992;326:242–250.

138. Davies MJ. The contribution of thrombosis to the clinical expression of coronary atherosclerosis. *Thromb Res* 1996;82:1–32.

139. Braunwald E, Antman EM, Beasley JW. et al. ACC/AHA 2002 guideline update for the management of patients with unstable angina and non-ST-segment elevation myocardial infarction: A report of the American College of Cardiology/American Heart Association Task Force on Practice Guidelines (Committee on the Management of Patients With Unstable Angina). *Am Coll Cardiol* 2003;2:27.

140. Gibbons RJ, Abrams J, Chatterjee K, et al. ACC/AHA 2002 guideline update for the management of patients with chronic stable angina—summary article: A report of the American College of Cardiology/American Heart Association Task Force on Practice Guidelines (Committee on the Management of Patients With Chronic Stable Angina). *Circulation* 2003;107:149–158.

141. DiMatteo MR, Lepper HS, Croghan TW. Depression is a risk factor for noncompliance with medical treatment: Meta-analysis of the effects of anxiety and depression on patient adherence. *Arch Intern Med* 2000;160:2101–2107.

142. Wang PS, Bohn RL, Knight E, et al. Noncompliance with antihypertensive medications: The impact of depressive symptoms and psychosocial factors. *J Gen Intern Med* 2002;17:504–511.

143. Blumenthal JA, Williams RS, Wallace AG, et al. Physiological and psychological variables predict compliance to prescribed exercise therapy in patients recovering from myocardial infarction. *Psychosom Med* 1982;44:519–527.

144. Glazer KM, Emery CF, Frid DJ, et al. Psychological predictors of adherence and outcomes among patients in cardiac rehabilitation. *J Cardiopulm Rehabil* 2002;22:40–46.

145. Evangelista LS, Berg J, Dracup K. Relationship between psychosocial variables and compliance in patients with heart failure. *Heart Lung* 2001;30:294–301.

146. Yusuf S. Two decades of progress in preventing vascular disease. *Lancet* 2002;360:2–3.

147. Butler J, Arbogast PG, BeLue R, et al. Outpatient adherence to beta-blocker therapy after acute myocardial infarction. *J Am Coll Cardiol* 2002;40:1589–1595.

148. Jackevicius CA, Mamdani M, Tu JV. Adherence with statin therapy in elderly patients with and without acute coronary syndromes. *JAMA* 2002;288:462–467.

149. Influence of adherence to treatment and response of cholesterol on mortality in the coronary drug project. *N Engl J Med* 1980;303:1038–1041.

150. Horwitz RI, Viscoli CM, Berkman L, et al. Treatment adherence and risk of death after a myocardial infarction. *Lancet* 1990;336:542–545.

151. McDermott MM, Schmitt B, Wallner E. Impact of medication nonadherence on coronary heart disease outcomes. A critical review. *Arch Intern Med* 1997;157:1921–1929.

152. Lustman PJ, Griffith LS, Clouse RE, et al. Effects of nortriptyline on depression and glycemic control in diabetes: Results of a double-blind, placebo-controlled trial. *Psychosom Med* 1997;59:241–250.

153. Lustman PJ, Griffith LS, Freedland KE, et al. Cognitive behavior therapy for depression in type 2 diabetes mellitus. A randomized, controlled trial. *Ann Intern Med* 1998;129:613–621.

154 Rich MW, Gray DB, Beckham V, et al. Effect of a multidisciplinary intervention on medication compliance in elderly patients with congestive heart failure. *Am J Med* 1996;101:270–276.

155. Penninx BW, van Tilburg T, Boeke AJ, et al. Effects of social support and personal coping

resources on depressive symptoms: Different for various chronic diseases? *Health Psychol* 1998;17:551–558.

156. Wade TD, Kendler KS. The relationship between social support and major depression: Cross-sectional, longitudinal, and genetic perspectives. *J Nerv Ment Dis* 2000;188:251–258.

157. Bosworth HB, Hays JC, George LK, et al. Psychosocial and clinical predictors of unipolar depression outcome in older adults. *Int J Geriatr Psychiatry* 2002;17:238–246.

158. Hays JC, Steffens DC, Flint EP, et al. Does social support buffer functional decline in elderly patients with unipolar depression? *Am J Psychiatry* 2001;158:1850–1855.

159. Colantonio A, Kasl SV, Ostfeld AM, et al. Psychosocial predictors of stroke outcomes in an elderly population. *J Gerontol* 1993;48:S261–S268.

160. Kwakkel G, Wagenaar RC, Kollen BJ, et al. Predicting disability in stroke: A critical review of the literature. *Age Ageing* 1996;25:479–489.

161. Berkman LF, Leo-Summers L, Horwitz RI. Emotional support and survival after myocardial infarction. A prospective, population-based study of the elderly. *Ann Intern Med* 1992;117:1003–1009.

162. Gorkin L, Schron EB, Brooks MM, et al. Psychosocial predictors of mortality in the Cardiac Arrhythmia Suppression Trial-1 (CAST-1). *Am J Cardiol* 1993;71:263–267.

163. Williams RB, Barefoot JC, Califf RM, et al. Prognostic importance of social and economic resources among medically treated patients with angiographically documented coronary artery disease. *JAMA* 1992;267:520–524.

164. Case RB, Moss AJ, Case N, et al. Living alone after myocardial infarction. Impact on prognosis. *JAMA* 1992;267:515–519.

165. Kawachi I, Colditz GA, Ascherio A, et al. A prospective study of social networks in relation to total mortality and cardiovascular disease in men in the USA. *J Epidemiol Community Health* 1996;50:245–251.

166. Krumholz HM, Amatruda J, Smith GL, et al. Randomized trial of an education and support intervention to prevent readmission of patients with heart failure. *J Am Coll Cardiol* 2002;39: 83–89.

167. Frasure-Smith N, Prince R. Long-term follow-up of the Ischemic Heart Disease Life Stress Monitoring Program. *Psychosom Med* 1989;51: 485–513.

168. Black PH, Garbutt LD. Stress, inflammation and cardiovascular disease. *J Psychosom Res* 2002; 52:1–23.

169. Brown GW, Harris TO. *Social Origins of Depression: A Study of Psychiatric Disorder in Women.* New York: Free Press. 1978.

170. Harris T. Recent developments in understanding the psychosocial aspects of depression. *Br Med Bull* 2001;57:17–32.

171. Kessler RC. The effects of stressful life events on depression. *Annu Rev Psychol* 1997;48:191–214.

172. Lora A, Fava E. Provoking agents, vulnerability factors and depression in an Italian setting: A replication of Brown and Harris's model. *J Affect Disord* 1992;24:227–235.

173. Monroe SM, Bellack AS, Hersen M, et al. Life events, symptom course, and treatment outcome in unipolar depressed women. *J Consult Clin Psychol* 1983;51:604–615.

174. Monroe SM, Harkness K, Simons AD, et al. Life stress and the symptoms of major depression. *J Nerv Ment Dis* 2001;189:168–175.

175. Ravindran AV, Griffiths J, Waddell C, et al. Stressful life events and coping styles in relation to dysthymia and major depressive disorder: Variations associated with alleviation of symptoms following pharmacotherapy. *Prog Neuropsychopharmacol Biol Psychiatry* 1995;19:637–653.

176. Kendler KS, Kessler RC, Neale MC, et al. The prediction of major depression in women: Toward an integrated etiologic model. *Am J Psychiatry* 1993;150:1139–1148.

177. Chevalier A, Bonenfant S, Picot MC, et al. Occupational factors of anxiety and depressive disorders in the French National Electricity and Gas Company. The Anxiety-Depression Group. *J Occup Environ Med* 1996;38:1098–1107.

178. Paterniti S, Niedhammer I, Lang T, et al. Psychosocial factors at work, personality traits and depressive symptoms. Longitudinal results from the GAZEL Study. *Br J Psychiatry* 2002;181: 111–117.

179. Bosworth HB, Steffens DC, Kuchibhatla M, et al. The relationship of social support, social networks and negative events with depression in patients with coronary artery disease. *Aging Ment Health* 2000;4:253–258.

180. Iso H, Date C, Yamamoto A, et al. Perceived mental stress and mortality from cardiovascular disease among Japanese men and women: The Japan Collaborative Cohort Study for Evaluation

of Cancer Risk Sponsored by Monbusho (JACC Study). *Circulation* 2002;106:1229–1236.

181. Rosengren A, Tibblin G, Wilhelmsen L. Self-perceived psychological stress and incidence of coronary artery disease in middle-aged men. *Am J Cardiol* 1991;68:1171–1175.

182. Tennant CC, Palmer KJ, Langeluddecke PM, et al. Life event stress and myocardial reinfarction: A prospective study. *Eur Heart J* 1994; 15:472–478.

183. Jenkinson CM, Madeley RJ, Mitchell JR, et al. The influence of psychosocial factors on survival after myocardial infarction. *Public Health* 1993;107:305–317.

184. Welin C, Lappas G, Wilhelmsen L. Independent importance of psychosocial factors for prognosis after myocardial infarction. *J Intern Med* 2000;247:629–639.

185. Bairey Merz CN, Dwyer J, Nordstrom CK, et al. Psychosocial stress and cardiovascular disease: Pathophysiological links. *Behav Med* 2002;27: 141–147.

186. Chrousos GP, Gold PW. The concepts of stress and stress system disorders. Overview of physical and behavioral homeostasis. *JAMA* 1992;267: 1244–1252.

187. Esch T, Stefano GB, Fricchione GL, et al. Stress in cardiovascular diseases. *Med Sci Monit* 2002; 8:RA93–RA101.

188. Yeung AC, Vekshtein VI, Krantz DS, et al. The effect of atherosclerosis on the vasomotor response of coronary arteries to mental stress. *N Engl J Med* 1991;325:1551–1556.

189. Blumenthal JA, Jiang W, Waugh RA, et al. Mental stress-induced ischemia in the laboratory and ambulatory ischemia during daily life. Association and hemodynamic features. *Circulation* 1995;92:2102–2108.

190. Jiang W, Babyak M, Krantz DS, et al. Mental stress-induced myocardial ischemia and cardiac events. *JAMA* 1996;275:1651–1656.

191. Sheps DS, McMahon RP, Becker L, et al. Mental stress-induced ischemia and all-cause mortality in patients with coronary artery disease: Results from the Psychophysiological Investigations of Myocardial Ischemia study. *Circulation* 2002;105:1780–1784.

192. McEwen BS. The neurobiology of stress: From serendipity to clinical relevance. *Brain Res* 2000;886:172–189.

193. Song C, Kenis G, Van Gastel A, et al. Influence of psychological stress on immune-inflammatory variables in normal humans. Part II. Altered serum concentrations of natural anti-inflammatory agents and soluble membrane antigens of monocytes and T lymphocytes. *Psychiatry Res* 1999; 85:293–303.

194. Uchakin PN, Tobin B, Cubbage M, et al. Immune responsiveness following academic stress in first-year medical students. *J Interferon Cytokine Res* 2001;21:687–694.

195. Andrews TC, Parker JD, Jacobs S, et al. Effects of therapy with nifedipine GITS or atenolol on mental stress-induced ischemic left ventricular dysfunction. *J Am Coll Cardiol* 1998;32:1680–1686.

196. Blumenthal JA, Babyak M, Wei J, et al. Usefulness of psychosocial treatment of mental stress-induced myocardial ischemia in men. *Am J Cardiol* 2002;89:164–168.

197. Fuster V, Gotto AM, Libby P, et al. 27th Bethesda Conference: Matching the intensity of risk factor management with the hazard for coronary disease events. Task Force 1. Pathogenesis of coronary disease: The biologic role of risk factors. [Review] [82 refs]. *J Am Coll Cardiol* 1996;27: 964–976.

198. Wilson PW, D'Agostino RB, Levy D, et al. Prediction of coronary heart disease using risk factor categories. *Circulation* 1998;97:1837–1847.

199. Severus WE, Littman AB, Stoll AL. Omega-3 fatty acids, homocysteine, and the increased risk of cardiovascular mortality in major depressive disorder. *Harv Rev Psychiatry* 2001;9:280–293.

200. Multiple Risk Factor Intervention Trial Research Group: Relationship between baseline risk factors and coronary heart disease and total mortality in the Multiple Risk Factor Intervention Trial. *Prev Med* 1986;15:254–273.

201. Quattrocki E, Baird A, Yurgelun-Todd D. Biological aspects of the link between smoking and depression. *Harv Rev Psychiatry* 2000;8:99–110.

202. Breslau N, Peterson EL, Schultz LR, et al. Major depression and stages of smoking. A longitudinal investigation. *Arch Gen Psychiatry* 1998;55: 161–166.

203. Anda RF, Williamson DF, Escobedo LG, et al. Depression and the dynamics of smoking. A national perspective. *JAMA* 1990;264:1541–1545.

204. Hall SM, Munoz RF, Reus VI, et al. Nicotine, negative affect, and depression. *J Consult Clin Psychol* 1993;61:761–767.

205. Shinn EH, Poston WS, Kimball KT, et al. Blood pressure and symptoms of depression and

anxiety: A prospective study. *Am J Hypertens* 2001;14:660–664.

206. Jonas BS, Lando JF. Negative affect as a prospective risk factor for hypertension. *Psychosom Med* 2000;62:188–196.

207. Davidson K, Jonas BS, Dixon KE, et al. Do depression symptoms predict early hypertension incidence in young adults in the CARDIA study? Coronary Artery Risk Development in Young Adults. *Arch Intern Med* 2000;160: 1495–1500.

208. Garcia MJ, McNamara PM, Gordon T, et al. Morbidity and mortality in diabetics in the Framingham population. Sixteen year follow-up study. *Diabetes* 1974;23:105–111.

209. Anderson RJ, Freedland KE, Clouse RE, et al. The prevalence of comorbid depression in adults with diabetes: A meta-analysis. *Diabetes Care* 2001;24:1069–1078.

210. Eaton WW, Armenian H, Gallo J, et al. Depression and risk for onset of type II diabetes. A prospective population-based study. *Diabetes Care* 1996;19:1097–1102.

211. Lustman PJ, Anderson RJ, Freedland KE, et al. Depression and poor glycemic control: A meta-analytic review of the literature. *Diabetes Care* 2000;23:934–942.

212. de Groot M, Anderson R, Freedland KE. Association of depression and diabetes complications: A meta-analysis. *Psychosom Med* 2001;63: 619–630.

213. Anderson KM, Castelli WP, Levy D. Cholesterol and mortality. 30 years of follow-up from the Framingham study. *JAMA* 1987;257:2176–2180.

214. Horsten M, Wamala SP, Vingerhoets A, et al. Depressive symptoms, social support, and lipid profile in healthy middle-aged women. *Psychosom Med* 1997;59:521–528.

215. Olusi SO, Fido AA. Serum lipid concentrations in patients with major depressive disorder. *Biol Psychiatry* 1996;40:1128–1131.

216. Steegmans PH, Fekkes D, Hoes AW, et al. Low serum cholesterol concentration and serotonin metabolism in men. *Br Med J* 1996;312:221.

217. Steegmans PH, Hoes AW, Bak AA, et al. Higher prevalence of depressive symptoms in middle-aged men with low serum cholesterol levels. *Psychosom Med* 2000;62:205–211.

218. Hyyppa MT, Kronholm E, Virtanen A, et al. Does simvastatin affect mood and steroid hormone levels in hypercholesterolemic men? A random-ized double-blind trial. *Psychoneuroendocrinology* 2003;28:181–194.

219. Wilson PW, D'Agostino RB, Sullivan L, et al. Overweight and obesity as determinants of cardiovascular risk: The Framingham experience. *Arch Intern Med* 2002;162:1867–1872.

220. Istvan J, Zavela K, Weidner G. Body weight and psychological distress in NHANES I. *Int J Obes Relat Metab Disord* 1992;16:999–1003.

221. Carpenter KM, Hasin DS, Allison DB, et al. Relationships between obesity and DSM-IV major depressive disorder, suicide ideation, and suicide attempts: Results from a general population study. *Am J Public Health* 2000;90:251–257.

222. Homocysteine Studies Collaboration: Homocysteine and risk of ischemic heart disease and stroke: A meta-analysis. *JAMA* 2002;288:2015–2022.

223. Schnyder G, Flammer Y, Roffi M, et al. Plasma homocysteine levels and late outcome after coronary angioplasty. *J Am Coll Cardiol* 2002;40: 1769–1776.

224. Klerk M, Verhoef P, Clarke R, et al. MTHFR 677C—>T polymorphism and risk of coronary heart disease: A meta-analysis. *JAMA* 2002;288: 2023–2031.

225. Coppen A, Bailey J. Enhancement of the antidepressant action of fluoxetine by folic acid: A randomised, placebo controlled trial. *J Affect Disord* 2000;60:121–130.

226. Guaraldi GP, Fava M, Mazzi F, et al. An open trial of methyltetrahydrofolate in elderly depressed patients. *Ann Clin Psychiatry* 1993;5:101–105.

227. Ormel J, Koeter MW, van den Brink W, et al. Recognition, management, and course of anxiety and depression in general practice. *Arch Gen Psychiatry* 1991;48:700–706.

228. Simon GE, VonKorff M. Recognition, management, and outcomes of depression in primary care. *Arch Fam Med* 1995;4:99–105.

229. Spitzer RL, Williams JB, Kroenke K, et al. Utility of a new procedure for diagnosing mental disorders in primary care. The PRIME-MD 1000 study. *JAMA* 1994;272:1749–1756.

230. Davidson JR, Meltzer-Brody SE. The underrecognition and undertreatment of depression: What is the breadth and depth of the problem? *J Clin Psychiatry* 1999;60(Suppl 7):4–9.

231. Goldman LS, Nielsen NH, Champion HC. Awareness, diagnosis, and treatment of depression. *J Gen Intern Med* 1999;14:569–580.

232. Kessler RC, Berglund P, Demler O, et al. The epidemiology of major depressive disorder:

Results from the National Comorbidity Survey Replication (NCS-R). *JAMA* 2003;289:3095–3105.

233. Olfson M, Marcus SC, Druss B, et al. National trends in the outpatient treatment of depression. *JAMA* 2002;287:203–209.

234. Hirschfeld RM, Keller MB, Panico S, et al. The National Depressive and Manic-Depressive Association consensus statement on the undertreatment of depression. *JAMA* 1997;277:333–340.

235. Alexopoulos GS, Borson S, Cuthbert BN, et al. Assessment of late life depression. *Biol Psychiatry* 2002;52:164–174.

236. Charlson M, Peterson JC. Medical comorbidity and late life depression: What is known and what are the unmet needs? *Biol Psychiatry* 2002;52:226–235.

237. Whooley MA, Avins AL, Miranda J, et al. Case-finding instruments for depression. Two questions are as good as many. *J Gen Intern Med* 1997;12:439–445.

238. Juenger J, Schellberg D, Kraemer S, et al. Health related quality of life in patients with congestive heart failure: Comparison with other chronic diseases and relation to functional variables. *Heart* 2002;87:235–241.

239. Avorn J, Everitt DE, Weiss S. Increased antidepressant use in patients prescribed beta-blockers. *JAMA* 1986;255:357–360.

240. Thiessen BQ, Wallace SM, Blackburn JL, et al. Increased prescribing of antidepressants subsequent to beta-blocker therapy. *Arch Intern Med* 1990;150:2286–2290.

241. Ko DT, Hebert PR, Coffey CS, et al. Beta-blocker therapy and symptoms of depression, fatigue, and sexual dysfunction. *JAMA* 2002;288:351–357.

242. Bright RA, Everitt DE. Beta-blockers and depression. Evidence against an association. *JAMA* 1992;267:1783–1787.

243. Kohn R. Beta-blockers an important cause of depression: A medical myth without evidence. *Med Health R I* 2001;84:92–95.

244. Koenig HG, George LK, Peterson BL, et al. Depression in medically ill hospitalized older adults: Prevalence, characteristics, and course of symptoms according to six diagnostic schemes. *Am J Psychiatry* 1997;154:1376–1383.

245. Freedland KE. The Depression Interview and Structured Hamilton (DISH): Rationale, development, characteristics, and clinical validity. *Psychosom Med* 2002;64:897–905.

246. Pignone MP, Gaynes BN, Rushton JL, et al. Screening for depression in adults: A summary of the evidence for the U.S. Preventive Services Task Force. *Ann Intern Med* 2002;136:765–776.

247. Writing Committee for the ENRICHD Investigators: The Effects of Treating Depression and Low Perceived Social Support on Clinical Events After Myocardial Infarction: The Enhancing Recovery in Coronary Heart Disease Patients (ENRICHD) Randomized Trial. *JAMA* 2003;289:3106–3116.

248. Frasure-Smith N, Lesperance F, Prince RH, et al. Randomised trial of home-based psychosocial nursing intervention for patients recovering from myocardial infarction. *Lancet* 1997;350:473–479.

249. Sheps DS. ENRICHD and SADHART: Implications for future biobehavioral intervention efforts. *Psychosom Med* 2003;65:1–2.

250. Swenson JR, O'Connor CM, Barton D, et al. Influence of depression and effect of treatment with sertraline on quality of life after hospitalization for acute coronary syndrome. *Am J Cardiol* 2003;92:1271–1276.

251. Walsh BT, Seidman SN, Sysko R, et al. Placebo response in studies of major depression: Variable, substantial, and growing. *JAMA* 2002;287:1840–1847.

252. Serebruany VL, Glassman AH, Malinin AI, et al. Platelet/endothelial biomarkers in depressed patients treated with the selective serotonin reuptake inhibitor sertraline after acute coronary events: The Sertraline AntiDepressant Heart Attack Randomized Trial (SADHART) Platelet Substudy. *Circulation* 2003;108:939–944.

253. van den Brink RH, van Melle JP, Honig A, et al. Treatment of depression after myocardial infarction and the effects on cardiac prognosis and quality of life: Rationale and outline of the Myocardial INfarction and Depression-Intervention Trial (MIND-IT). *Am Heart J* 2002;144:219–225.

254. Dobson KS. A meta-analysis of the efficacy of cognitive therapy for depression. *J Consult Clin Psychol* 1989;57:414–419.

255. Robinson LA, Berman JS, Neimeyer RA. Psychotherapy for the treatment of depression: A comprehensive review of controlled outcome research. *Psychol Bull* 1990;108:30–49.

256. Blumenthal JA, Jiang W, Babyak MA, et al. Stress management and exercise training in cardiac patients with myocardial ischemia. Effects on

prognosis and evaluation of mechanisms. *Arch Intern Med* 1997;157:2213–2223.

257. Linden W, Stossel C, Maurice J. Psychosocial interventions for patients with coronary artery disease: A meta-analysis. *Arch Intern Med* 1996;156:745–752.

258. Jones DA, West RR. Psychological rehabilitation after myocardial infarction: Multicentre randomised controlled trial. *Br Med J* 1996;313: 1517–1521.

259. Maeland JG, Havik OE. The effects of an in-hospital educational programme for myocardial infarction patients. *Scand J Rehabil Med* 1987;19: 57–65.

260. Carney RM, Blumenthal JA, Catellier D, et al. Depression as a risk factor for mortality after acute myocardial infarction. *Am J Cardiol* 2003; 92:1277–1281.

261. Heiligenstein JH, Ware JE Jr, Beusterien KM, et al. Acute effects of fluoxetine versus placebo on functional health and well-being in late-life depression. *Int Psychogeriatr* 1995;7(Suppl): 125–137.

262. Fortner MR, Brown K, Varia IM, et al. Effect of bupropion SR on the quality of life of elderly depressed patients with comorbid medical dis-

orders. *Prim Care Companion J Clin Psychiatry* 1999;1:174–179.

263. Judd LL, Akiskal HS, Maser JD, et al. A prospective 12-year study of subsyndromal and syndromal depressive symptoms in unipolar major depressive disorders. *Arch Gen Psychiatry* 1998; 55:694–700.

264. Beekman AT, Geerlings SW, Deeg DJ, et al. The natural history of late-life depression: A 6-year prospective study in the community. *Arch Gen Psychiatry* 2002;59:605–611.

265. Costello EJ, Pine DS, Hammen C, et al. Development and natural history of mood disorders. *Biol Psychiatry* 2002;52:529–542.

266. Jiang W, Alexander J, Christopher E, et al. Relationship of depression to increased risk of mortality and rehospitalization in patients with congestive heart failure. *Arch Intern Med* 2001; 161:1849–1856.

267. Puzynski S. Placebo in the investigation of psychotropic drugs, especially antidepressants. *Sci Eng Ethics* 2004;10:135–142.

268. Baldwin D, Broich K, Fritze J, et al. Placebo-controlled studies in depression: Necessary, ethical and feasible. *Eur Arch Psychiatry Clin Neurosci* 2003;253:22–28.

CHAPTER 11

Mood Disorders Following Stroke

Oladipo A. Kukoyi and Robert G. Robinson

▶ **INTRODUCTION**

Stroke represents a major public health problem in many countries throughout the world. In the United States, there are approximately 500,000 new strokes and 200,000 recurrent strokes each year. It is the most common serious neurologic disorder in the United States and the third leading cause of death.[1] Stroke is the number one source of significant disability with up to a third of survivors having significant residual impairment and 20% requiring institutional care in the 3 months following the stroke.[2] It is second only to dementia as a cause for nursing home placement. The incidence is expected to rise as the percent of elderly in the United States increases in the next 20 years. Furthermore, the incidence of stroke doubles each decade after age of 55 and 62% of the strokes each year occur in persons over the age of 65.[3] The American Heart Association estimates that there are currently about 4.8 million stroke survivors.[4]

For more than 20 years, systematic studies have documented the high incidence of mood disorders following stroke and their impact on recovery and survival. This chapter will discuss the prevalence, diagnosis, differential diagnosis, pathogenesis, and treatment of both depression and bipolar disorders following stroke.

▶ **HISTORY**

Early reports of depression after brain damage (such as in the poststroke period) were made by neurologists and psychiatrists in case descriptions. Adolf Meyer warned that new discoveries of cerebral localization in the early 1900s such as language function led to an over hasty identification of centers and functions of the brain. He identified several disorders such as delirium, dementia, and aphasia which were the direct result of brain injury.[5] In keeping with his view of biopsychosocial causes of most mental "reactions," however, he saw manic-depressive illness and paranoiac conditions as arising from a combination of brain injury (specifically citing left frontal lobe and cortical convexities) as well as a family history of psychiatric disorder and premorbid personal psychiatric disorders to produce the specific mental reaction.[5] Bleuler noted that after stroke "melancholic moods lasting for months and sometimes longer appear frequently."[6] Kraepelin recognized an association between manic-depressive insanity and cerebrovascular disease. He stated "the diagnosis of states of depression may offer difficulties, especially when arteriosclerosis is involved." Kraepelin concluded that cerebrovascular disorder may be an accompanying phenomenon of manic-depressive disease or may itself produce depressive disorder.[7]

▶ POSTSTROKE DEPRESSION

Prevalence

Numerous studies have examined the prevalence of poststroke depression (PSD). A summary of these studies is shown in Table 11-1. As is obvious from this table, there is a wide variation in the estimated prevalence of PSD and this largely depends upon whether patients were examined in hospital or in community surveys, whether they were studied during the acute poststroke period or many months following stroke, whether "minor" depression was included and whether severity measures with cutoff scores were used to define the existence of PSD, rather than the "gold standard" of structured interviews in combination with established diagnostic criteria.

Based on the data from the above studies, the mean prevalence of major depression (MDD) in patients hospitalized for acute stroke or rehabilitation services was 22% while minor depression (i.e., subsyndromal major depression by DSM-IV criteria) occurred in 17%. In outpatient stroke populations, the mean prevalence was 23% for MDD, and 35% for minor depression. In community samples, the mean prevalence was 13% for MDD and 10% for minor depression.

Diagnosis

Making the diagnosis of PSD is often complicated in the stroke survivor. For example, the presence of language or speech difficulties (aphasia), marked cognitive impairment, unawareness of sad feelings (anosognosia) and inability to move the facial muscles that convey sadness may make it hard to reliably ascertain the presence of depression. For example, a patient with aprosodia has difficulty matching words with their emotional affect. Receptive aprosodia, associated with right parietal lesions, disables the patients from telling whether a phrase sounds happy, sad, or angry. Expressive aprosodias, linked with right frontal lesions, lead to emotionally uninflected words. Thus, a patient is unable to say words as if they were angry, sad, or happy, leaving the words flat and devoid of emotional inflection.

Based on the *Diagnostic and Statistical Manual of Mental Disorders, Fourth Edition Text-Revision* (DSM-IV-TR),[8] the diagnosis for stroke-related depression is mood disorder due to stroke with (a) depressive features; (b) major depressive-like episode; (c) manic features; (d) mixed features.

Some investigators, however, have suggested that several somatic symptoms used by DSM-IV-TR for the diagnosis of major depression, such as loss of energy, poor appetite, weight loss, and insomnia, are also found among stroke patients with no mood disturbance due to their hospital environment, use of medications, associated medical conditions, or the stroke itself.[9] DSM-IV-TR addresses this issue explicitly, directing that the clinician should count all such symptoms toward the diagnosis of a major depressive episode, except in cases where one can clearly and convincingly show that the symptoms are secondary to the stroke.

Notwithstanding DSM-IV-TR recommendations, many researchers in the field of psychosomatic medicine continue to debate the most appropriate method for the diagnosis of depression when some symptoms (e.g., sleep, energy, or appetite disturbance) could result from the physical illness. Four approaches have been proposed to assess depression in the physically ill.[9] These approaches are the "inclusive approach" in which depressive diagnostic symptoms are counted regardless of whether they may be related to physical illness, the "etiologic approach" in which a symptom is counted only if the diagnostician feels that it is not caused by the physical illness, the "substitutive approach" in which other psychologic symptoms of depression replace the vegetative symptoms, and the

▶ **TABLE 11-1** PREVALENCE STUDIES OF POSTSTROKE DEPRESSION

Investigators	Patient Population	N	Criteria	% Major	% Minor	Total(%)
Wade et al. (1987)[38]	Community	379	Cutoff score			30
House et al. (1991)[55]	Community	89	PSE-DSM-III	11	12	23
Burvill et al. (1995)[56]	Community	294	PSE-DSM-III	15	8	23
Kotila et al. (1998)[57]	Community	321	Cutoff score			44
Pooled data means for community studies total N = 1083				14.1	9.1	31.8
Robinson et al. (1983)[25]	Acute hosp	103	PSE-DSM-III	27	20	47
Ebrahim et al. (1987)[58]	Acute hosp	149	Cutoff score			23
Fedoroff et al. (1991)[59]	Acute hosp	205	PSE-DSM-III	22	19	41
Castillo et al. (1995)[60]	Acute hosp	291	PSE-DSM-III	20	18	38
Starkstein et al. (1992)[61]	Acute hosp	80	PSE-DSM[III	16	13	29
Astrom et al. (1993)[16]	Acute hosp	80	DSM-III	25	NR	25*
Herrmann et al. (1993)[62]	Acute hosp	21	RDC	24	14	38
Singh et al. (2000)[63]	Acute hosp	81	Cutoff score			36
Andersen et al. (1994)[64]	Acute hosp or outpatient	285	HDRS cutoff	10	11	21
Gainotti et al. (1999)65	Acute or rehab hosp	153	PSDRS			31
	<2 months	27%				
	2–4 months	27%				
	>4 months	40%				
Folstein et al. (1977)[66]	Rehab hosp	20	PSE & items			45
Finklestein et al. (1982)[67]	Rehab hosp	25	Cutoff score			48
Sinyor et al. (1986)[68]	Rehab hosp	35	Cotoff score			36
Finset et al. (1989)[69]	Rehab hosp	42	Cutoff score			36
Eastwood et al. (1989)[22]	Rehab hosp	87	SADS-RDC	10	40	50
Morris et al. (1990)[14]	Rehab hosp	99	CIDI-DSM-III	14	21	35
Schubert et al. (1992)[29]	Rehab hosp	18	DSM-III-R	28	44	72
Schwartz et al. (1993)[70]	Rehab hosp	91	DSM-III	40		40*
Pooled data for all acute and rehab hospital studies				19.3	18.5	35.5†
Pohjasvaara et al. (1998)[26]	Outpatient	277	PSE-DSMIIIR	26	14	40
Feibel et al. (1982)[71]	Outpatient (6 months)	91	Nursing eval			26
Robinson et al. (1982)[72]	Outpatient (6 months to 10 years)	103	Cutoff score			29
Herrmann et al. (1998)[27]	Outpatient (3 months)	150	Cutoff score			27
	(1 year)	136	Cutoff score			22
Vataja et al. (2001)[73]	Outpatient (3 months)	275	PSE-DSMIIIR	26	14	40
Collin et al. (1987)[74]	Outpatient	111	Cutoff score			42

(*Continued*)

▶ **TABLE 11-1** PREVALENCE STUDIES OF POSTSTROKE DEPRESSION (*CONTINUED*)

Investigators	Patient Population	N	Criteria	% Major	% Minor	Total (%)
Astrom et al. (1993)[16]	Outpatient (3 months)	77	DSM-III	31	NR	31*
	(1 year)	73	DSM-III	16	NR	16*
	(2 years)	57	DSM-III	19	NR	19*
	(3 years)	49	DSM-III	29	NR	29*
Castillo et al. (1995)[60]	Outpatient (3 months)	77	PSE-DSM-III	20	13	33
	(6 months)	80	PSE-DSM-III	21	21	42
	(1 year)	70	PSE-DSM-III	11	16	27
	(2 years)	67	PSE-DSM-III	18	17	35
Pooled data for outpatient studies				23.3	15.0	32.9†

Abbreviations: PSE = present state examination; RDC = research diagnostic criteria; HDRS = Hamilton depression rating scale; SADS = schedule for affective disorders and schizophrenia; CIDI = composite international diagnostic interview; PSDRS = poststroke depression rating scale; NR = not reported.

*Because minor depression was not included, these values may be low.
†Pooled data mean is low because some studies excluded frequency of minor depression.

"exclusive approach" in which symptoms are removed from the diagnostic criteria if they are not found to be more frequent in depressed than nondepressed patients.

Paradiso et al. looked at these various approaches to the diagnosis of depression in the first 2 years following a stroke.[10] Among 142 patients who were examined in hospital and followed-up for examination at 3, 6, 12, or 24 months following stroke, 60 (42%) reported the presence of a depressed mood (depressed group) while they were in hospital and the remaining 82 patients were nondepressed. There were no significant differences in the background characteristics between the depressed and nondepressed groups except that the depressed group was younger and had a higher frequency of personal history of psychiatric disorder. Throughout the 2-year follow-up, depressed patients showed a higher frequency of both vegetative and psychologic symptoms compared with the nondepressed patients (Table 11-2). The only symptoms which were not more frequent in the depressed compared to nondepressed patients were weight loss and early awakening at the initial evaluation; weight loss and early morning awakening at 6 months;

weight loss, early morning awakening, anxious foreboding, and loss of libido at 1 year; and weight loss and loss of libido at 2 years. Among the psychologic symptoms, the depressed patients had a higher frequency of most psychologic symptoms throughout the 2-year follow-up. The only psychologic symptoms that were not significantly more frequent in the depressed than in the nondepressed group were suicidal plans, simple ideas of reference and pathologic guilt at 3 months; pathologic guilt at 6 months; pathologic guilt, suicidal plans, guilty ideas of reference and irritability at 1 year; and pathologic guilt and self-deprecation at 2 years.[10]

The effect of using each of the proposed alternative diagnostic methods for PSD using DSM-IV criteria was examined. Compared to gold standard diagnoses based solely on the existence of five or more specific symptoms (i.e., symptoms that were significantly more common in depressed than nondepressed patients for the diagnosis of DSM-IV major depression), diagnoses based on unmodified symptoms (i.e., early awakening and weight loss included) had a specificity of 98% and a sensitivity of 100%.

Similar results were found at 3, 6, 12, and 24 months follow-up. The sensitivity of unmodified

▶ **TABLE 11-2** NUMBER OF PATIENTS WITH VEGETATIVE DEPRESSIVE SYMPTOMS AT EACH POSTSTROKE EVALUATION

	Initial Evaluation		3-Month Follow-up		6-Month Follow-up		1-Year Follow-up		2-Year Follow-up	
	Depressive Mood	Nondepressive Mood	Depressive Mood	Nondepressive Mood	Depressive Mood	Nondepressive Mood	Depressive Mood	Nondepressive Mood	Depressive Mood	Nondepressive Mood
Autonomic anxiety	23 (39)	4 (5)*	15 (52)	5 (11)*	18 (58)	7 (15)*	9 (45)	6 (12)*	16 (64)	8 (20)*
Anxious foreboding	21 (36)	8 (10)*	13 (46)	3 (6)*	9 (29)	7 (15)	4 (20)	4 (8)	11 (44)	2 (5)*
Morning depression	38 (63)	4 (5)*	17 (67)	2 (4)*	20 (65)	2 (4)*	11 (55)	2 (4)*	17 (68)	0 (0)*
Weight loss	20 (34)	16 (20)	6 (22)	3 (6)	10 (32)	11 (24)	4 (20)	2 (4)	7 (28)	6 (15)
Delayed sleep	24 (40)	12 (15)*	10 (36)	9 (19)	15 (48)	7 (15)*	8 (40)	5 (10)*	11 (44)	2 (5)*
Subjective anergia	35 (58)	16 (20)*	17 (61)	12 (28)*	19 (61)	10 (22)*	10 (50)	8 (16)*	15 (60)	10 (24)*
Early awakening	16 (27)	13 (16)	9 (32)	8 (17)	4 (13)	7 (15)	3 (15)	3 (6)	11 (44)	5 (12)*
Loss of libido	16 (27)	7 (9)*	12 (46)	12 (11)*	12 (39)	6 (14)*	5 (25)	7 (14)	11 (44)	10 (24)

*Number and percentage (in parentheses) of patients with or without depressed mood who had specific symptoms of depression.

Source: Adapted from Paradiso et al., Int J Psychiatry Med 1997, reprinted with permission.

281

DSM-IV criteria consistently showed a sensitivity of 100% and a specificity that ranged from 95 to 98% compared to criteria only using specific symptoms.[10] Thus, one could reasonably conclude that modifying DSM-IV-TR criteria because of the existence of cerebrovascular disease is unnecessary, in accordance with DSM-IV-TR recommendations.[11]

While DSM-IV-TR minor depression is a research diagnosis, it is similar to "mood disorder due to stroke with depressive features." Minor depression, however, has a more precise definition than mood disorder due to stroke with depressive features. Minor depression requires the presence of depressed mood or loss of interest and at least one other symptom, but less than five total symptoms of major depression. It is a subsyndromal form of major depression and is associated with a number of general medical conditions, including stroke, cancer, and diabetes. Family studies suggest that relatives of probands with MDD have an increased incidence of minor depression.[8]

In an effort to determine whether minor depression is a distinct entity or whether it is part of continuum, Paradiso and Robinson[12] compared major and minor PSD. Patients with minor depression ($n = 30$) were compared to patients with major depression ($n = 24$) and no mood disorder ($n = 87$). Minor depression was associated with left hemisphere injury (67%) compared with nondepressed (37%). Patients with minor depression had a lower frequency of prior psychiatric history (3%) and more posterior lesions (43%) compared to patients with major depression (30%) and (17%), respectively. In addition, among patients with minor depression and no mood disorder, the distance of the posterior border of the lesion from the frontal pole was significantly correlated with severity of depression as measured by the Hamilton depression scale (Spearman's rho = 0.27, $P < 0.005$).

A study published in 2000 illustrates the effect of depressive symptoms on the risk for stroke.[13] This was a prospective cohort study that followed 6095 healthy adults, aged 25–74 in the early 1970s, for an average of 16 years in which they were assessed periodically with instruments that asked them detailed questions about their medical and psychologic histories. Even after adjusting for known risk factors such as age, gender, sex, education, smoking status, body mass index, alcohol use, blood pressure, physical activity, and cholesterol levels, their results showed that compared to nondepressed people:

- Patients with the highest levels of depression had a 73% increase in stroke
- Patients with an intermediate level of depression had a 25% increase in stroke
- Blacks with high levels of depression had a 160% increase in risk while White men and White women had increased risks of 68% and 52%, respectively

Duration

Several prospective studies have examined the duration of depressive episodes in the poststroke population.[14] We followed 142 patients with acute stroke at 3, 6, 12, and 24 months follow-up.[15] Of 27 patients with major depression in hospital, 38% still had major depression at 3 months and 47% had major depression at 6 months, but only 10% had major depression at 12 months and none at 24 months (Fig. 11-1). Thus, there appears to be a natural history to major depression with most patients improving between 6 and 12 months poststroke. Minor depression, however, in our sample, was more persistent. Although 70% of the patients with in-hospital minor depression no longer had the diagnosis at 3 months, 25% had switched to major depression and at 12 months follow-up 35% had minor and 25% had major depression. At 2 years follow-up, 25% had minor depression and 43% had major depression.

Morris et al.[14] found that the mean duration of poststroke major depression was 34 weeks while the mean duration of minor depression was only 13 weeks. Aström et al.[16] also found that the majority of major depressions remitted

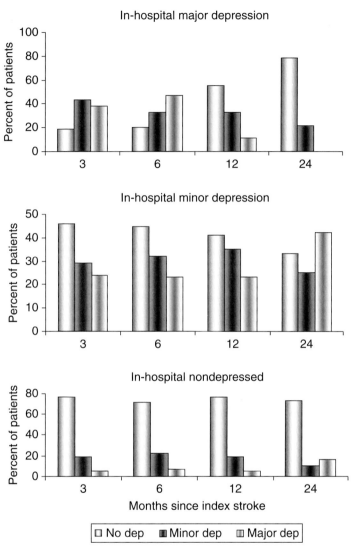

Figure 11-1. Diagnostic outcome at 3, 6, 12, and 24 months follow-up for 142 patients based on their in-hospital diagnoses of DSM-IV major depression (n = 27), DSM-IV minor depression (n = 36), or no mood disorder (n = 79). Among the patients with major depression at the in-hospital evaluation (top panel), note the increase in the percentage of patients with no depression at 12 and 24 months. This is not seen in the group of patients with an in-hospital diagnosis of minor depression patients (middle panel). About 25% of the initially nondepressed patients were found to have a diagnosis of depression at follow-up. (Source: Reprinted with permission from Robinson RG. *The Clinical Neuropsychiatry of Stroke.* Cambridge: Cambridge University Press, 1998, p. 79.)

by 1-year follow-up. However, 30% of patients with in-hospital major depression remained depressed at 1-year follow-up, 25% were depressed at 2-year follow-up, and 20% were still depressed at 3-year follow-up.

Thus, although the mean duration of major depression appeared to be about 9 months, there were about 20% of patients with major depression in-hospital who remained depressed for at least 3 years following stroke. Minor depression appeared to be more variable with more than half of our patients with in-hospital minor depression having a diagnosis of major or minor depression at 2 years follow-up. Other investigators have found minor depression to be less persistent.

Anatomic and Clinical Correlates

Lesion Location

There are several interesting hypotheses as to why depressive syndromes are so common in stroke survivors. One is that the location of the ischemic lesion is associated with both the presence and severity of the depression. For example, in 1984 we found that in the acute poststroke period, patients with left anterior lesions (left frontal cortex or left basal ganglia) had the highest frequency of depression and the closer the lesion was to the frontal pole, the more severe the depression.[17] Although the association of depression with left hemisphere lesions has been replicated by other authors, numerous studies have not found this relationship between lesion location and depression. Longitudinal studies of PSD and lesion location have generally found that these laterality effects are present only during the first 2 months following stroke. Furthermore, we have undertaken a meta-analysis of all published data which test the hypothesis that within 2 months after stroke, major depression is more frequent following left frontal or left basal ganglia stroke than following comparable lesions of the right hemisphere or posterior lesions of the left hemisphere.[18] Analysis of 7 studies (only 2 were independent

samples of ours) including 128 patients showed that the relative risk of major depression following left anterior versus left posterior lesions was 2.29 (95% CI 1.6–3.4) ($P < 0.001$) and for left anterior versus right anterior lesions was 2.18 (95% CI 1.4–3.3) ($P < 0.001$).[18] Thus, in spite of some investigators failure to replicate these findings, the consensus of data supports the conclusion that within the first 2 months poststroke, lesions involving the left frontal or left basal ganglia are associated with a significantly greater frequency of major depression than comparable lesions of the right hemisphere or posterior lesions of the left hemisphere.

This reanalysis also suggests that the failure of other investigators to replicate the association of left anterior lesion location with increased frequency of depression, in most cases, is probably related to time since stroke.[19]

Premorbid Risk Factors

The studies just reviewed indicate that although a significant proportion of patients with left anterior lesions developed PSD, not every patient with a lesion in these locations developed a major depression. This observation raises the question of why clinical variability occurs and why some but not all patients with lesions in these locations develop depression.

Starkstein et al.[20] examined this issue by comparing 13 patients with major PSD with 13 stroke patients without depression, all of whom had lesions of the same size and location. Eleven pairs of patients had left hemisphere lesions, and two pairs had right hemisphere lesions. Damage was cortical in 10 pairs and subcortical in 3 pairs. The groups did not differ on important demographic variables, such as age, sex, socioeconomic status, or education. They also did not differ on family or personal history of psychiatric disorders or neurologic deficits. Patients with major PSD, however, had significantly more subcortical atrophy ($P < 0.05$), as measured both by the ratio of third ventricle to brain (i.e., the area of the third ventricle divided by the area of the brain at the same level) and by the ratio of lateral ventricle to brain (i.e., the area of the body of the lateral ventricle contralateral to the brain lesion divided by the brain area at the same level). It is likely that the subcortical atrophy preceded the stroke because acute stroke would not likely increase the ventricular size in patients with depression but not identical strokes in patients without depression. Thus, a mild degree of subcortical atrophy may be a premorbid risk factor that increases the risk of developing major depression following a stroke.

Among patients with right hemisphere lesions, Starkstein et al.[21] found that patients who developed major depression after the occurrence of a right hemisphere lesion had a significantly higher frequency of family history of psychiatric disorders than did either nondepressed patients with right hemisphere lesions or patients with major depression following the occurrence of left hemisphere lesions. This finding suggests that a genetic predisposition for depression may play an important role after the occurrence of right hemisphere lesions. Eastwood et al.[22] and Morris et al.[14] have also reported that depressed patients were more likely than nondepressed patients to have either a personal or family history of psychiatric disorders. Other premorbid risk factors for PSD are high neuroticism personality trait[14,23] and major life events within 6 months of stroke.[24]

Activities of Daily Living

Even though the relationship between PSD and activities of daily living (ADL) is complicated by many variables that may influence this association, most investigators have been able to demonstrate a significant relationship. For example, we reported that the severity of depressive symptoms as measured by the Zung self-rating depression scale (ZDS), the Hamilton depression rating scale (HDRS), or the present state examination (PSE) was significantly correlated with the severity of impairment in ADL, i.e., the patients' ability to dress and feed themselves, walk, find their way around, express needs, read and write, and keep their room in order.[25] The strength of the correlation in most studies, however, was not very strong ranging from about 0.2

to 0.4. This would explain no more than about 16% in the variance of depression severity.

Several investigators have studied the effect of PSD on recovery in ADL.[26,27] Parikh et al.[28] in 1990 followed 63 neurologically comparable stroke patients and compared the course of recovery among 28 patients with PSD to that of 35 patients without depression. At 2-year follow-up, the depressed group was more impaired than the nondepressed group in both physical activities and language functions (Fig. 11-2).

A logistic regression analysis showed that severity of in-hospital depression was a significant independent factor in ADL recovery at 2 years even after other factors such as age, education, lesion volume, intellectual impairment, social functioning, hours of rehabilitation therapy, severity of in-hospital ADL impairment, and type of stroke were corrected ($r = 0.42$, $P < 0.05$).

The only other significant correlate was in-hospital ADL scores. Interestingly, in-hospital ADL scores did not correlate significantly with

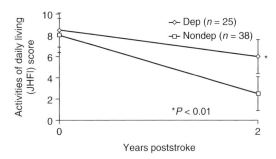

Figure 11-2. Johns Hopkins functioning inventory (JHFI) scores among patients with an acute in-hospital diagnosis of post-stroke major or minor depression or no mood disorder. Higher scores (mean + SEM shown) indicate greater impairment. There was a significant group-by-time interaction, demonstrating that depressed patients had less recovery in terms of activities of daily living than nondepressed patients. (Source: Reprinted with permission from Robinson RG. *The Clinical Neuropsychiatry of Stroke.* Cambridge: Cambridge University Press, 1998, p. 217.)

depression scores at 2 years follow-up.[15] Schubert et al.[29] examined 21 patients with PSD and reported that the severity of depression, measured by the Beck Depression Inventory (BDI), was associated with the severity of ADL, measured by the Barthel's index (BI) and that patients with PSD improved their ADL more slowly than nondepressed patients.[29] These findings suggest that in-hospital depression is one of the strongest predictors of recovery in ADL over 2 years and that the initial ADL impairment has no significant effect on depression at 2 years poststroke.

Since PSD impairs recovery in ADL, it makes sense to assume that recovery from PSD would be expected to improve recovery in ADL.

Several studies have reported that antidepressant treatment improved poststroke patients' ADL.[30–32] Reding et al.[30] studied 27 patients with stroke and found that patients with abnormal dexamethasone suppression tests (DST) showed significantly greater improvement in the BI, if they were given trazodone over 4–5 weeks compared with placebo. Similar results were reported by Gonzales-Torrecillas et al.[31] among 37 patients with PSD receiving open-label antidepressants (26 fluoxetine, 11 nortriptyline) compared to 11 poststroke depressed patients who remained untreated. Both nortriptyline and fluoxetine improved depression as measured by the HAM-D ADL as measured by the BI, and neurologic function assessment by the Orgogozo's scale. These differences between treated and nontreated patients were statistically significant from the third week to the end of the 6-week treatment trial.

Chemerinski et al. have reported similar findings.[33] Twenty-one depressed patients, whose mood improved between in-hospital evaluation and 3 or 6 months after stroke, had significantly greater recovery in ADL, at follow-up than did 34 patients whose mood did not improve (Fig. 11-3).[32] Interestingly, patients with either major or minor depression showed the same amount of recovery in ADL. This finding that major and minor depression did not differ in their relationship to recovery in ADL suggests that the effect may not be mediated by biologic or

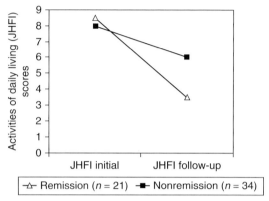

Figure 11-3. Poststroke patients with remission of depression showed significantly greater recovery in ADL than nonremitted patients at 3- or 6-month follow-up ($F = 6.37$; df = 1; 53, $P = 0.015$). (Source: Reprinted with permission from Chemerinski E, Robinson RG, Kosier JT. Improved recovery in activities of daily living associated with remission of poststroke depression. *Stroke* 2001;32:113–117.)

physiologic mechanisms but rather by psychologic mechanisms such as poor motivation or social withdrawal.

Chemerinski et al.[32] also conducted a merged analysis of patients who were treated in one of two double-blind trials of nortriptyline versus placebo for the treatment of PSD. There were 10 patients whose depression responded to treatment and who were matched in severity of initial ADL impairment to another 10 patients who failed to respond to treatment. At a dose of 100 mg/day, the patients who responded to treatment had significantly lower (i.e., less impaired) ADL scores at 6 or 9 weeks of treatment compared to the 10 patients who failed to respond at the same time and dose.[33]

Cognitive Impairment

Cognitive impairment is recognized as one of the most common consequences of stroke. Depression also causes cognitive impairment in patients with no known brain injury. The relationship between PSD and the degree of cognitive impairment has been examined by several groups.

In the section on "Premorbid Risk Factors" we discussed the study by Starkstein et al.[20] comparing 13 patients who developed major depression within 2 years following stroke with 13 patients who did not become depressed in the same period but who were matched for both size and location of lesion as the depressed group. The depressed group showed a significantly lower mean minimental state examination (MMSE) score and higher frequency of abnormal MMSE scores (i.e., MMSE score of 23 or below) than the lesion-matched nondepressed group. This finding lends credence to the idea that PSD might produce an intellectual impairment independent of the stroke lesion itself.

In another study, Bolla-Wilson et al.[34] administered a comprehensive neuropsychologic battery and found that patients with major depression and left hemisphere lesions had significantly greater cognitive impairments than did nondepressed patients with comparable left hemisphere lesions ($P < 0.05$). These cognitive deficits involved tasks of temporal orientation, language, and executive motor and frontal lobe functions (Fig. 11-4). On the other hand, among patients with right hemisphere lesions, patients with major depression did not differ from nondepressed patients on any of the measures of cognitive impairment. This finding indicated that the dementia of poststroke major depression was related to mechanisms induced by left hemisphere injury and right hemisphere injury leading to depression did not provoke the same mechanisms.

The association of PSD with cognitive impairment has also been demonstrated by other investigators.[35] Kauhanen et al. examined 106 patients with stroke using not only the MMSE but also other neuropsychologic examinations (i.e., two subtests of the Wechsler memory scale and the visual recognition memory task). In this study, PSD was associated with impairments in memory, nonverbal problem solving, attention, and psychomotor speed. The association between PSD and cognitive impairment has been reported in the acute stroke period,[15] at short-term follow-up,[35] and at long-term follow-up.[35]

The effect of PSD on the recovery from cognitive impairment has been examined in several

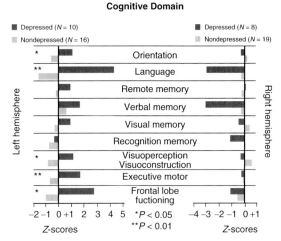

Cognitive Domain

Figure 11-4. The results of neuropsychologic testing in patients with major depression (Dep) or no mood disturbance (Nondep) following a single lesion of the left or right hemisphere. Scores in each cognitive domain were converted to Z scores so that comparisons could be made across domains. A more positive Z score indicates a greater degree of impairment. Note that among patients with left hemisphere strokes, patients with major depression were more impaired than the nondepressed in every cognitive domain. Five of these domains reached statistical significance, indicated by asterisks. None of the domains reached significance in the patients with right hemisphere stroke. (Source: Reprinted with permission from Robinson RG. *The Clinical Neuropsychiatry of Stroke.* Cambridge: Cambridge University Press, 1998, p. 157.)

studies. Downhill et al.[36] examined 309 patients with acute stroke and assessed the longitudinal course of cognitive impairment associated with in-hospital major PSD among 142 patients who were prospectively studied over 2 years. Patients with in-hospital major depression following a left hemisphere stroke were significantly more cognitively impaired than initially nondepressed patients at 3, 6, and 12 months follow-up. At 24 months, however, there was no difference in cognitive function between patients with major depression and nondepressed patients with either right or left hemisphere injury. This finding suggests that cognitive impairment produced by left hemisphere stroke and major depression lasts for 1 year, which is the usual course of major depression.

The treatment of cognitive impairment associated with stroke was examined in a merged analysis of our prior treatment studies.[37] We examined 47 patients with PSD (major n = 33; minor n = 14), divided into those who responded to depression treatment (n = 24) and those who failed to respond (n = 23). Although there was no significant difference between the responder and nonresponder group in their baseline depression scores, repeated-measures ANOVA of the MMSE scores demonstrated a significant time-by-response interaction (i.e., MMSE scores in the responder group improved more over the course of double-blind treatment than MMSE scores in the nonresponder group) (Fig. 11-5). The responder group improved in

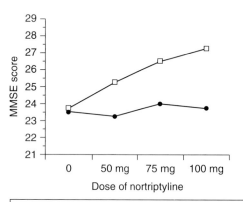

-□- Responders (n = 13)   -●- Nonresponders (n = 18)

Figure 11-5. Change of MMSE scores in patients with poststroke major depression during treatment study. Treatment responders (n = 13) showed significantly greater improvement in cognitive function than nonresponders (n = 18) (F3; 126 = 4.98, group by time interaction P = 0.002 at 25 mg group diff P = 0.036, at 100 mg group diff P = 0.024). Error bars represent standard errors on the mean (SE). (Source: Reprinted with permission from Kimura et al. Treatment of cognitive impairment after post stroke depression. *Stroke*, 2004;31(7):1482–1486,2000.)

both attention-calculation and recall items more than the nonresponder group.

Mortality

In a study looking at 976 patients with acute stroke, it was discovered that patients with depression, assessed at 3 weeks poststroke using the Wakefield self-assessment depression inventory, had 50% higher mortality at 1 year compared to nondepressed patients who were otherwise clinically comparable.[38] Our group has also replicated and extended this finding. We examined this association among 103 acute stroke patients followed for 10 years.[39] Although the in-hospital background characteristics were not significantly different between depressed and nondepressed patients, major or minor depression during in-hospital evaluation was significantly associated with an increased mortality rate over the next 6–7 years. The mortality rate among patient with major or minor depression were 71% and 70%, respectively, significantly higher than in patients without depression who had a mortality rate of 41%. The relative risk of depression for mortality was 3.4 (95% CI 1.4–8.4, P = 0.007). Using a logistic regression to assess the contribution of depression, social function, medical illness, age, sex, social class, physical and cognitive impairment, and size and location of stroke, we found depression remained an independent risk factor odds ratio (3.7, 95% CI 1.1–12.2, P = 0.03) (Fig. 11-6). Similar findings have been reported by Morris et al.[40] in an Australian study of 93 patients over 15 months and by House et al.[41] examining 448 hospitalized patients using the General Health Questionnaire (GHQ). Logistic regression showed that more severe depression on the GHQ, older age, lower mini-mental, and lower function on ADL were all independently associated with increased mortality.

If PSD is associated with increased mortality, it is possible that treatment or prevention of depression would lead to decreased mortality. We examined this hypothesis in a 9-year follow-up of

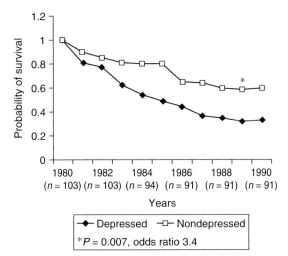

Figure 11-6. Survival curves over 10 years for 37 patients with major or minor depression at the time of in-hospital poststroke evaluation compared to 54 patients without an in-hospital diagnosis of depression. By 10 years follow-up, 14 of the 20 patients with major depression and 12 of the 17 with minor depression had died compared to only 22 of 54 nonepressed (odds ratio = 3.4, CI 1.4–8.4). (Source: Reprinted with permission from Morris PLP,[39] et al.)

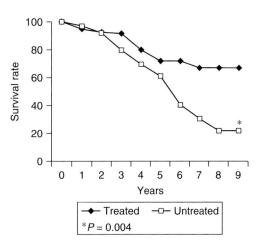

Figure 11-7. Survival rates over 9-year follow-up of acute stroke patients who received a 12-week poststroke course of antidepressants or placebo. Probability of survival was significantly greater in the patients receiving antidepressants ($\chi^2 = 8.2$, df = 1, $P = 0.004$, Kaplan-Meier survival analysis, log-rank test). (Source: Reprinted with permission from Jorge RE, Robinson RG, Arndt S, et al. Mortality and poststroke depression: A placebo-controlled trial of antidepressants. *Am J Psychiatry* 2003;160: 1823–1829.)

a PSD treatment study that will be discussed in detail in the section on "treatment."[42] This study found that active treatment with nortriptyline or fluoxetine over 12 weeks ($n = 53$) within the first 3 months following stroke resulted in increased probability of survival, compared to those who received placebo ($n = 28$) ($P = 0.005$) (Fig. 11-7). This was true even after we accounted for the effects of age, existence of diabetes, severity of ADL impairment, and volume of stroke lesion. Of the patients treated with 12 or more weeks of medication, 67.9% were alive at follow-up (mean 7.1 + 1.2 years), compared with only 35.7% of those who received placebo or who received less than 2 weeks of medication. Logistic regression examining age, stroke type, comorbid diabetes, relapsing depression, and antidepressant use found that antidepressant use ($P = 0.03$) and diabetes ($P = 0.02$) were independent predictors of mortality status at 7–9 years follow-up.

Mechanisms by Which Depression May Affect Stroke Outcomes

Given the dramatic effects of treatment of depression on recovery of ADLs cognitive function and mortality, one might wonder why depression affects recovery and survival following stroke. Although we don't know the answer, the following is a list of possible contributing factors to recovery or mortality:

1. Behavioral factors: Depressed patients are less likely to comply with treatment recommendations, follow-up, rehabilitation, or health-promoting behaviors. This puts them at risk of worse outcomes.
2. Comorbidities: Depressed patients are more likely to have comorbid medical conditions than nondepressed patients. It is known, for

example, that patients with depression have an average of 3.4 more chronic conditions than nondepressed patients. This includes conditions such as hypertension and coronary heart disease, which are known risk factors for stroke and poor stroke outcomes.

3. Decreased parasympathetic tone: There is a decrease in parasympathetic tone which leads to decreased beat-to-beat variability and an increase in susceptibility to arrhythmias and sudden death.

4. Sympathetic nervous system activation: This leads to a release of catecholamines which causes increased resistance in blood vessels.

5. Altered hypothalamic-pituitary-adrenal axis (HPA) function: Depression is frequently associated with a significant rise in cortisol production which leads to atherosclerosis, hypertension, hyperlipidemia, and poor sugar control in diabetics.

6. Altered platelet function: There is increased platelet activation and platelet aggregation as a result of increased platelet-derived growth factor. As a result of the increase in coagulation factors, there is an increase in thrombus formation which can increase the risk of a fatal MI.

Treatment

There are currently eight double-blind studies, which have examined the efficacy of antidepressant medication in PSD (Table 11-3).

The first controlled treatment trial of PSD was reported in 1984.[43] In this study, 39 patients with stroke who met the diagnostic criteria for major or minor depressive disorder were enrolled in a double-blind placebo-controlled study of the efficacy of nortriptyline among this population. Of the 39 patients entered in the study, five dropped out within 1 week. Of the 34 remaining patients, 14 received nortriptyline (20 mg week 1, 50 mg weeks 2 and 3, 70 mg week 4, 100 mg weeks 5 and 6) and 20 received placebo. Using either intention to treat analysis or efficacy analysis, repeated-measures analysis of variance of depression scores and posthoc tests

demonstrated that the nortriptyline group had significantly greater improvement than the placebo group at 4 and 6 weeks of treatment. Intention to treat analysis found response to treatment (i.e., >50% reduction in Ham-D score) and remission rate (Ham-D score <8) was 14 of 17 (82%) for nortriptyline while the placebo response rate and remission rate was 36% ($P = 0.002$).

In a controlled study by Reding et al.,[30] 7 PSD patients with an abnormal DST treated with trazodone had a significantly greater improvement in ADL at 2–3 months following stroke measured by the Barthel ADL scale, compared to 9 comparable patients treated with placebo.

Andersen et al.[44] assessed the efficacy and tolerability of the selective serotonin reuptake inhibitor antidepressant citalopram in a controlled study of 66 patients with stroke. The HAM-D and the Melancholia scale (MES) were significantly better at both 3 and 6 weeks of treatment among patients who received citalopram (20 mg throughout for patients <65 years old, 10 mg throughout for patients 65 or older) compared to patients given placebo.

Our second treatment study compared nortriptyline and fluoxetine in the treatment of depression using an entirely different socioeconomic population than our original study.[45] A total of 56 patients with acute stroke and major depression were randomized to receive nortriptyline, fluoxetine, or placebo over 12 weeks of treatment. Using an intention to treat analyses, patients treated with nortriptyline (25 mg week 1, 50 mg week 2, 75 mg weeks 3–6, and 100 mg weeks 7–12) had a significantly greater decline in HDRS scores than either fluoxetine (10 mg weeks 1–3, 20 mg weeks 4–6, 30 mg weeks 7–9, and 40 mg weeks 10–12) or placebo treated patients at 12 weeks of treatment ($F = 3.73$, df = 2.53; $P = <0.031$) (Fig. 11-8). There were no significant differences between fluoxetine and placebo treated patients. Intention to treat analysis showed that the response rate for nortriptyline was 63% and the remission rate was 50% while the response rates for fluoxetine and placebo were 9% and 24% and the remission rates were 0% and 6%, respectively (Fisher's

► TABLE 11-3 RANDOMIZED DOUBLE-BLIND STUDIES FOR THE TREATMENT OF POSTSTROKE DEPRESSION

Trial	Inclusion Diagnosis	Drugs	No. of Patients	Cardiovascular Adverse Effects	Psychiatric Outcome
Fruehwald et al. (2003)[75]	Moderate to severe depression by standard questionnaire	Fluoxetine vs. placebo	50	None reported	Improvement in depression scores at 4 weeks in both groups. Fluoxetine superior in open-label follow-up
Wiart et al. (2000)[46]	Major depression	Fluoxetine vs. placebo	31	No significant cardiovascular effects reported	Fluoxetine significantly more effective than placebo for depression
Robinson et al. (2000)[45]	Major or minor depression	Fluoxetine vs. nortriptyline vs. placebo	56	Increase in heart rate significantly greater in nortriptyline group than in placebo group	Nortriptyline significantly more effective than placebo or fluoxetine for depression
Dam et al. (1996)[76]	Depressed and nondepressed	Fluoxetine vs. maprotiline vs. placebo	52	No cardiovascular effects reported	Fluoxetine and maprotiline associated with significant improvement in depression Fluoxetine group superior to maprotiline and placebo groups in functional indices
Grade et al. (1998)[47]	Depressed and nondepressed	Methylphenidate vs. placebo	21	No serious cardiovascular side-effects reported	Methylphenidate treated patient had greater decline in Ham-D scores
Andersen et al. (1994)[77]	Moderate to severe depression by standard questionnaire	Citalopram vs. placebo	66	No serious cardiovascular side-effects reported	Better outcome in citalopram group
Reding et al. (1986)[30]	Depressed patients with an abnormal dexamethasone suppression test	Trazodone vs. placebo	16	None	
Lipsey et al. (1984)[43]	Major or minor depression	Nortriptyline vs. placebo	39		Nortriptyline was superior to placebo

Source: Adapted from Davies et al. Treatment of anxiety and depressive disorders in patients with cardiovascular disease. Br Med J, 2004;328:939–943.

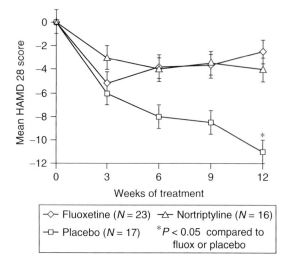

Figure 11-8. Intention-to-treat analysis. Change in (28-item) Hamilton rating scale for depression score over 12 weeks of treatment for all patients who were entered in the study. A repeated-measures ANOVA demonstrated a significant time-by-treatment interaction ($F = 3.45$, df = 8, 212, $P = 0.004$) with nortriptyline treated being significantly better than fluoxetine or placebo. (Source: Reprinted with permission from Robinson RG, Schultz SK, Castillo C, et al. Nortriptyline vs. fluoxetine in the treatment of depression and in short-erm recovery after stroke: A placebo-controlled, double-blind study. *Am J Psychiatry* 2000;157:351–359.)

exact test, $P = 0.0012$ for response and $P = 0.0003$ for remission).

Gastrointestinal side effects, insomnia, and headache were significantly more frequent in the fluoxetine treated group. In addition, fluoxetine led to an average 14 lb weight loss over 12 weeks that was not seen with the other treatments.[45]

Although this study failed to show a significant antidepressant effect of fluoxetine, a study by Wiart et al.[46] treated 16 patients with major depression following stroke and 15 major depressed stroke patients with placebo over 6 weeks. The fluoxetine patients showed significantly greater decline in Montgomery Asberg depression score than the placebo treated patients

and the response rate was 62% in the fluoxetine group and 33% in the placebo group ($P = 0.1$-NS). There is a placebo-controlled trial that shows fluoxetine to be effective in treating PSD.

It is reasonable to conclude that there is evidence from placebo-controlled randomized trials that citalopram is effective in the treatment of PSD. Lower doses should be used in the elderly. Nortriptyline has been shown to produce the largest treatment effects and appears to be a first-line agent, based on our data. It should be emphasized, however, that there are contraindications to the use of nortriptyline including heart block, cardiac arrhythmia, narrow angle glaucoma, and in some cases coronary artery disease.

There is one double-blind study that compared methylphenidate and placebo [47]. Patients given up to 30 mg of methylphenidate per day ($N = 10$) showed significantly greater reductions in Ham-D scores than patients given placebo ($N = 11$) over 3 weeks. Response and remission rates, however, were not reported.

Uncontrolled evidence exists for the efficacy of electroconvulsive therapy (ECT).[48] Two retrospective studies found response rates of 86–95% while a review done almost 20 years ago found about 50 case reports of successful use of ECT for PSD.[48] Medical complications were uncommon in these retrospective studies.

While no absolute contraindications exist for ECT, the poststroke patient has some relative risk factors, which must be considered when making the decision to proceed to ECT. These include the presence of a space-occupying lesion, intracranial hemorrhage, or recent myocardial infarction. Reports of successful ECTs in patients with these risk factors exist and suggest that with careful monitoring, these people would be viable candidates for ECT should the severity of their depression warrant it.

There is only one large trial of psychologic treatment for PSD [49]. The study involved 123 patients of whom 39 received 10 sessions of cognitive behavioral therapy (CBT) over 3 months. There were 43 patients who had an individual meeting with investigators and 41 patients had no contact. Of the 123 patients,

60 had a diagnosis of depression. The change in Beck depression scores over 3 months was not significantly different among the three groups. The authors concluded CBT was not effective in PSD.

Prevention

Given the adverse effect of PSD on cognitive and physical recovery from stroke, it is logical to determine whether PSD could be prevented. In one such study, 137 consecutive, nondepressed patients with acute ischemic stroke were randomized to receive 12 months of double-blind treatment with either sertraline or placebo.[50] Sertraline was initiated at 50 mg/day and could be increased after 2 weeks in 50-mg increments (maximum dosage, 150 mg/day). Exclusion criteria included stroke >4 weeks before admission; current major depression or cardiovascular disease; significant aphasia or dementia; history of schizophrenia, psychosis, or drug abuse; preexisting neurologic illnesses; or antidepressant treatment in the previous 4 weeks.

The mean dosage of sertraline was 62.9 mg/day, although more than 75% of the patients received only 50 mg/day. Dropout rates were approximately 50% but were similar in the two groups. Using a HDRC score of 18 or higher to indicate depression, the incidence of depression after 52 weeks was 8.2% (95% CI 2.2–13.9) in the sertraline group and 22.8% (95% CI 13.7–32.0) in the placebo group (P = NS). Between weeks 21 and 52, Ham-D scores, however, were significantly lower in the sertraline compared with the placebo group. Furthermore, there was a significantly higher frequency of adverse cardiovascular events and rehospitalization for physical illness among patients given placebo compared to those given sertraline. The drug was tolerated well, and the two groups showed no differences in side effects.[50] These data demonstrate that pretreatment with the SSRI sertraline is effective in preventing PSD and suggest that prophylaxis may be beneficial to patients with acute stroke.

▶ MANIA

Prevalence

Mania occurs much less frequently than depression following stroke (only three cases were identified among a consecutive series of more than 300 acute stroke patients including 143 patients with longitudinal assessment).[15] Although numerous case reports and empirical studies document that stroke is associated with mania, there are no epidemiologic studies which document the incidence or prevalence of this condition. About half of the reported cases involve single or repeated manic episodes without major depression. The best estimate is that it occurs in less than 1% of all strokes. Symptoms are similar to that of primary mania and include distractibility, talkativeness, reckless behavior, hyposomnia, ideas that race, grandiosity, and hypersexuality. Often times, mania is the presenting symptom of a stroke that is otherwise silent. In patients over 50 presenting with their first episode of mania, a thorough search for causes of secondary mania should be undertaken, including brain imaging to rule out a stroke.

Anatomic Correlates

We concluded a study of 17 patients with mania due to brain injury.[51] Among this group, 12 had unilateral right hemisphere lesions, which were significantly greater than right hemisphere lesions among 31 patients with major depression, who tended to have left frontal or basal ganglia lesions or 28 patients with no mood disorder following stroke (Fig. 11-9). Lesions associated with mania were either cortical (basotemporal cortex or orbitofrontal cortex) or subcortical (frontal white matter, basal ganglia, or thalamus). Positron emission tomographic (PET) scans using [^{18}F] fluorodeoxyglucose (FDG) were conducted on three patients with mania after brain injury and compared with seven age comparable normal controls.[52] Results showed focal hypometabolism in the right basotemporal

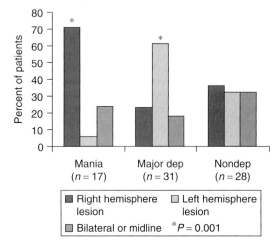

Figure 11-9. Frequency of right or left hemisphere lesion location in patients with mania following stroke ($n = 9$), tumors ($n = 6$), or traumatic brain injury ($n = 2$) compared to patients with acute poststroke major depression (major dep) or no mood disturbance (nondep) following stroke. Mania was strongly associated with a right hemisphere lesion location while major depression following acute stroke was associated with left hemisphere lesions. The association of diagnosis with lesion location was highly significant ($P = 0.0001$). (Source: Reprinted with permission from Robinson RG. *The Clinical Neuropsychiatry of Stroke*. Cambridge: Cambridge University Press, 1998, p. 308.)

cortex in all three patients with right subcortical lesions not seen in controls.

Thus, mania appears to be provoked by injury to specific right hemisphere structures that have connections to the limbic system. The right basotemporal cortex may be particularly important because direct lesions as well as distant hypometabolic effects (diaschisis) of this cortical region were associated with secondary mania.

Not every patient with a lesion in limbic areas of the right hemisphere, however, develops secondary mania. Therefore, there must be risk factors for this disorder. The study previously described, comparing mania with depression[53] found that patients with secondary mania had a significantly higher frequency of positive

family history of affective disorders than did depressed patients or patients with no mood disturbance (Fig. 11-10).

Another risk factor for poststroke mania was identified by comparing patients with secondary mania to patients with no mood disturbance who were matched for size, location, and etiology of brain lesion.[54] Patients with secondary mania had a significantly greater degree of subcortical atrophy, as measured by bifrontal and third ventricular to brain ratios. This subcortical atrophy probably preceded the stroke lesion and mania because it was found on both the sides of the brain only one side having been injured. Moreover, of the patients who developed secondary mania, those who had a positive family history of psychiatric disorders had significantly less atrophy than those without

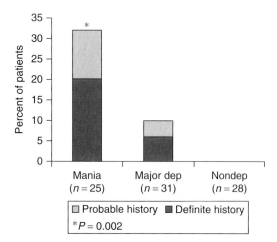

Figure 11-10. The frequency of family history (definite or probable) of mood disorder in the primary relatives of patients with mania following stroke ($n = 15$), tumors ($n = 6$), or trauma ($n = 4$) compared to poststroke major depression (major dep) or no mood disorder (nondep) following stroke. Patients with mania were significantly more likely to have a family history of mood disorders than the other two groups. (Source: Reprinted with permission from Robinson RG. *The Clinical Neuropsychiatry of Stroke*. Cambridge: Cambridge University Press, 1998, p. 305.)

such a family history, suggesting that a genetic predisposition to affective disorders and brain atrophy may be independent risk factors for poststroke mania.

Mechanism

Although the mechanism of secondary mania remains unknown, both lesion studies and metabolic studies have suggested that the right basotemporal cortex may plan an important role. The basotemporal cortex has strong efferent connections to the orbital frontal cortex suggesting that the lateral orbital frontal circuit in the right hemisphere may play a role in the etiology of mania. A combination of biogenic amine system dysfunction and release of tonic inhibitory input to the orbital frontal-thalamic circuit may lead to the production of mania.

Symptoms

The symptoms of mania were examined in a series of 25 consecutive patients who met DSM-IV criteria for a mood disorder due to brain injury with manic features. These patients, who developed mania after a stroke, traumatic brain injury, or tumors, were compared to 25 patients with primary mania (i.e., no known neuropathology) (Fig. 11-11).[15] Both groups of patients showed similar frequencies of elation, pressured speech, flight of ideas, grandiose thoughts, insomnia, hallucinations, and paranoid delusions.

Duration and Treatment

The course of mania following stroke has not been systematically examined. Anecdotal cases have been reported indicating that recurrent episodes of mania or depression may occur in these patients.[54]

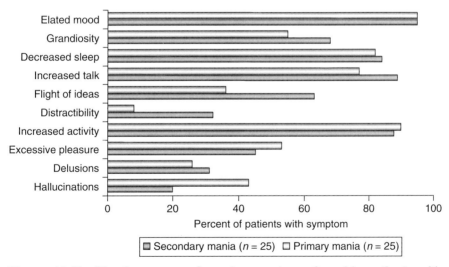

Figure 11-11. The frequency of manic symptoms found in patients with mania following brain injury (secondary) compared to patients with mania not associated with brain injury (primary). There were no significant differences in the frequency of any of the symptoms, which suggests that the clinical presentation of secondary mania is very similar to that of primary mania. (Source: Reprinted with permission from Robinson RG. *The Clinical Neuropsychiatry of Stroke*. Cambridge: Cambridge University Press, 1998, p. 299.)

The course of this disorder for individual patients with single or recurrent episodes of mania suggests that most patients respond to lithium, although some fail to respond to either lithium or carbamazepine.[54] Depakote and antipsychotics would also be an option, though no controlled trials exist.

▶ CONCLUSION

Currently more than 4 million people living in the United States have suffered a stroke. PSD has been recognized by clinicians for many years and represents one of the major complications of stroke. Two forms of depression are diagnosed in patients with stroke; mood disorder due to stroke with major depressive-like episode and a subsyndromal form of major depression termed minor depression. Studies of PSD have indicated that the prevalence rate depends on whether hospitalized patients or those living in the community are examined. The mean worldwide prevalence rate for major depression is 20% and for minor depression is 18%. During the acute period following stroke, major depression is significantly associated with left frontal and left basal ganglia lesions, premorbid mild brain atrophy, as well as personal and family history of psychiatric disorders. Recovery in ADL has been shown in numerous studies to be impaired by the existence of PSD. The degree of cognitive impairment is also increased by the existence of major depression. In addition to the effect of depression on physical and intellectual recovery from stroke, numerous studies have demonstrated that patients with acute PSD are more likely to die between 12 months and 10 years following stroke than patients who are acutely nondepressed. Numerous studies have also demonstrated that PSD can be effectively treated using several different classes of antidepressant medication including nortriptyline, trazodone, and citalopram. Recent data also indicate that PSD may be prevented using sertraline and this represents one of the first efforts at primary prevention in psychiatry.

Although mania is not as common as PSD, it does occur in approximately 1% of stroke patients and appears to involve dysfunction of the right basal temporal cortex in combination with a family history of mood disorder or mild subcortical atrophy. Although no controlled treatment studies are available, the existing literature from small case series suggests that mood stabilizing medications such as lithium or Depakote may also be used effectively in poststroke mania.

Future research should examine the mechanism of depression and mania following stroke with the hope of identifying more specific focused treatments for these disorders. In addition, further research is needed to identify the most effective, currently available, treatments for the prevention or early treatment of these disorders which lead to impaired recovery and increased mortality.

REFERENCES

1. Hachinski V, Norris JW. *The Acute Stroke.* Philadelphia, PA: F.A. Davis, 1985.
2. Broderick J, Brott T, Kothari R, et al. The greater Cincinnati/Northern Kentucky Stroke Study: Preliminary first-ever and total incidence rates of stroke among blacks. *Stroke* 1998;29:415–421.
3. Bonita R. Epidemiology of stroke. *Lancet* 1992;339:342–344.
4. Kelly-Hayes M, Robertson JT, Broderick JP, et al. The American Heart Association stroke outcome classification: Executive summary. *Circulation* 1998;97:2474–2478.
5. Meyer A. The anatomical facts and clinical varieties of traumatic insanity. *Am J Insanity* 1904;60:373.
6. Bleuler EP. *Textbook of Psychiatry.* New York: Macmillan, 1951, pp. 131–197.
7. Kraepelin E. *Manic Depressive Insanity and Paranoia.* Edinburgh: E & S Livingstone, 1921.
8. AmericanPsychiatricAssociation. *Diagnostic and Statistical Manual of Mental Disorder-DSM-IV-TR.* Washington, DC: American Psychiatric Association, 2000.
9. Cohen-Cole SA, Kauffman KG. Major depression in physical illness: Diagnosis, prevalence, and antidepressant treatment. *Depression* 1993;2:281–294.
10. Paradiso S, Ohkubo T, Robinson RG. Vegetative and psychological symptoms associated with depressed mood over the first two years after stroke. *Int J Psychiatry Med* 1997;27:137–157.

11. Harrington C, Salloway S. The diagnosis and treatment of post-stroke depression. *Med Health* 1997; 80:181–187.

12. Paradiso S, Robinson RG. Minor depression after stroke. An initial validation of the DSM-IV construct. *Am J Geriatr Psychiatry* 1999;7:244–251.

13. Jonas BS, Mussolino ME. Symptoms of depression as a propsective risk factor for stroke. *Psychosom Med* 2000;62:463–471.

14. Morris PLP, Robinson RG, Raphael B. Prevalence and course of depressive disorders in hospitalized stroke patients. *Intl J Psychiatr Med* 1990;20:349–364.

15. Robinson RG. *The Clinical Neuropsychiatry of Stroke*. Cambridge: Cambridge University Press, 1998, p. 491.

16. Astrom M, Adolfsson R, Asplund K. Major depression in stroke patients: A 3-year longitudinal study. *Stroke* 1993;24:976–982.

17. Robinson RG, Kubos KL, Starr LB, et al. Mood disorders in stroke patients: Importance of location of lesion. *Brain* 1984;107:81–93.

18. Robinson RG. The controversy over post-stroke depression and lesion location. *Psychiatr Times* 2003;20:39–40.

19. Carson AJ, MacHale S, Allen K, et al. Depression after stroke and lesion location: A systematic review. *Lancet* 2000;356:122–126.

20. Starkstein SE, Robinson RG, Price TR. Comparison of patients with and without post-stroke major depression matched for size and location of lesion. *Arch Gen Psychiatry* 1988;45:247–252.

21. Starkstein SE, Robinson RG, Honig MA, et al. Mood changes after right hemisphere lesion. *Br J Psychiatry* 1989;155:79–85.

22. Eastwood MR, Rifat SL, Nobbs H, et al. Mood disorder following cerebrovascular accident. *Br J Psychiatry* 1989;154:195–200.

23. Aben I, Verhey F, Lousberg R, et al. Validity of the Beck depression inventory, Hospital anxiety and depression scale, SCL-90, and Hamilton depression rating scale as screening instruments for depression in stroke patients. *Psychosomatics* 2002;43:386–393.

24. Bush BA. Major life events as risk factors for post-stroke depression. *Brain Inj* 1999;13:131–137.

25. Robinson RG, Starr LB, Kubos KL, et al. A two year longitudinal study of post-stroke mood disorders: Findings during the initial evaluation. *Stroke* 1983;14:736–744.

26. Pohjasvaara T, Leppavuori A, Siira I, et al. Frequency and clinical determinants of poststroke depression. *Stroke* 1998;29:2311–2317.

27. Herrmann N, Black SE, Lawrence J, et al. The Sunnybrook stroke study. A prospective study of depressive symptoms and functional outcome. *Stroke* 1998;29:618–624.

28. Parikh RM, Robinson RG, Lipsey JR, Starkstein et al. The impact of post-stroke depression on recovery in activities of daily living over two year follow–up. *Arch Neurol* 1990;47:785–789.

29. Schubert DSP, Taylor C, Lee S, et al. Physical consequences of depression in the stroke patient. *Gen Hosp Psychiatry* 1992;14:69–76.

30. Reding MJ, Orto LA, Winter SW, Fortuna IM, DiPonte P, McDowell FH. Antidepressant therapy after stroke: A double-blind trial. *Arch Neurol* 1986;43:763–765.

31. Gonzalez-Torrecillas JL, Mendlewicz J, Lobo A. Effects of early treatment of poststroke depression on neuropsychological rehabilitation. *Int Psychogeriatr* 1995;7:547–560.

32. Chemerinski E, Robinson RG, Kosier JT. Improved recovery in activities of daily living associated with remission of post-stroke depression. *Stroke* 2001;32:113–117.

33. Chemerinski E, Robinson RG, Arndt S, et al. The effect of remission of poststroke depression on activities of daily living in a double-blind randomized treatment study. *J Nerv Ment Dis* 2001; 189:421–425.

34. Bolla-Wilson K, Robinson RG, Starkstein SE, et al. Lateralization of dementia of depression in stroke patients. *Am J Psychiatry* 1989;146:627–634.

35. Kauhanen M, Korpelainen JT, Hiltunen P, et al. Poststroke depression correlates with cognitive impairment and neurological deficits. *Stroke* 1999; 30:1875–1880.

36. Downhill JE, Jr, Robinson RG. Longitudinal assessment of depression and cognitive impairment following stroke. *J Nerv Ment Dis* 1994;182:425–431.

37. Kimura M, Robinson RG. Treatment of poststroke generalized anxiety disorder comorbid with post-stroke depression. Merged analysis of nortriptyline trials. *Am J Geriatr Psychiatry* 2003;11:320–327.

38. Wade DT, Legh-Smith J, Hewer RA. Depressed mood after stroke, a community study of its frequency. *Br J Psychiatry* 1987;151:200–205.

39. Morris PLP, Robinson RG, Andrezejewski P, et al. Association of depression with 10-year post-stroke mortality. *Am J Psychiatry* 1993;150:124–129.

40. Morris PL, Robinson RG, Samuels J. Depression, introversion and mortality following stroke. *Aust N Z J Psychiatry* 1993;27:443–449.

41. House A, Knapp P, Bamford J, et al. Mortality at 12 and 24 months after stroke may be associated with depressive symptoms at 1 month. *Stroke* 2001;32:696–701.

42. Jorge RE, Robinson RG, Arndt S, et al. Mortality and post-stroke depression: A placebo controlled trial of antidepressants. *Am J Psychiatry* 2003;160: 1823–1829.

43. Lipsey JR, Robinson RG, Pearlson GD, et al. Nortriptyline treatment of post-stroke depression: A double–blind study. *Lancet* 1984;i:297–300.

44. Andersen G, Vestergaard K, Riis J. Citalopram for post-stroke pathological crying. *Lancet* 1993; 342(8875):837–839.

45. Robinson RG, Schultz SK, Castillo C, et al. Nortriptyline versus fluoxetine in the treatment of depression and in short term recovery after stroke: A placebo controlled, double-blind study. *Am J Psychiatry* 2000;157:351–359.

46. Wiart L, Petit H, Joseph PA, et al. Fluoxetine in early poststroke depression: A double-blind placebo-controlled study. *Stroke* 2000;31:1829–1832.

47. Grade C, Redford B, Chrostowski J, et al. Methylphenidate in early poststroke recovery: A double-blind, placebo-controlled study. *Arch Phys Med Rehabil* 1998;79:1047–1050.

48. Huffman J, Stern TA. Acute psychiatric manifestations of stroke: A clinical case conference. *Psychosomatics* 2003;44:65–75.

49. Lincoln NB, Flannaghan T. Cognitive behavioral psychotherapy for depression following stroke: A randomized controlled trial. *Stroke* 2003;34:111–115.

50. Rasmussen A, Lunde M, Poulsen DL, et al. A double-blind, placebo-controlled study of sertraline in the prevention of depression in stroke patients. *Psychosomatics* 2003;44:216–21.

51. Robinson RG, Boston JD, Starkstein SE, et al. Comparison of mania with depression following brain injury: Causal factors. *Am J Psychiatry* 1988; 145:172–178.

52. Starkstein SE, Mayberg HS, Berthier ML, et al. Mania after brain injury: Neuroradiological and metabolic findings. *Ann Neurol* 1990;27:652–659.

53. Starkstein SE, Pearlson GD, Boston J, et al. Mania after brain injury: A controlled study of causative factors. *Arch Neurol* 1987;44:1069–1073.

54. Starkstein SE, Fedoroff JP, Berthier MD, et al. Manic depressive and pure manic states after brain lesions. *Biol. Psychiatry* 1991;29:149–158.

55. House A, Dennis M, Mogridge L, et al. Mood disorders in the year after first stroke. *Br J Psychiatry* 1991;158:83–92.

56. Burvill PW, Johnson GA, Jamrozik KD, et al. Prevalence of depression after stroke: The Perth Community Stroke Study. *Br J Psychiatry* 1995; 166:320–327.

57. Kotila M, Numminen H, Waltimo O, et al. Depression after stroke. Results of the FINNSTROKE study. *Stroke* 1998;29:368–372.

58. Ebrahim S, Barer D, Nouri F. Affective illness after stroke. *Br J Psychiatry* 1987;151:52–56.

59. Fedoroff JP, Starkstein SE, Parikh RM, et al. Are depressive symptoms non-specific in patients with acute stroke? *Am J Psychiatry* 1991;148:1172–1176.

60. Castillo CS, Schultz SK, Robinson RG. Clinical correlates of early-onset and late-onset poststroke generalized anxiety. *Am J Psychiatry* 1995;152: 1174–1179.

61. Starkstein SE, Fedoroff JP, Price TR, et al. Anosognosia in patients with cerebrovascular lesions. A study of causative factors. *Stroke* 1992;23: 1446–1453.

62. Herrmann M, Bartles C, Wallesch C-W. Depression in acute and chronic aphasia: Symptoms, pathoanatomical-clinical correlations and functional implications. *J Neurol Neurosurg Psychiatry* 1993; 56:672–678.

63. Singh A, Black SE, Herrmann N, et al. Functional and neuroanatomic correlations in poststroke depression: The Sunnybrook Stroke Study. *Stroke* 2000;31:637–644.

64. Andersen G, Vestergaard K, Riis JO, et al. Incidence of post-stroke depression during the first year in a large unselected stroke population determined using a valid standardized rating scale. *Acta Psychiatr Scand* 1994;90:190–195.

65. Gainotti G, Azzoni A, Marra C. Frequency, phenomenology and anatomical-clinical correlates of major post-stroke depression. *Br J Psychiatry* 1999;175:163–167.

66. Folstein MF, Maiberger R, McHugh PR. Mood disorder as a specific complication of stroke. *J Neurol Neurosurg Psychiatry* 1977;40:1018–1020.

67. Finklestein S, Benowitz LI, Baldessarini RJ, et al. Mood, vegetative disturbance, and dexamethasone suppression test after stroke. *Ann Neurol* 1982;12:463–468.

68. Sinyor D, Amato P, Kaloupek P. Post-stroke depression: Relationship to functional impairment, coping strategies, and rehabilitation outcome. *Stroke* 1986; 17:112–117.

69. Finset A, Goffeng L, Landro NI, et al. Depressed mood and intra-hemispheric location of lesion in right hemisphere stroke patients. *Scand J Rehabil Med* 1989;21:1–6.

70. Schwartz JA, Speed NM, Brunberg JA, et al. Depression in stroke rehabilitation. *Biol Psychiatry* 1993;33:694–699.

71. Feibel JH, Springer CJ. Depression and failure to resume social activities after stroke. *Arch Phys Med Rehabil* 1982;63:276–278.

72. Robinson RG, Price TR. Post-stroke depressive disorders: A follow-up study of 103 outpatients. *Stroke* 1982;13:635–641.

73. Vataja R, Pohjasvaara T, Leppavuori A, et al. Magnetic resonance imaging correlates of depression after ischemic stroke. *Arch Gen Psychiatry* 2001; 58:925–931.

74. Collin SJ, Tinson D, Lincoln NB. Depression after stroke. *Clin Rehabil* 1987;1:27–32.

75. Fruehwald S, Gatterbauer E, Rehak P, et al. Early fluoxetine treatment of post-stroke depression—a three-month double-blind placebo-controlled study with an open-label long-term follow up. *J Neurol* 2003;250:347–351.

76. Dam M, Tonin P, De Boni A, et al. Effects of fluoxetine and maprotiline on functional recovery in poststroke hemiplegic patients undergoing rehabilitation therapy.[comment]. *Stroke* 1996;27: 1211–1214.

77. Andersen G, Vestergaard K, Lauritzen L. Effective treatment of poststroke depression with the selective serotonin reuptake inhibitor citalopram. *Stroke* 1994;25:1099–1104.

SECTION IV

Neurologic Disorders

CHAPTER 12

Depression in Alzheimer's Disease

PAUL B. ROSENBERG AND CONSTANTINE G. LYKETSOS

▶ INTRODUCTION

Clinicians have long struggled with the problem of how to help patients with Alzheimer's disease (AD) and their families in the absence of a definitive and curative treatment. In order to optimize current treatment one must recognize the salience of neuropsychiatric complications of AD including depression, agitation, hallucinations, delusions, insomnia, and others. Depression is one of the most troubling and prominent symptoms in this spectrum and clearly worth diagnosing and treating given its substantial adverse effects on patient and caregiver quality of life. There is a growing body of evidence that the symptoms of depression in AD are different than those of a typical major depressive episode. In addition, results from an increasing number of treatment trials are available to guide the clinician in choosing medications and psychosocial treatments. In this chapter, we review AD in general, depression in AD in particular, and discuss current evidence regarding its presentation, etiology, diagnosis, and treatment.

▶ ALZHEIMER'S DISEASE

Epidemiology

Alzheimer's disease is a cognitive disorder associated with aging that is a major cause of disability and burden to society and caregivers.

There are currently an estimated 4.5 million patients with AD in the United States, a number predicted to increase to approximately 15 million by 2050.[1] AD patients become fully dependent for their activities of daily living (ADLs) as the disease progresses and many require institutional care. The combined costs of medical and family care for AD is estimated at $100 billion/year in the United States alone[2,3] with the greatest financial cost being the time spent on caregiving by families.[4] Moreover the emotional costs to caregivers are incalculable with the increasing burden of caregiving leading to frail physical and mental health for the caregiver.[5]

Clinical Course

Alzheimer's disease is largely a disease of old age. Estimates of its prevalence increase from about 1% at ages 60–64 to 43–68% at ages >95.[6,7] Lower prevalence estimates in the very old were found in a population sample from Cache County, with a prevalence of 28% above age 90,[8] and there is evidence that incidence declines after age 90.[9] AD invariably presents slowly and insidiously, and families often interpret cognitive changes as changes in personality, mood, or attitude. In fact, in the clinic the chief complaint is equally like to be mood disorder or cognitive change. Typical neuropsychologic findings in early AD include deficits in verbal episodic memory and executive function[10,11] with accumulating deficits in verbal fluency, comprehension, gnosis, and praxis developing as the disease progresses.[12] Survival is relatively short after the onset of AD, with an estimated survival of 3–3.5 years at the population level, longer in clinical settings.[13] However, this may be an underestimate associated with delays in diagnosis as opposed to a more rapid course of disease. AD is often accompanied by neurologic symptoms including parkinsonism and frontal lobe reflexes (i.e., grasp, palmomental, snout, glabellar reflexes).

Neurobiologic Findings

The brain of AD patients is characterized by symmetrical cortical atrophy, deep cortical sulci, enlarged ventricles, and loss of total brain mass.[14,15] There is *extracellular* deposition of insoluble aggregates of β-amyloid fibrils in widespread cortical regions as well as intraneuronal accumulations of neurofibrillary tangles.[16] β-Amyloid fibrils are insoluble aggregates of amyloid-β, a 40-42 amino acid peptide product of the metabolism of amyloid precursor protein (APP). The latter can be cleaved by either β- or α-secretase cleavage followed by further cleavage by γ-secretase. The product of β-secretase cleavage is amyloid-β-1-42. This forms insoluble aggregates much more readily than the product of the α-pathway, amyloid-β-1-40. There are rare familial autosomal-dominant variants of AD in which the APP gene has a single base-pair mutation that leads to altered metabolic processing and a relative increase in the proportion of amyloid-β-1-42 compared to 1-40.[16] Depositing β-amyloid plaques are initially concentrated in temporal and parietal association cortices, but at later stages of AD are found throughout the cortex.

It is not definitely known whether the toxic moieties in AD are β-amyloid aggregates, amyloid-β monomers or oligomers.[16] There is increasing evidence that soluble amyloid-β oligomers may be more actively neurotoxic than aggregates and that by the time plaques appear neu-

ronal damage has already been done.[17] Neurofibrillary tangles consist of *intraneuronal* deposition of phosphorylated tau protein initially found in hippocampus, entorhinal cortex, and limbic areas, but spreading to many cortical areas in advanced disease.[18,19] In early stages of AD the density of tangles correlates better with cognitive impairment than density of plaques.[18]

The discovery of familial autosomal-dominant mutations in the APP gene with early-onset AD has led to the development of transgenic mouse models of AD that express mutant human APP genes.[20] These mice develop plaques and cognitive impairment as they age, although they lack neurofibrillary tangles, and in this respect are an incomplete model of AD. In these models, one mechanism of neurotoxicity appears to be activation of brain microglia by amyloid-β leading to release of proinflammatory cytokines such as interleukin (IL)-1-β, IL-6, and tissue necrosis factor-alpha (TNF-α).[21] In addition there is activation of the complement cascade not mediated by antibodies.[22] These findings suggest that neurotoxicity in AD is an inflammatory process, which has led to the study of anti-inflammatory drugs as potential AD therapies.[18,19,21,23,24]

In AD, there is loss of several neurotransmitter systems. Most well described is the dramatic decrease in the number of cholinergic neurons originating in the nucleus basalis of Meynert providing excitatory innervation throughout the cortex.[24,25] The latter finding provides the rationale for current treatment of AD with acetylcholinesterase inhibitors. In addition, there are changes in serotonergic, dopaminergic, and NMDA neurotransmission, which may make patients more vulnerable to neuropsychiatric symptoms of AD.[26]

AD brains have decreased volume in hippocampal and entorhinal cortex[27] and these structural changes may predate cognitive deficits in AD.[28] Functional imaging (single photon emission computed tomography [SPECT] and positron emission tomographic [PET] scans) studies show a pattern of temporo-parietal hypometabolism.[29] These changes may also predate cognitive deficits and are notable in cognitively intact patients with genetic susceptibility to AD.[30] These symmetrical and posterior deficits distinguish AD from fronto-temporal dementias, which have hypometabolic frontal cortices.[27]

▶ NEUROPSYCHIATRIC SYMPTOMS AND SYNDROMES IN ALZHEIMER'S DISEASE

While AD is often described as a purely cognitive disorder, patients frequently, almost universally, suffer from a multitude of neuropsychiatric symptoms as well. In our current state of practice, we have significantly greater success in treating these symptoms than in altering the course of cognitive decline. Thus, the clinician is well advised to incorporate these treatments into practice.

There are two recent population-based epidemiologic studies examining neuropsychiatric symptoms in AD. In the the Cache County study of memory and aging, 56% of demented participants and 53% of AD participants exhibited at least one neuropsychiatric disturbance on the Neuropsychiatric Inventory (NPI, reviewed below) in the past month.[31] Symptoms included (in order of prevalence) apathy, delusions, agitation/aggression, and depression. Similar results were seen in the Cardiovascular Health Study[32] with depression being the most prevalent neuropsychiatric symptom (32.3%). Comparable population-based studies in the United Kingdom found similar symptom frequencies.[33] The *incidence* of depression over an 18-month follow-up period in the Cache County study was comparably high (18%). The prevalence of neuropsychiatric disturbances by dementia severity remains controversial. The population studies above suggest that it differs by type of disturbance, with the overall prevalence being comparable across different stages of dementia. However, findings are different in clinical settings. For example, in a cross-sectional study at the University of Pittsburgh there were more neuropsychiatric symptoms at later stages of dementia.[34]

Neuropsychiatric symptoms in AD are not benign variants within a broader illness, but can lead to significant functional disability and caregiver stress above and beyond that caused by cognitive decline.[35] Patients with AD are struggling to make the best use of their remaining cognitive skills, but the development of depression, delusions, and anxiety limit their ability to utilize these skills in daily life. Similarly, there is no question that these neuropsychiatric symptoms detract from the quality of life for both patients and caregivers. Clearly they are a target for assessment and treatment of the patient and family in AD.

The differentiation of neuropsychiatric symptoms in AD is important to the targeting of therapies. Since agitation is most troubling to patients and caregivers it is has been the focus of much study. However, agitation, which is most frequent in later-stage dementia, is a nonspecific symptom that is usually reflective of a different disturbance. Several groups have reported on the use of factor analytic methods to subtype these neuropsychiatric symptoms. Most tend to agree that two groups of disturbance are distinguishable, one with predominately affective symptoms, and one with predominately psychotic symptoms (delusions and hallucinations).[36] Affective symptoms are most common and troubling to caregivers, especially, in earlier dementia.[35] Affective symptoms are often referred to using the term "depression" but in fact have a different mix of symptoms than that which is seen in depressed older patients. Specifically, those with dementia are more anxious, agitated, delusional, or inattentive, and have less guilt, less self-depreciation, and are rarely suicidal.

▶ EPIDEMIOLOGY OF DEPRESSION IN ALZHEIMER'S DISEASE

Mood disorders are the most common neuropsychiatric complications of dementia. Estimates of the prevalence of depressive symptoms in dementia range from 1.3 to 50% with modal estimates of about 20% for a depressive syndrome and >50% for any depressive symptom

▶ **TABLE 12-1** PREVALENCE OF DEPRESSION IN DEMENTIA

Reference	Estimated Prevalence of Depressive Symptoms in Dementia (%)	Methodological Comments
Garre-Olmo et al. (2003)[38]	50	NPI Depressive symptoms 55% persistence at 12-month follow-up Clinical sample
Migliorelli et al. (1995)[37]	51	28% dysthymia 23% major depression Clinical sample
Weiner et al. (1994)[131]	1.3–1.5	Strict criteria (DSM-III-R major depressive episode) Clinical sample
Cache County (2000)[31]	24 (20% for AD)	NPI Depressive symptoms Population sample
Cardiovascular Health Study (2002)[32]	32%	NPI Depressive symptoms Population sample
Burns et al. (2004)[33]	24	Trained observer 43% rated as depressed by relatives 63% had at least one depressive symptom Case registry sample

(Table 12-1). Risk factors for developing depression in AD include a prior history of depressive episodes,[37,38] family history of depression,[39,40] presenile onset of dementia,[41] and possibly low educational level.[42] There is one report that Blacks with dementia have a lower prevalence of depressive symptoms than Whites, although it is not known whether this represents differential vulnerability or differential access to diagnosis and treatment.[43] Depressive symptoms are relatively persistent with 55% of depressed demented patients remaining depressed at 12-month follow-up.[38]

▶ ASSESSMENT OF DEPRESSION IN ALZHEIMER'S DISEASE

Diagnostic Dilemmas

It is apparent from Table 12-1 that different criteria for depression in AD lead to widely varying prevalence estimates. Specifically, the one study using strict Diagnostic and Statistical Manual (DSM)-III-R criteria led to a very low estimate of prevalence at <2% while studies with broader criteria had much higher prevalence estimates. Applying strict DSM criteria for major depression to AD clearly excludes many patients with clinically significant depressive symptoms. For example, DSM criteria require that symptoms be present "most of the day, nearly every day," but AD patients' symptoms are prone to change throughout the day and a less restrictive time frame seems appropriate. Similarly, since depressed AD patients have more modest neurovegetative symptoms, such as insomnia, anorexia, or weight loss, requiring five of nine symptoms becomes very restrictive and few patients can meet these narrow standards.

In addition, AD patients have deficits in abstract thinking and executive functioning, which diminish their capacity to integrate emotions and behavioral reactions over time. Thus, they often have difficulty articulating a depressed mood even though they may have profound sadness or anhedonia. AD patients often answer questions about their mood with clichéd "empty" responses, possibly due to decreased verbal fluency.[44,45] This may account for AD patients' tendency to report fewer depressive symptoms than caregivers.

Another confound is the increased prevalence of chronic disease in any elderly population that tends to overlap with mood criteria that rely heavily on neurovegetative signs and symptoms of mood disorder such as insomnia, anorexia, weight loss, fatigue, and psychomotor retardation. DSM-IV and the Hamilton depression rating scale (HAM-D) tend to weight these symptoms relatively heavily. Although instructions for use of the criteria give the rater guidance as to how to judge whether a symptom is due to medical or psychologic factors, in practice this attribution judgment is often difficult. Given the prevalence of chronic illness, it is not clear that these neurovegetative symptoms have adequate specificity for diagnosis of depression in Alzheimer.[46,47]

The Differing Spectrum of Symptoms in Depression in AD and Elderly Without Dementia

Depression in AD has a different constellation of symptoms than major depressive disorder as defined in DSM-IV. Several studies have compared symptom clusters in depressed patients with and without dementia (Table 12-2). Janzing et al.[48] found that dementia patients had more "motivation" symptoms and fewer "mood" symptoms than a group without dementia, despite comparable severity of depressive symptoms. The motivation factor included fatigue, slowness of thinking and movement, lack of interest in activities, and decreased affective response to pleasurable activities. The mood factor included worry, depressed mood, tearfulness, hopelessness, and suicidal thoughts. Their cohort included patients with subsyndromal depression and is representative of patients typically seen in practice.

▶ **TABLE 12-2** SYMPTOM CONSTELLATION OF DEPRESSION IN ALZHEIMER'S DISEASE

More Common Symptoms of dAD	Less Common Symptoms of dAD
Anhedonia	Depressed mood
Anxiety	Guilt
Irritability	Hopelessness
Lack of motivation	Suicidality
Agitation	
Delusions	
Hallucinations	

Li et al.[49] similarly noted that motivational symptoms predominate among depressive symptoms of AD. Zubenko et al.[50] found depressed AD patients to be more likely than depressed nondemented patients to have delusions, hallucinations, and complaints of concentration difficulties and less likely to report guilt or suicidal ideation. Tractenberg et al.[51] and Bassiony et al.[52] concur that delusions and depression cluster together in AD, as do data from the Cache County cohort.[53] In the abovementioned studies insomnia and weight loss were equally common in AD and nondemented patients. However, Purandare et al.[54] reported differing results that neurovegetative signs did discriminate depressed AD patients from nondepressed. Rubin et al.[55] noted that indecision and fatigue are particularly helpful in discriminating depressed from nondepressed AD patients.

These converging results suggest that the symptom cluster of depression in AD has a different "flavor" to it than that seen in the elderly without dementia. Depressed AD patients are less likely to express typical mood complaints, including feeling sadness, hopelessness, guilt, suicidal, and so on. Rather, they tend to feel anxious, apathetic, unmotivated to participate in activities and do not feel pleasure when they do, and they complain of lack of concentration. For these reasons a revised set of diagnostic criteria incorporating these findings has recently been proposed for depression in AD.

Rating Scales

Since the symptom cluster of depression in AD differs from major depression it is not surprising that the use of rating scales to assess them must be carefully considered. The major rating scales for assessing depression in AD are summarized in Table 12-3. One approach to rating is to include depression in a general inventory of neuropsychiatric difficulties such as the Behavioral pathology in Alzheimer's Disease rating scale (BEHAVE-AD),[56] NPI,[57] and the Consortium to establish a register for Alzheimer's Disease (CERAD) behavior rating scale for AD.[58] These scales are particularly useful because they cover a broad range of problem behaviors and are designed to be administered to caregivers. As a group they are quite useful for screening but may not be sensitive enough to detect change with treatment.

A second approach is to use rating scales developed for a major depressive episode such as the Hamilton rating scale for depression (HAM-D),[59–61] geriatric depression scale (GDS),[62] Zung scale,[63] Montgomery-Asberg depression rating scale (MADRS),[64,65] and Beck depression inventory (BDI).[66] Each of these scales has been used with a reasonable degree of validity and reliability in mild-to-moderate AD. Disadvantages including (1) the scales are mostly designed for patient self-report which may underestimate symptoms[67,68]; (2) the HAM-D is substantially influenced by somatic symptoms which often overlap with medical illness in the elderly; (3) the items on several of the scales (particularly HAM-D and BDI) are phrased in relatively long sentences with abstract concepts that may be too difficult for patients with receptive language deficits which are common in AD.[69] Naarding et al. reported that to get the maximum specificity and sensitivity from the HAM-D requires different cutoffs for AD, stroke, and Parkinson's disease.[70] The MADRS has been developed to be sensitive to change and has shown treatment effects in medication trials, but its specific value in AD has not been fully demonstrated.[64,65]

The third approach is to develop scales specifically for depression in dementia. The most widely used scale is the Cornell Scale for Depression in Dementia (CSDD) which combines clinician observation, patient input, and caregiver input into a consensus determined by the interviewer.[71] The CSDD is relatively lightly weighted toward somatic symptoms, with only 7 of 19 items. It is easily administered to patients with a wide range of cognitive abilities and is sensitive to treatment effects[59,64,72] and is practical for screening for depression in nursing home populations.[73] A cutoff score of 13 or more is suggested for a major depressive episode, but clinicians should consider a lower cutoff of 6–7 for screening for depression in AD. The Dementia Mood Assessment Scale (DMAS)[74] is a similar scale with good reliability and face validity in demented patients, although it has not been widely used. The Clinical Assessment for Depression in Dementia (CADD)[50] is a promising new instrument that assesses both diagnosis and severity, incorporating items from the HAM-D and NPI, with good interrater reliability and robust face validity in that it incorporates items from two widely used scales.

Caregiver Input and Caregiver Bias in Depression Assessment

There is no doubt that caregiver input is essential for adequate assessment of depressive symptoms in AD. Deficits in short-term recall may rob a patient of the sense of time passing, of accurate recall of daily functioning, and of the severity of symptoms. The CSDD and NPI are rating scales that directly utilize caregiver input in the assessment. However, caregivers may tend to see the situation as "all bad" due to stress, just as patients may see the situation as "all good" due to lack of recall of problems. Thus, caregivers may over report and AD patients may underreport symptoms. Burke et al. administered a modified GDS to both patients and caregivers, and found that caregivers rated depressive symptoms higher on all items.[68] Teri and Truax found a moderate correlation between caregiver depression and patient depression.[67] Moreover, depressed caregivers nearly always rated the patient as depressed,

▶ **TABLE 12-3** INSTRUMENTS FOR ASSESSMENT OF DEPRESSION IN ALZHEIMER'S DISEASE

Instrument	Assessment	Rater	No. of Items	Range	Psychometric Properties in AD	Comments
Hamilton Depression Rating Scale (HAM-D)	Depression severity	Patient, interviewer	17 (most commonly used) or 21	0–50	Reliability approximately 0.9.[63] Sensitivity 90% but specificity varied 9–63% for diagnosis of depression in AD.[132,133]	Most widely used scale in nonelderly, but does not incorporate caregiver input. Optimal cutoff for depression in AD is >9.
Cornell Scale for Depression in Dementia (CSDD)	Depression severity	Patient, caregiver, interviewer	19	0–38	Reliability 0.63–0.84.[74] Correlation with HAM-D 0.86.[132] Sensitivity 90% and specificity 75% for diagnosis of depression in AD.[132]	Most widely used scale in AD due to incorporation of caregiver input
Geriatric Depression Scale (GDS)	Depression severity	Patient	15 (short version) 30 (long version)	0–15 (short version) 0–30 (long version)	Reliability > 0.9. Correlation with HAM-D > 0.8.[133]	Easy to administer but heavily dependent on patient comprehension of items
Montgomery-Asberg Depression Rating Scale (MADRS)	Depression severity	Patient, interviewer	10	0–60	Reliability 0.86. Correlation with HAM-D 0.82[134] (not specifically in demented subjects, however).	Designed to be sensitive to mood change. Minimal data for validity in depression in AD
Zung depression rating scale	Depression severity	Patient (self-administered)	20	0–80	Reliability 0.8–0.9.[63] Significant correlation with HAM-D but only for early stages of dementia.	Self-administered scale of questionable validity in dementia due to patients' tendency to underreport symptoms
Dementia Mood Assessment Scale	Depression severity	Patient, interviewer	17	0–112	Reliability 0.7.74 Correlation with HAM-D 0.47.[73]	Excellent face validity but only used in single study
Clinical Assessment of Depression in Dementia (CADD)	Depression severity, lifelong course of mood disorder	Patient, caregiver, interviewer	Not reported	Not reported	Reliability and validity > 0.9 for diagnosis of major depression. Correlation with HAM-D 0.94.[50]	Combines severity and diagnosis assessment

whereas nondepressed caregivers gave a more balanced assessment. Rubin et al. reported different symptom constellations arising out of factor analysis of caregiver and patient reports.[55]

These correlations between caregiver and patient mood are consistent enough to suggest a causal relationship. However, since there is no "gold standard" rating scale for depression of AD they do not clarify whether patients underreport or caregivers over report mood symptoms in AD. Thus, the clinician is advised to utilize *both* caregiver and patient input in assessing mood symptoms in AD, but not to take an average of the two. The clinician may need to factor in caregiver stress as a bias in reporting and utilize clinical judgment in how to incorporate caregiver input, patient report, and observation into a coherent whole. This complex process involves considerably more time and judgment than routine office management of major depressive episodes in adults. Later on, we discuss ways to get around this through the application of the "depression of Alzheimer's disease (dAD)" diagnostic criteria in an effort to clarify the diagnostic process.

Apathy Versus Depression

Apathy is an evolving concept in psychiatry referring to states in which patients have deficits in motivation without appearing sad or depressed. Patient apathy is a common presenting complaint by caregivers who feel frustrated and upset that the patient "just doesn't want to do anything." In institutional settings there is a converse problem, where apathy, which can lead to serious deconditioning, may remain undiagnosed because patients are passive and easier to manage. The distinction between apathy and depression is less clear; in practice, apathy is often treated as a symptom of mood disorder rather than a separate syndrome. In the Cache County study it was the most frequent neuropsychiatric symptom of dementia and was often present in the absence of depressive symptoms or other typical symptoms in the depres-

sion of AD constellation.[75] Starkstein et al. reported that 37% of a large clinical sample of AD patients were significantly apathetic.[76] Many (24%) but not all had apathy coexisting with major depression. Marin et al. reported that in AD patients the correlation between apathy and depressive symptoms was higher than in major depression or hemispheric strokes.[77] Apathy is associated with poorer cognitive functioning and worse ADL impairment,[78] and may be a symptom of preclinical AD.[79] Since apathy is better associated with measures of executive dysfunction than with mood measures,[80] it has not been included as a diagnostic criterion for dAD.

Depression of AD Diagnostic Criteria

Given the data supporting the idea that depression in AD has a unique symptom constellation, the National Institutes of Mental Health convened a consensus conference of experts in the field to develop coherent diagnostic criteria.[81,82] Table 12-4 presents the proposed NIMH criteria for dAD incorporating the phenomenology noted above and avoiding criteria that have notable overlap with cognitive deficits and/or chronic medical illness.[83] The table also presents a discussion of the criteria in hopes of helping clinicians better detect and diagnose depression in this context.

► CAUSES OF DEPRESSION IN ALZHEIMER'S DISEASE

Depression usually appears to have multiple risk factors rather than a single unitary cause. AD patients are no exception and there are significant psychosocial and biologic factors that increase risk for depression. Knowledge of these risk factors may present opportunities for early intervention and education in depression of AD.

▶ **TABLE 12-4** OPERATIONALIZED CRITERIA FOR DEPRESSION OF AD (DAD)

Criterion	Comment
1. Clinically significant depressed mood (e.g., depressed, sad, hopeless, discouraged, tearful)	The rater may distinguish between "not caring" (apathy) from more acute/distressed sad mood (depression), and may need to distinguish the patient's statements from behavior observed by others. The transient affective lability of "emotional incontinence" probably should not lead to a positive rating if it is not associated with changes in mood outside the periods of mood "incontinence."
2. Decreased positive affect or pleasure in response to social contacts and usual activities	To illustrate this item, the examiner might wish to elicit examples from the patient and caregiver of activities that the patient has usually found pleasurable in the past or that most people find pleasurable (i.e., a good meal, visiting with grandchildren, attending a family event, and so on). Reports of behavior tend to be most important in rating this item, often contradicting patient's recall of events. Useful questions include whether the participant is still "having as much fun as he/she used to," "still enjoying life," or "has a zest for life."
3. Social isolation or withdrawal	The examiner assesses both the patient's desire to seek out people and her sociability with other people. Social isolation/withdrawal do not lead to an positive rating if they are lifelong traits or appear to be motivated by an effort to avoid tasks that challenge cognition.
4. Disruption in appetite	Because a patient's cognitive deficits may especially interfere with recall and interpretation of appetite or weight change, it is essential to corroborate information on this item with caregiver reports and if possible documentation of weight changes.
5. Disruption in sleep	The examiner rates change from usual sleep habits and/or a sense of poor quality of sleep. It may be difficult to accurately assess sleep if the patient sleeps alone. Awakenings solely for purposes of toileting or hygiene if the patient is able to fall back to sleep rapidly (within 30 min) are best not used to make a positive rating.
6. Psychomotor changes (e.g., agitation or retardation)	**Agitation:** This may include inability to sit still, pacing, and/or hand wringing. This does not imply disruptive or oppositional behavior or combativeness/violent behavior. Agitation and irritability (criterion 7) are often seen together. Efforts are best made to distinguish agitation from anxiety, the latter being common but not specifically part of the dAD criteria. Note that agitation can coexist with fatigue/loss of energy. **Retardation:** The rater will need to assess the contribution of medical conditions to this item.
7. Irritability	Irritability is rated when it represents a change from the patient's usual personality traits. Typical descriptions include having a short temper, "flying off the handle," or "going off over little things." This item particularly requires sensitivity to cultural differences and diverse use of language. It excludes simple frustration over cognitive deficits or difficulties performing daily tasks. Delirium can mimic this symptom.
8. Fatigue or loss of energy	This symptom may be most apparent after taking a medical review of systems, and is often mimicked by medical illnesses. The examiner has to judge whether the degree of fatigue seems out of proportion to the burden of medical illness.

(Continued)

▶ **TABLE 12-4** OPERATIONALIZED CRITERIA FOR DEPRESSION OF AD (DAD) (*CONTINUED*)

Criterion	Comment
9. Feelings of worthlessness, hopelessness, or excessive or inappropriate guilt	Feelings of pessimism, negativity, lowered self-esteem, a sense of foreshortened future, self-blame, decreased confidence, and delusional guilt might be included in this rating. These feelings may be elicited when patients encounter their cognitive limitations during mental status examination. It is best to confirm that they are present at other times, so as to avoid making a positive rating entirely based on frustration with failing cognitive testing.
10. Recurrent thoughts or death, suicidal intention, plan, or attempt	This rating includes thoughts of wanting to die whether or not the patient appears to have "intent." It is important to distinguish desire to die from a decision to forego aggressive medical care in accordance with spiritual, moral, and ethical beliefs.

Psychosocial Factors

"Who wouldn't be depressed if they had AD?" It is often assumed that the diagnosis itself should lead to depression, particularly if the patient is aware of the diagnosis. But since even the highest prevalence estimates for depression of AD are 50% an equal number of AD patients lack mood disorder. The relationship between awareness of deficits and depression is complex. For example, it is often assumed that awareness of deficits is a major risk for depression, and that lack of awareness in advanced disease is protective against depression. AD patients tend to have insight into their cognitive deficits early in the course of disease,[84] yet several studies report no association between insight into AD and depression[85] with two studies reporting association with depression[86] and hopelessness.[87] Thus, the verdict is not in on whether awareness of deficits leads to depression in AD or not.

AD patients have major social stresses early in the illness, particularly involving loss of occupational function and diminished ability to socialise. Families may make strenuous efforts to minimize the impact of these changes and to keep them out of the patient's awareness so as not to confront the patient with his/her functional deficits. For example, many patients with AD will sign checks that their spouses have made out to maintain the illusion that they are still in charge of the finances. There are instances where patients maintain the illusion of working even with significant cognitive deficits, for example going to the office daily to "work" at his/her old desk even if the patient no longer can perform any functional work. Another stressor is the AD patient's knowledge, however cloudy, that they have increased dependency needs. Even patients with advanced stages of AD will frequently resist care because of denial and anger regarding their functional dependency.

Beyond these general stressors of dependency and functional decline, specific cognitive deficits may be detrimental to patients' self-image and self-esteem. One common and poignant example is diminished verbal fluency as evidenced by word-finding deficits.[44,45] When patients cannot speak fluently they often feel frustrated and embarrassed in social situations, and may avoid social contacts to avoid these conflicts. In more advanced stages of dementia AD patients frequently suffer from agnosia.[45] Patients may wander hazardously due to lack of cognizance of the distinction between different rooms in a facility or between indoors and outdoors, and may require placement in a locked dementia unit. Even patients with fairly advanced disease are often aware of the locked nature of the facility and become demoralized as a result. Disorientation to time, date, and situation can lead to profound mood changes. It is not uncommon for an AD patients to be tearful, sad, and beseeching because they cannot fathom where they live, or why they live there, or what the purpose of living there is, particularly if they are in a dementia unit or skilled nursing setting. The clinician should be sensitive to the interaction between the patient's awareness of functional limitations and vulnerability to depression.

Biologic Factors

Neurochemistry

There are several pathologic studies which suggest that neuronal degeneration in monoaminergic (serotoninergic and norepinephrinergic) brainstem nuclei is associated with depression in AD. Zubenko et al. studied 37 brains from patients with pathologic diagnoses of AD and found that depressive symptoms in these patients were associated with decreased numbers of pigmented cell bodies in the locus coeruleus (LC) and substantia nigra (SN), which supply the majority of the monoaminergic innervation to the brain.[88] Indeed these changes in cell number were associated with a marked decrease in norepinephrine in the neocortex and hippocampus as well.[89] There are two comparable studies supporting these findings in LC though not SN.[90,91] These findings were considered supportive of the hypothesis that depression was due to decreased monoaminergic activity. However, a recent report does not replicate these findings and highlights the methodologic problems of earlier studies.[92] These results may be due to cell loss in LC and SN being associated with cognitive decline in AD rather than specifically with depression. Thus, the monoaminergic theory of depression in AD is uncertain.

Genetics

Cognitive and mood symptoms of AD appear to have different genetic vulnerabilities and differ from the genetic vulnerabilities to depression in younger life. The e4 allele of the apolipoprotein E gene has been well established as a risk factor for the development of AD and for earlier age

of onset of AD.[93,94] The presence of apoe4 alleles has been reported to affect the time course of response to antidepressant treatment in nondemented elderly patients, with a more rapid response to mirtazapine and slower response to paroxetine.[95] However, it does not appear to increase vulnerability to depression in AD[96,97] and to have only minimal effect on depressive symptoms when viewed throughout the spectrum of neuropsychiatric symptoms of AD.[98] Although the apoe2 allele appears to protect against development of both AD and lifetime unipolar depressive disorder, it is associated with vulnerability to depression in AD.[99]

Neuroimaging

There is increasing evidence from functional imaging studies of depression in neurologic disease that frontal lobe hypometabolic changes may be associated with depression; preliminary findings in dAD are similar. O'Brien et al. noted a correlation between frontal lobe white matter hypointensities and depression in AD.[100] Hirono et al.[101] reported that frontal lobe hypometabolism was associated with depressive symptoms in 53 patients with AD. In addition, anterior cingulate hypometabolism was also associated with depressive symptoms, similar to Migneco et al.'s report associating apathy with depression in AD.[102] Further imaging studies suggest that depressive mood symptoms are associated with frontal lobe hypometabolism[103] while apathy is associated with decreased metabolism in the anterior cingulate cortex.[104]

Inflammatory Markers

The potential connection between inflammatory markers and dAD is intriguing though still entirely speculative. Given the growing evidence that neurotoxicity in AD is mediated by inflammatory mechanisms in the brain, including the release of proinflammatory cytokines by activated microglia,[21] and given the association of elevated serum levels of these cytokines with depressed mood in a large elderly community sample,[105] it is conceivable that these cytokines mediate both cognitive impairment and mood disorder in AD. CNS or peripheral cytokine synthesis and release may be a future target for treatment of AD and depression in AD.

▶ DIAGNOSIS AND TREATMENT OF DEPRESSION OF ALZHEIMER'S DISEASE

Diagnosis

Patients with dAD may present with a variety of complaints including depression, anxiety, "nerves," memory problems, lack of motivation, loss of interest, and so on. As noted above the complaints come more often from the family than from the patient. Given the insidious nature of the onset of both AD and depression, the clinician needs to tease out the time course and nature of both cognitive and mood symptoms.

It is clear from the literature that caregiver input is needed both for proper diagnosis and for treatment planning, and no evaluation should be considered complete without a caregiver interview. This may take various forms such as individual interviews with the patient and caregiver separately, telephone interview with the caregiver, or formal or informal treatment planning meetings with institutional staff (such as in an assisted living or nursing home environment). It is particularly valuable to interview the patient and caregiver separately whenever possible. This allows both to candidly express their feelings and concerns without worrying about causing greater conflict or friction, particularly in a family dyad. The very behaviors that a caregiver spouse might feel uncomfortable discussing in an interview with the couple—such as disrobing, inappropriate sexualizing, assaultiveness, or incontinence—are likely to be the behaviors causing maximal stress. The clinician should also be alert to the cultural and educational backgrounds of patients and caregivers, particularly in phrasing questions and interpreting responses. Some patients and families may be use terms such as "depression" and "anxiety"

with a meaning similar to the clinician's, but frequently the clinician needs to explore what the patient and family are trying to express. These communication issues may be due to cultural differences or to patients' cognitive deficits, and the clinician should be alert to either possibility.

The patient with dAD may have a presentation similar to major depressive episode in nondemented patients and including the typical signs and symptoms outlined in DSM-IV such as depressed mood, anhedonia, anorexia, fatigue, psychomotor agitation or retardation, difficulties concentrating, poor self-esteem, and suicidal ideation. But as noted above, the typical constellation of symptoms in dAD may be substantially different and lack obvious mood complaints. The patient may not present as sad, blue, tearful, guilty, or hopeless/suicidal as is typical of nondemented patients with depression. Rather, their symptoms may fit into the spectrum of affective symptoms of AD[75] including anxiety, agitation, apathy, anhedonia, decreased motivation, and difficulties in concentrating. These are often mistaken for pure cognitive symptoms and treated with cholinesterase inhibitors, or for nonspecific agitation and treated with antipsychotic medications. While both classes of medications may be useful adjuncts in dAD they are unlikely to be core treatments.

Many medical and neurologic conditions and medication toxicities can confound the diagnosis of dAD by mimicking depressive symptoms (Table 12-5). Common neurologic confounds including flat affect, bradykinesia and bradyphrenia of Parkinson's disease, pathologic tearfulness due to pseudobulbar palsy in multiple sclerosis, and "amotivation" from apraxia or executive dysfunction in many dementias. Psychomotor retardation is common to many medical conditions including congestive heart failure, chronic obstructive pulmonary disease, malignancy, and drug toxicity. Diminished concentration or sustained attention to task is common to many neurologic illnesses and delirium and is often misdiagnosed as depression.

The diagnostic workup for suspected depression of AD should be individualized to patient presentation but is based on routine

▶ **TABLE 12-5** MEDICAL CONDITIONS AND MEDICATIONS MIMICKING DEPRESSION OF AD

Medical Condition	Medication
Parkinson's disease	Corticosteroids
Multiple sclerosis	Benzodiazepines
Hypothyroidism	Chemotherapeutic agents
Neurosyphilis	Lithium toxicity
Cancer	Digitoxicity
Congestive heart failure	Phenytoin toxicity
Chronic obstructive pulmonary disease	Opioid analgesics
Delirium	Carbamazepine
Hyper- or hypoglycemia	Tricyclic antidepressants
Uremia	Anticholinergic medications (benztropine, antihistamines, chlorpromazine, thioridazine)
Hypernatremia	

evaluation for AD itself (Table 12-6). A thorough physical and neurologic examination is a must for clues to medical confounds, and a review of medications is equally essential. Clinicians should be particularly alert for the cognitive toxicity of anticholinergic medications[106,107] and sedation from benzodiazepines or opioid analgesics. If the mood change is relatively acute the clinician must rule out common causes of delirium in demented patients including urinary tract infection, pneumonia, metabolic disturbances, and recent medication changes.

When in doubt about the diagnosis or severity of depression, reliable and valid rating scales can help bring the clinical picture into focus. The authors recommend the CSDD as the most suitable scale for general clinical use. Administering the CSDD involves interviewing both patient and caregiver; the clinician then integrates observation and reports into item scores. In more advanced stages of dementia the patient's report becomes increasingly unreliable due to difficulties in comprehending the questions and responding with expressive language, and also due to difficulties with abstractions posed in questions

▶ **TABLE 12-6** DIAGNOSTIC WORKUP FOR SUSPECTED DEPRESSION OF AD

Diagnostic Test	Rationale
MRI or CT brain	Rule out CVA, subdural hematoma, brain tumor, occult closed-head injury
Lumbar puncture	Only if infection is suspected (TB, HIV, herpetic encephalitis)
Electroencephalogram	Only if seizure or delirium is suspected
Metabolic panel	Rule out hyperglycemia, hypernatremia, uremia
CBC	Rule out anemia (as cause of fatigue)
Thyroid panel	Rule out hypothyroidism
Serum B_{12}	Rule out B_{12} deficiency (usually from decreased absorption due to achlorhydria in elderly)
Urine toxicology screen	Rule out occult ingestion, sedative abuse
Serum drug levels (i.e., lithium phenytoin, carbamazepine, digoxin)	Rule out inattention/and reduced state of alertness due to toxicity

about the emotional state, and thus the clinician relies more on observations and caregiver report.

▶ TREATMENT

Medications

The results of controlled trials of antidepressant medications for depression in AD are summarized in Table 12-7. The efficacy of antidepressants in these studies is varied, replication studies are few, and there are several negative studies. Most of the "negative" studies reported substantial improvements in the patients in the placebo arms. One common problem is that unique criteria for dAD were not available when these trials were conducted, so that most studies used modified DSM-IV mood disorder criteria which may not be appropriate for this setting.

There is evidence to point toward choice of antidepressant but not a definitive first choice. For example, trials of tricyclic antidepressants (TCAs) note negative effects on cognition in AD patients. Selective serotonin reuptake inhibitors (SSRIs) appear better tolerated but not consistently effective. Comparisons of TCAs versus SSRIs generally note fewer side effects with SSRIs but mood symptoms respond equally well to either class of medication. There are no controlled studies of newer agents such as citalopram, venlafaxine, bupropion, or mirtazapine in dAD, but clinicians use them widely as second- or first-line agents in dAD.

Based on these results, the following approach to antidepressant medication treatment of depression in AD is recommended[108,109] (summarized in Table 12-8):

1. Start with an SSRI. There are more studies supporting the efficacy and safety of SSRIs in dAD than for any other class of medications. There is little evidence to prefer a single SSRI, but the authors recommend starting with sertraline, citalopram, or escitalopram because the first two have the best efficacy and safety data in AD and escitalopram is very similar to citalo-

pram. This was supported by a recent consenus expert panel.[108]. Dose recommendations are outlined in Table 12-8. One conclusion from clinical trials is that the doses of antidepressant to treat dAD are comparable to doses used in younger depressed patients; note that this finding is quite different from dosing strategies for other classes of psychotropic medications in the elderly. Paroxetine has some anticholinergic activity, which can lead to mild delirium, but has the advantage of being relatively sedating and helpful in particularly anxious patients. Fluoxetine has the longest half-life, with the disadvantage of prolonging side effects when present but the advantage of a once-weekly dosing alternative.

2. Titrate up from starting dose to maximal dose tolerated over 4 weeks if tolerated, but the clinician may proceed more cautiously in very elderly frail patients. If no response is seen at 4 weeks of maximum dose, consider changing medications or adding an antipsychotic or anticonvulsant. If partial response is seen at 4 weeks of maximum dose, up to 12 weeks may be needed to see a complete response.

3. Given the differing spectrum of symptoms from major depressive episode, the frequent presence of significant caregiver burden coloring assessment, and patient's difficulty with self-report, the clinician may have difficulty assessing initial response to treatment. The authors recommend using a rating scale such as the CSDD to clarify this assessment.

4. If response at 12 weeks is unsatisfactory the authors recommend tapering off the initial medication over 2 weeks and starting another agent from the list in Table 12-8.

5. If mood improves but the patients remain significantly agitated, consider adding an anticonvulsant such as Depakote. Initial doses of 250 mg bid or 500 mg q hs are recommended, titrating dose to reach treatment response or serum level of 50–100 μg/mL. Note that clinical response is often reached at levels below 50 μg/mL.[110]

6. The clinician need not prescribe antipsychotic medications for every report of delusions and

Reference	Design	N (Total)	Depression Diagnosis	Treatments	Effect of Treatment on Mood Outcomes	Effect of Treatment on Nonmood Outcomes	Safety Findings
Reifler et al. (1989)[135]	8-week, parallel, masked RCT	61	DSM-III major depression HAM-D > 14	Imipramine (Mean = 82–83 mg/day) Placebo	0	– Cognitive function declined with drug	Drowsiness and dizziness equally reported for both groups
Nyth and Gottfries (1990)[65]	4-week, parallel, masked RCT	98	None Baseline MADRS = 8.0	Citalopram (30 mg/day max) Placebo	0	+ Irritability improved with drug	Mild, expected side effects more common on citalopram
Nyth et al. (1992)[136]	6-week, parallel, masked RCT	149 (but only 29 with depression and AD)	HAM-D > 13 74% met criteria for DSM-III major depression (total sample)	Citalopram (30 mg/day max) Placebo	+	+ Cognitive function improved with drug	Side effects reported > 10% for entire sample: tiredness, sedation, tension
Petracca et al. (1996)[61]	12-week, crossover, RCT	21	DSM-III-R major depression or dysthymia HAM-D > 10	Clomipramine (100 mg/day max) Placebo	+	– Cognitive function declined with drug	Dry mouth, dizziness, sleep problems, tremor more frequent in clomipramine group
Roth et al. (1996)[60]	6-week, parallel, masked RCT	726	DSM-III major depressive episode HAM-D > 13	Moclobemide (400 mg/day max) Placebo	+	+ Cognitive function improved with drug	No significant differences in side effects, ECG, vital signs

(Continued)

317

Reference	Design	N (Total)	Depression Diagnosis	Treatments	Effect of Treatment on Mood Outcomes	Effect of Treatment on Nonmood Outcomes	Safety Findings
Magai et al. (2000)[137]	8-week, parallel, masked RCT	31	DSM-IV major or minor depression CSDD > 2 Gestalt scale > 0	Sertraline (100 mg/day max) Placebo	0	+ "Knit-brow face" improved with drug (trend)	Not reported
Petracca et al. (2001)[61]	6-week, parallel, masked RCT	41	DSM-IV major or minor depression HAMD > 13	Fluoxetine (40 mg/day max) Placebo	0	0	Mild tremor more common on fluoxetine
Lyketsos et al. (2003)[59]	12-week, parallel, masked RCT	44	DSM-IV major depressive episode	Sertraline (150 mg/day max) Placebo	+	+ Placebo group declined more than drug group in ADLs (trend)	No difference between sertraline and placebo
Taragano et al. (1997)[138]	45-day, parallel, masked RCT	37	DSM-III major depressive episode	Fluoxetine (25 mg/day max) Amitriptyline (10 mg/day max)	+ (No difference between drugs)	+ Cognitive function improved in both groups	42% completion for amitriptyline; 78% for fluoxetine
Katona et al. (1998)[64]	8-week, parallel, masked RCT	198	RDC major or minor depression MADRS > 19	Paroxetine (40 mg/day max) Imipramine (100 mg/day max)	+ (No difference between drugs)	N/A	Paroxetine better tolerated, but marginally so

318

Study	Design	N	Criteria	Intervention				
Teri et al. (1997)[116]	Parallel, RCT	72	DSM-III-R major depressive disorder or minor depressive disorder	(1) Patient intervention: "Pleasant events" (2) Caregiver intervention: "Problem solving" (3) Wait-list control (4) Typical care	+	Behavioral treatments both better than wait-list or typical care	+ Caregiver depression symptoms improved with both behavioral treatments	0
Teri et al. (2003)[72]	Parallel, RCT	153 total AD Unknown # in depressed subgroup	CSDD > 5	Behavioral intervention with caregivers + exercise program vs. usual care	+	N/A		0

Abbreviations: RCT: randomized-controlled trial; ADLs: activities of daily living.

▶ **TABLE 12-8** ANTIDEPRESSANT MEDICATIONS FOR DEPRESSION IN AD

Drug	Initial Dose	Maximum Dose	Comments
Fluoxetine	10 mg	20–40 mg	SSRIs in general: widely used due to favorable safety profile and effect on anxiety. Side effects include GI distress, anxiety, insomnia, medication interactions. FDA warning concerning emerging suicidality suggests careful monitoring in initial 10 days of treatment. Fluoxetine has long half-life with weekly preparation available but prolonged side effects.
Sertraline	25 mg	150 mg	(see fluoxetine)
Paroxetine	10 mg	20–40 mg	(see fluoxetine) May be calming and helpful for sleep.
Citalopram	10 mg	20–40 mg	(see fluoxetine)
Escitalopram	5 mg	20 mg	(see fluoxetine) Enantiomer of citalopram.
Venlafaxine (long-acting)	37.5 mg	225 mg	Side effect of hypertension (3%). More stimulating than SSRIs.
Bupropion (long-acting)	75 mg	450 mg	Side effect of seizures (at supra-therapeutic doses only). Dopaminergic effect may also be more stimulating than SSRIs.
Mirtazapine	7.5 mg	30 mg	Side effect of weight gain, sedation. Use at bedtime. Widely used as hypnotic.
Nortriptyline	10 mg	100 mg	Side effect of constipation, dry mouth. Best choice among tricyclic antidepressants due to favorable side effects profile.
Methylphenidate	5 mg in the morning	10 mg at breakfast and lunch	Side effects of insomnia, dyskinetic movements. May be helpful for apathy and fatigue. Limited research base.
Duloxetine	20 mg twice daily	40–60 mg twice daily	Side effect of hypertension less common than venlafaxine, sexual side effects less common than SSRIs. May be helpful for pain and somatizing syndromes.

hallucinations, particularly if they seem less prominent than the core mood syndrome. For example, a randomized clinical trial of citalopram versus perphenazine demonstrated comparable efficacy in treating agitation and psychosis in demented nursing home patients.[111]

7. Psychostimulants may be quite helpful for the apathetic, amotivated patient, but their niche has not been well defined due to lack of controlled data. The authors recommend short-acting methylphenidate given at breakfast and lunch, rather than long-acting preparations, because of the safety of short-acting drugs and ability to titrate finely to response. The advantage of psychostimulants is that patients respond very rapidly (within days) if they are responders.

8. Electroconvulsive therapy (ECT) may be effective for the treatment-refractory dAD patient. In a case series of 31 patients with depression and dementia, ECT improved mood to a clinically significant extent with minimal reports of worsening cognition or prolonged postictal delirium.[112]

Behavioral and Cognitive Therapies

Optimal care of depression in AD starts with good dementia care.[5] The mixed results from controlled trials of medications are in part related to substantial improvements in the patients on placebo. This probably reflects the responsiveness of depression in AD, at least in its milder forms, to nonpharmacologic interventions. In addition, medication therapies alone are often not always acceptable to patients. For example, in a medication-alone study of fluoxetine no patients completed the trial.[113] Thus, the clinician should consider a wide range of psychosocial interventions and individualize the treatment plan according to the patient's and caregiver's needs and strengths. However, traditional psychotherapy is clearly not directly applicable to cognitively impaired patients, since most models of psychotherapy depend on the patient's ability to recall insights from session to session. A popular strategy is to combine behavioral interventions for the patient and education, with problem-solving strategies for the caregiver.[114]

Table 12-7 summarizes findings from two controlled trials of behavioral treatments for depression in AD. Teri et al. found that two behavioral treatment programs, one based on problem-solving strategies and the other using the Pleasant Events Schedule,[115] both led to greater mood improvement in patients and controls as opposed to a waiting-list control group.[116] Similar results were seen with a similar intervention combining an individualized exercise program for the AD patient with problem-solving strategies for the caregiver; mood improvement was reported both in a general AD population and in a dAD subgroup.[72]

These intriguing findings suggest that in treating dAD, there may be value to therapeutic activities such as reminiscence therapy, focusing on pleasant events such as with the Pleasant Events Schedule,[115] music, and so on. A good alternative may also be an individualized exercise program designed to suit the patient's degree of mobility. These may be best implemented in the context of adult day health care or a senior citizens' center. It is sensible to target the activities to a patient's cognitive strengths and work around cognitive deficits (i.e., patients with language deficits may respond better to nonverbal programs involving music and exercise).

In addition, in treating dAD, a program directed at caregivers should also be considered. Important components include teaching caregivers the skills of caregiving, including practical approaches to handling problem behaviors. We present a sample caregiver targeted intervention developed for use in the depression in AD-2 controlled trial of sertraline treatment for dAD (Table 12-9). Note that this intervention covers problem behaviors, social issues, and addressing the emotional needs of the caregiver. Other aspects of this interventions include:

1. Validating the caregiver's accomplishments and altruism.
2. Encouraging realistic expectations.
3. Addressing safety issues such as wandering, driving, leaving the stove on, and so on. It is clear that patients with AD become significant driving risks as dementia advances[117] and timely referrals to a formal occupational therapy/driving evaluation may help guide the decision about whether a patient can still safely drive within a limited geographic distance.
4. Giving caregivers' permission to ventilate their feelings of grief, disappointment, and anger in the context of a safe, therapeutic interaction.
5. Planning placement to a higher level of care such as an assisted living or skilled nursing home. Most caregivers feel very conflicted about placement, and express fears that they are abandoning their loved ones and will no longer be involved in their care. In fact, caregivers continue to feel involved and stressed after placement in a nursing home[118] and the transition process continues throughout life. In many cases placement is the best solution to relieve the stress of a seemingly impossible care situation,

▶ **TABLE 12-9** SAMPLE CAREGIVER INTERVENTION IN DEPRESSION OF AD*

First Visit (up to 30 min)
1. Explain the purpose of the intervention:

   To improve the day-to-day quality of life of Mr./Ms. X (person with dementia)
   To improve the caregiver's ability to care for them, and
   To help sustain the caregiver in her/his difficult task.

2. Overview of the intervention: A brief counseling session lasting up to 30 min today, and then at all follow-up visits up to 20 min. At each session, the clinician will review and update the care plan using the patient and caregiver checklists, provide educational materials, discuss specific issues in depth, work on caregiving skills, and make any necessary referrals (e.g., PT, support groups, home health, and so on)
3. Provide information in writing as to how to reach the care team on a 24 × 7 basis to deal with crises (see example "Availability Form" provided).
4. Provide and discuss caregiver educational materials: (a) 36-h day[139] and (b) JHU Family Guidelines.
5. Review systematically the "JHU Supportive Care Checklists" first for patient and then for caregiver. Record the elements of the plan on the checklist.
6. Provide illness teaching about depression in AD, its recognition, causes, and treatment. Hand out the article from the Johns Hopkins Memory Bulletin on *Depression in AD*.
7. Special topic of the day: Choose a care problem (or issue) to focus on during this visit. Begin by asking: "What is the biggest care problem you are having right now?" Might also focus the discussion around one of the JHU Family Guidelines, parts of the Supportive Care checklists, or from the recent history that the caregiver provided. Discuss this topic in depth with the caregiver with an eye to teaching caregiving skills and problem-solving strategies. Tailor to the caregiver's level of sophistication.
8. Document duration of the intervention, the topics covered, and place the completed checklists in the source document.

Follow-up Visit (up to about 20–30 min)
1. Remind of the purpose and overview of the ongoing intervention.
2. Remind of team's 24 × 7 availability and how to access it.
3. Prompt for and answer questions about any of the written materials provided in the past (e.g., 36-h day, JHU Guidelines, Memory Bulletin article on depression in AD) or any other issues the caregiver has questions about.
4. Review and update the "JHU Supportive Care Checklists" first for patient and then for caregiver. Update as necessary the elements of the plan on the checklist.
5. Update, as needed, illness teaching about depression in AD, its recognition, causes, and treatment.
6. Special topic of the day: Choose a care problem (or issue) to focus on during this visit. Begin by asking: "What is the biggest care problem you are having right now?" Might also focus the discussion around one of the JHU Family Guidelines, parts of the Supportive Care checklists, or from the recent history that the caregiver provided. Discuss this topic in depth with the caregiver with an eye to teaching caregiving skills and problem-solving strategies. Tailor to the caregiver's level of sophistication.
7. Document duration of the intervention, the topics covered, and place the completed checklists in the source document.

Supportive Care Checklist: Caregiver

PATIENT_____ DATE___/___/___
CAREGIVER_____ RELATIONSHIP_____

Who are caregivers?
___Primary(-ies):_____
___Back-up plan:_____

Topic	Y/N	Date Completed	Intervention	Comment
Education			__Verbal (specify) __The 36-Hour Day[138] __Dementia Care Family Guidelines __Resource list and telephone numbers __Inventory of important documents	
Resource referral			__Alzheimer Association __Eldercare Attorney __Office on Aging/Social Services __Geriatric Case Management	
Caregiver mental health assessment			__Network/activity encouragement __Support group __Counseling referral __Psychiatric referral	
Caregiver physical health assessment			__Primary care	
Caregiver skills counseling			__Activities __Meds/side effects __Supervision __Night time __Behaviors __ADLs __Skills lab referral	
Respite counseling			__Other caregivers __Family/friends __Professional aides __Weekly time off __Monthly time off __Annual vacation	

Supportive Care Checklist: Patient

PATIENT_____ DATE___/___/___
CAREGIVER_____ RELATIONSHIP_____

Topic	Date Y/N	Completed	Intervention	Comment
Diagnostic awareness __Patient aware __Patient not aware				
Advanced directives __Healthcare agent: __Other POA __Will				
Illness education targeted at the patient			Topics covered: 1. 2. 3.	
Daily life schedule review			__Sample calendar	Schedule in place
Safety review Driving Wandering risk Level of care issues Home safety issues Fall risk Medication administration			__Advised to stop __Driving eval. __Level of care eval. __Home safety eval. __PT referral __Devise (specify) __Supervision __Administration	
General medical care			Primary care: Last seen:	
Referrals			__OT __PT __Speech __Home health __Dental __Vision __Hearing	

*It is recognized that not all caregivers need detailed counseling at every visit and that many refuse to be counseled at specific time points. Such refusals should be honored. All caregivers should be offered the educational materials and information about the study team's 24-h availability. As well, occasional visits will be short, lasting much less than the suggested time frame. This too is appropriate. It is left to clinical judgment to determine the exact length of each counseling session. If a caregiver requires more support or counseling than can be provided during these sessions, they should be referred to the appropriate resources in the area, as usual care would dictate.

Source: From *Depression in Alzheimer's Disease Study-2* [DIADS-2] Handbook, version 1.0, 2004.

and the role of the clinician is to give the caregiver permission and professional validation to "let go."

▶ SPECIAL CONSIDERATIONS FOR INSTITUTIONAL SETTINGS

Assisted Living Facilities and Skilled Nursing Facilities

The majority of residents of institutional facilities suffer from cognitive impairment; the prevalence of dementia in both assisted living and nursing home facilities is be about 65–70%.[119,120] Mood disorders in institutional settings can be particularly deleterious in impairing functional abilities in patients who are already highly dependent.

There may be environmental and architectural features of nursing facilities that impact on residents' mood. For example, a multicenter study of dementia unit design found that camouflaging exits was associated with less depression.[121] The authors suggest that this environmental feature reduces staff anxieties about residents eloping, leading to staff allowing residents greater freedom of movement and perhaps improving residents' sense of autonomy and empowerment. One can imagine similar interventions in other aspects of daily life in institutional settings that might improve this sense of autonomy; for example, allowing more latitude in daily planning, setting out a daily schedule to give a sense of purpose and direction to the day, and allowing more outings outdoors or off the premises.

Assessment of dAD in Institutional Settings

Mood disorders in institutional setting are likely to be underdiagnosed; for example, mandatory screening with the minimal data set (MDS) has less than half the yield of a geriatric psychiatrist's evaluation, but even the latter misses many patients with significant mood symptoms assessed on CSDD. Several rating scales have been shown to have good reliability and validity in nursing home populations, including the GDS, CSDD, and HAM-D.[122,123] From a practical standpoint, in institutional environments it is particularly important to utilize a multidisciplinary approach to assessment, including nurses, aides, families, occupational and physical therapists, recreational therapists, and so on.

The goal is to develop an integrated picture of how the patient reacts and interacts with the events and activities of a typical day, particularly with regard to assessing spontaneous interest in activities, need for cuing, exhibiting pleasure in social and recreational activities, and so on. Since physical and occupational therapies often require sustained effort, skilled therapists utilize a cognitive-behavioral approach to motivate the reluctant patient. These efforts are not only therapeutic in dAD but assess the patient's capacity to sustain motivation toward a goal. In other words, a patient who participates well in physical therapy is often demonstrating improvement in mood. In addition, patients often make self-deprecating comments when faced with their functional limitations, and documenting these comments can shed light on self-esteem issues. For severely impaired patients the clinicians should assess what tasks are appropriate to functional level try to get a sense of whether the patient is making an effort to perform at a maximum functional level. The guiding principle in assessment is that depression leads to decreased effort due to a sense of futility and hopelessness. Calorie counts, input from nutritionists, and weighing patients can quantitate decreased appetite when present. Medical confounds are particularly prevalent in institutional settings due to significant burdens of chronic illness and the clinician must have the same cautious approach to diagnosis mentioned above. Personality traits and issues can persist into advanced stages of dementia, and it is important to distinguish life-long issues of feeling victimized, for example, from a new onset of mood disorder.

Treatment

Medication treatment trials of depression in nursing home residents have yielded similar results to dAD patients as a group, and there are no significant modifications to the above recommendation except for the caveat to medicate cautiously given the high burden of chronic illness and polypharmacy in this population. Behavioral interventions that have been reported to improve mood in controlled trials of depressed nursing home residents include a supervised peer volunteer program,[124] group cognitive intervention,[125] therapeutic exercise with wheelchair biking,[126] and recreation therapy in general.[127,128] It is apparent from this diversity of approaches that a creative approach is needed in utilizing the particular strengths of the patient and facility.

In one randomized-controlled trial improved screening led to increase in the use of antidepressants and improved mood outcomes.[129] Even in this study, however, doses were often not increased over 12 weeks and patients seemed significantly underdosed, significant because antidepressant doses are best started very low and titrated up in this population.

One of the most challenging tasks facing the clinician is whether to discontinue antidepressant medications in euthymic patients when the history of antidepressant response is not well documented, usually in the context where the medication was started by a different clinician. There is evidence that discontinuation can be considered among treatment options. For example in one randomized trial of SSRI discontinuation in NH patients in Sweden, there was no significant decline in mood in patients who had been randomized to discontinuation, with about 25% requiring the restart of SSRI (also with no adverse consequences).[130]

► CONCLUSION

Depression is a major neuropsychiatric complication of AD and a source of distress to patients and caregivers alike. Depression in AD has a unique constellation of symptoms that differs from depression in other populations, with more motivational and less overt mood complaints. We present proposed criteria for this atypical depressive syndrome termed dAD. Caregiver input is essential in the assessment process but caregiver depression and burden must be taken into account as possible biases in reporting. The neurobiologic bases of depression in AD are not identical to the bases of the cognitive symptoms. Antidepressant medications show promise of improving mood in dAD but psychosocial interventions are equally necessary.

REFERENCES

1. Hebert LE, Scherr PA, Bienias JL, et al. Alzheimer's disease in the US population: Prevalence estimates using the 2000 census. *Arch Neurol* 2003;60:1119–1122.
2. Schumock GT. Economic considerations in the treatment and management of Alzheimer's disease. *Am J Health Syst Pharm* 1998;55(Suppl 2):17–21.
3. Fillit HM. The pharmacoeconomics of Alzheimer's disease. *Am J Manag Care* 2000;6:S1139–1144.
4. Souetre E, Thwaites RM, Yeardley HL. Economic impact of Alzheimer's disease in the United Kingdom. Cost of care and disease severity for non-institutionalised patients with Alzheimer's disease. *Br J Psychiatry* 1999;174: 51–55.
5. Rabins PV, Lyketsos CG, Steele CD. *Practical Dementia Care.* New York, NY: Oxford University Press, 1999.
6. Kukull WA, Bowen JD. Dementia epidemiology. *Med Clin North Am* 2002;86:573–590.
7. Franceschi M, Colombo B, Rossi P, et al. Headache in a population-based elderly cohort. An ancillary study to the Italian Longitudinal Study of Aging (ILSA). *Headache* 1997;37:79–82.
8. Breitner JC, Wyse BW, Anthony JC, et al. APOE-epsilon4 count predicts age when prevalence of AD increases, then declines: The Cache County Study. *Neurology* 1999;53:321–331.
9. Miech RA, Breitner JC, Zandi PP, et al. Incidence of AD may decline in the early 90s for men, later for women: The Cache County study. *Neurology* 2002;22:209–218.
10. Collie A, Maruff P. The neuropsychology of preclinical Alzheimer's disease and mild cognitive

impairment. *Neurosci Biobehav Rev* 2000;24: 365–374.

11. Binetti G, Magni E, Padovani A, et al. Executive dysfunction in early Alzheimer's disease. *J Neurol Neurosurg Psychiatry* 1996;60:91–93.

12. Petersen RC, Smith GE, Waring SC, et al. Mild cognitive impairment: Clinical characterization and outcome. *Arch Neurol* 1999;56:303–308.

13. Wolfson C, Wolfson DB, Asgharian M, et al. Clinical Progression of Dementia Study Group. A reevaluation of the duration of survival after the onset of dementia. *N Engl J Med* 2001;344: 1111–1116.

14. Petrella JR, Coleman RE, Doraiswamy PM. Neuroimaging and early diagnosis of Alzheimer's disease: A look to the future. *Radiology* 2003;226: 315–336.

15. Rombouts SA, Barkhof F, Witter MP, et al. Unbiased whole-brain analysis of gray matter loss in Alzheimer's disease. *Neurosci Lett* 2000;19(285): 231–233.

16. Selkoe DJ. Deciphering the genesis and fate of amyloid β-protein yields novel therapies for Alzheimer's disease. *J Clin Invest* 2002;110: 1375–1381.

17. Kim HJ, Chae SC, Lee DK, et al. Selective neuronal degeneration induced by soluble oligomeric amyloid beta protein. *FASEB J* 2003;17: 118–120.

18. Guillozet AL, Weintraub S, Mash DC, et al. Neurofibrillary tangles, amyloid, and memory in aging and mild cognitive impairment. *Arch Neurol* 2003;60:729–736.

19. Haroutunian V, Purohit DP, Perl DP, et al. Neurofibrillary tangles in nondemented elderly subjects and mild Alzheimer's disease. *Arch Neurol* 1999;56:713–718.

20. Gotz J, Streffer JR, David D, et al. Transgenic animal models of Alzheimer's disease and related disorders: Histopathology, behavior and therapy. *Mol Psychiatry* 2004;9:664–683.

21. McGeer PL, McGeer EG. Inflammation, autoxicity, and Alzheimer's disease. *Neurobiol Aging* 2001;22:799–809.

22. McGeer PL, McGeer EG. Inflammation of the brain in Alzheimer's disease: Implications for therapy. *J Leukoc Biol* 1999;65:409–415.

23. Szekely CA, Thorne JE, Zandi PP, et al. Nonsteroidal anti-inflammatory drugs for the prevention of Alzheimer's disease: A systematic review. *Neuroepidemiology* 2004;23:159–169.

24. Gomez-Isla T, Hollister R, West H, Mui et al. Neuronal loss correlates with but exceeds neurofibrillary tangles in Alzheimer's disease. *Ann Neurol* 1997;41:17–24.

25. Terry AV Jr, Buccafusco JJ. The cholinergic hypothesis of age and Alzheimer's disease-related cognitive deficits: Recent challenges and their implications for novel drug development. *J Pharmacol Exp Ther* 2003;306:821–827.

26. Meltzer CC, Price JC, Mathis CA, et al. PET imaging of serotonin type 2A receptors in late-life neuropsychiatric disorders. *Am J Psychiatry* 1999;156:1871–1878.

27. Good DC. Dementia and aging. *Br Med Bull* 2003;65:159–168.

28. Albert MS. Detection of very early Alzheimer's disease through neuroimaging. *Alz Dis Assoc Dis* 2003;17:S63–S65.

29. Jelic V, Nordberg A. Early diagnosis of Alzheimer's disease with positron emission tomography. *Alz Dis Assoc Disord* 2000; 14:S109–S113.

30. Small GW, Komo S, La Rue A, et al. Early detection of Alzheimer's disease by combining apolipoprotein E and neuroimaging. *Ann N Y Acad Sci* 1996;802:70–78.

31. Lyketsos CG, Steinberg M, Tschantz J, et al. Mental and behavioral disturbances in dementia: Findings from the Cache County Study on Memory in Aging. *Am J Psychiatry* 2000;157:708–714.

32. Lyketsos CG, Lopez O, Jones B, et al. Prevalence of neuropsychiatric symptoms in dementia and mild cognitive impairment: Results from the cardiovascular health study. *JAMA* 2002;288: 1475–1483.

33. Burns A, Jacoby R, Levy R. Psychiatric phenomena in Alzheimer's disease III: Disorders of mood. *Br J Psychiatry* 1990;157:81–86.

34. Lopez OL, Becker JT, Sweet RA, et al. Psychiatric symptoms vary with the severity of dementia in probable Alzheimer's disease. *J Neuropsychiatry Clin Neurosci* 2003;15:346–353.

35. Schulz R, Martire LM. Family caregiving of persons with dementia: Prevalence, health effects, and support strategies. *Am J Geriatr Psychiatry* 2004;12:240–249.

36. Lyketsos CG, Sheppard JM, Steinberg M, et al. Neuropsychiatric disturbance in Alzheimer's disease clusters into three groups: The Cache County study. *Int J Geriatr Psychiatry* 2001;16:1043–1053.

37. Migliorelli R, Teson A, Sabe L, et al. Prevalence and correlates of dysthymia and major depression

among patients with Alzheimer's disease. *Am J Psychiatry* 1995;152:37–44.

38. Garre-Olmo J, Lopez-Pousa S, Vilalta-Franch J, et al. Evolution of depressive symptoms in Alzheimer's disease: One-year follow-up. *Alz Dis Assoc Disord* 2003;17:77–85.

39. Pearlson GD, Ross CA, Lohr WD, et al. Association between family history of affective disorder and the depressive syndrome of Alzheimer's disease. *Am J Psychiatry* 1990;147:452–456.

40. Lyketsos CG, Tune LE, Pearlson G, et al. Major depression in Alzheimer's disease. An interaction between gender and family history. *Psychosomatics* 1996;37:380–384.

41. Loreck DJ, Folstein MF. Depression in Alzheimer's disease. In: Starkstein SC, Robinson RG (eds.), *Depression in Neurologic Disease*. Baltimore, MD: Johns Hopkins University Press, 1993.

42. Hargrave R, Reed B, Mungas D. Depressive syndromes and functional disability in dementia. *J Geriatr Psychiatry Neurol* 2000;13:72–77.

43. Cohen CI, Magai C. Racial differences in neuropsychiatric symptoms among dementia outpatients. *Am J Geriatr Psychiatry* 1999;7:57–63.

44. Cerhan JH, Ivnik RJ, Smith GE, et al. Diagnostic utility of letter fluency, category fluency, and fluency difference scores in Alzheimer's disease. *Clin Neuropsychol* 2002;16:35–42.

45. Storey E, Slavin MJ, Kinsella GJ. Patterns of cognitive impairment in Alzheimer's disease: Assessment and differential diagnosis. *Front Biosci* 2002;7:155–184.

46. Buysse DJ. Insomnia, depression and aging. Assessing sleep and mood interactions in older adults. *Geriatrics* 2004;59:47–51.

47. Grimby A, Svanborg A. Morbidity and health-related quality of life among ambulant elderly citizens. *Aging (Milano)* 1997;9:356–364.

48. Janzing JG, Hooijer C, van't Hof MA, et al. Depression in subjects with and without dementia: A comparison using GMS-AGECAT. *Int J Geriatr Psychiatry* 2002;17:1–5.

49. Li YS, Meyer JS, Thornby J. Longitudinal follow-up of depressive symptoms among normal versus cognitively impaired elderly. *Int J Geriatr Psychiatry* 2001;16:718–727.

50. Zubenko GS, Zubenko WN, McPherson S, et al. A collaborative study of the emergence and clinical features of the major depressive syndrome of Alzheimer's disease. *Am J Psychiatry* 2003;160: 857–66.

51. Tractenberg RE, Weiner MF, Patterson MB, et al. Comorbidity of psychopathological domains in community-dwelling persons with Alzheimer's disease. *J Geriatr Psychiatry Neurol* 2003;16: 94–99.

52. Bassiony MM, Warren A, Rosenblatt A, et al. The relationship between delusions and depression in Alzheimer's disease. *Int J Geriatr Psychiatry* 2002;17:549–56.

53. Lyketsos CG, Breitner JC, Rabins PV. An evidence-based proposal for the classification of neuropsychiatric disturbance in Alzheimer's disease. *Int J Geriatr Psychiatry* 2001;16:1037–1042.

54. Purandare N, Burns A, Craig S, et al. Depressive symptoms in patients with Alzheimer's disease. *Int J Geriatr Psychiatry* 2001;16:960–964.

55. Rubin EH, Veiel LL, Kinscherf DA, et al. Clinically significant depressive symptoms and very mild to mild dementia of the Alzheimer type. *Int J Geriatr Psychiatry* 2001;16;694–701.

56. Reisberg B, Auer SR, Monteiro M. Behavioral pathology in Alzheimer's disease (BEHAVE-AD) rating scale. *Int Psychogeriatr* 1996;3: 301–308.

57. Cummings JL, Mega M, Gray K, et al. The Neuropsychiatric Inventory: Comprehensive assessment of psychopathology in dementia. *Neurology* 1994;44:2308–2314.

58. Weiner MF, Doody RS, Sairam R, et al. Prevalence and incidence of major depressive disorder in Alzheimer's disease: Findings from two databases. *Dement Geriatr Cogn Disord* 2002;13:8–12.

59. Lyketsos CG, DelCampo L, Steinberg M, et al. Treating depression in Alzheimer's disease. Efficacy and safety of sertraline therapy and the benefits of depression reduction: The DIADS. *Arch Gen Psychiatry* 2003;60:737–746.

60. Roth M, Mountjoy CQ, Amrein R, and the International Collaborative Study Group. Moclobemide in elderly patients with cognitive decline and depression. *Br J Psychiatry* 1996;168: 149–157.

61. Petracca GM, Chemerinski E, Starkstein SE. A double-blind, placebo-controlled study of fluoxetine in depressed patients with Alzheimer's disease. *Int Psychogeriatr* 2001;13:233–240.

62. Parmelle, PA, Lawton MP, Katz IR. Psychometric properties of the Geriatric Depression Scale among the institutionalized aged. *Psychol Asses* 1989;1:331–338.

63. Gottlieb Gl, Gur RE, Gur RC. Reliability of psychiatric scales in patients with dementia of the Alzheimer type. *Am J Psychiatry* 1988;145:857–860.

64. Katona CL, Hunter BN, Bray J. A double-blind comparison of the efficacy and safely of paroxetine and imipramine in the treatment of depression with dementia. *Int J Geriatr Psychiatry* 1998;13:100–108.

65. Nyth AL, Gottfries CG. The clinical efficacy of citalopram in treatment of emotional disturbances in dementia disorders. A Nordic multicentre study. *Br J Psychiatry* 1990;157:894–901.

66. Wagle AC, Ho LW, Wagle SA, et al. Psychometric behaviour of BDI in Alzheimer's disease patients with depression. *Int J Geriatr Psychiatry* 2000;15:63–69.

67. Teri L, Truax P. Assessment of depression in dementia patients: Association of caregiver mood with depression ratings. *Gerontologist* 1994;34:231–234.

68. Burke WJ, Roccaforte WH, Wengel SP, et al. Disagreement in the reporting of depressive symptoms between patients with dementia of the Alzheimer type and their collateral sources. *Am J Geriatr Psychiatry* 1998;6:308–319.

69. Padovani A, Di Piero V, Bragoni M, et al. Patterns of neuropsychological impairment in mild dementia: A comparison between Alzheimer's disease and multi-infarct dementia. *Acta Neurol Scand* 1995;92:433–442.

70. Naarding P, Leentjens AFG, van Kooten F, et al. Disease-specific properties of the Hamilton rating scale for depression in patients with stroke, Alzheimer's dementia, and Parkinson's disease. *J Neuropsychiatry Clin Neurosci* 2002;14:329–334.

71. Alexopoulos GS, Abrams RC, Young RC, et al. Cornell scale for depression in dementia. *Biol Psychiatry* 1988;23:271–284.

72. Teri L, Gibbons LE, McCurry SM, et al. Exercise plus behavioral management in patients with Alzheimer's disease: A randomized controlled trial. *JAMA* 2003;290:2015–2022.

73. Kurlowicz LH, Evans LK, Strumpf NE, et al. A psychometric evaluation of the Cornell Scale for Depression in Dementia in a frail, nursing home population. *Am J Geriatr Psychiatry* 2002;10:600–608.

74. Sunderland T, Alterman IS, Yount D, et al. A new scale for the assessment of depressed mood in demented patients. *Am J Psychiatry* 1988;145:955–959.

75. Steinberg MS, Sheppard JM, Tschumg JT, et al. The incidence of mental and behavioral disturbances in dementia: The Cache County Study. *J Neuropsychiatry Clin Neurosci* 2003;15:340–345.

76. Starkstein SE, Petracca G, Chemerinski E, et al. Syndromic validity of apathy in Alzheimer's disease. *Am J Psychiatry* 2001;158:872–877.

77. Marin RS, Firinciogullari S, Biedrzycki RC. Group differences in the relationship between apathy and depression. *J Nerv Ment Dis* 1994;182:235–239.

78. Landes AM, Sperry SD, Strauss ME, et al. Apathy in Alzheimer's disease. *J Am Geriatri Soc* 2001;49:1700–1707.

79. Berger AK, Fratiglioni L, Forsell Y, et al. The occurrence of depressive symptoms in the preclinical phase of AD: A population-based study. *Neurology* 1999;53:1998–2002.

80. Stout JC, Wyman MF, Johnson SA, et al. Frontal behavioral syndromes and functional status in probable Alzheimer's disease. *Am J Geriatr Psychiatry* 2003;11:683–686.

81. Olin JT, Katz IR, Meyers BS, et al. Provisional diagnostic criteria for depression of Alzheimer's disease: Rationale and background. *Am J Geriatr Psychiatry* 2002;10:129–141.

82. Olin JT, Schneider LS, Katz IR, et al. Provisional diagnostic criteria for depression of Alzheimer's disease. *Am J Geriatr Psychiatry* 2002;10:125–128.

83. Rosenberg PB, Onyike CU, Katz I, et al for the Depression in Alzheimer's Disease Study-2. Clinical application of operationalized criteria for Depression of Alzheimer's Disease. *Int J Geriatric Psychiatry*, in press.

84. McDaniel KD, Edland SD, Heyman A. Relationship between level of insight and severity of dementia in Alzheimer's disease. CERAD Clinical Investigators. Consortium to establish a registry for Alzheimer's disease. *Alz Dis Assoc Disord* 1995;9:101–104.

85. Verhey FR, Ponds RW, Rozendaal N, et al. Depression, insight, and personality changes in Alzheimer's disease and vascular dementia. *J Geriatr Psychiatry Neurol* 1995;8:23–27.

86. Harwood DG, Sultzer DL, Wheatley MV. Impaired insight in Alzheimer's disease: Association with cognitive deficits, psychiatric symptoms, and behavioral disturbances. *Neuropsychiatry Neuropsychol Behav Neurol* 2000;13:83–88.

87. Harwood DG, Sultzer DL. Life is not worth living: Hopelessness in Alzheimer's disease. *J Geriatr Psychiatry Neurol* 2002;15:38–43.

88. Zubenko GS, Moosy J. Major depression in primary dementia: Clinical and neuropathological correlates. *Arch Neurol* 1988;45:1182–1186.

89. Zubenko GS, Moossy J, Kopp U. Neurochemical correlates of major depression in primary dementia. *Arch Neurol* 1990;47:209–214.

90. Forstl H, Burns A, Luthert P, et al. Clinical and neuropathological correlates of depression in Alzheimer's disease. *Psychol Med* 1992;22; 877–884.

91. Zweig RM, Ross CA, Hedreen JC, et al. The neuropathology of aminergic nuclei in Alzheimer's disease. *Ann Neurol* 1988;24:233–242.

92. Hoogendijk WJ, Sommer IE, Pool CW, et al. Lack of association between depression and loss of neurons in the locus coeruleus in Alzheimer's disease. *Arch Gen Psychiatry* 1999;56:45–51.

93. Tanzi RE, Bertram L. New frontiers in Alzheimer's disease genetics. *Neuron* 2001;32:181–184.

94. Khachaturian AS, Corcoran CD, Mayer LS, et al. Cache County Study Investigators. Apolipoprotein E epsilon4 count affects age at onset of Alzheimer's disease, but not lifetime susceptibility: The Cache County Study. *Arch Gen Psychiatry* 2004;61:518–524.

95. Murphy GM, Kremer C, Rodrigues H, et al. Mitrazapine versus paroxetine Study Group. The apolipoprotein E epsilon4 allele and antidepressant efficacy in cognitively intact elderly depressed patients. *Biol Psychiatry* 2003;54: 665–673.

96. Butters MA, Sweet RA, Mulsant BH, et al. APOE is associated with age-of-onset, but not cognitive functioning, in late-life depression. *Int J Geriatr Psychiatry* 2003;18:1075–1081.

97. Hirono N, Mori E, Yasuda M, et al. Lack of effect of apolipoprotein E E4 allele on neuropsychiatric manifestations in Alzheimer's disease. *J Neuropsychiatry Clin Neurosci* 1999;11: 66–70.

98. Cacabelos R, Rodriguez B, Carrera C, et al. Behavioral changes associated with different apolipoprotein E genotypes in dementia. *Alz Dis Assoc Disord* 1997;11:S27–S34.

99. Holmes C, Russ C, Kirov G, et al. Depressive illness, depressive symptoms, and Alzheimer's disease. *Biol Psychiatry* 1998;43:159–164.

100. O'Brien J, Perry R, Barber R, et al. The association between white matter lesions on magnetic resonance imaging and noncognitive symptoms. *Ann N Y Acad Sci* 2000;903:482–489.

101. Hirono N, Mori E, Ishii K, et al. Frontal lobe hypometabolism and depression in Alzheimer's disease. *Neurology* 1998;50:380–383.

102. Migneco O, Benoit M, Koulibaly PM, et al. Perfusion brain SPECT and statistical parametric mapping analysis indicate that apathy is a cingulate syndrome: A study in Alzheimer's disease and nondemented patients. *Neuroimage* 2001;13: 896–902.

103. Lai T, Payne ME, Byrum CE, et al. Reduction of orbital frontal cortex volume in geriatric depression. *Biol Psychiatry* 2000;48:971–975.

104. Sewards TV, Sewards MA. Representations of motivational drives in mesial cortex, medial thalamus, hypothalamus and midbrain. *Brain Res Bull* 2003;61:25–49.

105. Penninx BW, Kritchevsky SB, Yaffe K, et al. Inflammatory markers and depressed mood in older persons: Results from the health, aging and body composition study. *Biol Psychiatry* 2003;54:566–572.

106. Mulsant BH, Pollock BG, Kirshner M, et al. Serum anticholinergic activity in a community-based sample of older adults: Relationship with cognitive performance. *Arch Gen Psychiatry* 2003;60:198–203.

107. Sunderland T, Tariot PN, Cohen RM, et al. Anticholinergic sensitivity in patients with dementia of the Alzheimer type and age-matched controls. A dose-response study. *Arch Gen Psychiatry* 1987;44:418–426.

108. Alexopoulos GS, Katz IR, Reynolds CF, et al. Pharmacotherapy of depressive disorders in older adults. A Postgraduate Medicine Special Report. Minneapolis, Minn: McGraw-Hill 2001.

109. Lyketsos CG, Lee HB. Diagnosis and treatment of depression in Alzheimer's disease. *Dement Geriatr Cogn Disord* 2004;17:55–64.

110. Porsteinsson AP, Tariot PN, Jakimovich LJ, et al. Valproate therapy for agitation in dementia: Open-label extension of a double-blind trial. *Am J Geriatr Psychiatry* 2003;11:434–440.

111. Pollock BG, Mulsant BH, Rosen J, et al. Comparison of citalopram, perphenazine, and placebo for the acute treatment of psychosis and behavioral disturbances in hospitalized, demented patients. *Am J Psychiatry* 2002;159: 460–465.

112. Rao V, Lyketsos CG. The benefits and risks of ECT for patients with primary dementia who

also suffer from depression. *Int J Geriatr Psychiatry* 2000;15:729–735.

113. Stevens T, Katona C, Manela M, et al. Drug treatment of older people with affective disorders in the community: Lessons from an attempted clinical trial. *Int J Geriatr Psychiatry* 1999;14:467–472.

114. Teri L, Logsdon RG, McCurry SM. Nonpharmacologic treatment of behavioral disturbance in dementia. *Med Clin North Am* 2002;86:641–656.

115. Logsdon RG, Teri L. The Pleasant Events Schedule-AD: Psychometric properties and relationship to depression and cognition in Alzheimer's disease patients. *Gerontologist* 1997;37:40–45.

116. Teri L, Logsdon RG, Uomoto J, et al. Behavioral treatment of depression in dementia patients: A controlled clinical trial. *J Gerontol B Psychol Sci Soc Sci* 1997;52:159–166.

117. Dubinsky RM, Stein AC, Lyons K. Practice parameter: Risk of driving and Alzheimer's disease (an evidence-based review): Report of the quality standards subcommittee of the American Academy of Neurology. *Neurology* 2000;54:2205–2211.

118. Schulz R, Belle SH, Czaja SJ, et al. Long-term care placement of dementia patients and caregiver health and well-being. *JAMA* 2004;292:961–967.

119. Rosenblatt A, Samus QM, Steele CD, et al. The Maryland Assisted Living Study: Prevalence, recognition, and treatment of dementia and other psychiatric disorders in the assisted living population of central Maryland. *J Am Geriatr Soc* 2004;52:1618–1625.

120. Rovner BW, German PS, Broadhead J, et al. The prevalence and management of dementia and other psychiatric disorders in nursing homes. *Int Psychogeriatr* 1990;2:13–24.

121. Zeisel J, Silverstein NM, Hyde J, et al. Environmental correlates to behavioral health outcomes in Alzheimer special care units. *Gerontologist* 2003;43:697–711.

122. McGivney SA, Mulvihill M, Taylor B. Validating the GDS depression screen in the nursing home. *J Am Geriatr Soc* 1994;42:490–492.

123. Gerety MB, Williams JW, Mulrow CD, et al. Performance of case-finding tools for depression in the nursing home: Influence of clinical and functional characteristics and selection of optimal threshold scores. *J Am Geriatr Soc* 1994;42:1103–1109.

124. McCurren C, Dowe D, Rattle D, et al. Depression among nursing home elders: Testing an intervention strategy. *Appl Nurs Res* 1999;12:185–195.

125. Zerhusen JD, Boyle K, Wilson W. Out of the darkness: Group cognitive therapy for depressed elderly. *J Psychosoc Nurs Ment Health Serv* 1991;29:16–21.

126. Fitzsimmons S. Easy rider wheelchair biking. A nursing-recreation therapy clinical trial for the treatment of depression. *J Gerontol Nurs* 2001;5:14–23.

127. Rosen J, Rogers JC, Marin RS, et al. Control-relevant intervention in the treatment of minor and major depression in a long-term care facility. *Am J Geriatr Psychiatry* 1997;5:247–257.

128. Snowden M, Sato K, Roy-Byrne P. Assessment and treatment of nursing home residents with depression or behavioral symptoms associated with dementia: A review of the literature. *J Am Geriatr Soc* 2003;51:1305–1317.

129. Cohen CI, Hyland K, Kimhy D. The utility of mandatory depression screening of dementia patients in nursing homes. *Am J Psychiatry* 2003;160:2012–2017.

130. Ulfvarson J, Adami J, Wredling R, et al. Controlled withdrawal of selective serotonin reuptake inhibitor drugs in elderly patients in nursing homes with no indication of depression. *Eur J Clin Pharmacol* 2003;59:735–740.

131. Weiner MF, Edland SD, Luszczynski H. Prevalence and incidence of major depression in Alzheimer's disease. *Am J Psychiatry* 1994;151:1006–1009.

132. Vida S, Des Rosiers P, Carrier L, et al. Depression in Alzheimer's disease: Receiver operating characteristic analysis of the Cornell scale for depression in dementia and the Hamilton depression scale. *J Geriatr Psychiatry Neurol* 1994;7:159–162.

133. Lichtenberg PA, Marcopulos BA, Steiner DA, et al. Comparison of the Hamilton depression rating scale and the geriatric depression scale: Detection of depression in dementia patients. *Psychol Rep* 1992;70:515–521.

134. Korner A, Nielsen BM, Eschen F, et al. Quantifying depressive symptomatology: Inter-rater reliability and inter-item correlations. *J Affect Disord* 1990;20:143–149.

135. Reifler BV, Teri L, Raskind M, et al. Double-blind trial of imipramine in Alzheimer's disease patients with and without depression. *Am J Psychiatry* 1989;146;45–49.

136. Nyth AL, Gottfries CG, Lyby K, et al. A controlled multicenter clinical study of citalopram and placebo in elderly depressed patients with and without comcomitant dementia. *Acta Psychiatr Scand* 1992;86:138–145.

137. Magai C, Kennedy G, Cohen CI, et al. A controlled clinical trial of sertraline in the treatment of depression in nursing home patients with late-stage Alzheimer's disease. *Am J Geriatr Psychiatry* 2000;8:66–74.

138. Taragano FE, Lyketsos CG, Mangone CA, et al. A double-blind, randomized, fixed-dose trial of fluoxetine vs. amitriptyline in the treatment of major depression complicating Alzheimer's disease. *Psychosomatics* 1997;38:246–252.

139. Mace NL, Rabins PV. *The 36-Hour Day: A Family Guide to Caring for Persons with Alzheimer's Disease, Related Dementing Illnesses, and Memory Loss in Later Life*, 3rd ed. Baltimore, MD: Johns Hopkins University Press, 1999.

CHAPTER 13

Diagnosis and Treatment of Mood Disorders in Parkinson's Disease

PAUL E. HOLTZHEIMER III, WILLIAM M. MCDONALD,
AND MAHLON R. DELONG

► INTRODUCTION

Mood disorders are common in Parkinson's disease (PD), and contribute significantly to the distress and disability associated with the illness. The high incidence of mood disorders likely reflects a shared pathophysiology with PD, although "reactive depression" can also occur. Despite the importance of recognizing and treating mood disorders in PD patients, diagnosis can be difficult due to significant overlap of symptoms between depression and PD, the mood effects of concurrent PD treatments, and the presence of other comorbid medical and psychiatric illnesses. Treatment may be complicated by side effects of antidepressant medications and lack of efficacy data to guide treatment choices.

This chapter will highlight the prevalence of mood disorders in PD and discuss their impact on disability and quality of life for PD patients. The etiology and pathophysiology of mood disorders in PD will be reviewed, including the overlap of neuroanatomic changes and clinical presentations between PD and primary mood disorders. Next, an outline of the differential diagnosis of mood disorder symptoms and the importance of recognizing cooccurring disorders will be considered. Finally, the treatment of mood disorders in PD will be reviewed, with a focus on somatic treatments.

► EPIDEMIOLOGY

Depression

Depressive symptoms in PD have been recognized ever since James Parkinson described depression as one of the cardinal features of the illness in 1817. Using a national health registry-based approach, Leentjens et al. found that a diagnosis of depression was more than twice as likely to be present in patients with PD compared to age- and gender-matched controls without PD.[1] Reported prevalence rates for depression in PD have ranged from 2.7 to 70%.[2,3] This variability likely results from differences in sampling methods, assessment tools, and survey site. A meta-analysis of studies assessing prevalence of depression in PD (using any diagnostic method) found an overall rate of 31%.[4] For studies using structured depression rating instruments, the prevalence rate was 37.5%. For studies using clinical diagnosis based on Diagnostic and Statistical Manual (DSM) criteria, the rate was 42.4%.

Additionally, among studies using DSM criteria, rates for *major depression* comorbidity ranged from 2.7 to 39.6%,[2,5] while rates for *any* depressive syndrome ranged from 22.6 to 53.6%.[6,7] These differences highlight the fact that many PD patients with significant mood symptoms may not present with a classic major depressive episode, but rather with subsyndromal depression including minor depression or dysthymia.[7,8] Although studies have not been conducted in a population of patients with PD, subsyndromal depression in elderly patients can lead to significant disability and can increase the risk of developing major depression.[9,10]

Risk factors for depression in PD patients include being female[8,11,12] and having a history of depression,[13,14] although a family history of depression appears to confer no additional risk.[13,14] Some studies suggest patients with a younger age of onset of PD may be more likely to develop depression,[6,15–17] although the opposite pattern has also been found.[18] While severity of motor symptoms appears not to influence the prevalence of depression,[14,16,19–21] depression may be more common in PD patients with greater cognitive impairment.[12,18] Additionally, patients with greater right-sided motor symptoms (indicating greater left hemispheric dysfunction)[14] and akinetic-rigid PD (vs. more *classic* tremor-predominant PD)[7] appear more likely to develop depression.

Bipolar Disorders

There is little evidence to support an increased rate of mania or hypomania in patients with PD. While PD can clearly develop in patients with preexisting bipolar disorder, only isolated case reports suggest the later development of mania in PD patients.[22,23] The induction of manic symptoms has been reported in PD patients treated with subthalamic deep brain stimulation (DBS).[24–26] Transient manic symptoms following pallidotomy have also been described.[27]

Course

While there are few long-term studies, depression in PD is often a chronic illness.[28] One study followed PD patients over a 9-year period and found that only 35% of patients with depression at baseline showed an improvement in their symptoms.[12] Sixty-five percent remained stable or had worsening depression. However, the use and adequacy of antidepressant treatments were not assessed in that study. PD patients with major depression may also show greater cognitive decline, deterioration in ADLs, and faster progression of PD than patients with minor or no depression.[28] Comorbid depression has been shown to be associated with an increased risk of dementia in PD patients,[29] and may be a greater risk factor than dementia for the later development of psychosis, especially in younger patients.[30]

Impact of Comorbid Mood Disorders

As discussed above, depression may negatively impact nonmotor symptoms of PD, especially cognitive function.[28–34] Also, the psychomotor retardation associated with depression may worsen bradykinesia, and depression may impair fine motor skills in PD patients.[35] Not surprisingly, depression may negatively affect quality of life in PD patients.[36–39] Additionally, comorbid depression can greatly increase the burden on caregivers of PD patients.[40–44]

▶ ETIOLOGY AND PATHOPHYSIOLOGY

Parkinson's disease associated with depression may derive from: (1) a "reactive" process (i.e., a psychologic response to the psychosocial stress and disability associated with having PD) or (2) the neurodegenerative process of PD. These possible etiologies are not mutually exclusive and may coexist in the same patient.

Reactive Depression

Patients with PD must adjust to the reality of having a chronic, disabling illness with no known cure and progressive functional decline. Available treatments are largely palliative, with the exception of DBS. The psychologic impact of this reality is expected to be greater in younger patients, perhaps explaining the increased prevalence of depression in patients with earlier onset of PD.[6,15–17] Thus, depressive symptoms in PD may be reasonably explained, at least in part, as a reaction to the psychologic and functional losses associated with having the illness. Importantly though, reactive depression cannot explain the fact that patients with PD have a greater prevalence of depressive symptoms than patients with equally disabling illnesses.[19,45] As well, the degree of physical disability in PD does not appear to correlate with severity of depressive symptoms.[18,45]

Neurodegenerative Depression

Parkinson's disease is associated with the loss of dopaminergic neurons in the substantia nigra and ventral tegmental area (VTA), as well as degeneration and dysfunction of neurons in multiple other subcortical nuclei.[46] Recent evidence suggests that the pathophysiologic changes of PD first appear in the anterior olfactory and lower brainstem (glossopharyngeal and vagal nerve) nuclei, with ascending brainstem involvement of the locus ceruleus, nucleus gigantocellularis, and the raphé nuclei, followed by further extension into the magnocellular nuclei of the basal forebrain, the central nucleus of the amygdale, and the substantia nigra.[47] Thus, long before substantia nigra involvement in PD, many other subcortical nuclei are affected. It is highly likely that involvement of these nuclei plays a

significant role in the nonmotor (e.g., autonomic, sleep, emotional, cognitive) and refractory motor aspects (e.g., postural instability, gait and bulbar disturbances) of PD. Many of these brain areas have also been implicated in the pathophysiology of depression.[48] Studies showing more depressive symptoms in PD patients with greater left hemispheric dysfunction[3,14] and the akinetic-rigid subtype[7] further support a neuroanatomic/neurodegenerative etiology for depressive symptoms in PD.

Imaging studies of depressed PD patients support a neurodegenerative process in the development of depressive symptoms. Depressed PD patients have smaller subcortical nuclei than nondepressed controls and similar to depressed, non-PD patients.[49,50] Dysfunction in the subcortical nuclei may lead to disruption of a cortical-subcortical neuronal circuit involved in mood regulation,[48,51] resulting in symptoms of depression. Sheline points out that depression is common in neurologic diseases affecting the limbic-cortical-striatal-pallidal-thalamic circuits (e.g., PD, Huntington disease, stroke), and hypothesizes that this is due to damage of structures critical to emotional functioning, including frontal cortex, hippocampus, thalamus, amygdala, and basal ganglia.[51] PD patients with comorbid depression demonstrate decreased metabolic activity in orbitofrontal cortex, anterior temporal cortex, and caudate compared to nondepressed PD patients,[52] supporting cortical-subcortical dysfunction in the etiology of depression in PD.

▶ DIAGNOSIS

Presentation of Mood Disorders in PD

Data suggest depressed PD patients present with a different depressive symptom profile than depressed patients without PD. This profile includes increased anxiety, pessimism, irrationality, and increased suicidal ideation (without increased suicidal behavior).[3,4,53] As well, depressed PD patients may exhibit less guilt and self-blame.[3] Anxiety disorders, especially panic disorder, are relatively common in PD patients,[54–59] and depression and anxiety are often comorbid conditions in PD patients.[51] Such comorbidity may be more common in PD than in non-PD patients.[54,60] Menza et al. found that 92% of PD patients with an anxiety disorder diagnosis had depressive disorders or symptoms, and 67% of patients with depression had a comorbid anxiety disorder.[54] Thus, depressed patients with PD are likely to present with anxiety symptoms, and should be evaluated for comorbid anxiety disorders.

Suicidal ideation and risk must be carefully assessed in all depressed patients. Depressed PD patients may have increased suicidal ideation compared to depressed non-PD patients.[4] However, depressed PD patients may not be more likely to attempt or complete suicide.[3,61] One population-based study found the rate of suicide to be no greater in PD patients compared to the general population. This, however, does not lessen the importance of assessing suicidal thoughts in depressed PD patients. Suicidal ideation and risk should be carefully evaluated in all depressed PD patients, particularly because advanced age and chronic medical problems have been closely linked to increased risk of completed suicide.

Challenges in Diagnosing Mood Disorders in PD

Diagnosing depression in PD patients can be difficult. Nondepressed patients with PD often have sleep disturbance, psychomotor slowing, fatigue, apathy, and masked facies (which may mimic depressive affect). Due to disability from motor and cognitive symptoms, PD patients may exhibit withdrawal from social and occupational activities. PD patients may also rationally consider suicide due to the chronic and devastating course of their illness and the concern that they may burden their family. Also, mood and behavior must be evaluated within the context of PD treatments (which may have cognitive and emotional

effects) and patients' responses to these treatments (such as *on* and *off* periods—discussed in more detail below). Symptoms of dementia and other cooccurring illnesses may mimic symptoms of depression, further complicating the diagnosis.

Use of Specific Criteria to Diagnose Mood Disorders

In clinical settings, structured rating scales can be useful in confirming the diagnosis of mood disorders. Commonly used scales for diagnosing depression include the Hamilton depression rating scale (HDRS),[62] Beck depression inventory (BDI),[63] the Montgomery-Asberg depression rating scale (MADRS),[64] and the geriatric depression scale (GDS).[65] While each of these scales can be useful in making the diagnosis of depression, they all include at least some questions concerning somatic symptoms—symptoms that may be present with PD in the absence of depression. A discriminant analysis of the HDRS and MADRS showed that nonsomatic symptoms correlated most highly with a diagnosis of depression.[66] Except for decreased appetite and early morning awakening, somatic symptoms had relatively low correlation with a depression diagnosis.

Using rating scales with appropriate cutoffs may improve their accuracy. For example, Leentjens et al. found that cutoffs of 11/12 for the HDRS, 14/15 for the MADRS,[67] and 8/9 for the BDI[68] showed good sensitivity for screening for depression. Cutoffs of 16/17 for the HDRS, 17/18 for the MADRS,[67] and 16/17 for the BDI[68] gave the highest specificity in distinguishing depressed from nondepressed PD patients. An advantage of the BDI over the HDRS or MADRS is that it is subject-, rather than clinician-rated, thereby decreasing time needed during a clinical visit to complete the assessment. The GDS has also been used to diagnose depression in PD,[12,69,70] and cutoff scores have been suggested (with scores of 11–20 indicating mild to moderate depression, and scores greater than 20 indicating severe depression).[12] However, these cutoffs have not been rigorously validated in PD patients.

Many clinicians rely on criteria established by the American Psychiatric Association in the Diagnostic and Statistical Manual of Mental Disorders (DSM-IV) when diagnosing psychiatric illness.[71] While useful, these criteria are limited since they do not specifically address the diagnosis of mood disorders in the context of medical disorders. As with rating scales, these criteria include a number of somatic symptoms which may not be useful in distinguishing depressed from nondepressed medically ill patients. There currently exists no established method for using the DSM criteria to diagnose depression in medically ill patients, including those with PD. As well, these criteria are less useful in identifying the minor depressive syndromes commonly seen in PD patients.

In sum, no rating scales or specific criteria currently exist for diagnosing mood disorders in PD patients. However, using established rating scales with research-based scoring criteria can increase specificity and sensitivity. Using DSM-IV criteria can also be useful, but these criteria were developed to diagnose depression in nonmedically ill subjects. The DSM criteria may overestimate the incidence of depression in PD because certain somatic symptoms (e.g., anorexia and insomnia) are common in nondepressed PD patients. More research in this area would greatly increase the clinician's ability to accurately diagnose mood disorders in PD patients.

Effects of Parkinson's Disease Treatments on Mood and Behavior

When diagnosing mood symptoms in PD patients, it is important to recognize that many PD treatments can significantly influence mood and behavior. Both medications and surgical therapies have been associated with mood effects in at least some PD patients.

Medications

Medications used in the treatment of PD often affect mood and behavior. While dopamine agonists may have weak antidepressant properties,[72–74] they can cause a number of other psychiatric symptoms, including psychosis, agitation, and delirium. Levodopa, a mainstay of PD treatment, has little meaningful antidepressant activity, but is clearly associated with the development of psychosis and delirium.[75] Selegiline, a monoamine oxidase type B (MAO-B) inhibitor, can have antidepressant effects,[3] but is less effective for the motor symptoms of PD than nonspecific MAO inhibitors. Pramipexole, a D_2 dopamine receptor agonist, may have efficacy in treating depression in PD patients without negatively impacting the overall severity of the illness.[74,76,77] Anticholinergic agents used in PD can also cause and/or contribute to delirium, especially in older, medically ill patients.

Many PD patients experience "on" and "off" phases in their response to levodopa.[78] "On" states are characterized by an heightened responsiveness to levodopa leading to decreased bradykinesia and less rigidity, but may also result in drug-induced dyskinesias. "Off" states are characterized by increased rigidity and bradykinesia reflecting essentially no response to the medication. Many nondepressed patients will describe mood fluctuations that correlate with on and off periods. Patients evaluated in an "off" period may appear more depressed in that they will exhibit increased motor rigidity, masked facies, and psychomotor slowing. Depressed patients may have some improvement in their mood when they are "on," but clearly show depression in both on and off periods. As the severity of PD advances, "on" and "off" periods may increase in frequency and severity. Likewise, mood may fluctuate dramatically during on-off periods, with off-period depression/anxiety and on-period euphoria and agitation.[79–84] Use of other dopamine agonists early in the treatment of PD may decrease the need for levodopa and thereby limit the development of on-off phenomena.[85]

Ablative Surgery

Pallidotomy and thalamotomy are well-established ablative surgical treatments for PD. The surgeon performing a pallidotomy places a small lesion in the posteroventral portion of the globus pallidus interna (GPi), whereas a thalamotomy involves a lesion in the ventrolateral nucleus of the thalamus. Both surgical techniques have shown benefits for the motor symptoms of PD.[86,87] In general, pallidotomy and thalamotomy have few cognitive or psychiatric sequelae.[88–90] However, some data suggest that patients with a history of depression may be more likely to have a depressive episode following pallidotomy, although this may be a natural progression of their depressive illness.[90,91] Transient hypomania was reported in two patients following pallidotomy, although pallidotomy lesions in both patients were located in the anteromedial portion of the GPi, rather than the posteroventral portion.[27]

Deep Brain Stimulation

An important advancement in the treatment of PD is the development of nonablative DBS of subcortical structures. Targets for DBS in PD patients include the subthalamic nucleus (STN), GPi, and ventrointermedial (Vim) nucleus of the thalamus. Thalamic DBS has been most effective at reducing tremor in PD patients,[92] where STN and GPi DBS help reduce "off" period akinesias and dyskinesias.[93] A number of psychiatric side effects have been reported with STN DBS including depression, mania, psychosis, and delirium.[94,95] Recurrent manic episodes were reported in one patient receiving GPi DBS.[96]

Comorbid Medical Disorders

In evaluating PD patients with possible mood disorders, it is important to carefully assess for cooccurring disorders. Dementia, hypothyroidism, B_{12} or folate deficiency, elevated plasma homocysteine levels, and testosterone deficiency may each complicate the diagnosis of depression in PD patients. The presence of hypothyroidism, folate, B_{12}, or testosterone deficiency may also reduce or block the response to antidepressant therapy.

Dementia

PD patients with dementia have an increased risk of depression and depressed PD patients have an increased risk of developing dementia.[18,29,97] PD patients with depression should therefore be evaluated for signs of cognitive impairment. The mini-mental status examination (MMSE) is a useful screen for dementia, and is relatively quick and easy to perform. While comorbid depression may lead to lower MMSE scores, this screening tool can still be useful in depressed PD patients.[32] The workup for dementia might reasonably include a neuroimaging screen (usually with computed tomography [CT]), metabolic workup (including B_{12}, folate, thyroid function screen, serology, complete blood count, and basic chemistries), and substance abuse evaluation.

Hypothyroidism

Hypothyroidism is often associated with depression.[98] Hypothyroidism may also occur in PD, although the diagnosis may be confounded by shared symptomatology.[99–101] Therefore, the evaluation of depressive symptoms in PD patients should always include a screen for thyroid disease. It must be recognized, however, that some PD medications (such as levodopa) may inhibit secretion of thyroid stimulating hormone (TSH),[100,102] thus masking the laboratory diagnosis of hypothyroidism.

B_{12} Deficiency

B_{12} deficiency can be associated with neuropsychiatric symptoms including depression[103,104] and is relatively common in older patients.[105,106] Therefore, an evaluation of B_{12} status should be included in the workup of PD patients presenting with mood symptoms.

Homocysteinemia

Homocysteine levels have been shown to be increased in patients with depression,[107] dementia,[108] and PD.[109,110] Long-term treatment with levodopa (L-dopa) may also increase homocysteine levels in PD patients.[111,112] Given the association of elevated homocysteine levels with vascular disease,[113] it is important to monitor serum homocysteine levels. As well, treatment and/or augmentation with agents involved in the metabolism of homocysteine (e.g., S-adenosylmethionine [SAM]) may attenuate the effects of elevated homocysteine levels.[112] SAM may also have antidepressant effects in depressed patients with[114] and without PD.[115]

Testosterone Deficiency

Symptoms of testosterone deficiency (anhedonia, poor energy, sexual dysfunction, decreased mood) can overlap with symptoms of depression and PD. Testosterone deficiency has been associated with depressive symptoms in non-PD patients,[116,117] and testosterone supplementation may improve symptoms in these patients.[118] The depressive signs and symptoms associated with hypogonadism are generally mild with depressed libido, erectile dysfunction, and fatigue most prominent. Men with hypogonadism typically do not complain or admit to depression per se. Testosterone replacement therapy may also improve nonmotor symptoms in testosterone-deficient men with PD.[119] Therefore, an evaluation of testosterone status during the workup of depressive symptoms, especially in men with PD, is warranted.

Suggested Diagnostic Approach

Physicians must be vigilant for symptoms and signs of mood disorders. Like many patients with chronic medical conditions, depressed PD patients may be reluctant to talk about how they feel. PD patients often minimize depressive symptoms or attribute the symptoms to having PD, e.g., "Who wouldn't be depressed? I have Parkinson's disease." However, the severity of PD symptoms does not correlate with the degree of depression[15,16,20,21,120] and the risk for depression is associated with known risk factors (e.g., female gender and personal history of depression)[8,11–13,15] and neuroanatomic/neurophysiologic changes similar to those found in patients with primary depressive disorders.[51,52]

The clinician should use the diagnostic criteria for depression and treat patients who meet these criteria regardless of whether they attribute the depressive symptoms to PD or not. It may help in making a diagnosis to have additional family or caregivers present during the evaluation and to focus on nonsomatic symptoms of depression (e.g., crying spells, anhedonia, thoughts of death and suicide, hopelessness, worthlessness, and guilt) rather than relying entirely on the somatic symptoms that overlap with the PD syndrome (e.g., insomnia, decreased libido, decreased concentration).

Symptoms that may suggest depression in PD patients include poor treatment compliance (especially if this is a recent change), pessimistic outlook, "giving up," decreased attention to appearance and self-care, and increased social withdrawal. Depressed patients may develop a limited ability to experience pleasure in previously pleasurable activities (e.g., spending time with families or hobbies), and may become more irritable when pressed by friends or family to be more active. This irritability may be viewed by others as justified frustration at decreased functional capacity, but may also be a symptom of depression. Excessive guilt or ruminations may also indicate depression. Any evidence of suicidal thought or behavior should be followed up carefully.

When a diagnosis of depression is suspected, the clinician should begin with a careful history and physical examination. Past history of depression may be a predictor of future depression. Recent changes in mood and behavior should be assessed within the context of the patient's current PD treatment (e.g., potential on-off phenomena on levodopa or recent surgical intervention). A DSM-based evaluation of current depressive symptoms can be useful, especially if performed by a clinician that has known the patient over time. Collateral information/history from the caregiver and others who know the patient well are often essential in clarifying the diagnosis. Consultation with a geriatric or neuropsychiatrist should be considered in difficult cases.

Rating scales, especially the BDI or GDS, can also be helpful. The GDS is most useful as a screen for depression (using a fairly conservative cutoff of >9) and the BDI is useful for following the severity of symptoms during treatment. In demented patients with depression, the Cornell scale (which is completed by the family or a caregiver) has shown good reliability in non-PD populations.[121,122]

The diagnostic workup should include an assessment for cooccurring, and potentially confounding, illnesses. The MMSE is a useful screening tool for clinically significant cognitive impairment. Performing the MMSE regularly (e.g., once a year) can provide a baseline against which current results can be compared. If moderate to severe cognitive impairment is present, evaluation for potentially treatable causes should be considered. In all patients presenting with mood disorders symptoms, a basic chemistry panel, complete blood count, thyroid function testing, liver function testing, B_{12}/folate, and urinalysis should be performed. Testosterone levels should be checked in depressed men with PD. If hypogonadism is present, an evaluation for prostate cancer should be performed before replacing testosterone.

Neuroimaging should be considered in the workup of patients with unusual presentations (e.g., rapid onset of symptoms, concurrent worsening of motor symptoms, new neurologic symptoms). In general, a brain CT scan is sufficient to screen for intracranial disease that may be causing or contributing to mood and behavior changes. Magnetic resonance imaging (MRI), electroencephalography (EEG), nuclear imaging (e.g., single photon emission computed tomography [SPECT]) may provide additional diagnostic information in selected cases, such as patients presenting with features of normal pressure hydrocephalus or rapidly progressing cognitive impairment. Patients should also be evaluated for comorbid anxiety disorders. Panic symptoms and disorder may be more likely to occur in depressed PD patients than other depressed patients. The presence of comorbid anxiety disorders may influence treatment selection.

The impact depression in a PD patient can have on his or her caregiver should be considered. If possible, the clinician should assess caregiver well-being and health. Addressing relevant psychosocial concerns (e.g., support in the home, cost of medications and assistive devices, transportation) may help improve overall quality of life for the caregiver and patient.

▶ TREATMENT

Treating depression in PD patients can improve overall function and quality of life. However, managing depression in PD patients can be complex at times. Drug-drug interactions and side effects may limit the use of established antidepressant treatments in PD patients. Further, there are relatively few double-blind, placebo-controlled trials of antidepressant treatments in PD. More research is clearly needed to better define appropriate treatment strategies for PD patients with depression.

Somatic Treatments for Mood Disorders

Antidepressant Medications

The use of antidepressant medications in PD is limited by side effects and lack of placebo-controlled studies. A brief summary of the available data is given in Table 13-1. Tricyclic antidepressants (TCAs) have clear antidepressant efficacy in depressed non-PD patients, but have anticholinergic side effects including dry mouth, constipation, sedation, and confusion.[123–125] TCAs also have significant cardiovascular side effects including orthostatic hypotension and conduction disturbances. TCAs can be lethal in overdose due to the potential for third degree heart block and arrhythmias.

Selective serotonin reuptake inhibitors (SSRIs) have replaced TCAs as first-line agents in the treatment of depression. While no more efficacious than TCAs, SSRIs are better tolerated but can still have clinically significant side effects,

▶ **TABLE 13-1** OPEN AND CONTROLLED STUDIES OF ANTIDEPRESSANT MEDICATIONS IN DEPRESSED PATIENTS WITH IDIOPATHIC PARKINSON'S DISEASE

Medication	Study	Design	Outcome
SSRIs*			
Citalopram	Rampello et al. (2002)[148]	Open (N = 18 patients with depression [of 46 total])	Improvement in depression in 15 out of 18 patients
	Menza et al. (2004)[153]	Open (N = 10)	Significant improvements in depression, anxiety, and functional capacity
	Dell'Agnello et al. (2001)[145]	Citalopram vs. fluoxetine vs. fluvoxamine vs. sertraline (N = 62)	Significant improvement in depression in all groups; no significant difference between groups
	Wermuth et al. (1998)[151]	Citalopram vs. placebo (N = 37)	Significant improvement in depression in both groups at 6 and 52 weeks; no significant difference between groups
Fluoxetine	Serrano-Duenas et al. (2002)[124]	Low dose fluoxetine vs. low dose amitriptyline (N = 77)	Amitriptyline superior to fluoxetine at 3, 6, 9, and 12 months; significantly greater dropout in amitriptyline group
	Fregni et al. (2004)[200]	Fluoxetine vs. rTMS† (N = 42)	Improvement in depression in both groups; no significant difference between groups
	Avila et al. (2003)[158]	Fluoxetine vs. nefazodone (N = 16)	Significant improvement in depression in both groups; no significant difference between groups
	Dell'Agnello et al. (2001)[145]	Citalopram vs. fluoxetine vs. fluvoxamine vs. sertraline (N = 62)	Significant improvement in depression in all groups; no significant difference between groups
Fluvoxamine	McCance-Katz et al. (1992)[154]	Case report (N = 1)	Patient showed an antidepressant response
	Rabey et al. (1996)[123]	Fluvoxamine vs. amitriptyline (N = 47)	60% response rate in the fluvoxamine group; 55% response rate in the amitriptyline group; statistical difference between groups not reported
	Dell'Agnello et al. (2001)[145]	Citalopram vs. fluoxetine vs. fluvoxamine vs. sertraline (N = 62)	Significant improvement in depression in all groups; no significant difference between groups
Paroxetine	Ceravolo et al. (2000)[144]	Open (N = 33)	Significant improvement in depression at 1, 3, and 6 months
	Tesei et al. (2000)[138]	Open (N = 65)	Significant improvement in depression in 52 patients that completed a mean 125.3 (SD 89.6) days of treatment
Sertraline	Hauser and Zesiewicz (1997)[146]	Open (N = 15)	Significant improvement in depression at 7 weeks

(Continued)

341

▶ **TABLE 13-1** OPEN AND CONTROLLED STUDIES OF ANTIDEPRESSANT MEDICATIONS IN DEPRESSED PATIENTS WITH IDIOPATHIC PARKINSON'S DISEASE (*CONTINUED*)

Medication	Study	Design	Outcome
	Dell'Agnello et al. (2001)[145]	Citalopram vs. fluoxetine vs. fluvoxamine vs. sertraline (*N* = 62)	Significant improvement in depression in all groups; no significant difference between groups
	Leentjens et al. (2002)[152]	Sertraline vs. placebo (*N* = 12)	Significant improvement in depression in both groups; no significant difference between groups
TCAs[‡]			
Amitriptyline	Rabey et al. (1996)[123]	Fluvoxamine vs. amitriptyline (*N* = 47)	60% response rate in the fluvoxamine group; 55% response rate in the amitriptyline group; statistical difference between groups not reported
	Serrano-Duenas et al. (2002)[124]	Low dose fluoxetine vs. low dose amitriptyline (*N* = 77)	Amitriptyline superior to fluoxetine at 3, 6, 9, and 12 months; significantly greater dropout in amitriptyline group
Nortriptyline	Andersen et al. (1980)[125]	Nortriptyline vs. placebo (*N* = 22)	Significant improvement in depression in the nortriptyline group; statistical difference between groups not reported
Others			
Bupropion	Goetz et al. (1984)[160]	Open (*N* = 12 patients with depression of 20 total))	Improvement in depression in 5 of 12 patients
Nefazodone	Avila et al. (2003)[158]	Fluoxetine vs. nefazodone (*N* = 16)	Significant improvement in depression in both groups; no significant difference between groups

*Selective serotonin reuptake inhibitors.

[†]*Repetitive transcranial magnetic stimulation.*

[‡]*Tricyclic antidepressants.*

342

including bradycardia, sleep disturbance, sexual dysfunction, agitation, anxiety, headaches, weight gain, and gastrointestinal (GI) symptoms. Some side effects (e.g., agitation, anxiety, headaches, and GI symptoms) may be limited by slowly titrating the medication to target dose and will diminish with continued treatment. Other side effects (e.g., sleep disturbance and sexual dysfunction) may continue to cause distress for patients and interfere with treatment compliance.

Another potential SSRI side effect in PD patients is exacerbation of motor symptoms,[126] perhaps due to modulation of serotonin-mediated dopamine release in nigrostriatal pathways.[127,128] Extrapyramidal side effects (EPS) have been reported with SSRIs.[128–138] However, the occurrence of EPS with SSRIs appears to be relatively rare[139–141] and a number of studies suggest this side effect may not be clinically relevant for most patients, including those with PD.[142–149]

The combination of SSRIs (and potentially TCAs) with the MAO-B inhibitor selegiline can cause a potentially fatal "serotonin syndrome." Since selegiline can nonspecifically inhibit both MAO-A and MAO-B when given at high doses, an interaction with SSRIs and TCAs is theoretically possible. In practice, this concern may relatively be minor since the doses of selegiline used to treat PD are relatively low. One study found the use of selegiline with antidepressant medications led to symptoms consistent with serotonin syndrome in only 11 (0.24%) of 4568 patients treated with the combination.[126] Only 2 (0.04%) experienced serious symptoms, and no deaths were reported.

The data supporting the efficacy of antidepressant medications in PD are limited by small sample size, heterogeneous populations, inadequate antidepressant dosing, or inconsistent use of rating scales to document symptom change. A meta-analysis of antidepressant trials in PD found that only 3 of 43 studies were appropriate for analysis.[150] The most common reasons for exclusion included absence of a control group and inclusion of nondepressed PD patients. In one of the included studies, nortriptyline was more effective than placebo, but statistical significance was not reported.[125] A second study

found no statistically significant benefit for citalopram versus placebo.[151] The third study was not placebo-controlled, but showed improvements in depression with both fluvoxamine and amitriptyline with no significant difference between the two drugs.[123] A fourth placebo-controlled study, published after the meta-analysis was completed, demonstrated no statistically significant benefit for sertraline in depressed PD patients; however, the study was prematurely terminated due to extremely limited subject recruitment over the study period.[152]

The absence of well-designed placebo-controlled studies limits the conclusions about the efficacy of antidepressant medications in PD patients. However, a number of open studies do suggest some antidepressant efficacy for SSRIs.[138,144–148,153–155] SSRIs may also be especially useful in patients with comorbid anxiety symptoms and disorders.[156,157]

There are very little data to support the use of other antidepressant medications in PD. One study suggested that nefazodone, a mixed serotonin receptor antagonist and reuptake inhibitor, may be effective for treating depression and may potentially have a more favorable side effect profile (i.e., fewer EPS) than the SSRIs.[158] A case report suggested that mirtazapine, an alpha-2-receptor antagonist and serotonin receptor agonist and antagonist, appears to be safe in PD and may be effective in improving levodopa-associated dyskinesias[159]; however, there are no data on the antidepressant efficacy of mirtazapine in depressed PD patients. Bupropion, a weak reuptake inhibitor for dopamine and norepinephrine (although its exact mechanism of action is unknown), has been shown effective in some patients with depression, but its use may be limited by side effects, such as sleep disturbance, anxiety/agitation, and lowered seizure threshold.[160] There are currently no published data on venlafaxine, duloxetine, or escitalopram in PD patients. Although data from randomized, placebo-controlled trials are limited, modafinil may help treat the fatigue and daytime sleepiness common in PD patients, especially those with depression.[161–165]

Treatment of Psychosis

Psychosis in PD may occur as part of a mood syndrome but often is associated with the use of dopamine agonists. Psychosis is also more common in PD patients with cognitive disturbance. Patients should be educated that PD medications may cause hallucinations and to contact their physician if this occurs. The initial strategy should be to determine if there is a correlation between the onset of psychosis and the initiation of a specific medication, and whether that medication can be stopped. Clinically, patients may develop psychosis on one medication and not others. In general, anticholinergics and amantadine should be eliminated first. If hallucinations continue, some dopaminometics may have to be reduced or eliminated. The following order for eliminating medications is suggested: selegiline, nocturnal doses of dopamine agonists, Sinemet CR, daytime doses of dopamine agonists, and finally daytime doses of carbidopa/levodopa.

If parkinsonian symptoms worsen or psychotic symptoms persist with lowering of dopaminomimetic therapy, antipsychotic treatment should be initiated. Atypical antipsychotics are generally considered first-line treatments for psychosis in PD patients, due to their lower dopamine D_2 receptor blockade.[166] Clozapine has the strongest database supporting its safety and antipsychotic efficacy in PD patients, but use may be limited by its potential to cause agranulocytosis.[166–169] Data also support the use of quetiapine, although a mild worsening of motor symptoms may occur in more demented patients.[170–175] Olanzapine and risperidone have shown antipsychotic efficacy in PD patients, but can have significant side effects, including motor worsening.[166] Ziprasidone and aripiprazole have not been adequately studied in psychotic PD patients.[176–178] In PD patients with psychosis and dementia, anticholinesterase inhibitors may be beneficial.[179–183]

Electroconvulsive Therapy

Electroconvulsive therapy (ECT) can be effective in treating depression, psychosis, and motor symptoms in PD patients.[184–188] ECT may also be helpful in treating drug-induced psychosis in levodopa-treated patients.[188,189] While ECT is recognized as a safe, effective treatment,[190] it can have significant side effects, including confusion, memory disturbance, headaches, fatigue, and cardiovascular complications.[190–192] In elderly patients, ECT may also be associated with an increased risk of falls and interictal delirium.[193,194] Despite these limitations, ECT should be considered as a treatment option for PD patients with severe and/or treatment-resistant depression.

Repetitive Transcranial Magnetic Stimulation

Repetitive transcranial magnetic stimulation (rTMS) has been shown to have statistically significant antidepressant effects in non-PD patients.[195–198] A small open study suggested rTMS may have antidepressant benefits in PD patients as well,[199] and another suggested that rTMS was as effective as fluoxetine for the treatment of depression in PD patients.[200] rTMS may also improve motor symptoms of PD,[201–208] although other studies have found no benefit.[209–212] Interestingly, rTMS has been shown to induce subcortical dopamine release in both animals and humans.[213–217]

Psychotherapy in Parkinson's Disease

Cognitive behavioral therapy (CBT) and interpersonal psychotherapy (IPT), either alone or in combination with pharmacotherapy, are established treatment options for depression.[218–224] In combination with antidepressant medications, psychotherapy may be useful for any level of depression severity and can even be helpful in cognitively impaired patients.[220,221,225,226] However, no studies of psychotherapy in depressed PD patients have been published. Given the established efficacy of these psychotherapy techniques in treating depression, it would seem reasonable to consider these as viable treatment options for depressed PD patients.

Suggested Treatment Approach

Despite the lack of double-blind, placebo-controlled data, beginning treatment with an SSRI is a reasonable first step in the treatment of depression in PD. Starting at a low dose and titrating up slowly can help limit the severity of side effects. Still, medications should be titrated to established therapeutic doses if tolerated and used for appropriate duration to determine potential benefit (i.e., 4–6 weeks). Cooccurring disorders should be identified and treated when possible. Psychotic symptoms should be treated with an atypical antipsychotic. Daytime fatigue and sleepiness may be treated with modafinil. At any point, consultation with a geriatric or neuropsychiatrist can be helpful.

If the initial antidepressant medication is not tolerated, switching to another SSRI may provide a more acceptable side effect profile; however, many patients have similar side effects with several medications within a class. If the initial SSRI is partially effective, an attempt should be made to maximize the dose (within safe and tolerable limits) and duration of the treatment. If SSRIs are not tolerated or are ineffective, switching to venlafaxine, duloxetine, or mirtazapine should be considered.

Despite their side effect profile, TCAs should be considered in depressed patients who do not tolerate or respond to other antidepressant medications. Patients taking TCAs should be carefully monitored for side effects and suicide risk. In patients with treatment-resistant or extremely severe depression, a referral for ECT should be considered.

Although there are no trials specifically in PD to support its use, psychotherapy may be beneficial and should have few, if any, adverse effects. The addition of psychotherapy can occur at any stage in the treatment of depression (except perhaps with severely cognitively impaired patients), and should especially be considered in treatment-resistant cases.

▶ CONCLUSION

Mood disorders, especially depression, commonly occur in PD patients. Mood disorders are a significant cause of distress and decreased quality of life for patients and their caregivers. However, diagnosing and treating mood disorders in PD patients can be complicated. An effective diagnostic approach should include a careful history, physical, and workup for cooccurring illnesses. An attempt should be made to separate symptoms related to PD, PD treatments, and cooccurring illnesses from symptoms attributable to a primary mood disorder. There are very limited database to help guide the treatment of mood disorders in PD. However, available data provide some support for the use of several antidepressant medications. ECT should be considered for patients with severe or treatment-refractory symptoms. More research should help improve the diagnosis and treatment of mood disorders in PD.

REFERENCES

1. Leentjens AF, Van den Akker M, Metsemakers JF, et al. Higher incidence of depression preceding the onset of Parkinson's disease: A register study. *Mov Disord* 2003;18(4):414–418.
2. Hantz P, Caradoc-Davies G, Caradoc-Davies T, et al. Depression in Parkinson's disease. *Am J Psychiatry* 1994;151(7):1010–1014.
3. Cummings JL. Depression and Parkinson's disease: A review. *Am J Psychiatry* 1992;149(4): 443–454.
4. Slaughter JR, Slaughter KA, Nichols D, et al. Prevalence, clinical manifestations, etiology, and treatment of depression in Parkinson's disease. *J Neuropsychiatry Clin Neurosci* 2001;13(2): 187–196.
5. Sano M, Stern Y, Williams J, et al. Coexisting dementia and depression in Parkinson's disease. *Arch Neurol* 1989;46(12):1284–1286.
6. Cole SA, Woodard JL, Juncos JL, et al. Depression and disability in Parkinson's disease. *J Neuropsychiatry Clin Neurosci* 1996;8(1):20–25.
7. Starkstein SE, Petracca G, Chemerinski E, et al. Depression in classic versus akinetic-rigid Parkinson's disease. *Mov Disord* 1998;13(1):29–33.

8. Tandberg E, Larsen JP, Aarsland D, et al. The occurrence of depression in Parkinson's disease. A community-based study. *Arch Neurol* 1996; 53(2):175–179.

9. Lyness JM, Bruce ML, Koenig HG, et al. Depression and medical illness in late life: Report of a symposium. *J Am Geriatr Soc* 1996;44(2):198–203.

10. Horwath E, Johnson J, Klerman GL, et al. Depressive symptoms as relative and attributable risk factors for first-onset major depression. *Arch Gen Psychiatry* 1992;49(10):817–823.

11. Meara J, Mitchelmore E, Hobson P. Use of the GDS-15 geriatric depression scale as a screening instrument for depressive symptomatology in patients with Parkinson's disease and their carers in the community. *Age Ageing* 1999;28(1):35–38.

12. Rojo A, Aguilar M, Garolera MT, et al. Depression in Parkinson's disease: Clinical correlates and outcome. *Parkinsonism Relat Disord* 2003;10(1):23–28.

13. Mayeux R, Stern Y, Rosen J, et al. Depression, intellectual impairment, and Parkinson's disease. *Neurology* 1981;31(6):645–650.

14. Starkstein SE, Preziosi TJ, Bolduc PL, et al. Depression in Parkinson's disease. *J Nerv Ment Dis* 1990;178(1):27–31.

15. Starkstein SE, Berthier ML, Bolduc PL, et al. Depression in patients with early versus late onset of Parkinson's disease. *Neurology* 1989; 39(11):1441–1445.

16. Santamaria J, Tolosa E, Valles A. Parkinson's disease with depression: A possible subgroup of idiopathic parkinsonism. *Neurology* 1986;36(8): 1130–1133.

17. Kostic VS, Filipovic SR, Lecic D, et al. Effect of age at onset on frequency of depression in Parkinson's disease. *J Neurol Neurosurg Psychiatry* 1994;57(10):1265–1267.

18. Tandberg E, Larsen JP, Aarsland D, et al. Risk factors for depression in Parkinson's disease. *Arch Neurol* 1997;54(5):625–630.

19. Ehmann TS, Beninger RJ, Gawel MJ, et al. Depressive symptoms in Parkinson's disease: A comparison with disabled control subjects. *J Geriatr Psychiatry Neurol* 1990;3(1):3–9.

20. Kostic VS, Djuricic BM, Covickovic-Sternic N, et al. Depression and Parkinson's disease: Possible role of serotonergic mechanisms. *J Neurol* 1987;234(2):94–96.

21. Vogel HP. Symptoms of depression in Parkinson's disease. *Pharmacopsychiatria* 1982;15(6):192–196.

22. Keshavan MS, David AS, Narayanen HS, et al. "On-off" phenomena and manic-depressive mood shifts: Case report. *J Clin Psychiatry* 1986;47(2):93–94.

23. Cannas A, Spissu A, Floris GL, et al. Bipolar affective disorder and Parkinson's disease: A rare, insidious and often unrecognized association. *Neurol Sci* 2002;23(Suppl 2):S67–68.

24. Kulisevsky J, Berthier ML, Gironell A, et al. Mania following deep brain stimulation for Parkinson's disease. *Neurology* 2002;59(9):1421–1424.

25. Romito LM, Raja M, Daniele A, et al. Transient mania with hypersexuality after surgery for high frequency stimulation of the subthalamic nucleus in Parkinson's disease. *Mov Disord* 2002;17(6):1371–1374.

26. Herzog J, Reiff J, Krack P, et al. Manic episode with psychotic symptoms induced by subthalamic nucleus stimulation in a patient with Parkinson's disease. *Mov Disord* 2003;18(11): 1382–1384.

27. Okun MS, Bakay RA, DeLong MR, et al. Transient manic behavior after pallidotomy. *Brain Cogn* 2003;52(2):281–283.

28. Starkstein SE, Mayberg HS, Leiguarda R, et al. A prospective longitudinal study of depression, cognitive decline, and physical impairments in patients with Parkinson's disease. *J Neurol Neurosurg Psychiatry* 1992;55(5):377–382.

29. Stern Y, Marder K, Tang MX, et al. Antecedent clinical features associated with dementia in Parkinson's disease. *Neurology* 1993;43(9): 1690–1692.

30. Giladi N, Treves TA, Paleacu D, et al. Risk factors for dementia, depression and psychosis in long-standing Parkinson's disease. *J Neural Transm* 2000;107(1):59–71.

31. Starkstein SE, Bolduc PL, Mayberg HS, et al. Cognitive impairments and depression in Parkinson's disease: A follow up study. *J Neurol Neurosurg Psychiatry* 1990;53(7):597–602.

32. Starkstein SE, Rabins PV, Berthier ML, et al. Dementia of depression among patients with neurological disorders and functional depression. *J Neuropsychiatry Clin Neurosci* 1989; 1(3):263–268.

33. Starkstein SE, Preziosi TJ, Berthier ML, et al. Depression and cognitive impairment in Parkinson's disease. *Brain* 1989;112(Pt 5):1141–1153.

34. Troster AI, Stalp LD, Paolo AM, et al. Neuropsychological impairment in Parkinson's disease with

and without depression. *Arch Neurol* 1995; 52(12):1164–1169.

35. Kuhn W, Heye N, Muller T, et al. The motor performance test series in Parkinson's disease is influenced by depression. *J Neural Transm* 1996; 103(3):349–354.

36. Kuopio AM, Marttila RJ, Helenius H, et al. The quality of life in Parkinson's disease. *Mov Disord* 2000;15(2):216–223.

37. Phillips P. Keeping depression at bay helps patients with Parkinson's disease. *JAMA* 1999; 282(12):1118–1119.

38. Troster AI, Fields JA, Wilkinson S, et al. Effect of motor improvement on quality of life following subthalamic stimulation is mediated by changes in depressive symptomatology. *Stereotact Funct Neurosurg* 2003;80(1–4):43–47.

39. Global Parkinson's Disease Study Steering Committee. Factors impacting on quality of life in Parkinson's disease: Results from an international survey. *Mov Disord* 2002;17(1):60–67.

40. Thommessen B, Aarsland D, Braekhus A, et al. The psychosocial burden on spouses of the elderly with stroke, dementia and Parkinson's disease. *Int J Geriatr Psychiatry* 2002;17(1):78–84.

41. Carter JH, Stewart BJ, Archbold PG, et al. Living with a person who has Parkinson's disease: The spouse's perspective by stage of disease. Parkinson's Study Group. *Mov Disord* 1998; 13(1): 20–28.

42. Aarsland D, Larsen JP, Karlsen K, et al. Mental symptoms in Parkinson's disease are important contributors to caregiver distress. *Int J Geriatr Psychiatry* 1999;14(10):866–874.

43. Caap-Ahlgren M, Dehlin O. Factors of importance to the caregiver burden experienced by family caregivers of Parkinson's disease patients. *Aging Clin Exp Res* 2002;14(5):371–377.

44. Pal PK, Thennarasu K, Fleming J, et al. Nocturnal sleep disturbances and daytime dysfunction in patients with Parkinson's disease and in their caregivers. *Parkinsonism Relat Disord* 2004; 10(3):157–168.

45. Menza MA, Mark MH. Parkinson's disease and depression: The relationship to disability and personality. *J Neuropsychiatry Clin Neurosci* 1994;6(2):165–169.

46. Jellinger KA. Post mortem studies in Parkinson's disease—is it possible to detect brain areas for specific symptoms? *J Neural Transm Suppl* 1999;56:1–29.

47. Braak H, Del Tredici K, Rub U, et al. Staging of brain pathology related to sporadic Parkinson's disease. *Neurobiol Aging* 2003;24(2):197–211.

48. Mayberg HS. Modulating dysfunctional limbic-cortical circuits in depression: Towards development of brain-based algorithms for diagnosis and optimised treatment. *Br Med Bull* 2003;65: 193–207.

49. Lisanby SH, McDonald WM, Massey EW, et al. Diminished subcortical nuclei volumes in Parkinson's disease by MR imaging. *J Neural Transm Suppl* 1993;40:13–21.

50. McDonald WM, Krishnan KR. Magnetic resonance in patients with affective illness. *Eur Arch Psychiatry Clin Neurosci* 1992;241(5):283–290.

51. Sheline YI. Neuroimaging studies of mood disorder effects on the brain. *Biol Psychiatry* 2003;54(3):338–352.

52. Mayberg HS, Starkstein SE, Sadzot B, et al. Selective hypometabolism in the inferior frontal lobe in depressed patients with Parkinson's disease. *Ann Neurol* 1990;28(1):57–64.

53. Richard IH, Schiffer RB, Kurlan R. Anxiety and Parkinson's disease. *J Neuropsychiatry Clin Neurosci* 1996;8(4):383–392.

54. Menza MA, Robertson-Hoffman DE, Bonapace AS. Parkinson's disease and anxiety: Comorbidity with depression. *Biol Psychiatry* 1993; 34(7): 465–470.

55. Nuti A, Ceravolo R, Piccinni A, et al. Psychiatric comorbidity in a population of Parkinson's disease patients. *Eur J Neurol* 2004;11(5):315–320.

56. Marinus J, Leentjens AF, Visser M, et al. Evaluation of the hospital anxiety and depression scale in patients with Parkinson's disease. *Clin Neuropharmacol* 2002;25(6):318–324.

57. Shulman LM, Taback RL, Bean J, et al. Comorbidity of the nonmotor symptoms of Parkinson's disease. *Mov Disord* 2001;16(3):507–510.

58. Lauterbach EC, Freeman A, Vogel RL. Correlates of generalized anxiety and panic attacks in dystonia and Parkinson's disease. *Cogn Behav Neurol* 2003;16(4):225–233.

59. Lauterbach EC, Freeman A, Vogel RL. Differential DSM-III psychiatric disorder prevalence profiles in dystonia and Parkinson's disease. *J Neuropsychiatry Clin Neurosci* 2004;16(1):29–36.

60. Shiba M, Bower JH, Maraganore DM, et al. Anxiety disorders and depressive disorders preceding Parkinson's disease: A case-control study. *Mov Disord* 2000;15(4):669–677.

61. Stenager EN, Wermuth L, Stenager E, et al. Suicide in patients with Parkinson's disease. An epidemiological study. *Acta Psychiatr Scand* 1994;90(1):70–72.

62. Hamilton M, White J. Factors related to the outcome of depression treated with ECT. *J Ment Sci* 1960;106:1031–1041.

63. Beck AT, Ward CH, Mendelsohn M, et al. An inventory for measuring depression. *Arch Gen Psychiatry* 1961;4:561–571.

64. Montgomery SM. Depressive symptoms in acute schizophrenia. *Prog Neuropsychopharmacol* 1979;3(4):429–433.

65. Yesavage JA, Brink TL, Rose TL, et al. Development and validation of a geriatric depression screening scale: A preliminary report. *J Psychiatr Res* 1982;17(1):37–49.

66. Leentjens AF, Marinus J, Van Hilten JJ, et al. The contribution of somatic symptoms to the diagnosis of depressive disorder in Parkinson's disease: A discriminant analytic approach. *J Neuropsychiatry Clin Neurosci* 2003;15(1):74–77.

67. Leentjens AF, Verhey FR, Lousberg R, et al. The validity of the Hamilton and Montgomery-Asberg depression rating scales as screening and diagnostic tools for depression in Parkinson's disease. *Int J Geriatr Psychiatry* 2000;15(7):644–649.

68. Leentjens AF, Verhey FR, Luijckx GJ, et al. The validity of the Beck Depression Inventory as a screening and diagnostic instrument for depression in patients with Parkinson's disease. *Mov Disord* 2000;15(6):1221–1224.

69. Errea JM, Ara JR. Depression and Parkinson's disease. *Rev Neurol* 1999;28(7):694–698.

70. Caap-Ahlgren M, Dehlin O. Insomnia and depressive symptoms in patients with Parkinson's disease. Relationship to health-related quality of life. An interview study of patients living at home. *Arch Gerontol Geriatr* 2001; 32(1):23–33.

71. American Psychiatric Association. *Diagnostic and Statistical Manual of Mental Disorders.* 4th ed. Washington, DC: APA press; 1994.

72. Jouvent R, Abensour P, Bonnet AM, et al. Antiparkinsonian and antidepressant effects of high doses of bromocriptine. An independent comparison. *J Affect Disord* 1983;5(2):141–145.

73. Maricle RA, Nutt JG, Valentine RJ, et al. Dose-response relationship of levodopa with mood and anxiety in fluctuating Parkinson's disease: A double-blind, placebo-controlled study. *Neurology* 1995;45(9):1757–1760.

74. Rektorova I, Rektor I, Bares M, et al. Pramipexole and pergolide in the treatment of depression in Parkinson's disease: A national multicentre prospective randomized study. *Eur J Neurol* 2003;10(4):399–406.

75. Young BK, Camicioli R, Ganzini L. Neuropsychiatric adverse effects of antiparkinsonian drugs. Characteristics, evaluation and treatment. *Drugs Aging* 1997;10(5):367–383.

76. Biglan KM, Holloway RG. A review of pramipexole and its clinical utility in Parkinson's disease. *Expert Opin Pharmacother* 2002;3(2):197–210.

77. Lattanzi L, Dell'Osso L, Cassano P, et al. Pramipexole in treatment-resistant depression: A 16-week naturalistic study. *Bipolar Disord* 2002;4(5):307–314.

78. Friedenberg DL, Cummings JL. Parkinson's disease, depression, and the on-off phenomenon. *Psychosomatics* 1989;30(1):94–99.

79. Lees AJ. The on-off phenomenon. *J Neurol Neurosurg Psychiatry* 1989;(Suppl):29–37.

80. Hardie RJ, Lees AJ, Stern GM. On-off fluctuations in Parkinson's disease. A clinical and neuropharmacological study. *Brain* 1984;107(Pt 2):487–506.

81. Nissenbaum H, Quinn NP, Brown RG, et al. Mood swings associated with the 'on-off' phenomenon in Parkinson's disease. *Psychol Med* 1987;17(4):899–904.

82. Racette BA, Hartlein JM, Hershey T, et al. Clinical features and comorbidity of mood fluctuations in Parkinson's disease. *J Neuropsychiatry Clin Neurosci* 2002;14(4):438–442.

83. Menza MA, Sage J, Marshall E, et al. Mood changes and "on-off" phenomena in Parkinson's disease. *Mov Disord* 1990;5(2):148–151.

84. Maricle RA, Nutt JG, Carter JH. Mood and anxiety fluctuation in Parkinson's disease associated with levodopa infusion: Preliminary findings. *Mov Disord* 1995;10(3):329–332.

85. Shults CW. Treatments of Parkinson's disease: Circa 2003. *Arch Neurol* 2003;60(12):1680–1684.

86. Vitek JL, Bakay RA, Freeman A, et al. Randomized trial of pallidotomy versus medical therapy for Parkinson's disease. *Ann Neurol* 2003; 53(5): 558–569.

87. Burchiel KJ. Thalamotomy for movement disorders. *Neurosurg Clin North Am* 1995;6(1): 55–71.

88. York MK, Levin HS, Grossman RG, et al. Neuropsychological outcome following unilateral pallidotomy. *Brain* 1999;122(Pt 12):2209–2220.

89. Alegret M, Valldeoriola F, Tolosa E, et al. Cognitive effects of unilateral posteroventral pallidotomy: A 4-year follow-up study. *Mov Disord* 2003;18(3):323–328.

90. Green J, Barnhart H. The impact of lesion laterality on neuropsychological change following posterior pallidotomy: A review of current findings. *Brain Cogn* 2000;42(3):379–398.

91. Green J, McDonald WM, Vitek JL, et al. Neuropsychological and psychiatric sequelae of pallidotomy for PD: Clinical trial findings. *Neurology* 2002;58(6):858–865.

92. Limousin P, Speelman JD, Gielen F, et al. Multicentre European study of thalamic stimulation in parkinsonian and essential tremor. *J Neurol Neurosurg Psychiatry* 1999;66(3):289–296.

93. The Deep Brain Stimulation for Parkinson's Disease Study Group. Deep-brain stimulation of the subthalamic nucleus or the pars interna of the globus pallidus in Parkinson's disease. *N Engl J Med* 2001;345(13):956–963.

94. Bejjani BP, Damier P, Arnulf I, et al. Transient acute depression induced by high-frequency deep-brain stimulation. *N Engl J Med* 1999; 340(19):1476–1480.

95. Herzog J, Volkmann J, Krack P, et al. Two-year follow-up of subthalamic deep brain stimulation in Parkinson's disease. *Mov Disord* 2003;18(11): 1332–1337.

96. Miyawaki E, Perlmutter JS, Troster AI, et al. The behavioral complications of pallidal stimulation: A case report. *Brain Cogn* 2000;42(3): 417–434.

97. Hughes TA, Ross HF, Musa S, et al. A 10-year study of the incidence of and factors predicting dementia in Parkinson's disease. *Neurology* 2000;54(8):1596–1602.

98. Haggerty JJ, Jr., Prange AJ, Jr. Borderline hypothyroidism and depression. *Annu Rev Med* 1995;46:37–46.

99. Garcia-Moreno JM, Chacon-Pena J. Hypothyroidism and Parkinson's disease and the issue of diagnostic confusion. *Mov Disord* 2003;18(9): 1058–1059.

100. Tandeter HB, Shvartzman P. Parkinson's disease camouflaging early signs of hypothyroidism. *Postgrad Med* 1993;94(5):187–190.

101. Otake K, Oiso Y, Mitsuma T, et al. Hypothalamic dysfunction in Parkinson's disease patients. *Acta Med Hung* 1994;50(1–2):3–13.

102. Lefebvre J, Loeuille GA, Steinling M, et al. [Comparative action of L-dopa and bromocriptine on thyreostimulating hormone (T.S.H.) in primary hypothyroidism (author's transl)]. *Nouv Presse Med* 1979;8(38):3033–3036.

103. Lindenbaum J, Healton EB, Savage DG, et al. Neuropsychiatric disorders caused by cobalamin deficiency in the absence of anemia or macrocytosis. *N Engl J Med* Jun 30 1988;318(26): 1720–1728.

104. Dharmarajan TS, Norkus EP. Approaches to vitamin B12 deficiency. Early treatment may prevent devastating complications. *Postgrad Med* Jul 2001;110(1):99–105; quiz 106.

105. Dharmarajan TS, Ugalino JT, Kanagala M, et al. Vitamin B12 status in hospitalized elderly from nursing homes and the community. *J Am Med Dir Assoc* Jan-Feb 2000;1(1):21–24.

106. Dharmarajan TS, Adiga GU, Norkus EP. Vitamin B12 deficiency. Recognizing subtle symptoms in older adults. *Geriatrics* Mar 2003;58(3):30–34, 37–38.

107. Bottiglieri T, Laundy M, Crellin R, et al. Homocysteine, folate, methylation, and monoamine metabolism in depression. *J Neurol Neurosurg Psychiatry* 2000;69(2):228–232.

108. Reutens S, Sachdev P. Homocysteine in neuropsychiatric disorders of the elderly. *Int J Geriatr Psychiatry* 2002;17(9):859–864.

109. Kuhn W, Roebroek R, Blom H, et al. Hyperhomocysteinaemia in Parkinson's disease. *J Neurol* 1998;245(12):811–812.

110. Kuhn W, Roebroek R, Blom H, et al. Elevated plasma levels of homocysteine in Parkinson's disease. *Eur Neurol* 1998;40(4):225–227.

111. Muller T, Werne B, Fowler B, et al. Nigral endothelial dysfunction, homocysteine, and Parkinson's disease. *Lancet* 1999;354(9173):126–127.

112. Muller T, Woitalla D, Hauptmann B, et al. Decrease of methionine and S-adenosylmethionine and increase of homocysteine in treated patients with Parkinson's disease. *Neurosci Lett* 2001;308(1):54–56.

113. Hankey GJ, Eikelboom JW. Homocysteine and vascular disease. *Lancet* 1999;354(9176): 407–413.

114. Di Rocco A, Rogers JD, Brown R, et al. S-Adenosyl-Methionine improves depression in patients with Parkinson's disease in an open-label clinical trial. *Mov Disord* 2000;15(6):1225–1229.

115. Mischoulon D, Fava M. Role of S-adenosyl-L-methionine in the treatment of depression: A review of the evidence. *Am J Clin Nutr* 2002;76(5):1158S–1161S.

116. Barrett-Connor E, Von Muhlen DG, Kritz-Silverstein D. Bioavailable testosterone and depressed mood in older men: The Rancho Bernardo Study. *J Clin Endocrinol Metab* 1999; 84(2):573–577.

117. Okun MS, McDonald WM, DeLong MR. Refractory nonmotor symptoms in male patients with Parkinson's disease due to testosterone deficiency: A common unrecognized comorbidity. *Arch Neurol* 2002;59(5):807–811.

118. Seidman SN, Rabkin JG. Testosterone replacement therapy for hypogonadal men with SSRI-refractory depression. *J Affect Disord* 1998; 48(2–3):157–161.

119. Okun MS, Walter BL, McDonald WM, et al. Beneficial effects of testosterone replacement for the nonmotor symptoms of Parkinson's disease. *Arch Neurol* 2002;59(11):1750–1753.

120. Ehmann TS, Beninger RJ, Gawel MJ, et al. Coping, social support, and depressive symptoms in Parkinson's disease. *J Geriatr Psychiatry Neurol* 1990;3(2):85–90.

121. Alexopoulos GS, Abrams RC, Young RC, et al. Cornell Scale for Depression in Dementia. *Biol Psychiatry* 1988;23(3):271–284.

122. Kurlowicz LH, Evans LK, Strumpf NE, et al. A psychometric evaluation of the Cornell Scale for Depression in Dementia in a frail, nursing home population. *Am J Geriatr Psychiatry* 2002;10(5): 600–608.

123. Rabey JM, Orlov E, Korczyn AD. Comparison of fluvoxamine versus amitriptyline for treatment of depression in Parkinson's disease. *Neurology* 1996;46:A374.

124. Serrano-Duenas M. [A comparison between low doses of amitriptyline and low doses of fluoxetin used in the control of depression in patients suffering from Parkinson's disease]. *Rev Neurol* Dec 1–15 2002;35(11):1010–1014.

125. Andersen J, Aabro E, Gulmann N, et al. Antidepressive treatment in Parkinson's disease. A controlled trial of the effect of nortriptyline in patients with Parkinson's disease treated with L-DOPA. *Acta Neurol Scand* 1980;62(4): 210–219.

126. Richard IH, Kurlan R. A survey of antidepressant drug use in Parkinson's disease. Parkinson's Study Group. *Neurology* 1997;49(4):1168–1170.

127. Jimenez-Jimenez FJ, Tejeiro J, Martinez-Junquera G, et al. Parkinsonism exacerbated by paroxetine. *Neurology* 1994;44(12):2406.

128. Meltzer HY, Young M, Metz J, et al. Extrapyramidal side effects and increased serum prolactin following fluoxetine, a new antidepressant. *J Neural Transm* 1979;45(2):165–175.

129. Lambert MT, Trutia C, Petty F. Extrapyramidal adverse effects associated with sertraline. *Prog Neuropsychopharmacol Biol Psychiatry* 1998; 22(5):741–748.

130. Leo RJ. Movement disorders associated with the serotonin selective reuptake inhibitors. *J Clin Psychiatry* 1996;57(10):449–454.

131. Jones-Fearing KB. SSRI and EPS with fluoxetine. *J Am Acad Child Adolesc Psychiatry* 1996; 35(9): 1107–1108.

132. Simons JA. Fluoxetine in Parkinson's disease. *Mov Disord* 1996;11(5):581–582.

133. Coulter DM, Pillans PI. Fluoxetine and extrapyramidal side effects. *Am J Psychiatry* 1995;152(1): 122–125.

134. Bouchard R, Pourcher E, Vincent P. Fluoxetine and extrapyramidal side effects. *Am J Psychiatry* 1989;146(10):1352–1353.

135. Hesselink JM. Serotonin and Parkinson's disease. *Am J Psychiatry* 1993;150(5):843–844.

136. Steur EN. Increase of Parkinson's disability after fluoxetine medication. *Neurology* 1993;43(1): 211–213.

137. Tate JL. Extrapyramidal symptoms in a patient taking haloperidol and fluoxetine. *Am J Psychiatry* 1989;146(3):399–400.

138. Tesei S, Antonini A, Canesi M, et al. Tolerability of paroxetine in Parkinson's disease: A prospective study. *Mov Disord* 2000;15(5):986–989.

139. Schillevoort I, van Puijenbroek EP, de Boer A, et al. Extrapyramidal syndromes associated with selective serotonin reuptake inhibitors: A case-control study using spontaneous reports. *Int Clin Psychopharmacol* 2002;17(2):75–79.

140. Lane RM. SSRI-induced extrapyramidal side-effects and akathisia: Implications for treatment. *J Psychopharmacol* 1998;12(2):192–214.

141. Gony M, Lapeyre-Mestre M, Montastruc JL. Risk of serious extrapyramidal symptoms in patients with Parkinson's disease receiving antidepressant drugs: A pharmacoepidemiologic study comparing serotonin reuptake inhibitors and other antidepressant drugs. *Clin Neuropharmacol* 2003;26(3):142–145.

142. Mamo DC, Sweet RA, Mulsant BH, et al. Effect of nortriptyline and paroxetine on extrapyramidal signs and symptoms: A prospective double-blind

study in depressed elderly patients. *Am J Geriatr Psychiatry* 2000;8(3):226–231.

143. Caley CF, Friedman JH. Does fluoxetine exacerbate Parkinson's disease? *J Clin Psychiatry.* 1992;53(8):278–282.

144. Ceravolo R, Nuti A, Piccinni A, et al. Paroxetine in Parkinson's disease: Effects on motor and depressive symptoms. *Neurology* 2000;55(8): 1216–1218.

145. Dell'Agnello G, Ceravolo R, Nuti A, et al. SSRIs do not worsen Parkinson's disease: Evidence from an open-label, prospective study. *Clin Neuropharmacol* 2001;24(4):221–227.

146. Hauser RA, Zesiewicz TA. Sertraline for the treatment of depression in Parkinson's disease. *Mov Disord* 1997;12(5):756–759.

147. Montastruc JL, Fabre N, Blin O, et al. Does fluoxetine aggravate Parkinson's disease? A pilot prospective study. *Mov Disord* 1995;10(3): 355–357.

148. Rampello L, Chiechio S, Raffaele R, et al. The SSRI, citalopram, improves bradykinesia in patients with Parkinson's disease treated with L-dopa. *Clin Neuropharmacol* 2002;25(1):21–24.

149. Richard IH, Maughn A, Kurlan R. Do serotonin reuptake inhibitor antidepressants worsen Parkinson's disease? A retrospective case series. *Mov Disord* 1999;14(1):155–157.

150. Chung TH, Deane KH, Ghazi-Noori S, et al. Systematic review of antidepressant therapies in Parkinson's disease. *Parkinsonism Relat Disord* 2003;10(2):59–65.

151. Wermuth L, Sorensen PS, Timm B, et al. Depression in idiopathic Parkinson's disease treated with citalopram - a placebo controlled trial. *Nord J Psychiatry* 1998;52(2):163–169.

152. Leentjens AF, Vreeling FW, Luijckx GJ, et al. SSRIs in the treatment of depression in Parkinson's disease. *Int J Geriatr Psychiatry* 2003;18(6):552–554.

153. Menza M, Marin H, Kaufman K, et al. Citalopram treatment of depression in Parkinson's disease: The impact on anxiety, disability, and cognition. *J Neuropsychiatry Clin Neurosci* Summer 2004;16(3):315–319.

154. McCance-Katz EF, Marek KL, Price LH. Serotonergic dysfunction in depression associated with Parkinson's disease. *Neurology* Sep 1992;42(9): 1813–1814.

155. Meara J, Hobson P. Sertraline for the treatment of depression in Parkinson's disease. *Mov Disord* 1998;13(3):622.

156. Vaswani M, Linda FK, Ramesh S. Role of selective serotonin reuptake inhibitors in psychiatric disorders: A comprehensive review. *Prog Neuropsychopharmacol Biol Psychiatry* 2003;27(1): 85–102.

157. Zohar J, Westenberg HG. Anxiety disorders: A review of tricyclic antidepressants and selective serotonin reuptake inhibitors. *Acta Psychiatr Scand Suppl* 2000;403:39–49.

158. Avila A, Cardona X, Martin-Baranera M, et al. Does nefazodone improve both depression and Parkinson's disease? A pilot randomized trial. *J Clin Psychopharmacol* 2003;23(5):509–513.

159. Meco G, Fabrizio E, Di Rezze S, et al. Mirtazapine in L-dopa-induced dyskinesias. *Clin Neuropharmacol* 2003;26(4):179–181.

160. Goetz CG, Tanner CM, Klawans HL. Bupropion in Parkinson's disease. *Neurology* 1984;34(8): 1092–1094.

161. Rabinstein A, Shulman LM, Weiner WJ. Modafinil for the treatment of excessive daytime sleepiness in Parkinson's disease: A case report. Oct 2001;7(4):287–288.

162. Happe S, Pirker W, Sauter C, et al. Successful treatment of excessive daytime sleepiness in Parkinson's disease with modafinil. *J Neurol* Jul 2001;248(7):632–634.

163. Nieves AV, Lang AE. Treatment of excessive daytime sleepiness in patients with Parkinson's disease with modafinil. *Clin Neuropharmacol* Mar-Apr 2002;25(2):111–114.

164. Hogl B, Saletu M, Brandauer E, et al. Modafinil for the treatment of daytime sleepiness in Parkinson's disease: A double-blind, randomized, crossover, placebo-controlled polygraphic trial. *Sleep* Dec15 2002;25(8):905–909.

165. Adler CH, Caviness JN, Hentz JG, et al. Randomized trial of modafinil for treating subjective daytime sleepiness in patients with Parkinson's disease. *Mov Disord* Mar 2003;18(3): 287–293.

166. Fernandez HH, Trieschmann ME, Friedman JH. Treatment of psychosis in Parkinson's disease: Safety considerations. *Drug Saf* 2003;26(9): 643–659.

167. Trosch RM, Friedman JH, Lannon MC, et al. Clozapine use in Parkinson's disease: A retrospective analysis of a large multicentered clinical experience. *Mov Disord* 1998;13(3):377–382.

168. The Parkinson's Study Group. Low-dose clozapine for the treatment of drug-induced psychosis in

Parkinson's disease. *N Engl J Med* March 11, 1999 1999;340(10):757–763.

169. The French Clozapine Parkinson's Study Group. Clozapine in drug-induced psychosis in Parkinson's disease. *Lancet* 1999;353(9169): 2041–2042.

170. Fernandez HH, Trieschmann ME, Burke MA, et al. Long-term outcome of quetiapine use for psychosis among Parkinsonian patients. *Mov Disord* 2003;18(5):510–514.

171. Reddy S, Factor SA, Molho ES, et al. The effect of quetiapine on psychosis and motor function in parkinsonian patients with and without dementia. *Mov Disord* 2002;17(4):676–681.

172. Bullock R, Saharan A. Atypical antipsychotics: Experience and use in the elderly. *Int J Clin Pract* 2002;56(7):515–525.

173. Morgante L, Epifanio A, Spina E, et al. Quetiapine versus clozapine: A preliminary report of comparative effects on dopaminergic psychosis in patients with Parkinson's disease. *Neurol Sci* 2002;23(Suppl 2):S89–90.

174. Wijnen HH, van der Heijden FM, van Schendel FM, et al. Quetiapine in the elderly with parkinsonism and psychosis. *Eur Psychiatry* 2003; 18(7):372–373.

175. Juncos JL, Roberts VJ, Evatt ML, et al. Quetiapine improves psychotic symptoms and cognition in Parkinson's disease. *Mov Disord* 2004; 19(1):29–35.

176. Connemann BJ, Schonfeldt-Lecuona C. Ziprasidone in Parkinson's disease psychosis. *Can J Psychiatry* 2004;49(1):73.

177. Schonfeldt-Lecuona C, Connemann BJ. Aripiprazole and Parkinson's disease psychosis. *Am J Psychiatry* Feb 2004;161(2):373–374.

178. Fernandez HH, Trieschmann ME, Friedman JH. Aripiprazole for drug-induced psychosis in Parkinson's disease: Preliminary experience. *Clin Neuropharmacol* Jan-Feb 2004;27(1):4–5.

179. McKeith IG, Grace JB, Walker Z, et al. Rivastigmine in the treatment of dementia with Lewy bodies: Preliminary findings from an open trial. *Int J Geriatr Psychiatry* 2000;15(5): 387–392.

180. Bullock R, Cameron A. Rivastigmine for the treatment of dementia and visual hallucinations associated with Parkinson's disease: A case series. *Curr Med Res Opin* 2002;18(5):258–264.

181. Bergman J, Lerner V. Successful use of donepezil for the treatment of psychotic symptoms in patients with Parkinson's disease. *Clin Neuropharmacol* 2002;25(2):107–110.

182. Fabbrini G, Barbanti P, Aurilia C, et al. Donepezil in the treatment of hallucinations and delusions in Parkinson's disease. *Neurol Sci* 2002;23(1): 41–43.

183. Reading PJ, Luce AK, McKeith IG. Rivastigmine in the treatment of parkinsonian psychosis and cognitive impairment: Preliminary findings from an open trial. *Mov Disord* 2001;16(6):1171–1174.

184. Pridmore S, Pollard C. Electroconvulsive therapy in Parkinson's disease: 30 month follow up. *J Neurol Neurosurg Psychiatry* 1996;60(6):693.

185. Friedman J, Gordon N. Electroconvulsive therapy in Parkinson's disease: A report on five cases. *Convuls Ther* 1992;8(3):204–210.

186. Fall PA, Ekman R, Granerus AK, et al. ECT in Parkinson's disease. Changes in motor symptoms, monoamine metabolites and neuropeptides. *J Neural Transm Park Dis Dement Sect* 1995; 10(2–3):129–140.

187. Moellentine C, Rummans T, Ahlskog JE, et al. Effectiveness of ECT in patients with parkinsonism. *J Neuropsychiatry Clin Neurosci* 1998;10(2): 187–193.

188. Factor SA, Molho ES, Brown DL. Combined clozapine and electroconvulsive therapy for the treatment of drug-induced psychosis in Parkinson's disease. *J Neuropsychiatry Clin Neurosci* 1995; 7(3):304–307.

189. Hurwitz TA, Calne DB, Waterman K. Treatment of dopaminomimetic psychosis in Parkinson's disease with electroconvulsive therapy. *Can J Neurol Sci* 1988;15(1):32–34.

190. van der Wurff FB, Stek ML, Hoogendijk WJ, et al. The efficacy and safety of ECT in depressed older adults: A literature review. *Int J Geriatr Psychiatry* 2003;18(10):894–904.

191. Datto CJ. Side effects of electroconvulsive therapy. *Depress Anxiety* 2000;12(3):130–134.

192. Zielinski RJ, Roose SP, Devanand DP, et al. Cardiovascular complications of ECT in depressed patients with cardiac disease. *Am J Psychiatry* 1993;150(6):904–909.

193. Salzman C, Wong E, Wright BC. Drug and ECT treatment of depression in the elderly, 1996–2001: A literature review. *Biol Psychiatry* 2002/8/1 2002;52(3):265–284.

194. Figiel GS, Hassen MA, Zorumski C, et al. ECT-induced delirium in depressed patients with Parkinson's disease. *J Neuropsychiatry Clin Neurosci* 1991;3(4):405–411.

195. Holtzheimer PE, IIIrd, Russo J, et al. A meta-analysis of repetitive transcranial magnetic stimulation in the treatment of depression. *Psychopharmacol Bull* 2001;35(4):149–169.

196. Burt T, Lisanby SH, Sackeim HA. Neuropsychiatric applications of transcranial magnetic stimulation: A meta-analysis. *Int J Neuropsychopharmacol* 2002;5(1):73–103.

197. Kozel FA, George MS. Meta-analysis of left prefrontal repetitive transcranial magnetic stimulation (rTMS) to treat depression. *J Psychiatr Pract* 2002;8(5):270–275.

198. Martin JL, Barbanoj MJ, Schlaepfer TE, et al. Repetitive transcranial magnetic stimulation for the treatment of depression: Systematic review and meta-analysis. *Br J Psychiatry* 2003;182: 480–491.

199. Dragasevic N, Potrebic A, Damjanovic A, et al. Therapeutic efficacy of bilateral prefrontal slow repetitive transcranial magnetic stimulation in depressed patients with Parkinson's disease: An open study. *Mov Disord* 2002;17(3):528–532.

200. Fregni F, Santos CM, Myczkowski ML, et al. Repetitive transcranial magnetic stimulation is as effective as fluoxetine in the treatment of depression in patients with Parkinson's disease. *J Neurol Neurosurg Psychiatry* 2004;75(8): 1171–1174.

201. Pascual-Leone A, Valls-Sole J, Brasil-Neto JP, et al. Akinesia in Parkinson's disease. II. Effects of subthreshold repetitive transcranial motor cortex stimulation. *Neurology* 1994;44(5):892–898.

202. Siebner HR, Mentschel C, Auer C, et al. Repetitive transcranial magnetic stimulation has a beneficial effect on bradykinesia in Parkinson's disease. *Neuroreport* 1999;10(3):589–594.

203. Siebner HR, Rossmeier C, Mentschel C, et al. Short-term motor improvement after sub-threshold 5-Hz repetitive transcranial magnetic stimulation of the primary motor hand area in Parkinson's disease. *J Neurol Sci* 2000;178(2): 91–94.

204. de Groot M, Hermann W, Steffen J, et al. Contralateral and ipsilateral repetitive transcranial magnetic stimulation in Parkinson's patients. *Nervenarzt* 2001;72(12):932–938.

205. Sommer M, Kamm T, Tergau F, et al. Repetitive paired-pulse transcranial magnetic stimulation affects corticospinal excitability and finger tapping in Parkinson's disease. *Clin Neurophysiol* 2002;113(6):944–950.

206. Shimamoto H, Takasaki K, Shigemori M, et al. Therapeutic effect and mechanism of repetitive transcranial magnetic stimulation in Parkinson's disease. *J Neurol* 2001;248(Suppl 3):III48–52.

207. Mally J, Stone TW. Therapeutic and "dose-dependent" effect of repetitive microelectroshock induced by transcranial magnetic stimulation in Parkinson's disease. *J Neurosci Res* 1999;57(6): 935–940.

208. Mally J, Stone TW. Improvement in Parkinsonian symptoms after repetitive transcranial magnetic stimulation. *J Neurol Sci* 1999;162(2):179–184.

209. Boylan LS, Pullman SL, Lisanby SH, et al. Repetitive transcranial magnetic stimulation to SMA worsens complex movements in Parkinson's disease. *Clin Neurophysiol* 2001;112(2):259–264.

210. Okabe S, Ugawa Y, Kanazawa I. 0.2-Hz repetitive transcranial magnetic stimulation has no add-on effects as compared to a realistic sham stimulation in Parkinson's disease. *Mov Disord* 2003;18(4):382–388.

211. Tergau F, Wassermann EM, Paulus W, et al. Lack of clinical improvement in patients with Parkinson's disease after low and high frequency repetitive transcranial magnetic stimulation. *Electroencephalogr Clin Neurophysiol Suppl* 1999;51: 281–288.

212. Ghabra MB, Hallett M, Wassermann EM. Simultaneous repetitive transcranial magnetic stimulation does not speed fine movement in PD. *Neurology* 1999;52(4):768–770.

213. Ohnishi T, Hayashi T, Okabe S, et al. Endogenous dopamine release induced by repetitive transcranial magnetic stimulation over the primary motor cortex: An [11C]raclopride positron emission tomography study in anesthetized macaque monkeys. *Biol Psychiatry* 2004;55(5): 484–489.

214. Kanno M, Matsumoto M, Togashi H, et al. Effects of acute repetitive transcranial magnetic stimulation on dopamine release in the rat dorsolateral striatum. *J Neurol Sci* 2004;217(1):73–81.

215. Strafella AP, Paus T, Fraraccio M, et al. Striatal dopamine release induced by repetitive transcranial magnetic stimulation of the human motor cortex. *Brain* 2003;22:22.

216. Keck ME, Welt T, Muller MB, et al. Repetitive transcranial magnetic stimulation increases the release of dopamine in the mesolimbic and mesostriatal system. *Neuropharmacology* 2002; 43(1):101–109.

217. Strafella AP, Paus T, Barrett J, et al. Repetitive transcranial magnetic stimulation of the human

prefrontal cortex induces dopamine release in the caudate nucleus. *J Neurosci* 2001;21(15): RC157.

218. DeRubeis RJ, Gelfand LA, Tang TZ, et al. Medications versus cognitive behavior therapy for severely depressed outpatients: Mega-analysis of four randomized comparisons. *Am J Psychiatry* 1999;156(7):1007–1013.

219. Scott J. Cognitive therapy for depression. *Br Med Bull* 2001;57:101–113.

220. Gloaguen V, Cottraux J, Cucherat M, et al. A meta-analysis of the effects of cognitive therapy in depressed patients. *J Affect Disord* 1998; 49(1): 59–72.

221. Thase ME, Greenhouse JB, Frank E, et al. Treatment of major depression with psychotherapy or psychotherapy-pharmacotherapy combinations. *Arch Gen Psychiatry* 1997;54(11):1009–1015.

222. Browne G, Steiner M, Roberts J, et al. Sertraline and/or interpersonal psychotherapy for patients with dysthymic disorder in primary care: 6-month comparison with longitudinal 2-year follow-up of effectiveness and costs. *J Affect Disord* 2002;68(2–3):317–330.

223. Reynolds CF 3rd, Frank E, Perel JM, et al. Nortriptyline and interpersonal psychotherapy as maintenance therapies for recurrent major depression: A randomized controlled trial in patients older than 59 years. *JAMA* 1999;281(1):39–45.

224. Frank E, Kupfer DJ, Wagner EF, et al. Efficacy of interpersonal psychotherapy as a maintenance treatment of recurrent depression. Contributing factors. *Arch Gen Psychiatry* 1991;48(12): 1053–1059.

225. Cole MG, Elie LM, McCusker J, et al. Feasibility and effectiveness of treatments for depression in elderly medical inpatients: A systematic review. *Int Psychogeriatr* 2000;12(4):453–461.

226. Miller MD, Cornes C, Frank E, et al. Interpersonal psychotherapy for late-life depression: Past, present, and future. *J Psychother Pract Res* 2001;10(4):231–238.

CHAPTER 14

Depression in Epilepsy

ANDRES M. KANNER

► INTRODUCTION

Depressive disorders (DD) are the most common comorbid psychiatric conditions associated with epilepsy[1]; however, its real incidence and prevalence have yet to be established. The diversity in methodologies and sample populations across studies, the under-reporting of symptoms of depression by patients and families and the under-diagnosis by clinicians are three of the primary reasons for the absence of these data. However, there is a consensus among various authors that the prevalence of depression in epilepsy is higher than in a matched population of healthy controls, ranging from 3 to 9% in patients with controlled epilepsy and 20 to 55% in patients with recurrent seizures.[1–5]

Epidemiologic Aspects

Research on the concerns of living with epilepsy demonstrated that about one-third of patients spontaneously label mood as a significant issue.[6] To provide typical data, four of the largest studies are briefly examined below. Jacoby et al.,[2] in a community-based study that used the hospital anxiety and depression scale, reported that of 168 patients with recurrent seizures, 21% were depressed. Using the same scale, O'Donoghue et al.[3] showed that, of a group of 155 patients identified through two large primary care prac-

tices in the United Kingdom, 33% with recurrent seizures and 6% of those in remission had depression. Edeh and Toone[4] used the Clinical Interview Schedule to demonstrate a depressive disorder in 22% of 88 epilepsy patients identified from general practices in the United Kingdom. In a population-based survey that investigated a life-time prevalence of depression, epilepsy, diabetes, and asthma in close to 181,000 individuals, Blum et al. found that among the 2281 patients with epilepsy, 29% reported having experienced at least one episode of depression.[5] This contrasted with 8.7% prevalence in healthy respondents and with 17% and 16% in patients with diabetes and asthma, respectively. It is worth noticing the lack of gender difference in the prevalence rates of depression among patients with epilepsy. Additionally, 9.8% of these patients reported symptoms of manic-depressive illness.

No one doubts the higher prevalence in patients with epilepsy compared to healthy controls; however, there is an ongoing debate as to whether depression is more frequent among patients with epilepsy than in patients with other neurologic disorders. In fact, four controlled studies comparing the prevalence of depression between patients with epilepsy and other neurologic diseases, including traumatic brain injury, neuromuscular diseases, and multiple sclerosis failed to demonstrate any difference in the rates of depression[6–9,18,19,22,23]; although, in general, both groups seem to be at increased risk for depression compared to healthy controls. On the other hand, three controlled studies argue that epileptics have a higher rate of depression than patients with nonepileptic neurologic diseases.[10–12,18,24,25] In a review of the literature, Dodrill and Batzel examined the prevalence rates of depression among patients with epilepsy, with neurologic (other than epilepsy) and nonneurologic illness and discovered increased rates of depression in epileptics as compared with nonneurologic disorders, but equivalent rates of depression in epilepsy and neurologic disorders.[13,19]

The comorbidity of depression in patients with epilepsy is of concern, given its association with an increased risk of suicidality among these patients. In a review of the literature, Gilliam and Kanner concluded that suicide has one of the highest standardized mortality rates (SMR) of all causes of death in persons with epilepsy.[14,26] In a review of 17 studies pertaining to mortality in epilepsy, Robertson found that suicide was 10 times more frequent than in the general population.[15,27] Similarly, Rafnsson et al.[16] reported the results of a population-based incidence cohort study from Iceland, which also showed that suicide had the highest SMR (5.8) of all causes of death. A Swedish study reported an SMR of 3.5 among 9000 previously hospitalized patients with epilepsy.[17,29] These results have not been replicated in other population-based studies, however. Hauser et al.,[18,] in a population-based study, found only 3 suicides, which did not exceed the expected figure. In another population study, from the United Kingdom, Cockerell et al.[19] reported only 1 suicide during follow up of 6.9 (median) years.

The Different Clinical Presentations of Depression in Epilepsy

Patients with epilepsy can suffer from forms of DD identical to those experienced by nonepileptic patients. However, a review of the literature of DD in epilepsy clearly reveals an atypical clinical presentation in a significant percentage of patients that fail to meet any of the Diagnostic and Statistical Manual (DSM) (be it III, III-R, or IV) axis I categories.[20] Recently, we have argued that DD in many patients with epilepsy is in fact different from that of nonepileptic patients.[21,118]

To understand the different clinical expressions of symptoms of depression and DD better, they have to be classified according to their temporal relation to seizure occurrence. Thus, symptoms can be recognized prior to the onset of seizures (preictal period), following seizures (during the postictal period, which may include time periods of up to 120 hours following the seizure), as an expression of the actual seizure (ictal depression) and completely unrelated to the seizure occurrence, that is, interictally.[1] As shown below, patients may experience symptoms of depression during periictal and interictal periods.

Symptoms that precede or follow seizures are referred to as periictal symptoms, are often unrecognized by clinicians, which accounts for the scarcity of data regarding their prevalence and response to treatment.

Depression During Periictal Periods: Don't Ask and They Won't Tell!

Preictal symptoms of depression generally manifest as a cluster of dysphoric symptoms for hours or even 1–3 days prior to the onset of a seizure. In one study, Blanchet and Frommer[22] examined mood changes over 56 days in 27 patients who were asked to rate their mood on a daily basis. These ratings pointed to symptoms of dysphoria, anxiety, and irritability 3 days prior to a seizure in 22 patients. Changes in mood were more significant during the 24 hours preceding the seizure. In children, these dysphoric moods typically declare as irritability, poor frustration tolerance, and aggressive behavior.

Ictal symptoms of depression are the clinical manifestation of a simple partial seizure. Estimates suggest that psychiatric symptoms occur in 25% of "auras," with 15% of these involving affect or mood changes.[23–25,119–123] Ictal depression, for instance, ranked second in one study[25,123] after anxiety/fear as the most common type of ictal affect. Occasionally, mood changes signify the only clinical expression of simple partial seizures, and therefore may be difficult to identify as epileptic phenomena. They are usually brief, stereotypical, develop out of context, and are affiliated with other ictal phenomena. Feelings of anhedonia (inability to experience pleasure in anything), guilt, and suicidal ideation represent the most prevalent symptoms. More often, however, ictal symptoms of depression are followed by an alteration of consciousness as the ictus advances from a simple to a complex partial seizure.

Postictal symptoms of depression have been identified for quite some time, but have been studied in a systematic manner in only one study.[26] Indeed, in a study at the Rush Epilepsy Center we investigated the prevalence and clinical characteristics of postictal symptoms of depression, anxiety, psychosis, hypomania, neurovegetative and cognitive symptoms in 100 consecutive patients with poorly controlled partial seizure disorders. Symptoms were identified with a 42-item questionnaire. The postictal period was defined as the 72 hours that followed recovery of consciousness from a seizure or cluster of seizures. The questions on depressive symptoms were intended to target symptoms of anhedonia, irritability, poor frustration tolerance, feelings of hopelessness and helplessness, suicidal ideation, feelings of guilt and self-deprecation, and crying bouts. Five neurovegetative symptoms including changes in patterns of sleep and appetite and in sexual drive and postictal fatigue were investigated but were not classified as symptoms of depression, since they are common postictal symptoms, and we did not want to falsely increase the prevalence of postictal symptoms of depression. Only those symptoms identified by patients during the postictal period *following more than 50% of their seizures* were made subject to analysis, which insured that we were targeting postictal symptoms of repeated

occurrence. We approximated the typical duration of each symptom, identified the symptoms that were *also* occurring during the interictal period, and compared their severity during interictal versus postictal periods.

Forty-three patients (47%) experienced a median of 5 postictal symptoms of habitual depression (range: 2–9). Two-thirds of symptoms had a median duration of 24 hours or longer. Thirty-five patients reported at least two postictal symptoms with a minimum duration of 24 hours, and 13 of these patients experienced at least 7 symptoms clustered to mimic symptoms of a major depression spanning 24 hours or longer.

We identified *postictal suicidal ideation* in 13 patients. Eight patients experienced passive and active suicidal thoughts, while five only reported passive suicidal ideation. Ten of these 13 patients (77%) had a past history of either major depression or bipolar disorder and this association was highly significant. Furthermore, the presence of postictal suicidal ideation was also significantly associated with a history of psychiatric hospitalization. Clearly, the presence of postictal suicidal ideation should alert the clinician on the existence of a current or past serious history of depression.

Postictal symptoms of depression often occurred with other psychiatric symptoms. In 23 patients we identified comorbid postictal symptoms of anxiety ($n = 23$) and in seven patients a combination of postictal symptoms of depression, psychosis, and anxiety. Also worth noting is the significant association between the presence of postictal depressive symptoms and greater postictal cognitive deficits. Clearly, postictal depressive symptoms seem to be fairly frequent in a sample of patients with poorly controlled epilepsy. Whether this is applicable to patients with rare seizures remains to be investigated. A few studies have argued that adverse life events may be associated with the presence of postictal depression; however, this suggestion is still unconfirmed.[27,28,130,131]

Clearly, postictal symptoms of depression are relatively frequent in patients with refractory epilepsy. Yet, despite this high prevalence, postictal symptoms of depression continue to be ignored. Typically, in the course of an evaluation clinicians inquire about postictal cognitive changes, motor deficits or headaches, and yet rarely ask about the presence of postictal psychiatric symptoms. Interestingly, of our 100 patients just 14% presented exclusively with cognitive deficits postictally.

The Different Expressions of Interictal Depression in Epilepsy

The *most commonly recognized* manifestation of affective disorders among patients with epilepsy is interictal depression.[1] As previously stated, DD may be identical to any of the mood disorders detailed in the DSM-IV classification (i.e., major depression [MDD], dysthymic [DyD], bipolar disorder [BPD], and so on). Referral to psychiatrists is typically initiated when a DD presents as a severe MDD; however, many cases of interictal DD fail to meet criteria of any of the DSM-IV affective disorders.[1,20] Mendez et al., for instance, found that 50% of depressive episodes identified in their study had to be classified as atypical depression, according to DSM-III criteria.[29]

It is our judgment, and that of others, that interictal depression in epileptics most frequently manifests as a pleomorphic cluster of symptoms of depression, irritability, anxiety, and neurovegetative symptoms with a chronic course that is interrupted by recurrent symptom-free periods of hours to several days duration. This mode of presentation of DD bears the closest resemblance to a dysthymic disorder; therefore, we have referred to it as dysthymic-like disorder of epilepsy (DLDE). In a study of 97 consecutive patients with a DD of enough severity to warrant pharmacotherapy, we found DLDE in 69 (70%) patients.[30] Further, we found that the failure to meet DSM-IV criteria of dysthymic disorder was due to the interrupted course of these symptoms. Overall, the potency of these DD was milder than that of a MDD; however, they were the cause of sizable disruptions in patients' daily activities, social relations, and quality of life.

In 1923, Kraepelin had published a description of interictal DD in epileptic patients suggesting the pleomorphic nature of its semiology.[31] Six decades later, Blumer expanded on Kraepelin observations and coined the term *interictal dysphoric disorder* (IDD) to refer to this type of DD.[31] Blumer suggested that IDD consist of the following eight affective-somatoform symptoms: irritability, depressive moods, anergia, insomnia, pains, anxiety, phobic fears, and euphoric moods presenting intermittently. In his opinion, the presence of three symptoms was sufficient to be associated with significant disability. IDD tend to develop 2 years or longer following the onset of epilepsy. Nearly one-third to one-half of patients with epilepsy seeking medical care suffer from IDD of sufficient degree to warrant pharmacologic treatment.

Depression in epilepsy has received scant attention from both patients and physicians and thus its timely diagnosis and treatment have generally been neglected. For example, in the study cited above, 60 of our 97 patients presented a depressive disorder of more than 1-year duration. Only one-third of these 60 patients had been treated within 6 months of the onset of their symptoms. The same proportion of patients with chronic MDD and DLDE failed to be started on AD for more than 1 year; therefore, the severity of the depressive disorder did not contribute to the delay in recognizing the need for therapy.[30]

Unless clinicians inquire about depressive symptoms *as an integral part of their evaluation of the seizure disorder*, these DD will continue to go undetected. The best available method for making an appropriate and early diagnosis continues to be a carefully obtained clinical history and patients need not present a full-blown MDD before therapy has to be considered. Also, the process of identification of depression cannot be restricted to the completion of a rating scale. We must recall that there are no specific diagnostic instruments developed for depression in epilepsy and the available rating scales and other standard diagnostic instruments were developed for DD in nonepileptic patients. Some of the often used scales in depression, such as the Hamilton scale for depression,[33,135] fail to ask about symptoms of irritability, which is very common in DLDE. The Beck depression inventory[34,136] may be a useful diagnostic tool for screening and identifying symptomatic patients in the office setting, but patients with "high" scores should undergo a more extensive and detailed evaluation.

Impact of Depression in Quality of Life

Depressive disorders have a significant negative impact on the quality of life of patients with epilepsy. For example, while investigating 56 consecutive patients with temporal lobe epilepsy (TLE), Lehrner et al.[35] measured health-related quality of life (HRQOL) and depression. Depression was shown to be the most powerful predictor for each domain of HRQOL. Even after controlling for seizure frequency and severity, and other psychosocial variables, there remained a significant association of depression with HRQOL. Another investigation of 257 epilepsy patients to identify the relationship of neuropsychologic function to HRQOL was conducted by Perrine et al.[36]. Mood, verbal memory, psychomotor function, visual-spatial functions, language, and cognitive inhibition, were some of the independent neuropsychologic variables included. The mood factor had the highest correlation with scales of the quality of life in epilepsy inventory-89 (QOLIE-89) and was the strongest predictor of quality of life in regression analyses. The mood factor was responsible for 46% of the variance in overall quality of life.

Likewise, studying a group of 125 patients more than 1 year after temporal lobe surgery, Gilliam et al. showed that mood status was the most significant predictor of the patients' assessment of their own health status.[37] Thus, these findings further suggest the significance of mood disorders in the subjective health status and quality of life of patients with epilepsy. In another investigation, Gilliamet al. examined the variables responsible for poor quality of life identified with the QOLIE-89 in 194 adult patients with refractory partial epilepsy,[38] and concluded that the only independent variables significantly related to poor quality of life scores on the QOLIE-89 summary score were high levels of depression and neurotoxicity from antiepileptic drugs (AEDs). Patients had a median 9.7 seizures/month (range: 0.3–51), but the authors saw no relationship between the type and or the frequency of seizures. Therefore, depression is one of the most important variables to have an impact on the quality of life in patients with refractory epilepsy, even greater than the seizure frequency and severity.

A Bidirectional Relationship between Depression and Epilepsy

Epilepsy as a Risk Factor for Depression

As already stated in our section on epidemiologic aspects of depression in epilepsy, depression is four to five times more frequent in these patients than in the general population, and rates of suicide are five times greater. Certain researchers have argued that 20% patients with TLE become depressed, while upward of 62% of patients with intractable complex partial seizures have had a history of a depressive episode, which, at times, may be recurrent.[39,40,13,14] In population-based studies, the frequency of mood disorders is lower, as shown in the study by Jacoby et al. cited in our introduction, who found a prevalence of depression of 10% among patients with less than one seizure/month, 21% in those whose seizure frequency was >1/month, and 4% in seizure-free patients, which is comparable to the incidence rate in the general population.[2]

Differences in the methodology used to target psychiatric symptomatology and to select the type of patient populations studied are responsible for the different prevalence rates cited in the literature. For instance, some researchers assessed data based on self-rating scales or personality inventories, while others obtained data from standardized psychiatric interviews. Most studies were conducted in specialty centers, because these tend to draw patients with more severe epileptic disorders, and thus more frequently report a higher prevalence of psychopathology. Results extracted from these studies cannot be generalized to all epileptic patients; however, there is still a consensus that depression is more prevalent among patients with poorly controlled seizures. The therapeutic implications of these conclusions are rigorously examined below.

History of Depression Preceding a Seizure Disorder

Twenty-six centuries ago, Hippocrates was the first one to suggest a bidirectional relationship between epilepsy and depression when he wrote: *"melancholics ordinarily become epileptics, and epileptics melancholics: what determines the preference is the direction the malady takes; if it bears upon the body, epilepsy, if upon the intelligence, melancholy."*[41,17] This 2600-year-old observation has been supported by three population-based controlled studies published in the past 10 years. Forsgren and Nystrom conducted a population-based, case-control study of patients with newly diagnosed onset epilepsy in Sweden, and discovered patients were seven times more likely to exhibit a history of depression than were controls. The history of depression was 17 times more prevalent among patients than controls when analyzes targeted patients with partial seizure disorders.[42] Hesdorffer et al.[43] conducted a second population-based, case-control investigation of the prevalence of new onset epilepsy among adults aged 55 and older, and showed that compared to controls, patients were 3.7 more likely to have had a history of depression prior to their first seizure. Unlike Forsgren and Nystrom, these authors controlled for medical therapies of depression. The same authors conducted similar research in Iceland, and found that depression (meeting DSM-IV criteria) was four times more frequent among

epileptic children than among controls matched for age and gender.[44,20,21]

From these findings, can it be hypothesized that depression is a risk for epilepsy and vice versa? Do any studies support a bidirectional interaction between epilepsy and depression? Are there any data that reflect both types of disorders sharing common pathogenic mechanisms? For example, are the same neurotransmitters affected in depression and epilepsy, which in turn, may explain the therapeutic effect of AEDs in the management of patients with affective disorders?[45,22] These questions will be explored in the following section.

Neurotransmitter Dysfunction in Epilepsy and Depression: Is there a Common Link?

The critical pathogenic mechanisms of depression have been identified as abnormal serotonergic, noradrenergic, dopaminergic, and GABAergic functions, and have provided the basis for antidepressant pharmacologic treatments.[46,23] Interestingly, a decreased activity of these same neurotransmitters has been demonstrated to contribute to the kindling process of seizure foci, to worsen seizure severity, and heighten seizure predisposition in some animal models of epilepsy.[47,24] Therefore, it is very likely that parallel changes of serotonin (5HT), noradrenaline (NE), dopamine (DA), and gamma-aminobutyric acid (GABA) may be working factors in the pathophysiology of DD and epilepsy. The monoamine hypothesis of depression will not be reviewed in this article.

The Role of Neurotransmitters in Animal Models of Epilepsy

The role of 5HT and NE in the pathogenic mechanisms of epilepsy has been investigated in various animal models of epilepsy, but it has been with two strains of genetic epilepsy prone rats (GEPR, GEPR-3, and GEPR-9) that the pathogenic role of NE and 5HT has been shown in a compelling manner.[47] Indeed, both strains of rats show inherent noradrenergic and serotonergic pre- and postsynaptic transmission deficits, which have been related to the predisposition to suffer from seizures. It is worth noting that GEPR-9s rats have a more significant NE transmission deficit and, in turn, exhibit more severe seizures than GEPR-3 rats.[47,40] Increments of either NE and/or 5HT transmission can halt seizure occurrence, while reduction will stimulate the opposite effect. Utilization of selective serotonin-reuptake inhibitors (SSRIs) and monoamino-oxidase inhibitors (MAOIs) has produced anticonvulsant effects in genetically prone epilepsy mice and baboons and in (non-genetically prone) cats, rabbits, and rhesus monkeys.[48–52,45]

The role of 5HT and NE in epilepsy can also be appreciated from research on the effect of AED on these two neurotransmitters. For example, carbamazepine (CBZ), lamotrigine (LTG), zonisamide (ZNS), valproic acid (VPA) have been shown to increase synaptic secretion of 5HT,[47,24] while LTG has been shown to block the synaptic reuptake of NE in rats.[53,47] In GEPRs, the anticonvulsant effect of CBZ can be prevented with 5HT depleting drugs[54,46]; however, AEDs that do not cause a release of 5HT, such as phenytoin (PHT), cannot replicate this result.

Furthermore, it has been argued that the anticonvulsant protection of the vagal nerve stimulator (VNS) could be partially mediated by the activation of monoaminergic transmission. VNS, in fact, has been shown to activate the locus coeruleus in the rat.[55,59] The anticonvulsant effect in the rat of VNS versus electroshock or pentylenetetrazol-induced seizures can be halted or significantly reduced by deletion of noradrenergic and serotonergic neurons.[56,60] Additionally, the antidepressant results of the VNS may be caused by its effect on the locus coeruleus.

Some Observations on the Role of 5HT and NE in Humans with Epilepsy

An increase in the prevalence and severity of seizures in epileptic patients has been related to depletion of monoamines with reserpine.[57,58,48,49]

Similarly, the use of reserpine in patients with schizophrenia at doses of 2–10 mg/day was demonstrated to lessen the electroshock seizure threshold and the severity of the proceeding seizures.[59–61]

The anticonvulsant effect of antidepressant drugs in humans is much less obvious than that shown in the animal models of epilepsy; however, certain data are worth citing. In a double-blind placebo-controlled study, imipramine, a tricyclic antidepressant (TCA) with reuptake inhibitory effects of NE and 5HT was demonstrated to suppress absence and myoclonic seizures.[62–64,54–56] In open trials, Ojemann et al. found a lessened seizure frequency of patients while on doxepin, trazodone, and desipramine,[65] and similarly, Favale et al. showed a seizure frequency reduction following the introduction of fluoxetine in an open study.[66]

Structural and Functional Abnormalities in Major Depression: Common Pathogenic Mechanisms to Epilepsy?

Mood disorders and certain types of epileptic syndromes are associated with structural and functional neuroimaging abnormalities of common neuroanatomic structures. With prevalence rates ranging from 19 to 65% in various patient series, depression has been recognized most often in patients with seizures of temporal and frontal lobe origin, such as seizures involving the limbic circuit, and these rates are greater than those of patients with generalized seizure disorders. For instance, Perini et al., found that patients with TLE have a greater prevalence of affective and personality disorders than patients with both, Juvenile Myoclonic Epilepsy (JME) and diabetes.[67] Additionally, patients with auras consisting of psychic symptoms (i.e., involving limbic structures) tend to have a greater prevalence of depression than patients with partial seizures without auras or whose auras consist of motor or sensory symptoms.[68,70] We will review these data in this section.

Hippocampal Atrophy

Temporal lobe epilepsy is the most frequent type of epilepsy among adults and the most frequent cause of epilepsy refractory to AEDs.[69] In 75–80% of patients with TLE, mesial structures (amygdala, hippocampal formation, entorhinal cortex, parahippocampal gyrus) are the site of the epileptogenic area[69,70] and hippocampal atrophy caused by mesial temporal sclerosis is the most frequent cause of TLE. By the same token, the prevalence of depression has been found to be significantly higher among patients with epilepsy that involve mesial temporal structures. For example, Gilliam et al.[71] produced some of the most persuasive results documenting the relationship between severity of depression and temporal lobe dysfunction. They conducted proton magnetic resonance spectroscopy (1HMRS) of the temporal lobes in 33 patients with refractory TLE, with a mean age of 35 years and a mean age of seizure onset of 15 years. Severity of 1HMRS correlated significantly with depression. In a study of 60 patients with TLE, Quiske et al. found that patients with mesial temporal sclerosis had significantly higher depression scores on the Beck depression inventory than other patients.[72] Furthermore, Schmitz et al. found that higher Beck depression inventory scores were correlated with decreased temporal lobe and frontal lobe perfusion on ^{99m}Tc-HMPAO SPECT scans in a study of 40 patients with TLE.[73]

In the last decade, functional and structural abnormalities have been identified in patients with MDD. Sheline et al. were among the initial researchers to demonstrate the existence of bilateral hippocampal atrophy in an analysis of 10 patients with recurrent MDD in remission.[74] They also showed that the total number of days depressed was corollary to the number of large ($\geq$4.5 mm in diameter) hippocampal low signal foci. Further, their results showed a significant inverse correlation between the duration of depression and left hippocampal volume; and therefore, the hippocampal atrophy was more typically recognized in patients with a more chronic and active disease. A larger investigation of 24 patients with remitted MDD compared to matched controls for age, sex, and height produced similar findings,[75,76] showing that the amygdala core nuclei volumes correlated with hippocampal volumes. Likewise, in a comparison of hippocampal volumes of 20 patients with treatment-resistant MDD to 20 patients that responded to therapy and 20 healthy controls, Shah et al. found that patients with treatment-resistant MDD were more likely to show hippocampal atrophy.[77]

Lower verbal memory scores proved a functional consequence of hippocampal damage. MacQueen et al. compared hippocampal volumes and hippocampal-dependent memory tests between 20 patients with an untreated first episode and normal age-matched controls,[78] while identical comparisons were conducted between a second group of 17 patients with recurrent depressive episodes, matched controls, and the patients with a single depressive episode. Only patients with multiple episodes had hippocampal atrophy; however, patients with both single and multiple episodes had verbal memory deficits. Similar to Sheline's research, there was a sizable relationship between the time span of the depressive illness and the severity of hippocampal atrophy. The volume of hippocampal formation and entorhinal cortex between 30 patients with MDD and 47 matched controls was compared by Bell-McGinty et al., who reported an inverse relationship between the volumes of hippocampus and entorhinal cortex and the time since the initial lifetime depressive episodes.[79]

Recently, Posener et al. highlighted the need to study the shape of the hippocampus as well as the measurement of its volume, since studying shape can reveal structural changes even in the absence of decreased volume.[80] In a study that compared high dimensional brain mapping of 27 patients with MDD and 42 healthy controls, these authors produced 10 variables or components of the hippocampal shape. While finding no differences in hippocampal volumes between the two groups, they were able to find in depressed patients hippocampal deformation suggestive of specific involvement of the subiculum.

Changes in Amygdala

There exist less consistent data on the volumetric changes of amygdala of patients with MDD than those of hippocampal formation. An obvious reason for this is that the amygdala and its nuclei are technically much more difficult than that of hippocampal structures. Sheline et al. compared the total volume of amygdala and that of its core nuclei in 20 patients with a history of MDD, free of any neurologic disorder, and 20 matched controls.[81] The core volumes of amygdala nuclei were decreased bilaterally among patients, but not its total volume.

We should point out that magnitude of hippocampal atrophy is significantly greater in TLE caused by mesial temporal sclerosis than in MDD.[82] Furthermore, there is evidence to suggest that hippocampal atrophy in MDD may be reversible or prevented with SSRI therapy,[83] while such is not the case in TLE. These differences strongly suggest different pathogenic mechanisms mediating hippocampal and amygdala atrophy in these two disorders.

In mesial temporal sclerosis, neuropathologic findings consist of astrocytosis and neuronal cell loss most prominent in CA1 and CA3 and to a lesser degree the dentate gyrus and subiculum, as well as in amygdala entorhinal cortex and parahippocampal gyrus.[82] Unfortunately, there have been very few neuropathologic studies of the human hippocampal formation in patients with primary MDD. Lucassen et al. carried out a neuropathologic study of 15 hippocampi of patients with a history of MDD and compared them to those of 16 matched controls, and 9 steroid-treated patients (since high steroids are associated with hippocampal atrophy). In 11 of 15 depressed patients, rare but convincing apoptosis was identified in entorhinal cortex, subiculum, dentate gyrus, CA1 and CA4. Apoptosis was also found in three steroid-treated patients and one control. However, no apoptosis of pyramidal cells in CA3 was identified.[84]

Sheline et al. verified the therapeutic impact of antidepressants in a recent analysis of 38 female outpatients with a history of MDD.[83] A significant relationship was demonstrated between reduction in hippocampal volume and the duration of untreated depression. However, hippocampal volume loss showed no correlation to the duration of time depressed while taking antidepressant medication or with lifetime exposure to antidepressants; therefore, these results may offer that antidepressants can have a neuroprotective effect during depression.

Bowley et al. conducted a neuropathologic investigation of amygdala and entorhinal cortex, performing a neuronal and glial cell count in brains from 7 patients with MDD, 10 with BPD, and 12 control cases.[85] There was a sizable reduction of glial cells and of the glial/neurons ratio in left amygdala, and to a lesser degree in the left entorhinal cortex, in the specimens of MDD patients and those of patients with BPD not treated with lithium and VPA.

Structural and Functional Abnormalities in Frontal Lobes

Frontal lobe epilepsy has also been associated with a higher prevalence of depression, not unlike TLE. This is not surprising given that the inferior frontal cortex is the main target of the meso-limbic dopaminergic neurons and gives input to the serotonergic neurons of the dorsal raphe nucleus. Thus, it appears that frontal lobe dysfunction may be related to a deficit in the serotonergic transmission, which can predispose to depression. In fact, functional disturbances of frontal lobe structures have been recognized in TLE and particularly among patients with TLE and comorbid depression, as they have been found to have bilateral reduction in infero-frontal metabolism.[86–95] Likewise, neuropsychologic testing with the Wisconsin Card Sorting Test, which is highly sensitive to executive dysfunction, has revealed poor performance in patients with TLE and comorbid depression.[91,92]

Functional neuroimaging and neuropsychologic research has identified the role of frontal lobes in primary depression.[96–98] Structural changes in certain structures of the frontal lobes including the prefrontal cortex, cingulate gyrus as well as in their white matter have been examined in various studies. Bremner et al. analyzed the volume of orbito-frontal cortex and other frontal cortical regions of 15 patients with MDD in remission versus 20 controls and found that patients with depression had notably smaller orbito-frontal cortical volumes.[99] Similarly, Coffey et al. identified smaller frontal lobe volumes in 48 inpatients with severe depression that had been referred for electroshock therapy compared to 76 controls.[100]

Likewise, neuropathologic research has noted structural cortical changes in frontal lobes of depressed patients. Rajkowska et al. found decreases in cortical thickness, neuronal sizes, and neuronal densities in layers II, III, and IV of the rostral orbito-frontal region in the brains of depressed patients.[101] There were sizable reductions in glial densities in cortical layers V and VI in the caudal orbito-frontal cortex that were also correlated with a lessoning of neuronal sizes. Lastly, the dorsolateral prefrontal cortex showed a decrease in neuronal and glial density and size in all cortical layers.

In elderly patients with depression, structural changes that have been noted deserve a brief review. Lai et al. found smaller bilateral orbito-frontal cortex volumes in 20 elderly patients with MDD than 20 matched controls.[102] Also, Taylor et al. reported smaller orbito-frontal cortex volumes in 41 elderly patients with MDD than 40 controls.[103] Additionally, these authors found that decreased volumes were independently associated with cognitive impairment.[104] In a study by Kumar et al., the magnitude of prefrontal volume changes was related to the severity of the depression, as elderly patients with MDD had greater changes than those with minor depression.[105]

Other Pathogenic Mechanisms of Depression in Epilepsy

A Genetic Predisposition

In patients without epilepsy, the most common risk to develop a depressive disorder is a family history of depression, and in turn, a family history of depression was typical among depressed patients with epilepsy. In fact, over 50% of epileptic patients suffering from depression have been found to show a family history of psychiatric illness, affective disorders being the most frequent condition.[106] Patients with epilepsy and MDD appear to be unipolar and to have a genetic predisposition comparable to that of primary or idiopathic affective disorder.[106,107]

Laterality of the Seizure Focus?

Despite having been raised as a potential pathogenic parameter, the question of the relevance of the laterality of the seizure focus remains a topic of debate. Certain authors suggest that a left hemispheric focus may be a predisposing factor of depression.[108,109] Functional neuroimaging research conducted with positron emission tomography (PET) and single photon emission tomography (SPECT) investigations have found lower metabolism and blood flow, respectively, in the left than right hemisphere in patients with partial epilepsy and a history of interictal depression.[110]

Depression as an Iatrogenic Process

Every AED, including those with positive psychotropic properties can trigger psychiatric symptoms in epileptic patients, some with a greater severity than others.[111,112] Phenobarbital can result in depression that may occasionally be related to the presence of suicidal ideation and of suicidal and parasuicidal behavior. Other AED reported to often trigger symptoms of depression include primidone,[96] tiagabine, vigabatrin,[98] felbamate,[99] topiramate, levetiracetam, and ZNS.[113–120]

Identifying any current or prior DD may have an important effect on the threat of developing adverse cognitive events when exposed to topiramate. In fact, cognitive adverse events were reported by 41% of 592 patients in a study on tropimate (TPM) polytherapy[119]; a history of DD was a significant predictor of these cognitive adverse events.

Depression Following Epilepsy Surgery

In the last two decades, there have been a growing number of reports of DD following an antero-temporal lobectomy.[121] It is common for patients to exhibit "mood lability" within the first 6 weeks after surgery, and usually these symptoms subside; however, overt depressive symptoms become clear within the initial 6 months in up to 30% of patients. Typically, symptoms of depression range in caliber from mild to very severe, including suicidal attempts. In general, pharmacologic treatment with antidepressant drugs is effective.[122] Patients with a past depressive history are at increased risk, and it should be noted that this risk is independent of the postsurgical control of seizures. Thus, all patients preparing for epilepsy surgery should be warned of this possible risk, prior to surgery.

A paradoxical "iatrogenic" cause of psychopathology among epileptic patients includes the phenomenon of "Forced Normalization," which consists of the development of psychiatric disorders following the cessation of epileptic seizures.[123] An interictal depression, therefore, may exacerbate or present de novo in patients as increased seizure control is attained; although, the frequency of this phenomenon remains to be established.

Psychosocial Causes of Depression

Patients with epilepsy have to confront and manage on a daily basis many psychosocial factors and obstacles. These include: (1) the patient's inability to accept and adjust to his condition.[124–128] (2) The stigma related to the diagnosis of epilepsy and the well-known discrimination patients face. (3) The lack of control in one's life resulting from the unpredictable occurrence of epileptic seizures.[129] (4) The patient's lack of social support, and the need to make major adjustments in life-style, such as giving-up driving privileges, or changing jobs to maximize seizure precautions.[130–134] Any one or combination of these factors could result in an *initial* adjustment reaction with depressive and anxiety features, but they are unlikely *on their own* to result in *chronic* DD. Also, patients displaying comorbid DD may have less ability to cope with these obstacles. Additionally, even epileptic patients with a normal intelligence have been found to show a lower degree of flexibility of mental processing compared with normal controls in neuropsychologic studies.[135,136]

For many years, clinicians and patients have, unfortunately, attributed and explained their patients' depressed mood as a "normal reaction" to the numerous social and personal obstacles resulting from epilepsy. As previously stated, however, an initial "reactive" episode is usually self-limited in time. Therefore, a depressed state that persists after several months can no longer be diagnosed from a clinical standpoint as a "normal" reactive process and warrants a detailed psychiatric evaluation.

Extensive research has been conducted on the evolution from a state of chronic stress to a DD. It has been suggested by several animal models of depression that the evolution of depressive symptoms proceeding a "chronic stress" paradigm can help demonstrate how exposure to random and repeated obstacles (akin to the pattern of seizure occurrence) can eventually lead to a depressive disorder in animals and probably in humans, as well.[137] Willner et al. illustrated the Chronic Mild Stress of Depression model, which is developed from applications of various random, stressful conditions to rats, including mild uncontrollable foot shock, forced swimming in cold water, changes in housing conditions, food and water deprivation, reversal of light/dark periods, and exposure to noise and bright light.[138] Proceeding 2–3 weeks of exposure to these stressors, the rats began exhibiting behavioral changes, including: (1) reduced open field activity; (2) a reduced sensitivity to rewards, such as a decrease in the consumption of sucrose solution, and (3) sleep alterations, including a decreased latency to the first REM period (a biologic marker of depression in humans). These behavior alterations continued for months and were seen as the equivalent of depressive symptoms, and logically, thus improved after treatment with antidepressant drugs.

Therefore, it is imperative that we move away from the idea that mood disorders are a "normal" phenomenon that require no treatment, even if we continue to explain the presence of a mood disorder as a "reactive" process to adverse events. If in addition to the impact of the exposure to chronic stress we take into account the behavioral consequences of the neurotransmitter changes related to the epileptic process, it could follow that seizure disorders involving limbic structures can *contribute* to the development of mood disorders.

Treatment of Depression in Epilepsy

Despite its relatively high prevalence, the treatment of depression in epilepsy is still "unexplored territory." In fact, the *untested* assumption "that patients with depression and epilepsy should respond to antidepressant drugs in the same manner as depressed nonepileptic patients" has been the basis for the treatment of these patients. Surprisingly, there has only been *one* double-blind placebo-controlled study, published in 1979, that compared the effectiveness of mianserin (which is no longer available in the United States), amytriptyline, and a placebo in epileptic patients with a MDD.[139]

It seems somewhat incredible that psychiatrists or neurologists, given the atypical clinical presentation of depression in a large number of patients, have not questioned the need to evaluate its management in a more scientific manner. This issue is further complicated by a certain level of reluctance to use psychotropic drugs in these patients, because of the reported "epileptogenic potential" of several antidepressants.[140–143]

The following causes of a depressive episode should be ruled out before beginning a patient's antidepressant drug (AD) therapy. (1) The depressive episode occurred after the discontinuation of an AED with mood-stabilizing properties such as CBZ, VPA, or LTG.[144] In this instance, reintroduction of that AED or of another mood-stabilizing agent may be enough

to reach a euthymic state. (2) The depressive episode occurred after the introduction or dose increment of an AED with known negative psychotropic properties. In these cases, lowering of the dose or discontinuation of the AED should facilitate symptom remission. However, if the AED has produced the most effective seizure control to date, clinicians may treat the depressive disorder symptomatically. Indeed, the triggering of a depressive episode by an AED with negative psychotropic properties, like phenobarbital, primidone, topiramate, and levetiracetam, can be counteracted with an AD. These patients are often treated with a SSRI, such as sertraline or paroxetine, for the depressive episode.

The variables related to a heightened risk of seizure development proceeding exposure to AD in nonepileptic patients include: (1) high plasma serum concentrations. In fact, there are no reports in the literature of TCA-induced seizures at therapeutic plasma concentration. Patients developing drug-induced seizures after ingesting therapeutic doses of TCA have been shown to be slow metabolizers of these drugs; (2) rapid dose increments; (3) the existence of other drugs with proconvulsant effects; and (4) the presence of CNS pathology, abnormal EEG, and personal and family history of epilepsy.[140–143] Therefore, patients should begin with low doses in small increments until the attainment of the objective clinical response, thereby minimizing the risk of producing and/or worsening seizures.

The actual threat of AD exacerbating seizures in epileptic patients is small, however, and should not slow or prevent the start of therapy. In a study at the Rush Epilepsy Center, sertraline was reported to *definitely* worsen seizures in just 1 out of 100 patients,[30] while in another 5 patients, a transient increment in seizure frequency was linked to this AD with a likely, but not definite, causality. Four of these five patients continued with sertraline therapy, and following an adjustment in the dose of their AED, no further seizure exacerbation was presented by any of these patients. Additionally, Blumer and

Zielinski have demonstrated the use of TCA alone and TCA in combination with SSRI in epileptic patients without a worsening of seizure.[40] Nonepileptic patients are not known to experience seizures from MAO-I. The antidepressant drugs with the severest proconvulsant effects are bupropion, maprotiline, and amoxapine, and should not be used to treat epileptic patients.[143,145]

Pharmacokinetic Interactions between AD and AED

Most AD are metabolized in the liver and their metabolism is hastened in the presence of AED with enzyme-inducing properties which include PHT, CBZ, phenobarbital, primidone, and topiramate and oxcarbazepine at high doses. This pharmacokinetic effect is not seen with the new AED such as gabapentin, LTG, though topiramate and oxcarbazepine can produce a mild inducing effect on liver enzymes. The dose of AD may need to be adjusted as needed. Conversely, certain AD may alter AED metabolism. Specifically, several AD of the SSRI family are inhibitors of one or more isoenzymes of the cytochrome P450 system. These include fluoxetine, paroxetine, and fluvoxamine and to a lesser degree, sertraline.[147–149] Citalopram, however, does not have pharmacokinetic interactions with AED.

Choice of AD

Before starting any AD, clinicians must be fully aware of whether their patient's depressive episode is part of a bipolar disease, as the introduction of such drugs may trigger a manic or hypomanic episode in these patients, and worsen the course of the bipolar disorder in the long term, particularly in those patients with rapid-cycling bipolar disease.[150] In patients with bipolar disease, a mood-stabilizing agent should be the first-line treatment. However, given the potential adverse events of lithium in patients with epilepsy, clinicians should consider the use of AEDs with mood-stabilizing properties such as LTG, which has been shown to have antidepressant properties in bipolar disease,[151–154] CBZ, or VPA.[151]

When the potential for adverse events of AD is being considered, the first-line treatment in depressed patients with epilepsy should be an SSRI. These are safe, regarding seizure propensity, are less likely to lead to death after an overdose, and have a favorable adverse effects profile. Additionally, positive results in dysthymic disorders and in symptoms of irritability and low frustration tolerance make this group of AD more appealing among patients with epilepsy. Citalopram or sertraline can be utilized as a first-line SSRI due to their minimal or absent pharmacokinetic interactions with AED.[155] Sertraline can be started at a daily dose of 25–50 mg, with 50 mg dosage increments at 3-week intervals until the desired therapeutic effects are achieved, a maximal dose of 200 mg/day has been reached, or negative effects begin to develop.

Recently, psychiatrists have argued for the use of AD with both, serotonergic and noradrenergic properties in the treatment of nonepileptic patients with depression.[155] At our center, we have conducted open trials with venlafaxine (Effexor), a reuptake inhibitor of NE and 5HT in patients with partial epilepsy and either dysthymic disorders or major depression. At doses ranging from 75 to 225 mg/day, we saw improvement in symptoms, including in patients that did not respond to trials with SSRIs, while none of the 76 patients treated experienced worsening of their seizures. However, these findings still need to be reproduced in double-blind placebo-controlled trials. Currently, this drug is being utilized as a first-line AD or if patients do not respond to SSRI.

The TCA produce strong clinical results, but the cardiotoxic effects and severe complications seen in overdoses render these drugs a second-line AD. Blumer has anecdotal reports of the utility of low dose TCA in patients with epilepsy and IDD.[32] In his research, he utilized TCA, usually imipramine at daily dosages of 100–150 mg. Additionally, Blumer has reported on the efficacy of "double-antidepressants" in depressed patients with epilepsy refractory to TCAs.[32] Also, he has noted that this is a rare clinical issue, even with low TCA dosages seen in ~15% of patients with an IDD.

Among other psychotropic drugs commonly used in the management of mood disorders special attention needs to be paid to the use of lithium when started in patients with epilepsy, as it is has been fraught with several problems.[156] These include changes in EEG recordings and proconvulsant properties at therapeutic serum concentrations in nonepileptic patients.[157] Lithium's neurotoxicity and related increase in seizure risk increases with the concurrent use of neuroleptic drugs, in the presence of EEG abnormalities and of a history of CNS disorder. Furthermore, lithium can be associated with neurotoxicity when given in combination with CBZ, even when the serum concentrations of both drugs are in the therapeutic range. This pharmacodynamic interaction presents as symptoms of dizziness, diplopia, blurred vision, and fatigue and requires the reduction in the dose of CBZ or a switch to another AED.

A well-kept secret in medicine is the safety on the use of electroconvulsive therapy (ECT) in patients with epilepsy: it is not contraindicated![158] ECT is worth considering in patients with epilepsy with very severe depression that fails to respond to AD, or in patients with rapid cycling bipolar disease that failed to respond to mood-stabilizing drugs.[157] Blackwood et al. found that the incidence of seizures in patients following treatment with ECT was no higher than in the general population.[158] In fact, several studies have shown that ECT increases seizure threshold by 50–100%.[159–165]

In addition to pharmacologic intervention, the value of psychotherapy for the treatment of depression in epileptic patients should not be overlooked. Counseling and psychotherapy can be very useful in helping the patient deal with the stressors and limitations of living with epilepsy. The type of psychotherapy used should be tailored to the individual patient's needs. Inclusion of the patient's family and significant others in the process may be of value.[166]

► CONCLUSION

Depression is a fairly frequent and important comorbidity of epilepsy that has a significant, adverse effect on the quality of life of these patients. The potential bidirectional relationship, or the existence of common pathogenic mechanisms, connecting these two disorders may also inform the efficacy of AEDs in the treatment of patients with affective disorders. We must explore whether the manifestation of depression is a "biologic marker" for a resistant epileptic seizure disorder, considering the data and given that a higher prevalence of depression has been consistently identified among patients with poorly controlled seizures.

Depression is under-identified and under-treated in epileptic patients. Not only are there little to no controlled data on the efficacy of pharmacologic and nonpharmacologic treatments, there are also many unfounded fears on the part of physicians to utilize psychotropic drugs in epileptic patients. A concerted and well-coordinated effort to develop research on the treatment of depression in epilepsy is overdue!

REFERENCES

1. Kanner AM, Balabanov A. Depression in Epilepsy: How closely related are these two disorders? *Neurology* 2002;58(Suppl 5):S27–S39.
2. Jacoby A, Baker GA, Steen N, et al. The clinical course of epilepsy and its psychosocial correlates: Findings from a U.K. Community study. Epilepsia 1996;37(2):148–161.
3. O'Donoghue MF, Goodridge DM, Redhead K, et al. Assessing the psychosocial consequences of epilepsy: A community-based study. *Br J Gen Pract* 1999;49(440):211–214.
4. Edeh J, Toone B. Relationship between interictal psychopathology and the type of epilepsy. Results of a survey in general practice. *Br J Psychiatry* 1987;151:95–101.
5. Blum D, Reed M, Metz A. Prevalence of major affective disorders and manic/hypomanic symptoms in persons with epilepsy: A community survey. *Neurology* 2002;(Suppl 3):A-175.

6. Indaco A, Carrieri P, Nappi C. Interictal depression in epilepsy. *Epilepsy Res* 1992;12:45–50.

7. Victoroff J, Benson F, Grafton S. Depression in complex partial seizures. Electroencephalography and cerebral metabolic correlates. *Arch Neurol* 1994;51:155–163.

8. Blumer D. Epilepsy and disorders of mood. In: Smith D, Treiman D, Trimble M (eds.), *Neurobehavioral Problems in Epilepsy*. New York: Raven Press, 1991, p. 185.

9. Robertson M. Depression in patients with epilepsy: An overview. *Sem Neurol* 1991;11:182–189.

10. Roy A. Some determinants of affective symptoms in epileptics. *Can J Psychiatry* 1979;24:554–556.

11. Altshuler L. Depression and epilepsy. In: Devinsky O, Theodore W (eds.), *Epilepsy and Behavior*. New York: Wiley-Liss, 1991, p. 47.

12. Dodrill C, Batzel L. Interictal behavioral features of patients with epilepsy. *Epilepsia* 1986;27:S64–S72.

13. Robertson M. Carbamazepine and depression. *Int Clin Psychopharmacol* 1987;2:23–35.

14. Gilliam F, Kanner AM. The treatment of depression in epilepsy. *Epilepsy* Behavior 2002;3:6.

15. Robertson MM. Suicide, parasuicide, and epilepsy. In: Engel J, Pedley TA (eds.), *Epilepsy: A Comprehensive Textbook*. Philadelphia, PA: Lippincott-Raven, 1997.

16. Rafnsson V, Olafsson E, Hauser WA, et al. Cause-specific mortality in adults with unprovoked seizures. A population-based incidence cohort study. *Neuroepidemiology* 2001;20(4):232–236.

17. Nilsson L, Tomson T, Farahmand BY, et al. Cause-specific mortality in epilepsy: A cohort study of more than 9,000 patients once hospitalized for epilepsy. Epilepsia 1997;38(10):1062–1068.

18. Hauser WA, Annegers JK, Elvenback IR. Mortality in patients with epilepsy. *Epilepsia.* 1980;21:399–412.

19. Cockerell OC, Johnson AL, Sander JWAS. Mortality from epilepsy: results from a prospective population-based study. *Lancet.* 1994;344:918–921.

20. *Diagnostic and Statistical Manual of Mental Disorders*, 4th ed. Washington, DC: American Psychiatric Press.

21. Kanner AM, Barry JJ. Depression and psychotic disorders associated with epilepsy: Are they unique? *Epilepsy Behav* 2001;2:170–186.

22. Blanchet P, Frommer GP. Mood change preceding epileptic seizures. *J Nerv Ment Dis* 1986;174:471–476.

23. Williams D. The structure of emotions reflected in epileptic experiences. *Brain* 1956;79:29–67.

24. Weil A. Depressive reactions associated with temporal lobe uncinate seizures. *J Nerv Ment Dis* 1955;121:505–510.

25. Daly D. Ictal affect. *Am J Psychiatry* 1958;115:97–108.

26. Kanner AM, Soto A, Gross-Kanner H. Prevalence and clinical characteristics of postictal psychiatric symptoms in partial epilepsy. *Neurology* 2004;62:708–713.

27. Hancock J, Bevilacqua A. Temporal lobe dysrhythmia and impulsive or suicidal behavior. *South Med J* 1971;64:1189–1193.

28. Anatassopoulos G, Kokkini D. Suicidal attempts in psychomotor epilepsy. *Behav Neuropsychiatry* 1969;1:11–16.

29. Mendez MF, Cummings J, Benson D, et al. Depression in epilepsy. Significance and phenomenology. *Arch Neurol* 1986;43:766–770.

30. Kanner AM, Kozak AM, Frey M. The use of sertraline in patients with epilepsy: Is it safe? *Epilepsy Behav* 2000;1(2):100–105.

31. Kraepelin E. Psychiatrie. Leipzig: Johann Ambrosius Barth, Vol. 3, 1923.

32. Blumer D, Altshuler LL. Affective disorders. In: Engel J, Pedley TA (eds.), Epilepsy: A Comprehensive Textbook. Philadelphia, PA: Lippincott-Raven, 1998, pp. 2083–2099.

33. Hamilton M. Development of a rating scale for primary depressive illness. *Br J Social Clin Psychol* 1967;6:278–269.

34. Beck AT, Ward CH, Mendelson M, et al. An inventory for measuring depression. *Arch Gen Psychiatry* 1961;4:561–571.

35. Lehrner J, Kalchmayr R, Serles W, et al. Health-related quality of life (HRQOL), activity of daily living (ADL) and depressive mood disorder in temporal lobe epilepsy patients. *Seizure* 1999;8(2):88–92.

36. Perrine K, Hermann BP, Meador KJ, et al. The relationship of neuropsychological functioning to quality of life in epilepsy [see comments]. *Arch Neurol* 1995;52(10):997–1003.

37. Gilliam F, Kuzniecky R, Faught E, et al. Patient-validated content of epilepsy-specific quality-of-life measurement. *Epilepsia* 1997;38(2):233–236.

38. Gilliam F. Optimizing health outcomes in active epilepsy. *Neurology* 2002;58(Suppl 5):S9–S19.

39. Currie S, Heathfield K, Henson R. Clinical course and prognosis of temporal lobe epilepsy. A survey of 666 patients. *Brain* 1971;92:173–190.

40. Blumer D, Zielinski J. Pharmacologic treatment of psychiatric disorders associated with epilepsy. *J Epilepsy* 1988;1:135–150.

41. Lewis A. Melancholia: A historical review. *J Mental Sci* 1934;80:1–42.

42. Forsgren L, Nystrom L. An incident case referent study of epileptic seizures in adults. *Epilepsy Res* 1990;6:66–81.

43. Hesdorffer DC, Hauser WA, Annegers JF, et al. Major depression is a risk factor for seizures in older adults. *Ann Neurol* 2000;47:246–249.

44. Hesdorffer DC, Ludvigsson P, Hauser WA, Olafsson E. Depression is a risk factor for epilepsy in children. *Epilepsia* 1998;39:222A.

45. Duman RS. The neurochemistry of depressive disorders. In: Charney DS, Nesler EJ, eds. *Neurobiology of Mental Illnesses*. 2nd ed. New York: Oxford University Press; 2004:421–439.

46. Schildkraut JJ. The catecholamine hypothesis of effective disorders: A review of supporting evidence. *Am J Psychiatry* 1965;122:509–522.

47. Jobe PC, Dailey JW, Wernicke JF. A noradrenergic and serotonergic hypothesis of the linkage between epilepsy and affective disorders. *Crit Rev Neurobiol* 1999;13:317–356.

48. Lehmann A. Audiogenic seizures data in mice supporting new theories of biogenic amines mechanisms in the central nervous system. *Life Sci* 1967;6:1423.

49. Meldrum BS, Anlezark GM, Adam HK, et al. Anticonvulsant and proconvulsant properties of viloxazine hydrohloride: Pharmacological and pharmacokinetic studies in rodents and epileptic baboon. *Psychopharmacology (Berlin)* 1982;76:212.

50. Polc P, Schneeberger J, Haefely, W. Effects of several centrally active drugs on the sleep wakefulness cycle of cats. *Neuropharmacology* 1979;18:259.

51. Piette Y, Delaunois AL, De Shaepdryver AF, et al. Imipramine and electroshock threshold. *Arch Int Pharmacodyn Ther* 1963;144:293.

52. Yanagita T, Wakasa Y, Kiyohara H. Drug-dependance potential of viloxazine hydrochloride tested in rhesus monkeys. *Pharmacol Biochem Behav* 1980;12:155.

53. Southam E, Kirkby D, Higgens GA, et al. Lamotrigine inhibits monoamine uptake in vitro and modulates 5-hydroxytriptamine uptake in rats. *Eur J Pharmacol* 1998;358:19.

54. Dailey JW, Reith MEA, Yan QS, et al. Anticonvulsant doses of carbamezapine increase hippocampal extracellular serotonin in genetically epilepsy-prone rats;dose response relationships. *Neurosci Lett* 1997;227:13.

55. Naritokku DK, Terry WJ, Helfert RH. Regional induction of fos immunoreactivity in the brain by anticonvulsant stimulation of the vagus nerve. *Epilepsy* Res 1995;22:53.

56. Browning Ra, Clark KB, Naritoku DK, et al. Loss of anticonvulsant effect of vagus nerve stimulation in the pentylenetetrazol seizure model following treatment with 6-hydroxydopamine or 5,7-dihydroxy-tryptamine. *Soc Neurosci* 1997;23:2424.

57. Maynert EW, Marczynski Tj, Browining RA. The role of the neurotransmitters in the epilepsies. In: Friedlander WJ (ed.), *Advance in Neurology*. New York: Raven Press, 1975, p. 79.

58. Naidoo D. The effects of reserpine (serpasil) on the chronic disturbed schizophrenic: A comparative study of rauwolfia alkaloids and electroconvulsive therapy. *J Nerv Ment Dis* 1956:123.

59. Noce RH, Williams DB,, Rapaport W. Reserpine (serpasil) in management of the mentally ill. *JAMA* 1955;158:11.

60. Tasher DC, Chermak MW. The use of reserpine in shock-reversible patients and shock-resistant patients. *Ann N Y Acad Sci* 1955;61:108.

61. Berg S, Gabriel, AR, Impastato DJ. Comparative evaluation of the safety of chlorpromazine and reserpine used in conjuction with ECT. *J Neuropsychiatry* 1959;1:104.

62. Fromm GH, Rosen JA, Amores CY. Clinical and experimental investigation of the effect of imipramine on epilepsy. *Epilepsia* 1971;12:282.

63. Fromm GH, Wessel HB, Glass JD, et al. Imipramine in absence and myoclonic-astatic seizures. *Neurology* 1978;28:953.

64. Fromm GH, Amores CY, Thies W. Imipramine in epilepsy. *Arch Neurol* 1972;27:198.

65. Ojemann LM, Friel PN, Trejo WJ, et al. Effect of doxepin on seizure frequency in depressed epileptic patients. *Neurology* 1983;33:66.

66. Favale E, Rubino V, Mainardi P, et al. The anticonvulsant effect of fluoxetine in humans. *Neurology* 1995;45:1926.

67. Perini GI, Tosiu C, Carraro C, et al. Interictal mood and personality disorder in temporal lobe epilepsy and juvenile myoclonic epilepsy. *J Neurol Neurosurg Psychiatry* 1996;61:601–605.

68. Mendez M, Engebrit D, Doss R. The relationship of epileptic auras and psychological attributes. *J Neuropsychiatry Clin Neurosci* 1996;8:287–292.

69. Semah F, Pierot MC, Adam C. Is the underlying cause of epilepsy a major prognostic factor for recurrrences? *Neurology.* 1998;51:1256–1262.

70. Kwan P, Brodie MJ. Early identification of refractory epilepsy. *N Engl J Med.* 2000;342:314–319.

71. Gilliam F, Maton B, Martin RC, et al. Extent of 1H spectroscopy abnormalities independently predicts mood status and quality of life in temporal lobe epilepsy. *Epilepsia* 2000;41(Suppl):54.

72. Quiske A, Helmstaedter C, Lux S, et al. Depression in patients with temporal lobe epilepsy is related to mesial temporal sclerosis. *Epilepsy Res* 2000;39(2):121–125.

73. Schmitz EB, Moriarty J, Costa JC, et al. Psychiatric profiles and patterns of cerebral blood flow in focal epilepsy: Interactions between depression, obsessionality, and perfusion related to the laterality of the epilepsy. *J Neurol Neurosurg Psychiatry* 1997;62(5):458–463.

74. Sheline YI, Wang PW, Gado MH, et al. Hippocampal atrophy in recurrent major depression. *Proc Natl Acad Sci USA* 1996;93(9):3908–3913.

75. Sheline YI, Sanghavi M, Mintun MA, et al. Depression duration but not age predicts hippocampal volume loss in medically healthy women with recurrent major depression. *J Neurosci* 1999;19(12):5034–5043.

76. Sheline YI, Sanghavi M, Mintun MA, et al. Depression duration but not age predicts hippocampal volume loss in medically healthy women with recurrent major depression. *J Neurosci* 1999;19(12):5034–5043.

77. Shah PJ, Ebmeier KP, Glabus MF, et al. Cortical grey matter reductions associated with treatment-resistant chronic unipolar depression. Controlled magnetic resonance imaging study. *Br J Psychiatry* 1998;172:527–532.

78. MacQueen GM, Campbell S, McEwen BS, et al. Course of illness, hippocampal function, and hippocampal volume in major depression. *Proc Natl Acad Sci USA* 2003;100(3):1387–1392.

79. Bell-McGinty S, Butters MA, Meltzer CC, et al. Brain morphometric abnormalities in geriatric depression: Long term neurobiological effects of illness duration. *Am J Psychiatry* 2002;159(8): 1424–1427.

80. Posener JA, Wang L, Price JL, et al. High-dimensional mapping of the hippocampus in depression. Am *J Psychiatry* 2003;160:83–89.

81. Sheline YI, Gado MH, Price JL. Amygdala core nuclei volumes are decreased in recurrent major depression. *Neuroreport* 1998;9(9):2023–2028.

82. Mathern GW, Babb TL, Armstrong DL. Hippocampal sclerosis. In: Engel J Jr, Pedley TA (eds.), *Epilepsy: A Comprehensive Textbook.* Philadelphia, PA: Lippincott-Raven, 1997, pp. 133–155.

83. Sheline YI, Gado MH, Kramer HC. Untreated depression and hippocampal volume loss. *Am J Psychiatry.* 2003;160:1516–1518.

84. Lucassen PJ, Muller MB, Holsboer F, et al. Hippocampal apoptosis in major depression is a minor event and absent from subareas at risk for glucocorticoid overexposure. *Am J Pathol* 2001; 158:453–468.

85. Bowley MP, Drevets WC, Ongur D, et al. Low Glial numbers in the amygdala in major depressive disorder. *Biol Psychiatry;* 2002;52(5):404–412.

86. Seidenberg M, Hermann BP, Noe A. Depression in temporal lobe epilepsy: A possible role for associated frontal lobe dysfunction? In: Sackellares JC, Berent S (eds.), *Psychological Disturbances in Epilepsy.* Newton, MA: Butterworth-Heinemann, 1996, pp. 143–157.

87. Hermann BP, Wyler AR, Richey ET. Epilepsy, frontal lobes and personality. *Biol Psychiatry* 1987;22:1055–1057.

88. Hermann BP, Wyler AR, Richey ET. Wisconsin card sorting test performance in patients with complex partial seizures of temporal-lobeorigin. *J Clin Exp Neuropsychol* 1988;10:467–476.

89. Hermann B, Seidenberg M. Executive system dysfunction in temporal lobe epilepsy: Effects of nociferous cortex versus hippocampal pathology. *J Clin Exp Neuropsychol* 1995;17: 809–819.

90. Hermann BP, Seidenberg M, Schoenfeld J, et al. Neuropsychological characteristics of the syndrome of mesial temporal lobe epilepsy. *Arch Neurol* 1997;54:369–376.

91. Corcoran R, Upton D. A role for the hippocampus in card sorting? *Cortex* 1993;29:293–304.

92. Horner MD, Flashman LA, Freides D, et al. Temporal lobe epilepsy and performance on the Wisconsin Card Sorting Test. *J Clin Exp Neuropsychol* 1996;18:310–113.

93. Hempel A, Risse GL, Mercer K, et al. Neuropsychological evidence of frontal lobe dysfunction in patients with temporal lobe epilepsy. *Epilepsia* 1996;37(Suppl 5):119.

94. Jokeit H, Seitz RJ, Markowitsch HJ, et al. Prefrontal asymmetric interictal glucosa hypometabolism and cognitive impairment in patients with temporal lobe epilepsy. *Brain* 1997;12: 2283–2294.

95. Menzel C, Grunwald F, Klemm E, et al. Inhibitory effect of mesial temporal partial seizures onto frontal neocortical structures. *Acta Neurol Belg* 1998;98:327–331.

96. Baxter LR, Phelps ME, Mazziotta JC, et al. Local cerebral glucose metabolic rates in obsessive-compulsive disorder: A comparison with rates in unipolar depression and in normal controls. *Arch Gen Psychiatry* 1987;44:211–218.

97. Baxter LR, Schawrtz JM, Phelps ME, et al. Reduction of the prefrontal cortex glucose metabolism common to three types of depression. *Arch Gen Psychiatry* 1989;46:243–250.

98. Starkstein SE, Robinson RG. Depression and frontal lobe disorders. In: Miller BL, Cummings JL (eds.), *The Human Frontal Lobes, Functions and Disorders*. New York: The Gilford Press, 1998, pp. 3–26, 537–546.

99. Bremner JD, Vithilingham M, Vermetten E, et al. Reduced volume of orbitofrontal cortex in major depression. *Biol Psychiatry* 2002;51:273–279.

100. Coffey CE, Wilkinson WE, Weiner RD, et al. Quantitative cerebral anatomy in depression: A controlled magnetic resonance imaging study. *Arch Gen Psychiatry* 1993;50:7–16.

101. Rajkowska G, Miguel-Hidalgo JJ, Wei J, et al. Morphometric evidence for neuronal and glial prefrontal cell pathology in major depression. *Biol Psychiatry* 1999;45(9):1085–1098.

102. Lai T, Payne ME, Byrum CE, et al. Reduction of orbital frontal cortex volume in geriatric depression. *Biol Psychiatry* 2000;48(10):971–975.

103. Taylor WD, Steffens DC, McQuoid DR, et al. Smaller orbital frontal cortex volumes associated with functional disability in depressed elders. *Biol Psychiatry* 2003;53(2):144–149.

104. Taylor WD, MacFall Jr, Steffens DC, et al. Localization of age-associated white matter hyperintensities in late-life depression. *Prog Neuropsychopharmacol Biol Psychiatry* 2003; 27(3):539–544.

105. Kumar A, Zhisong J, Warren B, et al. Late-onset minor and major depression: Early evidence for common neuroanatomical substrates detected by using MRI. *Proc Natl Acad Sci USA* 1998; 95(13):7654–7658.

106. Robertson M. Carbamazepine and depression. *Int Clin Psychopharmacol* 1987;2:23–35.

107. Indaco A, Carrieri P, Nappi C. Interictal depression in epilepsy. *Epilepsy Res* 1992;12:45–50.

108. Septien L, Giroud M, Didi-Roy R. Depression and partial epilepsy: Relevance of laterality of the epileptic focus. *Neurol Res* 1993;15:136–138.

109. Altshuler LL, Devinsky O, Post RM, et al. Depression, anxiety, and tempoal lobe epilepsy. *Arch Neurol* 1990;47:284–288.

110. Bromfield E, Altshuler L, Leiderman D. Cerebral metabolism and depression in patients with complex partial seizures. *Epilepsia* 1990;31:625.

111. Collaborative Group for Epidemiology of Epilepsy. Reactions to antiepileptic drugs: A multicenter survey of clinical practice. *Epilepsia* 1986;27:323–330.

112. McConnell H, Duncan D. Treatment of psychiatric comorbidity in epilepsy. In: McConnell H, Snyder P (eds.), *Psychiatric Comorbidity in Epilepsy*. Washington, DC: American Psychiatric Press, 1998, pp. 245.

113. Brent D, Crumrine P, Varma R. Phenobarbital treatment and major depressive disorder in children with epilepsy. *Pediatrics* 1987;80:909–917.

114. Ferrari N, Barabas G, Matthews W. Psychological and behavioral disturbance among epileptic children treated with barbiturate anticonvulsants. *Am J Psychiatry* 1983;140(1):112–113.

115. Smith D, Collins J. Behavioral effects of carbamazepine, phenobarbital, phenytoin and primidone. *Epilepsia* 1987;28:598.

116. Barabas G, Matthews W. Barbiturate anticonvulsants as a cause of severe depression. *Pediatrics* 1988;82:284–285.

117. Ring H, Reynolds E. Vigabatrin and behavior disturbance. *Lancet* 1990;335:970.

118. McConnell H, Duffy J, Cress K. Behavioral effects of felbamate. *J Neuropsychiatry Clin Neurosci* 1994;6:323.

119. Kanner AM, Faught E, French J, et al. Psychaitric adverse events caused by topiramate and lamotrigine: A postmarketing prevalence and risk factor study. *Epilepsia* 2000;41(Suppl 7):169.

120. Mula M, Trimble MR, Yuen A, et al. Psychiatric adverse events during levetiracetam therapy. *Neurology* 2003;61:704–706.

121. Savard G, Andermann LF, Reutens D, et al. Epilepsy, surgical treatment and postoperative

psychiatric complications: A re-evaluation of the evidence. In: Trimble MR, Schmitz B (eds.), *Forced Normalization and Alternative Psychosis of Epilepsy*. Petersfield: Writson Biomedical Publishing, 1998, pp. 179–192.

122. Blumer D, Wakhlu S, Davies K, et al. Psychiatric outcome for temporal lobectomy for epilepsy: Incidence and treatment of psychiatric complications. *Epilepsia* 1998;39:478–486.

123. Robertson M. Forced normalization and the aetiology of depression in epilepsy. In: Trimble MR, Schmitz B (eds.), *Forced Normalization and Alternative Psychosis of Epilepsy*. Petersfield: Writson Biomedical Publishing, 1998, pp. 143–168.

124. Chaplin J, Yepez R, Shorvon S. A quantitative approach to measuring the social effects of epilepsy. *Neuroepidemiology* 1990;9:151–158.

125. Dell J. Social dimension of epilepsy: Stigma and response. In: Whitman S, Hermann B (eds.), *Psychopathology in Epilepsy: Social Dimensions*. New York: Oxford University Press, 1986.

126. Jacoby A. Felt versus enacted stigma: A concept revisited. *Soc Sci Med* 1994;38:269–274.

127. Scambler G. Sociological aspects of epilepsy. In: Hopkins A (ed.), *Epilepsy*. New York: Demos, 1987.

128. DeVellis R, DeVellis B, Wallston B. Epilepsy and learned helplessness. *Basic Appl Soc Psychol* 1980;1:241–253.

129. Hermann B, Whitman S. Psychosocial predictors of interictal depression. *J Epilepsy* 1989;2:231–237.

130. Dodrill C. Neuropsychology. In: Laidlaw J, Richens A, Chadwick D (eds.), *A Textbook of Epilepsy*, 4th ed. London: Churchill Livingstone, 1993.

131. Craig C, Oxley J. Social aspects of epilepsy. In: Laidlaw J, Richens A, Oxley J (eds.), *A Textbook of Epilepsy*, 3rd ed. London: Churchill Livingstone, 1988.

132. Goldstein J, Seidenberg M, Peterson R. Fear of seizures and behavioral functioning in adults with epilepsy. *J Epilepsy* 1990;3:101–106.

133. Mittan R. Fear of seizures. In: Whitman S, Hermann B (eds.), *Psychopathology in Epilepsy: Social Dimensions*. New York: Oxford University Press, 1986.

134. Roth D, Goode K, Williams V. Physical exercise, stressful life experience, and depression in adults with epilepsy. *Epilepsia* 1994;35:1248–1255.

135. Brown S, Reynolds E. Cognitive impairment in epileptic patients. In: Reynolds E, Trimble M (eds.), *Epilepsy and Psychiatry*. Edinburgh: Churchill Livingstone, 1981, p. 147.

136. Sorensen A, Hansen H, Hogenhaven H. Ego functions in epilepsy. *Acta PsychiatrScand* 1988;78:211–221.

137. Holsboer F. Animal models of mood disorders. In: Charney DS, Nesler EJ, Bunney BS (eds.), *Neurobiology of Mental Illness*. New York: Oxford University Press, 1999, pp. 317–332.

138. Willner P, Muscat R, Papp M. Chronic mild stress-induced anhedonia: A realistic animal model of depression. *Neurosci Biobehav Rev* 1992;16:525–534.

139. Robertson M. Depression in patients with epilepsy: An overview and clinical study. In: Trimble M (ed.), *The Psychoopharmacology of Epilepsy*. New York: John Wiley and Sons, 1985, p. 65.

140. Rosenstein D, Nelson J, Jacobs S. Seizures associated with antidepressants: A review. *J Clin Psychiatry* 1993;54:289–299.

141. Preskorn S, Fast G. Tricyclic antidepressant induced seizures and plasma drug concentration. *J Clin Psychiatry* 1992;53:160–162.

142. Curran S, DePauw. Selecting an antidepressant for use in a patient with epilepsy. Safety considerations. *Drug Safety* 1998;18:125–133.

143. Swinkels J, Jonghe F. Safety of antidepressants. *Int Clin Psychopharmacol* 1995;9(Suppl 4):19–25.

144. Ketter TA, Malow BA, Flamini R, et al. Anticonvulsant withdrawal-emergent psychopathology. *Neurology* 1994;44:55–61.

145. Spiller H, Ramoska E, Krenzelok E. Bupropion overdose: A 3-year multicenter retrospective analysis. *Am J Emerg Med* 1994;12:43–45.

146. Grimsley S, Jann M, Carter J. Increased carbamazepine plasma concentration after fluoxetine co-administration. *Clin Pharmacol Ther* 1991;50:10–15.

147. Pearson H. Interaction of fluoxetine with carbamazepine. *J Clin Psychiatry* 1990;51:126.

148. Fritze J, Unsorg B, Lanczik M. Interaction between carbamazepine and fluvoxamine. *Acta Psychiatr Scand* 1991;84:583–584.

149. American Psychiatric Association. Guidelines for the treatment of bipolar disorders. *Am J Psychiatry* 2002;195(Suppl 4):1–50.

150. Anticonvulsants for the treatment of manic depression. *Cleve Clin J Med* 1989;56:756–761.

151. Fatemi SH, Rapport DJ, Calabrese JR, et al. Lamotrigine in rapid-cycling bipolar disorder. *J Clin Psychiatry* 1997;58:522–527.

152. Fogelson DL, Sternbach H. Lamotrigine treatment of refractory bipolar disorder. *J Clin Psychiatry* 1997;58:271–273.

153. Sporn J, Sachs G. The anticonvulsant lamotrigine in treatment-resistant manic-depressive illness. *J Clin Psychopharmacol* 1997;17:185–189.

154. Barry JJ, Lembke A, Huynh N. Affective disorders in epilepsy. In: Ettinger AB, Kanner AM (eds.), *Psychiatric Issues in Epilepsy: A Practical Guide to Diagnosis and Treatment*. Philadelphia, PA: Lippinkott Williams & Wilkins, 2001, pp. 45–72.

155. Schaztzberg AF, Cole JO, DeBattista C. Mood stabilizers. In: *Manual of Clinical Psychopabrmacology*. 5th ed. Washington, DC: American Psychiatric Publishing; 2005:237–243.

156. Bell AJ, Cole A, Eccleston D, et al. Lithium neurotoxicity at normal therapeutic levels. *Br J Psychiatry* 1993;162:688–692.

157. Post R, Putnam F, Uhde T. Electroconvulsive therapy as an anticonvulsant: Implications for its mechanisms of action in affective illness. In: Malitz S, Sackeim H (eds.), *Electroconvulsive Therapy: Clinical and Basic Research Issues*. New York: New York Academy of Sciences, 1986.

158. Blackwood DHR, Cull RE, Freeman CP, et al. A study of the incidence of epilepsy following ECT. *J Neurol Neurosurg Psychiatry* 1980;43:1098–1102.

159. Abrams R. Electroconvulsive therapy in the high-risk patient. In: Abrams R (ed.), *Electroconvulsive Therapy*. New York: Oxford University Press, 1997, pp. 81–113.

160. Sackeim HA. The anticonvulsant hypothesis of the mechanisms of action of ECT: Current status. *J ECT* 1999;15:5–26.

161. Viparelli U, Viparelli G. ECT and grand mal epilepsy. *Convulsive Ther* 1992;8:39–42.

162. Coffey CE, Lucke J, Weiner RD, et al. Seizure threshold in electroconvulsive therapy (ECT) II. The anticonvulsant effect of ECT. *Biol Psychiatry* 1995;37:777–788.

163. Sackeim HA, Decina P, Prohovnik I, et al. Anticonvulsant and antidepressant properties of electroconvulsive therapy: A proposed mechanism of action. *Biol Psychiatry* 1983;18: 1301–1310.

164. Regenold WT, Weintraub D, Taller A. Electroconvulsive therapy for epilepsy and major depression. *Am J Geriatr Psychiatry* 1998; 6: 180–183.

165. Fink M, Kellner C, Sackheim HA. Intractable seizures, status epilepticus and ECT. *JECT Lett* 1999;15:282–284.

166. Gilliam RA. Refractory epilepsy: An evaluation of psychological methods in outpatient management. *Epilepsia* 1990;31:427–432.

SECTION V

Immunologic and Infectious Diseases

CHAPTER 15

Depression in Cancer: Mechanisms, Consequences, and Treatment

CHARLES L. RAISON, JANINE GIESE-DAVIS, ANDREW H. MILLER, AND DAVID SPIEGEL

▶ INTRODUCTION

A diagnosis of cancer is one of life's most distressing events, frequently leaving in its wake the wreckage of once-taken-for-granted timetables and long-term life goals. In place of old certainties are the very real prospects of prolonged psychologic distress, physical suffering, and a foreshortened future. While only half of all people diagnosed with cancer will die of it, all face an existential crisis when diagnosed with it. These factors, combined with our own fear of cancer, promote the frequently unexamined assumption among clinicians that depression is a normal reaction to the disease. Remarkably, however, despite prevalence rates in excess of those seen in medically healthy individuals,[1] most patients with cancer do not develop major depression, suggesting that cancer is a risk factor and not a mandate for depression.[2] Rather than being excused or explained away as a natural reaction to the illness, the development of depression in patients with cancer should be a cause for clinical concern and an indication for timely intervention. Indeed, it is becoming increasingly clear that even mild depressive conditions negatively impact the quality of life, compliance with treatment, and morbidity in cancer patients. Moreover, data suggest that, above and beyond these concerns, depression may contribute to—or reflect—physiologic processes that hasten mortality in response to anticancer therapy.[1,3,4] Fortunately, increasing data demonstrate the efficacy of psychotherapeutic and pharmacologic treatments in treating depression in cancer patients.

This chapter will review the current state of our knowledge regarding bidirectional relationships between depression and cancer, focusing on recent theoretical developments that have practical therapeutic implications. Especially notable in this regard are emerging data on the role of physiologic processes (especially the inflammatory arm of the immune system and the hormonal stress response system) in the development of both the emotional and physical symptoms of depression. Following this discussion, pharmacologic and psychosocial interventions for depression and related symptoms (e.g., fatigue) will be discussed. However, prior to any discussion of etiologic mechanisms or treatment strategies, it will be necessary to review issues regarding how to best conceive of depression in the context of cancer, for, as will become apparent, how depression is defined in cancer patients significantly affects, and how commonly it is diagnosed and treated.

▶ DIAGNOSIS OF DEPRESSION IN CANCER PATIENTS

Inclusive Versus Exclusive Approach

Diagnosing depression in patients with cancer has long been recognized to be highly problematic as a result of the striking symptom overlap between sickness and depression.[2] Especially relevant in this regard are neurovegetative symptoms of depression that are often directly caused by pathophysiologic processes inherent to illness itself or by concurrent treatment modalities, such as chemotherapy or radiation. These symptoms include fatigue, anorexia, weight loss, loss of libido, sleep alterations, and psychomotor slowing. Thus, the question facing the clinician is when, if ever, should neurovegetative symptoms be counted as indicating a diagnosis of depression in cancer patients, and when may these symptoms simply be an indication that a patient is sick? How this question is answered significantly impacts the prevalence of depression in patients with cancer and affects when a clinician considers that treatment is appropriate.

Opposing strategies to resolve the issue have been proposed over the years (Table 15-1). In their simplest iteration, they take two forms: an inclusive approach that counts all depressive symptoms listed in the Diagnostic and Statistical Manual of Mental Disorders, Fourth Edition (DSM-IV)[5] toward a diagnosis of depression, regardless of putative etiology, and an exclusive approach that removes neurovegetative symptoms when these symptoms could likely be caused by the underlying illnesses.[6] Refinements of these simpler approaches include (1) replac-

ing the removed neurovegetative symptoms with alternate emotional symptoms (thus keeping the total number of required diagnostic symptoms the same) and (2) privileging the time course in determining whether neurovegetative symptoms are related to depression or illness. In terms of symptom replacement strategies, the oft-cited approach proposed by Endicott substitutes tearfulness/depressed appearance for changes in weight or appetite, social withdrawal/decreased talkativeness for sleep disturbance, brooding/self pity/pessimism for fatigue/loss of energy, and lack of reactivity to environmental events for diminished ability to think/concentrate or indecisiveness.[7] An alternate approach, based on the assumption that the temporal order of symptom development reveals something about etiology, only counts neurovegative symptoms toward a diagnosis of depression if these symptoms coincide with, or intensify after, the development of significant depressed mood, anhedonia, or helplessness.[8] Studies support the validity of both approaches; however, other data suggest that this type of substitution strategy under-diagnoses depression in the medically ill when compared to inclusive approaches.[9]

Inclusive approaches have the advantage of increasing the likelihood that all patients who have a depression will be identified, but run the risk of misclassifying patients with a mild mood or hedonic disturbance as having a full major depression when in fact they are only mildly depressed and very sick. Exclusive approaches increase diagnostic specificity (i.e., if a patient meets criteria they are very likely to have significant emotional symptoms over and above any sickness-neurovegetative symptoms), but are liable to remove from consideration many patients who might benefit from psychiatric interventions, especially given increasing evidence for the efficacy of these interventions in treating neurovegetative symptoms, even when these occur outside the context of a diagnosable mood disorder. Exclusive approaches that count or discount neurovegetative symptoms in cancer patients based on the putative etiology of these symptoms are especially problematic and

► TABLE 15-1 INCLUSIVE VS. EXCLUSIVE DIAGNOSTIC APPROACHES: ADVANTAGES AND DISADVANTAGES

Inclusive Approach	Exclusive Approach		
	Symptom Removal	Symptom Substitution	Time-Course-Based/Etiologic
Procedure: Count all DSM-IV symptoms that are present toward a diagnosis of major depression regardless of time course or putative etiology of symptoms	Procedure: Remove neurovegetative symptoms shared by illness and depression (i.e., fatigue, anorexia) from counting toward major depression diagnosis	Procedure: Substitutes neurovegetative symptoms shared by illness and depression with more depression-specific affective and cognitive symptoms Substitution scheme: 1. Tearfulness/depressed appearance substituted for changes in weight or appetite 2. Social withdrawal/decreased talkativeness substituted for sleep disturbance 3. Brooding/self pity/pessimism substituted for fatigue/loss of energy 4. Lack of reactivity to environmental events substituted for diminished ability to think/concentrate or indecisiveness	Procedure: Qualifying affective symptoms of depressed mood, anhedonia or hopelessness only counted toward major depression diagnosis if not easily explained by physical illness, treatments, or related environmental stressors. Associated depressive symptoms (i.e., anorexia, fatigue, sleep problems, and so on) only counted if they begin or worsen coincident with, or after, qualifying affective symptoms
Advantages: 1. Highly sensitive and reliable. Will identify all patients who are likely to have a depressive disorder. 2. Will identify a wider range of patients likely to benefit from psychosocial and/or pharmacologic therapy Disadvantages: 1. Not specific. May overdiagnose major depression in medically ill patients	Advantages: 1. Exclusive approaches have high specificity. Patients diagnosed are very likely to have significant depressive symptoms above and beyond any illness-related problems. Disadvantages: 1. Exclusive approaches may miss many patients with depressive syndromes and/or symptoms that would benefit from psychosocial and/or pharmacologic treatment 2. Exclusive approaches may overprivilege affective and cognitive symptoms at the expense of pain and neurovegetative symptoms that are also responsive to treatment		

run the risk of being overly subjective. How does a clinician know whether a patient with cancer is fatigued because of his disease or because he is losing sleep due to a recent job loss and a resultant "depression"? Such decisions are by nature ad hoc, because all patients with cancer, especially during periods of chemotherapy or worsening disease activity have a condition that qualifies them for a diagnosis of "Mood Disorder Secondary to a General Medical Condition" by DSM-IV criteria. For these reasons, and because many medically ill patients have neurovegetative symptoms without concomitant mood/anxiety disturbance, symptom-substitution schemes are probably a more logically consistent way to increase diagnostic specificity in cancer patients. Fortunately, recent data (detailed later) provide novel ways of synthesizing inclusive and exclusive approaches for diagnosing depression in the context of medical illness, allowing clinicians to draw from the strengths of each of these approaches in aiding cancer patients.

A second diagnostic complication in the context of cancer revolves around the issue of how much depression is enough to merit recognition and treatment. This question is embedded within the larger psychiatric issue of whether mood disorders are best understood as categorical entities with firm boundaries (i.e., either you have the disorder or you do not) or as spectrum phenomena that differ from "normalcy" only by matters of degree. Defining normalcy when one has just been diagnosed with cancer or informed of a tumor recurrence is a difficult proposition, given that grief, fear, and other symptoms that define or attend depression are extremely common under these circumstances. Many solutions have been proposed for determining when normal sadness has progressed to a clinically relevant condition, but the problem remains a vexing one with clear diagnostic and treatment implications. Much of the mood disturbance observed in studies of cancer patients falls under the rubric of "adjustment disorder,"[10] a label that bespeaks little need for treatment beyond reassurance, support, and clinical patience. On the other hand, studies increasingly point to the fact that even minor levels of

depressive symptoms (regardless of putative etiology) significantly impair quality of life and physical functioning and may increase mortality in the context of medical illness. Clearly, therapeutic errors can be committed on either side of the Scylla and Charybdis of under- and overtreatment, but most data indicate that patients with cancer and depressive symptoms receive inadequate treatment for their depression.[11,12] Combined with recent evidence that even mild cancer-related depressive syndromes respond to treatment and with data documenting the effectiveness of antidepressants in treating many disease-related symptoms (see later), the weight of the data support erring on the side of treating even milder depressive presentations, especially in patients who are open to—or request—treatment and in patients with persistent symptoms.

Rating Scales

The widespread tendency to excuse depression as a natural reaction to cancer and the overlap between sickness and depressive symptoms both point to the importance of accurately assessing depression in the context of neoplastic illness. Standardized instruments are especially valuable in this regard, whether they are valid and reliable self-report questionnaires, such as the Zung self-rating depression scale (SDS)[13] or the Beck depression inventory (BDI),[14] or interview-based assessments such as the Montgomery-Asberg depression rating scale (MADRS)[15] or the Hamilton depression rating scale (HAM-D).[16] Self-report questionnaires have the advantage of not requiring the presence of a trained psychiatric interviewer and can thus be completed by patients while waiting to see the physician. Having patients complete such scales prior to office visits often provides the clinician with additional key information that time pressures may have otherwise precluded. On the other hand, interviewer-based assessments benefit from the insight of a trained clinical interviewer and may avoid self-reporting biases. And while assessment interviews tend to define overlapping populations, specific instruments are more useful for identifying depression either exclusively or inclusively in patients with cancer. For example, the BDI emphasizes mood and cognitive symptoms that are more specific to depression than are neurovegetative symptoms shared by major depression and physical illness. Similarly, the MADRS was designed to reduce the impact of neurovegetative symptoms on the identification of depression in the context of medical illness. At the other end of the inclusive-exclusive spectrum, the neurotoxicity rating scale (NRS) (a 39-item self-report instrument) may be useful for assessing the full range of neurobehavioral symptoms that frequently afflict patients with cancer.[17] Nevertheless, further validation of the NRS in medically ill patients is required. Even if circumstances do not permit the administration of either self-report or clinician-conducted questionnaires, recent data suggest that simply asking cancer patients the single question "Do you feel depressed most of the time?" effectively identifies most subjects with clinically relevant mood disorders.[10] At the very least, such a simplified approach would identify patients in whom more careful evaluation is warranted.[18]

▶ PREVALENCE OF DEPRESSION IN CANCER

Patients with cancer face widely disparate physiologic and psychologic conditions, not only when compared to each other, but over the disease course of a single individual. Some patients diagnosed with cancer are essentially healthy and face the prospect of a full life span. Others are desperately ill, under intense psychosocial stress or facing an imminent death. Tumors vary in terms of location, tissue type, biochemical effects, and proclivity to produce illness and interfere with daily functioning. Add to these factors the multiple diagnostic schemes used to identify depression in the medically ill, and it should not be surprising that depression prevalence rates in patients with cancer vary widely:

from 1 to 50%.[1,2,10] Despite this wide range, however, the vast majority of studies indicate that rates of both major depression and depressive symptoms is elevated in cancer patients compared to healthy controls. Reviews of the literature place median point prevalence rates between 15 and 29%,[10,19] which is significantly higher than prevalence rates for major depression in the general U.S. population.[20] Recent studies continue to report widely divergent rates of major depression in cancer patients, but findings from these studies are generally consistent with earlier work in terms of risk factors (discussed further) and depression prevalence (i.e., rates between 3 and 37%). Moreover, even in studies with low rates of depression, prevalence was typically increased in cancer patients compared to rates in the general populations in the countries in which the studies were performed.

Variability in Prevalence Estimates

Rather than being an impediment to managing depression in the context of cancer, we suggest that a great deal of useful clinical information can be gleaned from the factors that underlie the tremendous variations in depression prevalence reported in the world literature (Table 15-2). We have already touched upon one such reason: the lack of uniformity in how depression is defined in the context of medical illness. In this regard, depression is more common in cancer patients when it is diagnosed via inclusive methods. Indeed, several studies show that rates of depression approximately double in the same group of patients depending on whether an inclusive or exclusive diagnostic approach is employed.[10,21] This finding suggests that many cancer patients are significantly troubled by depression-related neurovegetative symptoms, such as fatigue and poor sleep/appetite, even while not endorsing sadness or loss of interest in life. This observation has clinical relevance for at least two reasons. First, the presence of neurovegetative and other sickness-related symptoms are a risk factor for the development of full depression

▶ **TABLE 15-2** FACTORS ASSOCIATED WITH DEVELOPING DEPRESSION IN THE CONTEXT OF CANCER

- Past history of depression or anxiety disorder
- Current subsyndromal depressive and/or anxiety symptoms
- Lack of social support
- Recent diagnosis or recurrence of illness
- Type of cancer
  Pancreas > oropharynx > breast > colon > gynecologic > lymphoma > gastric > leukemia
- Severity of disease
- Uncontrolled pain
- Chemotherapeutic regimens associated with induction of depressive symptoms:
  Interferon-alpha, interleukin (IL)-2, amphotericin-B, cycloserine, glucocorticoids, L-asparaginase, leuprolide, procarbazine, tamoxifen, vinblastine, vincristine
- Surgery type
  Mastectomy > breast conservation
- Depression criteria employed for diagnosis
  Inclusive > exclusive
  Symptomatic > categorical

in patients receiving cancer treatment. For example, sleep disturbance has been repeatedly found to predict both the future development of new depression as well as depressive relapse in remitted patients. Second, increasing data demonstrate that antidepressants and related pharmacologic strategies effectively treat a number of sickness-related and neurovegetative symptoms, including sleep disturbance, decreased appetite, pain and fatigue (discussed further).

A second debate that affects the prevalence of depression in cancer centers around how much depression is enough to qualify as a clinically relevant entity. Studies suggest that the majority of cancer patients with mood disturbances meet criteria for conditions other than major depression. Consistent with this, a recent study found that although 23% of outpatients with cancer endorsed significant depressive

symptoms, only a third of these patients met criteria for major depression.[11] The most common mood-related DSM diagnosis in patients with cancer is adjustment disorder. The essential components of an adjustment disorder with depressed mood include (1) the presence of mood symptoms that do not meet criteria for major depression, (2) the mood symptoms arise in response to an identifiable psychosocial stressor, and (3) the mood symptoms impair functioning.[5] These symptoms can persist indefinitely if the stressor is chronic. Given overwhelming data that stressors of all types profoundly increase the risk of depression,[22] and given that many patients with cancer are, by definition, dealing with a severe and chronic stressor, the diagnosis of adjustment disorder seems impossible to credibly differentiate from a mild depression or dysthymic disorder. Increasing data consistently indicate that even mild depressions profoundly interfere with both functioning and quality of life and have adverse health consequences.[23] These considerations raise the question of why a depressive syndrome that arises from the known stressor of cancer (i.e., an adjustment disorder) should be treated differently from symptomatically similar syndromes that arise for other reasons, especially given ample data that depressive syndromes, even when not meeting criteria for major depression, are amenable to therapeutic intervention. On the other hand, the fact that most patients with mood symptoms meet adjustment disorder criteria also suggests that at least some of these patients may have a syndrome that will resolve in a reasonable time period without specific pharmacologic intervention. In this regard, accurate assessment of each patient will require some clinical judgment, but again, the fact that depression prevalence is greatly affected by where the lower limits are set has important and clinically meaningful treatment implications.

Vulnerability to Depression

In addition to diagnostic issues, prevalence rates of depression are affected by other factors, including premorbid patient characteristics, tumor characteristics, disease severity, and type of treatment administered. Several studies concur that patients with a history of psychiatric illness (including a past history of depression) are at increased risk of developing depression in the context of cancer. Similarly, a family history of mood disorder has also been observed to be a risk factor for cancer-related depression. Women appear more likely to develop mood disorders in the context of cancer, consistent with a world-wide body of literature suggesting that women are generally more prone to depression than men.[24] It is increasingly recognized that a patient's current mood and/or anxiety state strongly influences their emotional responses in the face of cancer's exigencies, both psychologic and physiologicl. So, for example, increased self-reported depression and anxiety at the time of cancer diagnosis (presumably caused or exacerbated by the psychologic stress attendant upon such a diagnosis) are associated with psychologic greater distress 6 months later,[25] and numerous studies demonstrate that increased depressive and/or anxiety symptoms just prior to treatment predict the development of depression during interferon-alpha-2b (IFN-alpha) therapy—a regimen known to activate inflammatory pathways and produce high rates of depression.[26] The clinical implications of these data are clear: patients recently diagnosed or about to undergo depressogenic treatments should be evaluated for past and current mood and anxiety symptoms, as well as for a family history of depression. Patients with positive histories in these domains will likely benefit from closer monitoring and in some cases (especially in the context of depressogenic treatments) may merit prophylactic antidepressant treatment, or treatment at the earliest signs of mood disturbance.

Type of Cancer and Depression

Prevalence of depression appears to vary with tumor type and location (Table 15-3). Depression rates are generally reported to be highest for pancreatic, oropharyngeal, and breast carcinomas, intermediate for gynecologic cancers,

▶ **TABLE 15-3** PREVALENCE OF MAJOR DEPRESSION IN DIFFERENT TYPES OF CANCER

Tumor Site	Prevalence of Major Depression (%)
Pancreas	50
Oropharynx	22–40
Colon	13–25
Breast	10–32
Gynecologic	23
Lymphoma	17
Gastric	11
Acute leukemia	1.5

and lowest for lymphoma, leukemia, and gastric cancers.[2,27] Brain tumors are also associated with high rates of depression, especially when tumors are located in the frontal lobe, especially on the left side—a brain area implicated in the genesis and treatment of depression in general. Delirium and seizures are also extremely common in these patients. Both of these conditions have high rates of associated mood disturbance and hence need to be evaluated and ruled out prior to ascribing mood or anxiety symptoms to a mood disorder diagnosis. As with medical illnesses in general,[23] rates of depression in cancer patients increase as disease severity intensifies.[1,28,29]

Cancer Treatment and Depression

The type of treatment patients undergo also affects the likelihood of developing depression. As discussed below, cytokines such as IFN-alpha or interleukin (IL)-2 that are used in the treatment of several malignancies are notorious for inducing depressive symptoms.[30] For example, rates of developing major depression approach 50% in patients receiving chronic, high-dose, IFN-alpha therapy.[31] Other cancer-related medications frequently associated with depression include amphotericin-B, cycloserine, glucocorticoids, L-asparaginase, leuprolide, procarbazine, tamoxifen, vinblastine, and vincristine.[32] Recent data suggest that in some instances chemotherapeutic regimens may have long-term effects on mood. In a large study of adults who had survived childhood leukemia, Hodgkin disease or non-Hodgkin lymphoma, depressive symptoms were significantly more common in cancer survivors than in nonaffected siblings.[33] Intensity of chemotherapeutic exposure in childhood predicted the prevalence of depressive symptoms in adulthood in these patients.[33] Finally, oncologic surgery may increase the risk of developing depression. A prospective study reported that depression is more common in women who undergo mastectomies compared to women who have breast-conserving treatment.[34] While this observation has been traditionally ascribed to psychologic stress resulting from an altered body image following mastectomy, more invasive surgical procedures also induce higher levels of IL-6 and C-reactive protein.[35,36] Hence, it is possible that surgery may promote depression in cancer patients at least in part via activation of the proinflammatory cytokine network (discussed in more detail below).[37] Consistent with this notion, increased serum concentrations of IL-6 have been reported to correlate with increasing depressive symptom scores in patients undergoing abdominal surgery.[38] It should be noted, however, that several studies have failed to replicate an association between mastectomy and increased depression.[39,40] In those studies, it was patient participation in decision-making regarding the choice of surgical approach that predicted better long-term emotional outcome. Moreover, the effects of surgery on immune function appear to be complex, and not all studies report increased proinflammatory cytokine activity postsurgery.[41,42]

▶ DEPRESSION AS A PREDICTOR OF CANCER PROGRESSION AND MORTALITY

Depression and Treatment Adherence

One pathway through which depression may influence cancer progression is by exerting a negative impact on treatment adherence. Depression may impair the motivation or ability to comply with treatment recommendations. Moreover, depressed cancer patients may lack the concentration required to remember complex treatment regimens or the energy to follow through with treatment requirements. Feelings of hopelessness in the context of depression may make it difficult to muster sufficient belief in proposed treatments. Depression may also disrupt the social relationships that would ordinarily encourage patients to comply with treatment and withstand the side effects and uncertainty often associated with chemotherapy and radiation.

In a meta-analysis of studies examining anxiety and depression and noncompliance with a medical regimen, a strong relationship was found between depression (but not anxiety) and noncompliance (odds ratio of 3.03 with more than 142 new studies finding no relation necessary to question the finding).[43] The studies entered into the meta-analysis examined a variety of medical conditions, but of the cancer studies that were included (3 of 12), all found that depression hampered treatment adherence.[44–46] "When patients are noncompliant, they do not take their medication correctly, forget or refuse to diet, do not engage in prescribed exercise, cancel or do not attend appointments, and persist in lifestyles that endanger health. Noncompliance can result in exacerbation of illness, incorrect diagnoses, and patient and physician frustration."[43] Not only does noncompliance reduce treatment effectiveness, it may make it more difficult for patients to express their needs to their physicians.

Depression can impact cancer treatment and screening compliance in a number of different ways. For example, depression may delay screening so that patients are diagnosed at later stages. In a study linking epidemiologic data on lifetime psychiatric history with records from a tumor registry, major depression predicted diagnosis of breast cancer at a later stage whereas phobia was related to diagnosis at an earlier stage. In the study the authors interpreted these results as indicating that distress may delay cancer screening and increase risk for mortality.[47] In a study of adolescent cancer patients, nonadherence with treatment was associated with higher concurrent depression and higher mortality rates 6 years later.[48] Depression may also increase if patients are unresponsive to treatment, which may increase patients' reluctance to follow future treatment recommendations.[49]

Depression or anxiety may also be associated with avoidance of screening procedures for people who have familial risk of cancer. In a cross-sectional study, breast cancer worries were associated with lower compliance with suggested mammography schedules in first-degree relatives of women with breast cancer.[50] In another study, Lerman et al. found that higher baseline stress predicted that first-degree relatives of women with breast cancer would not ask for DNA results for BRCA1 (a genetic marker for increased cancer risk).[51] A study of women who were at familial risk for breast cancer found that procedure-specific anxiety was associated with noncompliance with breast self-examinations, but not with pap smears or mammography.[52] Nevertheless, the literature in this area is small, and a number of studies have failed to find a relationship between depression and poor screening adherence. Indeed, some studies have found that depression and anxiety increased treatment or screening compliance. In a study of patients who were mostly minority or of low social economic status, compliance with chemotherapy in women with breast cancer was associated with greater depression and anxiety, as well as with greater fighting spirit and vigor symptoms. Noncompliance was associated with guilt and hostility.[53] Additionally, in a study of patients seeking information on familial-genetic ovarian cancer risk, depression measures were not predictive of adherence to screening. Instead, those who judged themselves to be at high familial risk were the most nonadherent to screening recommendations over 12–18 months.[54] In a prospective study of cancer patients recommended to receive postsurgical treatment, depression did not predict compliance.[55] In a prospective study of compliance with head and neck cancer treatment, neither depression nor anxiety was associated with later compliance.[56]

Some studies[57] have found that depression is associated with greater patient seeking of complementary or alternative medicine treatments; however, other studies,[58,59] do not arrive at the same conclusion. Moreover, patients undergoing bone marrow transplant were found to be more likely to volunteer for experimental adjunctive therapy if they were highly anxious and had experienced more stressful life events in the past year; but these patients were not significantly more depressed.[60]

Lastly, several psychosocial intervention trials that have reduced depression have been associated with greater compliance posttreatment. A nonrandomized study of a supportive-expressive intervention for women with at least one first-degree relative with breast cancer found that the intervention was significantly associated with reduced unresolved grief, depression, anxiety, and trauma symptoms and more accurate risk comprehension than at baseline.[61] In another intervention study to increase compliance with treatment for hematologic cancer, patients improved compliance in each of three different treatment arms of the study. Of note, depression was associated with decreased compliance with pill taking in this study.[62]

In summary, depression may complicate and impede the treatment of cancer. Although in some populations, fear and depression may motivate greater adherence with treatment, it is clear that depression-related nonadherence to treatment can have a significant impact on cancer progression. Psychosocial treatments to reduce depression and anxiety may increase compliance with treatment regimens as well as increase quality of life for people with cancer.

Depression, the HPA Axis, and Disease Progression

Depression and HPA Function

Depression has physiologic effects that may affect the course of cancer. Indeed, fifteen of twenty-four studies have found that depression was associated with more rapid progression of cancer.[1] These findings raise the obvious question of how the pathophysiology of depression may interact with that of cancer. The use of biomarkers for depression in cancer patients may be especially useful because of the ease with which depressive symptoms can be confounded with symptoms of cancer and the side effects of its treatment.[2] The cortisol profile is one of the best-studied indicators of hypothalamic-pituitary-adrenal (HPA) axis function in depressed populations. Cortisol is a glucocorticoid hormone produced by the adrenal cortex whose circulating levels and circadian rhythm are regulated by the hypothalamus and pituitary gland.[63] Cortisol is the classical stress hormone, mobilizing secretion of glucose into the blood to fuel the "fight or flight" reaction. Cortisol is also one of the most potent immunomodulatory hormones in the body. Cross-sectional comparisons of depressed and nondepressed individuals have identified elevated 24-hour mean cortisol levels and a flattened circadian cortisol rhythm in depressed subjects.[64–66]

Abnormalities in the circadian rhythm of cortisol have been observed in breast and ovarian cancer patients.[67] Among breast cancer patients, these abnormalities include high basal levels throughout a 24-hour period,[67,68] erratic peaks and troughs, and flattened circadian profiles.[67] There is also evidence that loss of normal circadian variation in cortisol, similar to that observed in depression, predicts earlier mortality among metastatic breast cancer patients.[69] This abnormality in HPA functioning involves peaks late in the day, rather than the typical early morning peak, or flat cortisol profiles throughout the day. Such dysregulation of diurnal cortisol is also stress-related, and has been associated with loss of marital support through bereavement or divorce. Other recent studies have shown that women who engage in night shift work are at higher risk for being diagnosed with breast cancer.[70,71] While these authors attribute this effect to suppressed melatonin levels,[72] disruption of circadian cortisol rhythms is another possible mechanism.[73] Of note, Mormont et al. failed to observe a significant effect of blunted diurnal cortisol rhythms in patients with gastrointestinal tumors.[74] Nevertheless, there was a trend in their data suggesting earlier mortality in patients with blunted rhythms. Moreover, they utilized a categorical rather than continuous test of significance, which may have limited statistical power. Recently, Filipski et al. dysregulated diurnal cortisol in an animal model.[75] They ablated the suprachiasmatic nucleus in mice, demonstrated that the circadian cortisol rhythm was blunted, and observed that implanted osteosarcomas and pancreatic adenocarcinomas grew significantly more rapidly than in sham-operated animals. Thus, the clinical observations in humans have been supported in laboratory animals.

Potential Mechanisms of Endocrine Effects on Disease Progression

A number of mechanisms have been proposed by which the neuroendocrine correlates of stress and depression may promote neoplastic growth. For example, glucocorticoids may have differential effects on gluconeogenesis in healthy versus tumor cells. Data suggest that tumor cells may become resistant to glucocorticoid signaling and the catabolic action of cortisol, which inhibits the uptake of glucose in numerous cell types. In such cases, energy would be preferentially shunted to the tumor and away from normal cells by cortisol.[76] Moreover, it appears that the androgen receptor in certain prostate cancer cell lines can become cortisol-sensitive, thereby allowing physiologic levels of cortisol to stimulate androgen-mediated tumor growth.[77] Several studies have also found an association between stress-related elevation of glucocorticoids and more rapid tumor growth in animals.[78–80] It has also been theorized that hormones of the HPA axis can promote the expression of breast cancer oncogenes by the activation of proopiomelanocortin (POMC) genes by corticotropin releasing hormone (CRH). The POMC promoter has homology with POMC transcription factors that bind to human MAT-1 breast cancer oncogenes.[81] Thus, there are a variety of means by which depression-related abnormalities in HPA function could affect the rate of cancer progression. One other major hypothesis posits an association between HPA axis and immune dysfunction, given that glucocorticoids are potently immunodulatory and may suppress relevant antitumor, host responses.

Depression and Immunity in Cancer

One link between depression and cancer progression is the effect of depression on the immune response. Depression is associated with reductions in both viral- and antigen-specific measures of cell-mediated immunity. Depression appears to be linked to poorer cell-mediated control over the steady state expression of latent Epstein-Barr virus (EBV), a measure of immunosurveillance. While depressed subjects do not appear to exhibit higher EBV antibody titers when compared to nondepressed controls, the severity of depressive symptoms has been associated with higher antibody titers to EBV capsid antigen (VCA).[82–85] Depression also affects antigen-specific cell-mediated immunity. Depressed individuals show evidence of poorer delayed-type hypersensitivity (DTH) skin test responses.[86] Decrements in the DTH response suggest poorer ability of T-cells to mount antigen-specific responses such as those necessary to combat viruses, bacteria, and possibly tumors.[87–89] Depression has also been repeatedly associated with decrements in natural killer (NK) cell functioning.[90,91]

The severity of depression (and related repressive coping in response to it) is associated with a deleterious effect on immunocompetence in cancer patients.[92] Clinician-rated symptoms of depression significantly predict both lower white blood cell counts and NK cell numbers in this population.[93] Symptoms of depression and a lack of social support predicted reduced NK cell cytotoxicity measured at a 3-month follow-up in breast cancer patients.[94] NK cells attack transformed or dying cells in the absence of any particular antigen, and are therefore thought to be involved in cancer surveillance. It has been established that a reduction in NK cytotoxicity is associated with more rapid progression of metastatic breast cancer.[88,94,95] There are, however, data suggesting that acute stress is associated with increased NK and T-cell responses in women with breast cancer.[96,97] Andersen et al. studied 116 breast cancer patients shortly after surgical treatment.[97] They found that the level of stress was associated with lower NK cell cytotoxicity, even when supplemented by gamma-interferon. Stress was also associated with lower lymphocyte proliferative responses.

In terms of the mechanisms by which stress may influence the immune system and possibly cancer progression, alterations in HPA axis hormones and the sympathetic nervous system (SNS) may be involved. HPA dysregulation may lead to depression-related immunosuppression. Stress hormones may suppress immune resistance to tumors.[98,99] Preclinical studies have documented suppressive effects of chronic HPA axis activation on T-cell-mediated immune responses.[63] In addition, because stress- and depression-related increases in SNS and HPA activity are known to have generally suppressive effects on immune function,[100] it is possible that immune functions important in resistance to breast tumor growth are thereby suppressed.[93,101–103]

Thus, depressive symptoms appear to be associated with poorer cellular immune function. Furthermore, the associations between depressive symptoms and immune system function are moderated by factors such as aging and gender.[104,105] Conditioning may also play a role in immunosuppressive effect of depression. It is well known that chemotherapy is powerfully immunosuppressive, since these cytotoxic agents are selected for their ability to kill rapidly proliferating cells. Indeed, cancer patients experience conditioned immunosuppression *prior* to receiving their next round of chemotherapy,[106] similar to the conditioned immunosuppression observed in animals.[107–109] Conditioning is an association of psychologic and somatic states. To the extent that the persistent state of depression is associated with decrements in specific types of immune function, it is possible that the depressive state itself evokes conditioned immunosuppression similar to that observed from the conditioned response to the chemotherapy environment. Or conversely, it is possible that depression merely potentiates the conditioned immunosuppression that occurs with chemotherapy, i.e., depressed patients associate chemotherapy with immunosuppression even more strongly because the depressive symptoms intensify the experience.

Depression can be understood as a chronic and maladaptive stress response which may have adverse effects on both endocrine and immune function.[110] Studies of depression provide preliminary evidence that depression may adversely affect both HPA and immune function, and that these effects are interactive. However, the link between such enumerative measures of immunity and clinically meaningful immune function related to cancer surveillance is still unclear. More research is needed which examines specific endocrine and immunologic correlates of depression for their effects on the health status of cancer patients.

▶ MECHANISMS OF DEPRESSION IN PATIENTS WITH CANCER

Psychologic Factors

Depression may be an acute reaction to the diagnosis and treatment of cancer as it is with other serious illnesses.[111–116] It can also occur in the course of coping with chronic illness.[117] Depression can also be an early indication of onset of diseases such as pancreatic cancer.[2] Even for patients who do not develop axis I psychiatric disorders, serious medical illness can be understood as a series of stressors that can elicit psychologic and physiologic stress responses.[118]

Cancer and depression can interact over the long term in such a way as to have a seriously deleterious effect on quality of life. More rapid cancer progression and increased symptoms, especially pain, are associated with more severe depression.[119–121] Comorbid depression is associated with declining function and poorer quality of life over the course of chronic illness,[122,123] and also reduces optimism about the effectiveness of medical treatment.[124]

Biologic Factors

Although the symptom overlap between sickness and depression complicates the task of identifying and treating patients with cancer, it also offers clues to mechanisms by which the physiology of illness contributes to the pathophysiology of depression. Moreover, as often happens, expanding knowledge has provided support for dichotomous positions previously perceived as being exclusive, in this case, giving credence to both inclusive and exclusive ways of understanding depression in the context of sickness. Indeed, accumulating data lend support for an emerging paradigm in which immune system activation is seen to induce physical and behavioral symptoms common to both illness and depression and to induce changes in central nervous and stress system pathways that additionally predispose vulnerable individuals to the development of profound mood and hedonic alterations in the context of sickness.

Cytokines, Sickness Behavior, and Symptom Complexes

While psychosocial factors undoubtedly contribute to the development of depression in patients with cancer (especially at times of greatest stress such as initial diagnosis and/or disease recurrence), recent advances in our understanding of biologic changes that occur with disease have prompted a shift in how depression in the context of cancer is conceptualized.[125] The immune system has received increasing attention as a potential contributor to the depressive symptoms often observed, not just in patients with cancer, but in the context of medical illness in general.

Most processes integral to illness, including neoplasia, infection, autoimmunity, and tissue trauma activate a network of functionally related proteins known as proinflammatory cytokines, the best described of which (in terms of the nervous system) are tumor necrosis factor-alpha (TNF-alpha), IL-1, and IL-6. In addition to local effects at the site of tumor, infection, or trauma, these cytokines profoundly influence both general physiologic functioning and behavior via effects on the central nervous system (CNS). Although too large to pass freely through the blood-brain barrier, proinflammatory cytokines gain access to the CNS through several means, including passage through leaky regions in the blood-brain barrier and active transport. In addition, cytokine signals from the periphery, signal the CNS via afferent nerve fibers (e.g., vagus).[126–128] Within the brain, a cytokine network has been described that consists of cell types that can both produce cytokines (glia/neurons) and receive their signals through relevant receptors.[129] Acting via these receptors, cytokines induce behavioral changes in humans and animals that have been characterized as "sickness behavior."[130–133] The symptoms of sickness behavior overlap strikingly with symptoms frequently observed in major depression and include anhedonia, cognitive dysfunction, anxiety/irritability, psychomotor slowing, anergia/fatigue, anorexia, loss of libido, sleep alterations, and increased sensitivity to pain.[130] Each of the proinflammatory cytokines has been shown to reproduce sickness behavior when administered individually or when induced in concert by immunologic stimuli such as the bacterial cell-wall product lipopolysaccharide.[37] Studies in animals demonstrate that this syndrome can be ameliorated or reversed by administering specific cytokine antagonists (e.g., IL-1 receptor antagonist) or anti-inflammatory cytokines (e.g., IL-10) directly into the brain.[134,135] Consistent with studies in animals, human data suggest that anti-TNF drugs (i.e., etanercept and infliximab) improve mood, energy, and other sickness type symptoms when compared to a placebo.[136]

The clinical relevance of these observations is underscored by studies linking increased cytokine activity with behavioral disturbance in the context of illness. For example, significantly increased plasma concentrations of IL-6 have been found in cancer patients with depression compared with cancer patients who do not have depression.[137] Consistent with this, depression scores have been reported to correlate with increased concentrations of the soluble receptor for the cytokine IL-2 in patients with metastatic colorectal cancer.[138] In cancer patients receiving cytokine therapy (IL-2 or IL-2 plus IFN-alpha), increases in proinflammatory activity, as assessed by the concomitant production of the anti-inflammatory cytokine IL-10, correlated with the development of depressive symptoms early in the course of treatment have been noted.[139] Finally, correlations have been observed between increased production of proinflammatory cytokines, such as IL-1 and IL-6, and fatigue (a common symptom of both major depression and medical illness) in cancer patients receiving chemotherapy or radiation treatment.[140,141]

At least five pathways have been identified by which proinflammatory cytokines may cause depression/sickness behavior. Cytokines have been shown to have potent stimulatory effects on the HPA axis, in large part through activation of CRH.[142,143] CRH has behavioral effects in animals that are similar to those seen in patients suffering from depression/sickness behavior, including alterations in activity, appetite, and sleep.[144] Moreover, patients with depression have been found to exhibit increased CRH activity as manifested by elevated concentrations of CRH in the cerebrospinal fluid (CSF), increased mRNA in the paraventricular nucleus of the hypothalamus and a blunted adrenocortiotropic hormone (ACTH) response to CRH challenge (likely reflecting down regulation of pituitary CRH receptors).[145,146] Reductions in receptors for CRH in the frontal cortex have been noted in suicide victims (presumably secondary to hypersecretion of CRH).[146]

Proinflammatory cytokines (especially IL-1, IL-6, and TNF-alpha) have been shown to alter the metabolism of the monoamines including norepinephrine, serotonin, and dopamine, all of which have been implicated in the pathophysiology of mood disorders.[131] Special interest has been paid to the ability of proinflammatory cytokines to reduce serum concentrations of L-tryptophan via induction of the enzyme indolamine 2,3-dioxygenase (IDO) that breaks down tryptophan (TRP) into kynurenine.[147–149] TRP is the primary precursor of serotonin, and depletion of TRP has been associated with the precipitation of mood disturbances in vulnerable patients.[150]

In vivo and in vitro studies suggest that proinflammatory cytokines, including IL-1, may induce resistance of nervous, endocrine, and immune system tissues to circulating glucocorticoid hormones through direct inhibitory effects on the expression and/or function of glucocorticoid receptors.[151] Glucocorticoid resistance has been repeatedly demonstrated in patients with depression (as reflected in nonsuppression on the dexamethasone suppression test),[151] and may contribute to impaired feedback regulation of CRH and the further release of proinflammatory cytokines.

Finally, proinflammatory cytokines have been associated with the euthyroid sick syndrome (ESS) that is characterized by normal TSH and T4 levels and reduced T3 levels in the early stages and by normal TSH and reduced T3 and T4 in the later stages.[152] Alterations in thyroid hormone availability are well known to influence mood regulation. The mechanism by which ESS occurs is believed to involve both direct effects of cytokines on thyroid gland function as well as inhibition of the metabolic enzymes (5′-deiodination) that convert peripheral T4 to T3 (the more biologically active form of thyroid hormone), especially in the liver.[152]

To aid in separating immune from psychosocial contributions to depression in the context of medical illness, researchers have employed treatment with IFN-alpha as a model system for cytokine-mediated behavioral disturbance. IFN-alpha is a cytokine released early in viral infection that has both antiviral and antiproliferative activities.[153] In addition to direct effects on the immune system, IFN-alpha also potently stimulates the production of proinflammatory cytokines including IL-6 and to a lesser extent, TNF-alpha and IL-1 alpha and beta.[154,155] Because of its antiproliferative/antiviral activities, IFN-alpha is currently used for the treatment of several malignancies and viral infections.[156] Although frequently of benefit in each of these conditions, IFN-alpha has been repeatedly observed to cause a variety of neuropsychiatric side effects that closely resemble sickness behavior in animals and that meet symptom criteria for major depression in many patients. Indeed, our group observed that nearly 50% of patients receiving high-dose IFN-alpha for malignant melanoma developed major depression over 3 months of treatment (although it should be noted that by strict DSM-IV criteria IFN-alpha-induced depression qualifies as a *substance-induced mood disorder*).[30] These results are especially striking given that depressive symptom scores were minimal in this population prior to treatment.

To evaluate the efficacy of antidepressants in patients exposed to an unambiguous immune stimulus, the possibility that antidepressant pretreatment might ameliorate neurobehavioral toxicity in patients receiving high doses of IFN-alpha for the treatment of malignant melanoma has been examined (Fig. 15-1).[31] In this study, 40 patients with nonmetastatic disease were randomized in a double-blind manner to receive either the selective serotonin reuptake inhibitor (SSRI) paroxetine or placebo. Antidepressant (or placebo) treatment was commenced 2 weeks prior to the initiation of IFN-alpha and continued for an additional 10 weeks of IFN-alpha therapy. At the end of this period only 11% of patients receiving paroxetine had developed symptoms sufficient to meet diagnostic criteria for major depression, compared to 45% of patients receiving placebo. Moreover, rates of discontinuation from IFN-alpha were significantly lower in paroxetine-treated patients: 5% versus 35% for patients receiving placebo.

A recent study in rodents suggested that the SSRI fluoxetine prevents cytokine-induced decrements in the gustatory hedonic domain, while having no impact on cytokine-induced

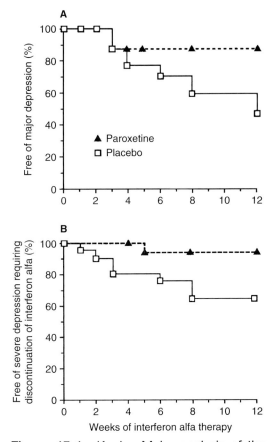

Figure 15-1. Kaplan-Meier analysis of the percentage of patients receiving paroxetine or placebo who remained free of major depression (Panel A) or of severe depression requiring treatment discontinuation (Panel B) during interferon (IFN)-alpha therapy for malignant melanoma. In Panel A, a comparison of the curves for the 20 patients in the placebo group and the 18 patients remaining in the paroxetine group shows a significant difference between the groups in the development of major depression (relative risk in the paroxetine group, 0.24; 95% confidence interval, 0.08–0.93; $P = 0.04$ by the log-rank test). In Panel B, a comparison of the curves for the 20 patients in the placebo group and the original 20 patients in the paroxetine group shows a significant difference between groups in the development of severe depression requiring the discontinuation of IFN-alpha before 12 weeks (relative risk in the paroxetine group, 0.14; 95% confidence interval, 0.05–0.85; $P = 0.03$ by the log-rank test).

anorexia.[157] Given that major depression is a syndrome consisting of both mood/hedonic and neurovegetative symptoms (like anorexia),[5] Capuron and colleagues examined whether paroxetine was equally effective in ameliorating all depressive symptoms in patients receiving INF-alpha or whether its ability to prevent major depression derived from a more limited spectrum of therapeutic efficacy. A dimensional analysis revealed that symptoms more commonly seen in depression than in sickness, including depressed mood, loss of interest, suicidal thoughts, guilt, and anxiety, as well as subjective cognitive complaints were prevented by SSRI pretreatment, whereas neurovegetative symptoms, including fatigue, anorexia, and psychomotor retardation, were minimally responsive to the antidepressant.[158] Additionally, neurovegetative and somatic symptoms were noted to develop early during treatment (within the first 2 weeks) in the majority of patients, whereas depression-specific and cognitive symptoms developed later and tended only to occur in patients who met DSM-IV criteria for major depression.

Similar patterns have been identified in the phenomenology and treatment response of behavioral disturbances in the context of cancer. In terms of phenomenology, a factor analysis in a large group of patients found that mood, anxiety, and cognitive symptoms clustered together, whereas fatigue, anorexia, and physical symptoms represented separate factors.[159] Consistent with SSRI response patterns during IFN-alpha treatment, paroxetine has been recently shown in a large double-blind, placebo-controlled trial to ameliorate depression, but not fatigue, in cancer patients undergoing chemotherapy.[160] Taken together, these findings reinforce the notion that depression during immune activation may represent an amalgam of at least two subsyndromes: a neurovegetative/somatic syndrome that develops in most sick individuals, appears early in the course of inflammation, and is minimally responsive to SSRI treatment and a mood/anxiety/cognition syndrome that occurs in a subset of patients (who are also most likely to meet full criteria for major depression).

This syndrome develops after more prolonged inflammatory exposure and responds to SSRI treatment.

The finding that both IFN-alpha-induced and cancer-related depression can be meaningfully subdivided on the basis of phenomenology and treatment response into a more depression-specific syndrome of mood, anxiety, and cognitive symptoms and a more generalized sickness syndrome comprised of neurovegetative and somatic symptoms strongly suggest that separate pathophysiologic mechanisms may underlie these syndromes, with the corollary that different symptoms may respond to different treatment strategies in depressed, medically ill patients.[158] Recent work aimed at delineating pathways by which immune activation produces behavioral disturbance supports this notion.

PATHWAYS ASSOCIATED WITH MOOD/ANXIETY AND COGNITIVE SYMPTOMS

As mentioned above, inflammatory stimuli (including IFN-alpha exposure) lead to a depletion of TRP via an immune-mediated induction of the enzyme IDO, which metabolizes TRP to kynurenine and hence reduces the amount of TRP that is available for the synthesis of serotonin.[148,161] It has been argued that IDO induction serves several adaptive purposes, including diminishing TRP availability for bacterial pathogens (for which TRP is also an essential amino acid) and promoting maternal T-cell tolerance toward the fetus during pregnancy.[162] Despite these evolutionary benefits, however, IDO induction might also be expected to increase the risk of developing depressive symptoms during conditions of immune activation, given evidence that TRP depletion is capable of rapidly inducing depressive symptoms in nondepressed but vulnerable individuals.[163,164] Data from patients receiving IFN-alpha suggest this is true: several studies report that treatment results in decreases in serum TRP and increases in kynurenine,[148,161,165] consistent with activation of IDO.[166] Moreover, the amount of reduction in TRP during treatment has been correlated with depressive symptom

severity scores.[148,165] Similarly, it has been observed that antidepressant-free patients who met criteria for major depression during IFN-alpha therapy for malignant melanoma demonstrated significantly larger increases in kynurenine and the ratio of kynurenine to TRP and prolonged decreases in TRP during treatment when compared to patients who did not develop major depression.[161]

A dimensional analysis demonstrated that the relationship between major depression and TRP depletion resulted from a significant correlation between decreases in serum TRP concentrations and the development of mood, anxiety, and cognitive symptoms. No association was seen between TRP metabolism and neurovegetative symptoms or pain complaints. That alterations in TRP metabolism correlated with the same symptoms that responded to treatment with paroxetine (and did not correlate with symptoms that were not responsive to the SRI)[158] strongly suggests that serotonergic mechanisms contribute significantly to the expression of mood, anxiety, and cognitive complaints in these patients. This possibility is strengthened by the fact that no such correlation was observed in patients pretreated with paroxetine, which might be expected, via effects of this medication on the serotonin reuptake pump, to compensate for IDO-induced decrements in serotonergic functioning. By the same logic, serotonergic mechanisms did not appear to play a central role in the mediation of neurovegetative or pain symptoms.

Because CRH hyperactivity is a frequently reported abnormality in major depression,[151] and because IFN-alpha robustly stimulates the HPA axis in animals and humans via stimulation of CRH, Capuron and colleagues examined whether patients who responded to IFN-alpha treatment with HPA axis hyperactivity would be at increased risk of developing depression during treatment. In antidepressant-free patients, those who developed major depression during IFN-alpha treatment exhibited increased CRH activity in response to the first dose of IFN-alpha (as assessed by postinjection increases in serum concentrations of ACTH and cortisol). Of note, none of the patients met criteria for depression at the time of the first injection.[155] Although the first dose of IFN-alpha also markedly increased serum concentrations of IL-6, no differences in this cytokine were observed between patients who did and did not develop major depression, suggesting that the vulnerability to depression was accounted for by preexisting sensitivity of CRH pathways to an immune stimulus and not by an abnormality within the proinflammatory cytokine network itself.

Interestingly, both CRH pathway and cytokine responses to IFN-alpha rapidly attenuated with repeated treatment, such that within a week of initiating therapy no differences were observed in postinjection ACTH or cortisol responses between patients who did and did not subsequently develop major depression.[155] This finding is quite different from the temporal pattern observed between IDO-induced TRP depletion and depression, where changes in TRP levels and the development of depressive symptoms were contemporaneous.[161] However, it is intriguing that patients who demonstrated CRH hyperactivity in response to an initial dose of IFN-alpha were also more likely to later demonstrate increased TRP depletion, indicating a possible link between CRH and serotonergic systems in the mediation of depressive symptoms in the context of immune activation. Moreover, as with IDO-induced TRP depletion, CRH hyperactivity predicted the subsequent development of major depression through an effect on mood, anxiety, and cognitive symptoms.[155] No correlation was observed between CRH hyperactivity and the later development of neurovegetative or somatic symptoms. Taken together these findings suggest that patients with preexisting super-sensitivity in CRH-mediated stress pathways may be at risk of developing mood, anxiety, and cognitive symptoms, not perhaps through ongoing abnormalities in stress system responses to immune stimulation, but rather through as yet unidentified functional connections between CRH and serotonergic metabolism. On the other hand, neurovegetative and physical symptoms that are frequent in the con-

text of illness, even when more depression-specific symptoms are absent, may not be as directly related to alterations in CRH and/or serotonergic systems.

POTENTIAL PATHWAYS FOR THE DEVELOPMENT OF CYTOKINE-INDUCED NEUROVEGETATIVE SYMPTOMS

A first clue to the neural mechanisms by which activation of the cytokine network promotes the development of neurovegetative symptoms such as fatigue or psychomotor slowing in patients with cancer is provided by data linking abnormalities in CNS dopamine with fatigue and psychomotor slowing in the context of medical illness. For example, human immunodeficiency virus (HIV) infection and Parkinson's disease, conditions in which fatigue and psychomotor slowing are prominent, are characterized by abnormalities in dopamine metabolism in basal ganglia and by extreme sensitivity to medications, such as antipsychotic agents, that further reduce dopaminergic signaling via postsynaptic receptor blockade.[167,168] Consistent with this, even in medically healthy depressed patients, affective flattening and psychomotor retardation are associated with evidence of altered dopaminergic functioning in the left caudate nucleus.[169] Finally, agents with dopaminergic activity have been repeatedly shown to effectively treat fatigue in a number of medical conditions.[170–172] Interestingly in this regard, increasing data suggest that dopamine receptor agonists are effective antidepressants in medically healthy subjects,[173,174] further supporting a role for dopaminergic abnormalities in major depression.

Chronic immune activation appears to inhibit dopamine signaling within fronto-striatal circuits within the CNS. Rodents treated chronically with IFN-alpha demonstrate inhibition of dopaminergic neural activity and CNS dopamine metabolism, with concomitant decrements in motor activity.[175] In humans, high-dose IFN-alpha reliably slows reaction time on standardized neuropsychologic tests and in extreme cases has been reported to produce frankly Parkinsonian states that are responsive to treatment with levodopa.[30,176]

These findings support the possibility that psychomotor retardation and fatigue observed during states of immune activation may be related in part to cytokine-induced reductions in dopamine activity. Cytokine receptors are expressed in abundance in key areas of the basal ganglia/thalamo-cortical circuitry including the striatum and cerebral cortex and therefore are uniquely poised to influence dopamine neuronal activity in these brain regions.[177] Moreover, chronic infusion of lipopolysaccharide (LPS) into rat brain leads to delayed and selective degeneration of dopaminergic neurons in the substantia nigra through microglial activation.[178] Finally, the targeting of basal ganglia and dopamine pathways during activation of the cytokine network is suggested by involvement of these pathways in infectious diseases associated with neuropsychiatric alterations including HIV.[168]

Taken together, these data suggest that alterations in basal ganglia, notably in dopamine neurotransmission, may contribute to the development of core neurovegetative symptoms of IFN-alpha-induced depression, including psychomotor slowing. Consistent with this, preliminary data from our group and others demonstrate altered glucose metabolism in the basal ganglia of IFN-alpha-treated patients.[179,180]

Diagnostic Implications

The concept of sickness behavior promotes awareness that many symptoms of both physical and emotional distress in cancer patients may have a significant biologic component, arising out of the body's own attempt to fight disease and at the same time maintain homeostatic balance. This perspective discourages simple dichotomies between emotional and physical suffering in the context of cancer and points to the clinical utility of extending therapeutic concerns beyond depression into the larger sickness syndrome of which depression in the medically ill is a component. Such a perspective argues for an inclusive approach to identifying patients with clinically relevant behavioral disturbances, even when these disturbances do not meet criteria for currently recognized DSM-IV

mood disorders. Moreover, recognizing that inflammation provides a physiologic substrate that promotes mood disturbance implies that markers of inflammation may provide an additional diagnostic tool to identify individuals at risk for developing depressive disorders. Such inflammatory risk markers have recently been identified for both diabetes and coronary artery disease—conditions which, like cancer, are associated with increased rates of depression. Relevant in this regard are data showing that patients with cancer who develop depression have significantly higher levels of IL-6 than cancer patients without depression.[181] Other abnormalities that may hold promise as predictive markers for depressive disorders include IDO-mediated decreases in plasma TRP and alterations in the production of HPA axis hormones, such as ACTH and cortisol, as discussed above. Similarly, imaging studies of patients undergoing cytokine exposure may in the future cast light on neural circuits that mediate both risk for, and expression of, behavioral toxicity.

However, if the elucidation of sickness behavior promotes an inclusive approach to behavioral symptoms in patients with cancer, findings on depressive subsyndromes and the pathways that underlie these different symptom dimensions argue for the wisdom inherent in exclusive approaches that privilege more depression-specific symptoms and downplay the importance of neurovegetative symptoms. Specifically, studies in patients undergoing immune activation strongly suggest that sickness symptoms, including fatigue and other neurovegetative symptoms, are widespread and serve as a physiologic base from which a smaller number of vulnerable individuals will progress to develop symptoms most classically associated with mood disturbances, including sadness, loss of pleasure, anxiety, hopelessness, helplessness, and suicidal ideation. A strong rationale for privileging these symptoms comes from studies over the last several years suggesting that these symptoms may be the primary mediators of the relationship between depression and poor health outcomes.[8]

► TREATMENT OF DEPRESSION IN PATIENTS WITH CANCER

Psychosocial Treatment of Depression in Cancer

Of the many approaches that are available to treat depression in medically ill patients, psychotherapy emphasizing social support, emotional expression, cognitive restructuring, and improved coping skills is effective in addressing the psychosocial problems of depressed patients with cancer.[182] Indeed, a supportive dynamic intervention reviewing the life lived, addressing depression and anxiety, loneliness, loss, or fears about protracted and painful death, discussing advance directives for medical care, and preparing for death, has been beneficial for many terminally ill patients.[183–186] Studies make it clear that facing rather than avoiding issues such as dying and death, which could be considered likely to exacerbate depression, actually helps to reduce it. This approach encourages patients to face what they most fear, and find some aspect of it they can do something about, e.g., control the process of dying when death is unavoidable. This helps patients to feel more active and less helpless, even in the face of dying. Others as well emphasize such a cognitive-existential approach with cancer patients,[187] which they find effective in reducing symptoms of distress.

Cognitive-behavioral treatments, frequently used to treat depression, have been applied in cancer patients.[188] In one trial with breast cancer patients, improvement in mood was found only in the near term.[189] One study with breast cancer patients found that such an approach to stress management resulted in improved mood and lower cortisol levels.[190] Similarly, van der Pompe and colleagues offered a 13-week experiential-existential group therapy treatment protocol to early-stage breast cancer patients.[191] At the end of treatment, patients in the treatment group showed lower levels of plasma cortisol and prolactin. A pilot study for an intervention with interpersonal psychotherapy (IPT), widely used

in depression treatment,[192,193] as adapted for cancer patients, indicates that it is helpful for patients and their partners.[194] Female outpatients undergoing aggressive treatment for metastatic breast cancer ($n = 14$), and their partners ($n = 11$), participated in individual telephone IPT sessions coinciding with chemotherapy and continuing for 4 weeks after treatment. Therapy focused on salient psychosocial issues such as distress, family concerns, coping with illness, treatment demands, and relationships with medical personnel. Overall, the patients rated the intervention from good to excellent. Partners reported that the telephone contact was their only outlet to help them cope with role transitions, anticipated losses, depression and anxiety, and feelings of fear, anger, and frustration.[194] Thus, a variety of standard psychotherapeutic interventions have been shown to be effective in treating depression and related symptoms among cancer patients.

Implications for Cancer Progression and Mortality

There is a small portion of literature that raises the possibility that psychotherapeutic intervention may affect survival time as well as quality of life.[195–199] Five of eleven published randomized trials demonstrate such an effect.[200] Spiegel and colleagues reported that a year (minimum) of supportive-expressive group psychotherapy resulted in a significant 18-month increase in survival time in metastatic breast cancer patients.[195] A 6-week cognitive-behavioral group intervention composed of education, stress management, coping skills training, and psychologic support for malignant melanoma patients found significantly lower death rates at 10-year follow-up in the treatment group.[201] Interestingly, in this study, patients with higher initial levels of distress seemed to experience lower rates of disease recurrence and death.[197] An educational intervention aimed at increasing compliance with cancer treatment also had beneficial effects on survival in patients with newly diagnosed hematologic cancers.[196] A study of individual psychotherapeutic support offered at the bedside early in the course of disease to a group of gastrointestinal cancer inpatients also had favorable results on survival.[198] Finally, in a 4-week intervention consisting of patient education, psychologic support, and implementation of a community-based network of support services, McCorkle and colleagues found improved survival in late-stage cancer patients, though no difference in survival time was found in early-stage patients.[199]

Six other trials found no enhanced survival with psychosocial intervention.[184,197–201] One excellent multicenter trial utilizing supportive-expressive group psychotherapy with metastatic breast cancer patients showed reduced distress and pain, but no survival advantage.[202] However, the controversy over whether or not psychotherapy can extend survival should not obscure the finding that essentially every well-conducted study of psychotherapy in cancer patients has resulted in improved quality of life or reduced distress. Nevertheless, the potential benefits of psychotherapeutic support on cancer progression remain an important but unresolved research question.

Antidepressants

Another major approach for addressing depression in the patient with cancer is the use of antidepressants (Fig. 15-2 for a treatment algorithm). It is becoming increasingly clear that as is the case with major depression in general, depression that arises in the context of cancer is responsive to antidepressant treatment.[32] Initial evidence that antidepressants were useful in depressed cancer patients came from an open trial of the tricyclic antidepressant imipramine by Evans and colleagues in the late 1980s.[203] Since that time, five controlled, randomized trials have been published. Three of these trials were placebo controlled,[204–206] and two of the trials utilized an active comparator without placebo.[207,208] Using various measures of depression and outcome, these studies indicate that paroxetine (1 study),[208] mianserin (2 studies),[204,206] fluoxetine (1

study),[205] amitriptyline (1 study),[208] and desipramine (1 study)[207] are useful in treating depression in patients with cancer. A recent open-label, crossover trial suggests that mirtazapine decreased depressive symptoms, improved functional capacity, and reduced cachexia.[209]

Recent studies provide intriguing evidence for a central argument of this chapter: that both inclusive and exclusive approaches to depression in patients with cancer have important clinical implications, and that, although apparently contradictory, both approaches should be held in mind for clinicians to optimally relieve suffering in the context of neoplasia. As discussed above, with the development of the concept of sickness behavior, a coherent rationale is provided for addressing a more inclusive range of emotional, neurovegetative, and physical symptoms than would be targeted under strict definitions of current DSM-IV mood disorders. One implication of this is that mild depressive syndromes, and even subsyndromic depressive symptoms, may be profitably addressed with antidepressant therapy. Two large recent controlled trials support this view. Fisch and colleagues found that treatment with fluoxetine significantly improved depressive symptoms and some measures of quality of life when compared to placebo in cancer patients with a variety of tumors with an expected survival of 3–24 months.[210] Importantly, these patients were recruited based on replies that they were bothered by depressed moods at a severity of "somewhat" or greater and not by meeting criteria for full major depression. A second large trial compared paroxetine to placebo in cancer patients with fatigue and found that the antidepressant significantly lowered depressive symptom scores, even though the mean scores in both groups at baseline were below the standard cutoff for clinically relevant depression.[160]

A second implication of an inclusive approach based on the concept of sickness behavior is that patients may benefit from symptom treatment even when these symptoms do not occur in the context of a mood disturbance.

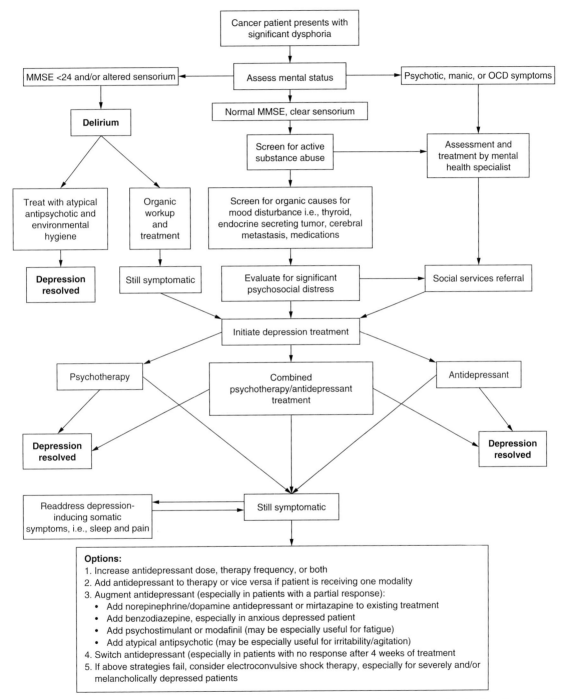

Figure 15-2. Suggested algorithm for the evaluation and pharmacologic treatment of depression in patients with cancer.

Although controversial, gathering data support this notion. In double-blind trials fluoxetine, paroxetine, and venlafaxine have been shown to reduce hot flashes, and have been reported to decrease pruritis in cancer patients.[211–213] Venlafaxine, bupropion, and the tricyclic antidepressants have been shown to relieve neuropathic pain, which frequently accompanies cancer and its treatment.[214–216] A recent open trial found that in cancer patients mirtazapine decreased pain, aided in weight gain, and improved sleep.[209]

While sickness behavior in general supports a broadening of the terrain that is appropriate for therapeutic intervention, recent evidence that cytokine-induced depression is not a unitary phenomenon, but rather represents an amalgam of at least two separable subsyndromes, provides a rationale for privileging depression-specific symptoms that are core features of exclusive diagnostic approaches to depression in the medically ill. Consistent with findings in patients receiving IFN-alpha, a large study has recently observed that depression-specific symptoms are more sensitive to treatment with paroxetine than is fatigue.[160] Specifically, in a large population of cancer patients undergoing several cycles of chemotherapy, paroxetine significantly decreased depression scores compared to placebo, but had no effect on fatigue. Interestingly, patients in this study were recruited based on complaints of fatigue and not depression. Combined with the IFN-alpha literature, this study strongly suggests that serotonergic antidepressants are remarkably effective in treating symptoms privileged by exclusive diagnostic approaches (i.e., symptoms more common in depression than sickness) and less effective in relieving the neurovegetative and physical symptoms shared by sickness and mood disorders. These data highlight the importance of carefully assessing sadness, hopelessness, anxiety, loss of pleasure, and related symptoms, because these symptoms appear to be especially amenable to antidepressant therapy. The urgency of recognizing and addressing these symptoms is also highlighted by increasing data that depression-specific symptoms may disproportionately contribute to the relationship between depression and morbidity/mortality in the context of medical illness.[8,217]

These findings may also provide an explanation for the oft repeated observation that agents with catecholaminergic activity are generally more effective than SSRIs in the treatment of neurovegetative and somatic symptoms, such as pain and fatigue, especially when these symptoms occur outside the context of a diagnosable mood disorder.[170–172,214,218–220] Consistent with this, animal studies suggest that norepinephrine reuptake inhibitors are more effective than serotonergic agents in blocking inflammatory activation and behavioral disturbances following an immune challenge.[221] Moreover, given evidence that proinflammatory cytokines contribute to the development of depression even in medically healthy individuals,[133] these findings may also provide a partial explanation for the growing dataset indicating that combined serotonin-norepinephrine/dopamine treatment strategies (such as adding desipramine or bupropion to an SSRI or using a serotonin-norepinephrine reuptake inhibitor, such as venlafaxine, duloxetine, or milnacipran) outperform serotonergic strategies in the treatment of major depression, even in medically healthy individuals.[222] This increased efficacy may occur, at least in part, because serotonergic and noradrenergic reuptake inhibition targets different symptom dimensions (i.e., by invoking both mechanisms, combined strategies address both depression-specific and neurovegetative symptoms). And indeed, some evidence suggests that combined serotonin-norepinephrine agents are more effective in treating both symptom domains, even in medically healthy individuals.[220,223]

Two implications emerge from these data. The first is that agents with both a broad spectrum of activity (i.e., with effects on serotonin and norepinephrine/dopamine) may be especially effective as first-line treatment in medically ill patients with depression, especially when symptoms such as sadness and loss of interest are combined with prominent fatigue and/or psychomotor slowing. A second implication is that medically ill patients with neurovegetative symptoms, but without prominent mood or anxiety symptoms, might be more parsimoniously treated with noradrenergic/dopaminergic agents, such as psychostimulants or modafinil that will target symptoms such as fatigue and psychomotor slowing, without the added side effect burden (especially sexual dysfunction) imposed by agents that block the reuptake of serotonin. Given their rapid onset of therapeutic action and benign side effects, psychostimulants are also the agents of choice for cancer patients with brief expected survival periods. Although less data are available, dopaminergic agonists may also hold promise for the treatment of cytokine-mediated fatigue and may be useful for the treatment of depression.

Future Considerations

Although not currently included in the standard treatment armamentarium for depression, an obvious first place to intervene in cytokine-induced behavioral disturbance is at the level of cytokine signaling itself. Accumulating data indicate that anticytokine agents effectively diminish a wide range of depressive and sickness symptoms in humans and animals. For example, etanercept (a soluble receptor for TNF-alpha) reduced circulating TNF-alpha in rats with experimentally induced heart failure and restored hedonic drive in a brain stimulation paradigm.[224] In patients with rheumatoid arthritis (RA), etanercept has been shown to significantly improve fatigue and reduce depressive and anxiety symptoms. Similar results have recently been observed in patients with Crohn disease receiving the anti-TNF-alpha antibody infliximab. When compared to placebo, treatment with infliximab significantly improved ability to work and pursue leisure activities and decreased fatigue, depression, and anger.[225] Animal studies suggest that the soluble receptor antagonist for IL-1 (IL-1ra) may also have potential as a treatment for cytokine-induced symptoms,[134,226,227] but little has been published regarding the effect of this agent on sickness/depressive symptoms

in humans. Despite their potential usefulness, however, the value of anticytokine therapies in the treatment of cytokine-induced depressive syndromes will need to be balanced against the potential for serious side effects posed by these agents, including an increased risk for infection and autoimmune conditions.[228–230]

The physiologic effects of proinflammatory cytokines are mediated by activation of intracellular second messenger systems, such as mitogen-activated protein kinase and nuclear factor-kappa-beta signaling pathways.[133] Studies evaluating the therapeutic potential of attenuating activity in these pathways are in their infancy. Nevertheless, agents that increase signaling in intracellular pathways known to inhibit inflammatory signaling may be of benefit in the treatment of immune-related depression. These agents include phosphodiesterase type 4 inhibitors, such as rolipram and ariflo, which decrease proinflammatory cytokine signaling by increasing signaling in cyclic adenosine monophosphate (c-AMP) pathways and possibly through enhancement of anti-inflammatory glucocorticoid pathways.[133,231]

Finally, although all antidepressants have the capacity to normalize functioning in CRH pathways, novel agents in development that directly target CRH type I receptors may hold additional promise for the treatment of depression in the context of cancer. Also, there is evidence that dysregulation of diurnal cortisol levels, which are mediated by CRH, predicts more rapid disease progression in metastatic breast cancer patients.[232] Thus, modulating CRH has the potential to affect both depressive symptoms and potentially could have an effect on disease progression as well.[233]

▶ SUMMARY

Depression is a common and serious problem complicating the lives of cancer patients. There is evidence that depression can be a response to cancer, that preexisting depression can be exacerbated by cancer, and that cancer and its treatment may induce or intensify depression.

Neural pathways involved include serotonergic, noradreneregic, CRH-ACTH-cortisol, and cytokine effects on all of these and others. The evidence is clear that psychopharmacologic treatments are highly effective in reducing depressive symptoms via these and other putative pathways. Similarly, psychotherapies aimed at aiding with the inevitable existential issues confronting cancer patients, along with enhancing active coping, altering depressive cognition, encouraging expression of emotion, and enhancing social support, are effective in reducing depression. Depression is a common but not inevitable complication of life with cancer. Cancer patients deserve vigorous treatment for it.

REFERENCES

1. Spiegel D, Giese-Davis J. Depression and cancer: Mechanisms and disease progression. *Biol Psychiatry* 2003;54:269–282.
2. McDaniel JS, Musselman DL, Porter MR, et al. Depression in patients with cancer; diagnosis, biology and treatment. *Arch Gen Psychiatry* 1995;52:89–99.
3. Colon EA, Callies AL, Popkin MK, et al. Depressed mood and other variables related to bone marrow tranplant survival in acute leukemia. *Psychosomatics* 1991;32:420–425.
4. Giese-Davis J, Spiegel D. Emotional expression and cancer progression. In: Davidson RJ, Scherer K, Hill Goldsmith H (eds.), *Handbook of Affective Sciences.* Oxford: Oxford University Press, 2003, pp. 1053–1082.
5. American Psychiatric Association. *Diagnostic and Statistical Manual of Mental Disorders.* Washington, DC: American Psychiatric Press, 1994.
6. Cohen-Cole SA, Brown FW, McDaniel JS. Diagnostic assessment of depresskon in the medically ill. In: Stoudemire A, Fogel B (eds.), *Psychiatric Care of the Medical Patient.* New York: Oxford University Press, 1993, pp. 53–70.
7. Endicott J. Measurement of depression in patients with cancer. *Cancer* 1984;53:2243–2249.
8. von Ammon Cavanaugh S, Furlanetto LM, Creech SD, et al. Medical illness, past depression, and present depression: A predictive triad for in-hospital mortality. *Am J Psychiatry* 2001;158:43–48.
9. Koenig HG, George LK, Peterson BL, et al. Depression in medically ill hospitalized older adults: Prevalence, characteristics, and course of symptoms according to six diagnostic schemes. *Am J Psychiatry* 154:1376–1383.
10. Chochinov HM. Depression in cancer patients. *Lancet Oncol* 2001;2:499–505.
11. Sharpe M, Strong V, Allen K, et al. Major depression in outpatient's attending a regional cancer centre: Screening and unmet treatment needs. *Br J cancer.* 2004;90:314–320.
12. Norton TR, Manne SL, Rubin S, et al. Prevalence and predictors of psychological distress among women with ovarian cancer. *J Clin Oncol* 2004; 22:919–926.
13. Zung WW. A self-rating depression scale. *Arch Gen Psychiatry* 1965;12:63–70.
14. Beck AT. Psychometric properties of the Beck Depression Inventory: Twenty-five years later. *Clin Psychol Rev* 1988;8:77–100.
15. Davidson J, Turnbull CD, Strickland R, et al. The Montgomery-Asberg depression scale: Reliability and validity. *Acta Psychiatr Scand* 1986;73: 544–548.
16. Hamilton MA. A rating scale for depression. *J Neurol Neurosurg Psychiatry* 1960;23:56–62.
17. Valentine AD, Meyers CA, Kling MA, et al. Mood and cognitive side effects of interferon-alpha therapy. *Semin Oncol* 1998;25:39–47.
18. Roth AJ, Kornblith AB, Batel-Copel L, et al. Rapid screening for psychologic distress in men with prostate carcinoma: A pilot study. *Cancer* 1998;82:1904–1908.
19. Hotopf M, Chidgey J, Addington-Hall J, et al. Depression in advanced disease: A systematic review Part 1. Prevalence and case finding. *Palliat Med* 2002;16:81–97.
20. Kessler RC, McGonagle KA, Zhao S, et al. Lifetime and 12-month prevalence of DSM-III-R psychiatric disorders in the United States. Results from the National Comorbidity Survey. *Arch Gen Psychiatry* 1994;51:8–19.
21. Silverstone PH. Concise assessment for depression (CAD): A brief screening approach to depression in the medically ill. *J Psychosom Res* 1996;41:161–170.
22. Handwerker WP. Cultural diversity, stress, and depression: Working women in the Americas. *J Womens Health* 1999;8:1303–1311.
23. Evans DL, Staab JP, Petitto JM, et al. Depression in the medical setting: Biopsychological interactions and treatment considerations. *J Clin Psychiatry* 1999;60:40–55; discussion 6.

24. Weissman MM, Bland RC, Canino GJ, et al. Cross-national epidemiology of major depression and bipolar disorder. *JAMA* 1996;276:293–299.

25. Akechi T, Okamura H, Nishiwaki Y, et al. Psychiatric disorders and associated and predictive factors in patients with unresectable nonsmall cell lung carcinoma: A longitudinal study. *Cancer* 2001;92:2609–2622.

26. Raison CL, Demetrashvili M, Capuron L, et al. Neuropsychiatric side effects of interferon-alpha: Recognition and management. *CNS Drugs*, in press.

27. Evans DL, McCartney CF, Nemeroff CB, et al. Depression in women treated for gynecological cancer: Clinical and neuroendocrine assessment. *Am J Psychiatry* 1986;143:447–452.

28. Moffic HS, Paykel ES. Depression in medical in-patients. *Br J Psychiatry* 1975;126:346–353.

29. Ciaramella A, Poli P. Assessment of depression among cancer patients: The role of pain, cancer type and treatment. *Psychoncology* 2001;10:156–165.

30. Capuron L, Ravaud A, Dantzer R. Timing and specificity of the cognitive changes induced by interleukin-2 and interferon-alpha treatments in cancer patients. *Psychosom Med* 2001;63:376–386.

31. Musselman DL, Lawson DH, Gumnick JF, et al. Paroxetine for the prevention of depression induced by high-dose interferon alfa. *N Engl J Med* 2001;344:961–966.

32. Raison CL, Nemeroff C. Cancer and depression: Prevalence, diagnosis and treatment. *Home Health Care Consultant* 2000;7:34–41.

33. Zebrack BJ, Zeltzer LK, Whitton J, et al. Psychological outcomes in long-term survivors of childhood leukemia, Hodgkin's disease, and non-Hodgkin's lymphoma: A report from the Childhood Cancer Survivor Study. *Pediatrics* 2002;110:42–52.

34. Omne-Ponten M, Holmberg L, Burns T, et al. Determinants of the psycho-social outcome after operation for breast cancer. Results of a prospective comparative interview study following mastectomy and breast conservation. *Eur J Cancer* 1992;28A:1062–1067.

35. Jakeways MS, Mitchell V, Hashim IA, et al. Metabolic and inflammatory responses after open or laparoscopic cholecystectomy. *Br J Surg* 1994;81:127–131.

36. Kristiansson M, Saraste L, Soop M, et al. Diminished interleukin-6 and C-reactive protein responses to laparoscopic versus open cholecystectomy. *Acta Anaesth Scand* 1999;43:146–152.

37. Yirmiya R, Weidenfeld J, Pollak Y, et al. Cytokines, "depression due to a general medical condition," and antidepressant drugs. *Adv Exp Med Biol* 1999;461:283–316.

38. Kudoh A, Katagai H, Takazawa T. Plasma inflammatory cytokine response to surgical trauma in chronic depressed patients. *Cytokine* 2001;13:104–108.

39. Fallowfield LJ, Hall A, Maguire GP, et al. Psychological outcomes of different treatment policies in women with early breast cancer outside a clinical trial. [see comments.]. *Br Med J* 1990;301:575–580.

40. Levy SM, Haynes LT, Herberman RB, et al. Mastectomy versus breast conservation surgery: Mental health effects at long-term follow-up [see comments]. *Health Psychol* 1992;11:349–354.

41. Kruimel JW, Pesman GJ, Sweep CG, et al. Depression of plasma levels of cytokines and ex-vivo cytokine production in relation to the activity of the pituitary-adrenal axis, in patients undergoing major vascular surgery. *Cytokine* 11:382–8, 1999.

42. Di Padova F, Pozzi C, Tondre MJ, et al. Selective and early increase of IL-1 inhibitors, IL-6 and cortisol after elective surgery. *Clin Exp Immunol* 1991;85:137–142.

43. DiMatteo MR, Lepper HS, Croghan TW. Depression is a risk factor for noncompliance with medical treatment: Meta-analysis of the effects of anxiety and depression on patient adherence. *Arch Intern Med* 2000;160:2101–2107.

44. Blotcky AD, Cohen DG, Conatser C, et al. Psychosocial characteristics of adolescents who refuse cancer treatment. *J Consult Clin Psychol* 1985;53:729–731.

45. Gilbar O, De-Nour AK. Adjustment to illness and dropout of chemotherapy. *J Psychosom Res* 1989;33:1–5.

46. Lebovits AH, Strain JJ, Schleifer SJ, et al. Patience noncompliance with self-administered chemotherapy. *Cancer* 1990;65:17–22.

47. Desai MM, Bruce ML, Kasl SV. The effects of major depression and phobia on stage at diagnosis of breast cancer. *Int J Psychiatry Med* 1999;29:29–45.

48. Kennard BD, Stewart SM, Olvera R, et al. Nonadherence in adolescent oncology patients: Preliminary data on psychological risk factors and

relationships to outcome., *J Clin Psychol Med Settings* 2004;11:30–39.

49. Miranda CR, de Resende CN, Melo CF, et al. Depression before and after uterine cervix and breast cancer neoadjuvant chemotherapy. *Int J Gynecol Cancer* 2002;12:773–776.

50. Lerman C, Daly M, Sands C, et al. Mammography adherence and psychological distress among women at risk for breast cancer. *J Natl Cancer Inst* 1993;85:1074–1080.

51. Lerman C, Narod S, Schulman K, et al. BRCA1 testing in families with hereditary breast-ovarian cancer. A prospective study of patient decision making and outcomes. *JAMA* 1996;275:1885–1892.

52. Lindberg NM, Wellisch D. Anxiety and compliance among women at high risk for breast cancer. *Ann Behav Med* 2001;23:298–303.

53. Ayres A, Hoon PW, Franzoni JB, et al. Influence of mood and adjustment to cancer on compliance with chemotherapy among breast cancer patients. *J Psychosom Res* 1994;38:393–402.

54. Ritvo P, Irvine J, Robinson G, et al. Psychological adjustment to familial-genetic risk assessment for ovarian cancer: Predictors of nonadherence to surveillance recommendations. *Gynecol Oncol* 2002;84:72–80.

55. Simmons K, Lindsay S. Psychological influences on acceptance of postsurgical treatment in cancer patients. *J Psychosom Res* 2001;51:355–360.

56. Girardi P, dePisa E, Cianfriglia F, et al. Compliance with treatment for head and neck cancer: The influence of psychologic and psychopathologic variables: A longitudinal study. *Eur J Psychiatry* 1992;6:45–50.

57. Burstein HJ, Gelber S, Guadagnoli E, et al. Use of alternative medicine by women with early-stage breast cancer. *N Engl J Med* 1999;340:1733–1739.

58. Sollner W, Maislinger S, DeVries AC, et al. Use of complementary and alternative medicine by cancer patients is not associated with perceived distress or poor compliance with standard treatment but with active coping behavior: A survey. *Cancer* 2000;89:873–880.

59. Verhoef MJ, Hagen N, Pelletier G, et al. Alternative therapy use in neurologic diseases: Use in brain tumor patients. *Neurology* 1999;52:617–622.

60. Mehta P, Rodrigue J, Nejame C, et al. Acquiescence to adjunctive experimental therapies may relate to psychological distress: Pilot data from a bone marrow transplant center. *Bone Marrow Transplant* 2000;25:673–676.

61. Esplen MJ, Toner B, Hunter J, et al. A supportive-expressive group intervention for women with a family history of breast cancer: Results of a phase 11 study. *Psychooncology* 2000;9:243–252.

62. Richardson JL, Marks G, Johnson CA, et al. Path model of multidimensional compliance with cancer therapy. *Health Psychol* 1987;6:183–207.

63. McEwen B. Influences of hormones and neuroactive substances on immune function. In: Cotman CW, Briton RE, Galaburda A, McEwen B, Schneider DM (eds.), *The Neuro-Immune-Endocrine Connection*. New York: Raven Press, 1987.

64. Deuschle M, Schweiger U, Weber B, et al. Diurnal activity and pulsatility of the hypothalamus-pituitary-adrenal system in male depressed patients and healthy controls. *J Clin Endocrinol Metab* 1997;82:234–238.

65. Thompson LM, Rubin RT, McCracken JT. Neuroendocrine aspects of primary endogenous depression: XII. Receiver operating characteristic and kappa analyses of serum and urine cortisol measures in patients and matched controls. *Psychoneuroendocrinology* 1992;17:507–515.

66. Yehuda R, Teicher MH, Trestman RL, et al. Cortisol regulation in posttraumatic stress disorder and major depression: A chronobiological analysis. *Biol Psychiatry* 1996;40:79–88.

67. Touitou Y, Levi F, Bogdan A, et al. Rhythm alteration in patients with metastatic breast cancer and poor prognostic factors. *J Cancer Res Clin Oncol* 1995;121:181–188.

68. vd Pompe G, Antoni M, Visser A, et al. Adjustment to breast cancer: The psychobiological effects of psychosocial interventions. *Patient Educ Couns* 1996;28:209–219.

69. Sephton SE, Sapolsky RM, Kraemer HC, et al. Early mortality in metastatic breast cancer patients with absent or abnormal diurnal cortisol rhythms. *J Nat Cancer Inst* 2000;92:994–1000.

70. Davis S, Mirick D, Stevens R. Night shift work, light at night, and risk of breast cancer. *J Nat Cancer Inst* 2001;93:1557–1562.

71. Schernhammer E, Laden F, Speizer F, et al. Rotating night shifts and risk of breast cancer in women participating in the nurses' health study. *J Nat Cancer Inst* 2001;93:1563–1568.

72. Shafii M, Shafii SL. *Melatonin in psychiatric and neoplastic disorders*. Washington, DC: American Psychiatric Press, 1998, Vol. xxiii, p. 314.

73. Spiegel D, Sephton S. Night shift work, light at night, and risk of breast cancer. *J Natl Cancer Inst* 2002;94:530; author reply 2–3.

74. Mormont MC, Bogdan A, Cormont S, et al. Cortisol diuranal variation in blood and saliva of patients with metastatic corectal cancer: Relevance for clinical outcome. *Anti Cancer Res* 2002;22:1243–1250.

75. Filipski E, King VM, Li X, et al. Host circadian clock as a control point in tumor progression. *J Nat Cancer Inst* 2002;94:690–7.

76. Romero L, Raley-Susman K, Redish D, et al. A possible mechanism by which stress accelerates growth of virally-derived tumors. *Proc Natl Acad Sci USA* 1992;89:11084.

77. Zhao X-Y, Malloy PJ, Krishnan AV, et al. Glucocorticoids can promote androgen-independent growth of prostate cancer cells through a mutated androgen receptor. *Nat Med* 2000;6:703–706.

78. Sapolsky RM, Donnelly TM. Vulnerability to stress-induced tumor growth increases with age in rats: Role of glucocorticoids. *Endocrinology* 1985;117:662–666.

79. Ben-Eliyahu S, Yirmiya R, Liebeskind JC, et al. Stress increases metastatic spread of a mammary tumor in rats: Evidence for mediation by the immune system. *Brain Behav Immun* 1991;5: 193–205.

80. Rowse GJ, Weinberg J, Bellward GD, et al. Endocrine mediation of psychosocial stressor effects on mouse mammary tumor growth. *Cancer Lett* 1992;65:85–93.

81. Licinio J, Gold PW, Wong ML. A molecular mechanism for stress-induced alterations in susceptibility to disease. *Lancet* 1995;346:104–106.

82. Maes M, Bosmans E, Meltzer HY. Immunoendocrine aspects of major depression. Relationships between plasma interleukin-6 and soluble interleukin-2 receptor, prolactin and cortisol. *Eur Arch Psychiatry Clin Neurosci* 1995;245: 172–178.

83. Maes M, Meltzer HY, Stevens W, et al. Natural killer cell activity in major depression: Relation to circulating natural killer cells, cellular indices of the immune response, and depressive phenomenology. *Prog Neuropsychopharmolacol Biol Psychiatry* 1994;18:717–730.

84. Allen AD, Tilkian SM. Depression correlated with cellular immunity in systemic immunodeficient Epstein-Barr virus syndrome (SIDES). *J Clin Psychiatry* 1986;47:133–135.

85. DeLisi LE, Nurnberger JS, Goldin LR, et al. Epstein-Barr virus and depression [letter]. *Arch Gen Psychiatry* 1986;43:815–816.

86. Hickie I, Hickie C, Lloyd A, et al. Impaired in vivo immune responses in patients with melancholia. *Br J Psychiatry* 1993;162:651–657.

87. Kniker WT. Multi-Test skin testing in allergy: A review of published findings. *Ann Allergy* 1993;71:485–491.

88. Levy SM, Herberman RB, Maluish AM, et al. Prognostic risk assessment in primary breast cancer by behavioral and immunological parameters. *Health Psychol* 1985;4:99–113.

89. Levy SM, Wise BD. *Psychosocial Risk Factors and Cancer Progression.* Chichester: John Wiley & Sons, 1988.

90. Evans DL, Folds JD, Petitto JM, et al. Circulating natural killer cell phenotypes in men and women with major depression. Relation to cytotoxic activity and severity of depression. *Arch Gen Psychiatry* 1992;49:388–395.

91. Herbert TB, Cohen S. Depression and immunity: A meta-analytic review. *Psychol Bull* 1993;113: 472–486.

92. Baltrusch HJ, Stangel W, Titze I. Stress, cancer and immunity. New developments in biopsychosocial and psychoneuroimmunologic research. *Acta Neurol* 1991;13:315–327.

93. Andersen BL, Kiecolt-Glaser JK, Glaser R. A biobehavioral model of cancer stress and disease course. *Am Psychol* 1994;49:389–404.

94. Levy S, Herberman R, Lippman M, et al. Correlation of stress factors with sustained depression of natural killer cell activity and predicted prognosis in patients with breast cancer. *J Clin Oncol* 1987;5:348–353.

95. Levy SM, Herberman RB, Lippman M, et al. Immunological and psychosocial predictors of disease recurrence in patients with early-stage breast cancer. *Behav Med* 1991;17:67–75.

96. Levy SM, Herberman RB, Whiteside T, et al. Perceived social support and tumor estrogen/progesterone receptor status as predictors of natural killer cell activity in breast cancer patients. *Psychosom Med* 1990;52:73–85.

97. Andersen BL, Farrar WB, Golden-Kreutz D, et al. Stress and immune responses after surgical treatment for regional breast cancer. *J Nat Cancer Inst* 1998;90:30–36.

98. Landmann RM, Muller FB, Perini C, et al. Changes of immunoregulatory cells induced by

psychological and physical stress: Relationship to plasma catecholamines. *Clin Exp Immunol* 1984;58:127–135.

99. Callewaert DM, Moudgil VK, Radcliff G, et al. Hormone specific regulation of natural killer cells by cortisol. *FEBS J* 1991;285:108–110.

100. Felten SY, Olschowka J. Noradrenergic sympathetic innervation of the spleen: II. Tyrosine hydroxylase (TH)-positive nerve terminals form synapticlike contacts on lymphocytes in the splenic white pulp. *J Neurosci Res* 1987;18:37–48.

101. Bovbjerg D. Psychoneruoimmunology and cancer. *Handbook Psychooncol* 1989:727–754.

102. Bergsma J. Illness, the mind, and the body: Cancer and immunology: An introduction. *Theor Med* 1994;15:337–347.

103. Souberbielle B, Dalgleish A. Anti-tumor immune mechanisms. In: Lewis CE, O'Sullivan C, Barraclough J (eds.), *The Psychoimmunology of Cancer: Mind and Body in the Fight for Survival*. Oxford: Oxford University Press, 1994, pp. 267–290.

104. Schleifer SJ, Keller SE, Bond RN, et al. Major depressive disorder and immunity. Role of age, sex, severity, and hospitalization. *Arch Gen Psychiatry* 1989;46:81–87.

105. Stein M, Miller AH, Trestman RL. Depression, the immune system, and health and illness. Findings in search of meaning. *Arch Gen Psychiatry* 1991;48:171–177.

106. Bovbjerg DH, Redd WH, Maier LA, et al. Anticipatory immune suppression and nausea in women receiving cyclic chemotherapy for ovarian cancer. *J Consult Clin Psychol* 1990;58:153–157.

107. Ader R, Felten D, Cohen N. Interactions between the brain and the immune system. *Annu Rev Pharmacol Toxicol* 1990;30:561–602.

108. Ader R, Cohen N. Psychoneuroimmunology: Conditioning and stress. *Annu Rev Psychol* 1993;44:53–85.

109. Ader R, Cohen N, Felten D. Psychoneuroimmunology: Interactions between the nervous system and the immune system. *Lancet* 1995;345:99–103.

110. Gold PW, Goodwin FK, Chrousos GP. Clinical and biochemical manifestations of depression. Relation to the neurobiology of stress. *N Engl J Med* 1988;319:348–353.

111. Alter CL, Pelcovitz D, Axelrod A, et al. Identification of PTSD in cancer survivors. *Psychometrics* 1996;37:137–143.

112. Andrykowski MA, Cordova MJ. Factors associated with PTSD symptoms following treatment for breast cancer: A test of the Andersen model. *J Traum Stress* 1998;11:189–203.

113. Andrykowski MA, Cordova MJ, Studts JL, et al. Posttraumatic stress disorder after treatment for breast cancer: Prevalence of diagnosis and use of the PTSD Checklist-Civilian Version (PCL-C) as a screening instrument. *J Consult Clin Psychol* 1998;66:586–590.

114. Green BL, Rowland JH, Krupnick JL, et al. Prevalence of posttraumatic stress disorder (PTSD) in women with breast cancer. *Psychometrics* 1998;32:102–111.

115. Smith MY, Redd W, DuHamel K, et al. Validation of the PTSD checklist-civilian version in survivors of bone marrow transplant. *J Traum Stress* 1999;12:485–499.

116. Spiegel D, Kato P. Psychosocial influences on concer incidence and progression. *Harv Rev Psychiatry* 1996;4:10–26.

117. Kaplan RM, Ries AL, Prewitt LM, et al. Self-efficacy expectations predict survival for patients with chronic obstructive pulmonary disease. *Health Psychol* 1994;13:366–368.

118. Koopman C, Hermanson K, Diamond S, et al. Social support, life stress, pain and emotional adjustment to advanced breast cancer. *Psychooncology* 1998;7:101–111.

119. Spiegel D, Bloom JR. Pain in metastatic breast cancer. *Cancer* 1983;52:341–345.

120. Bukberg J, Penman D, Holland JC. Depression in hospitalized cancer patients. *Psychosom Med* 1984;46:199–212.

121. Spiegel D, Sands S, Koopman C. Pain and depression in patients with cancer. *Cancer* 1994;74:2570–2578.

122. Katon W, Sullivan M. Depression and chronic medical illness. *J Behav Med* 1990;11:3–11.

123. Weitzner MA, Meyers CA, Stuebing KK, et al. Relationship between quality of life and mood in long-term survivors of breast cancer treated with mastectomy. *Support Care Cancer* 1997;5:241–248.

124. Cohen L, de Moor C, Amato RJ. The association between treatment-specific optimism and depressive symptomatology in patients enrolled in a Phase I cancer clinical trial. *Cancer* 2001;91:1949–1955.

125. Maier SF, Watkins LR. Cytokines for psychologists: Implications of bidirectional immune-to-brain

communication for understanding behavior, mood, and cognition. *Psychol Rev* 1998;105: 83–107.

126. Rivest S, Lacroix S, Vallieres L, et al. How the blood talks to the brain parenchyma and the paraventricular nucleus of the hypothalamus during systemic inflammatory and infectious stimuli. *Proc Soc Exp Biol Med* 2000;223:22–38.

127. Plotkin SR, Banks WA, Kastin AJ. Comparison of saturable transport and extracellular pathways in the passage of interleukin-1 alpha across the blood-brain barrier. *J Neuroimmunol* 1996;67: 41–47.

128. Watkins LR, Maier SF, Goehler LE. Cytokine-to-brain communication: A review & analysis of alternative mechanisms. *Life Sci* 1995;57:1011–1026.

129. Benveniste EN. Cytokine actions in the central nervous system. *Cytokine Growth Factor Rev* 1998;9:259–275.

130. Kent S, Bluthe RM, Kelley KW, et al. Sickness behavior as a new target for drug development. *Trends Pharmacol Sci* 1992;13:24–28.

131. Dunn AJ, Wang J, Ando T. Effects of cytokines on cerebral neurotransmission. Comparison with the effects of stress. *Adv Exp Med Biol* 1999; 461:117–127.

132. Dantzer R. Cytokine-induced sickness behavior: Where do we stand? *Brain Behav Immun* 2001; 15:7–24.

133. Raison CL, Miller AH. When not enough is too much: The role of insufficient glucocorticoid signaling in the pathophysiology of stress-related disorders. *Am J Psychiatry* 2003;160:1554–1565.

134. Maier SF, Watkins LR. Intracerebroventricular interleukin-1 receptor antagonist blocks the enhancement of fear conditioning and interference with escape produced by inescapable shock. *Brain Res* 1995;695:279–282.

135. Pugh CR, Nguyen KT, Gonyea JL, et al. Role of interleukin-1 beta in impairment of contextual fear conditioning caused by social isolation. *Behav Brain Res* 1999;106:109–118.

136. Mathias SD, Colwell HH, Miller DP, et al. Health-related quality of life and functional status of patients with rheumatoid arthritis randomly assigned to receive etanercept or placebo. *Clin Ther* 2000;22:128–139.

137. Musselman DL, Miller AH, Porter MR, et al. Higher than normal plasma interleukin-6 concentrations in cancer patients with depression: Preliminary findings. *Am J Psychiatry* 2001;158:1252–1257.

138. Allen-Mersh TG, Glover C, Fordy C, et al. Relation between depression and circulating immune products in patients with advanced colorectal cancer. *J Royal Soc Med* 1998;91:408–413.

139. Capuron L, Ravaud A, Gualde N, et al. Association between immune activation and early depressive symptoms in cancer patients treated with interleukin-2-based therapy. *Psychoneuroendocrinology* 2001;26:797–808.

140. Greenberg DB, Gray JL, Mannix CM, et al. Treatment-related fatigue and serum interleukin-1 levels in patients during external beam irradiation for prostate cancer. *J Pain Symp Manage* 1993;8:196–200.

141. Bower JE, Ganz PA, Aziz N, et al. Fatigue and proinflammatory cytokine activity in breast cancer survivors. *Psychosom Med* 2002;64: 604–611.

142. Besedovsky H, del Rey A, Sorkin E, et al. Immunoregulatory feedback between interleukin-1 and glucocorticoid hormones. *Science* 1986;233:652–654.

143. Rivier C. Influence of immune signals on the hypothalamic-pituitary axis of the rodent. *Front Neuroendocrinol* 1995;16:151–182.

144. Owens MJ, Nemeroff CB. Physiology and pharmacology of corticotropin-releasing factor. *Pharmacol Rev* 1991;43:425–473.

145. Holsboer F, Barden N. Antidepressants and hypothalamic-pituitary-adrenocortical regulation. *Endocrine Rev* 1996;17:187–205.

146. Owens MJ, Nemeroff CB. The role of corticotropin-releasing factor in the pathophysiology of affective and anxiety disorders: Laboratory and clinical studies. *Ciba Found Symp* 1993;172: 296–308; discussion 16.

147. Lestage J, Verrier D, Palin K, et al. The enzyme indoleamine 2,3-dioxygenase is induced in the mouse brain in response to peripheral administration of lipopolysaccharide and superantigen. *Brain Behav Immun* 2002;16:596–601.

148. Capuron L, Ravaud A, Neveu PJ, et al. Association between decreased serum tryptophan concentrations and depressive symptoms in cancer patients undergoing cytokine therapy. *Mol Psychiatry* 2002;7:468–473.

149. Liebau C, Baltzer AW, Schmidt S, et al. Interleukin-12 and interleukin-18 induce indoleamine 2,3-dioxygenase (IDO) activity in human osteosarcoma cell lines independently from interferon-gamma. *Anticancer Res* 2002;22:931–936.

150. Moore P, Landolt HP, Seifritz E, et al. Clinical and physiological consequences of rapid tryptophan depletion. *Neuropsychopharmolacol* 2000;23:601–622.

151. Pariante CM, Miller AH. Glucocorticoid receptors in major depression: Relevance to pathophysiology and treatment. *Biol Psychiatry* 2001;49:391–404.

152. Papanicolaou DA. Euthyroid sick syndrome and the role of cytokines. *Rev Endocr Metab Disord* 2000;1:43–48.

153. Abbas AK, Lichtman AH. *Cellular and Molecular Immunology.* Philadelphia, PA: W.B. Saunders, 2003.

154. Taylor JL, Grossberg SE. The effects of interferon-alpha on the production and action of other cytokines. *Semin Oncol* 1998;25:23–29.

155. Capuron L, Raison CL, Musselman DL, et al. Association of exaggerated HPA axis response to the initial injection of interferon-alpha with development of depression during interferon-alpha therapy. *Am J Psychiatry* 2003;160:1342–1345.

156. Schaefer M, Engelbrecht MA, Gut O, et al. Interferon alpha (IFNa) and psychiatric syndromes: A review. *Prog Neuropsychopharmolacol* 2002;26:731–746.

157. Merali Z, Brennan K, Brau P, et al. Dissociating anorexia and anhedonia elicited by interleukin-1beta: Antidepressant and gender effects on responding for "free chow" and "earned" sucrose intake. *Psychopharmacology* 2003;165:413–418.

158. Capuron L, Gumnick JF, Musselman DL, et al. Neurobehavioral effects of interferon-alpha in cancer patients: Phenomenology and paroxetine responsiveness of symptom dimensions. *Neuropsychopharmol* 2002;26:643–652.

159. Cleeland CS, Mendoza TR, Wang XS, et al. Assessing symptom distress in cancer patients: The M.D. Anderson Symptom Inventory. *Cancer* 2000;89:1634–1646.

160. Morrow GR, Hickok JT, Roscoe JA, et al. Differential effects of paroxetine on fatigue and depression: A randomized, double-blind trial from the university of Rochester Cancer Center community clinical oncology program. *J Clin Oncol* 2003;21:4635–4641.

161. Capuron L, Neurauter G, Musselman DL, et al. Interferon-alpha-induced changes in tryptophan metabolism: Relationship to depression and paroxetine treatment. *Biol Psychiatry* 2003;54:906–914.

162. Mellor AL, Munn DH. Tryptophan catabolism and T-cell tolerance: Immunosuppression by starvation? *Immunol Today* 1999;20:469–473.

163. Moreno FA, Gelenberg AJ, Heninger GR, et al. Tryptophan depletion and depressive vulnerability. *Biol Psychiatry* 1999;46:498–505.

164. Moreno FA, Heninger GR, McGahuey CA, et al. Tryptophan depletion and risk of depression relapse: A prospective study of tryptophan depletion as a potential predictor of depressive episodes. *Biol Psychiatry* 2000;48:327–329.

165. Bonaccorso S, Marino V, Puzella A, et al. Increased depressive ratings in patients with hepatitis C receiving interferon-alpha-based immunotherapy are related to interferon-alpha-induced changes in the serotonergic system. *J Clin Psychopharmacol* 2002;22:86–90.

166. Widner B, Ledochowski M, Fuchs D. Interferon-gamma-induced tryptophan degradation: Neuropsychiatric and immunological consequences. *Cur Drug Metab* 2000;1:193–204.

167. Cummings JL. Depression and Parkinson's disease: A review. *Am J Psychiatry* 1992;149:443–454.

168. Berger JR, Arendt G. HIV dementia: The role of the basal ganglia and dopaminergic systems. *J Psychopharmacol* 2000;14:214–221.

169. Martinot M, Bragulat V, Artiges E, et al. Decreased presynaptic dopamine function in the left caudate of depressed patients with affective flattening and psychomotor retardation. *Am J Psychiatry* 2001;158:314–316.

170. Sarhill N, Walsh D, Nelson KA, et al. Methylphenidate for fatigue in advanced cancer: A prospective open-label pilot study. *Am J Hospice Palliat Care* 2001;18:187–192.

171. Sugawara Y, Akechi T, Shima Y, et al. Efficacy of methylphenidate for fatigue in advanced cancer patients: A preliminary study. *Palliat Med* 2002;16:261–263.

172. Zifko UA, Rupp M, Schwarz S, et al. Modafinil in treatment of fatigue in multiple sclerosis. Results of an open-label study. *J Neurol* 2002;249:983–987.

173. Goldberg JF, Burdick KE, Endick CJ. Preliminary randomized, double-blind, placebo-controlled trial of pramipexole added to mood stabilizers for treatment-resistant bipolar depression. *Am J Psychiatry* 2004;161:564–566.

174. Corrigan MH, Denahan AQ, Wright CE, et al. Comparison of pramipexole, fluoxetine, and placebo in patients with major depression. *Depress Anxiety* 2000;11:58–65.

175. Shuto H, Kataoka Y, Horikawa T, et al. Repeated interferon-alpha administration inhibits dopaminergic neural activity in the mouse brain. *Brain Res* 1997;747:348–351.

176. Sunami M, Nishikawa T, Yorogi A, et al. Intravenous administration of levodopa ameliorated a refractory akathisia case induced by interferon-alpha. *Clin Neuropharmacol* 2000;23:59–61.

177. Haas HS, Schauenstein K. Neuroimmunomodulation via limbic structures: The neuroanatomy of psychoimmunology. *Progr Neurobiol* 1997;51:195–222.

178. Gao HM, Jiang J, Wilson B, et al. Microglial activation-mediated delayed and progressive degeneration of rat nigral dopaminergic neurons: Relevance to Parkinson's disease. *J Neurochem* 2002;81:1285–1297.

179. Juengling FD, Ebert D, Gut O, et al. Prefrontal cortical hypometabolism during low-dose interferon alpha treatment. *Psychopharmacol* 2000;152:383–389.

180. Capuron L, Pagnoni G, Lawson D, et al. Altered fronto-pallidal activity during high-dose interferon-alpha treatment as determined by positron emission tomography. *Soc Neurosci Abstract* 2002;498:5.

181. Musselman DL. Higher than normal plasma interleukin-6 concentrations in cancer patients with depression: Preliminary findings. *Am J Psychiatry* 2001;158:1252–1257.

182. Sutor B, Rummans TA, Jowsey SG, et al. Major depression in medically ill patients. *Mayo Clin Proc* 1998;73:329–337.

183. Spiegel D. Effects of psychotherapy on cancer survival. *Nat Rev Cancer* 2002;2:383–389.

184. Classen C, Butler LD, Koopman C, et al. Supportive-expressive group therapy reduces distress in metastatic breast cancer patients: A randomized clinical intervention trial. *Arch Gen Psychiatry* 2001;58:494–501.

185. Spiegel D, Classen C. *Group Therapy for Cancer Patients: A Research-Based Handbook of Psychosocial Care.* New York: Basic Books, 2000.

186. Spiegel D, Bloom JR, Yalom I. Group support for patients with metastatic cancer. A randomized outcome study. *Arch Gen Psychiatry* 1981;38:527–533.

187. Kissane DW, Bloch S, Miach P, et al. Cognitive-existential group therapy for patients with primary breast cancer: Techniques and themes. *Psychooncology* 1997;6:25–33.

188. Loscalzo M. Psychological approaches to the management of pain in patients with advanced cancer. *Hematol Oncol Clin North Am* 1996;10:139–155.

189. Edelman S, Lemon J, Bell DR, et al. Effects of group CBT on the survival time of patients with metastatic breast cancer. *Psychooncology* 1999;8:474–481.

190. Cruess DG, Antoni MH, McGregor BA, et al. Cognitive-behavioral stress management reduces serum cortisol by enhancing benefit finding among women being treated for early stage breast cancer. *Psychosom Med* 2000;62:304–308.

191. van der Pompe G, Duivenvoorden HJ, Antoni MH, et al. Effectiveness of a short-term group psychotherapy program on endocrine and immune function in breast cancer patients: An exploratory study. *J Psychosom Res* 1997;42:453–466.

192. Rounsaville B, Chevron E, Weissman M. *Specification of techniques in interpersonal psychotherapy.* New York: Guilford Press, 1984.

193. Elkin I, Shea MT, Watkins JT, et al. National Institute of Mental Health Treatment of Depression Collaborative Research Program. General effectiveness of treatments [see comments]. *Arch Gen Psychiatry* 1989;46:971–982; discussion 83.

194. Donnelly JM, Kornblith AB, Fleishman S, et al. A pilot study of interpersonal psychotherapy by telephone with cancer patients and their partners. *Psychooncology* 2000;9:44–56.

195. Spiegel D, Bloom JR, Kraemer HC, et al. Effect of psychosocial treatment on survival of patients with metastatic breast cancer. *Lancet* 1989;2:888–891.

196. Richardson JL, Shelton DR, Krailo M, et al. The effect of compliance with treatment on survival among patients with hematologic malignancies. *J Clin Oncol* 8:356–364.

197. Fawzy F, Fawzy N, Hyun C, et al. Malignant Melanoma: Effects of an early structural psychiatric intervention, coping and affective state on recurrence and survival 6 years later. *Arch Gen Psychiatry* 1993;50:681–689.

198. Kuchler T, Henne-Bruns D, Rappat S, et al. Impact of Psychotherapeutic support on gastrointestinal cancer patients undergoing surgery: Survival results of a trial. *Hepatogastroenterology* 1999;46:322–335.

199. McCorkle R, Strumpf NE, Nuamah IF, et al. A specialized home care intervention improves survival among older post–surgical cancer

patients. [see comments.]. *J Am Geriatr Soc* 2000; 48:1707–1713.

200. Giese-Davis J, Koopman C, Butler L, et al. Change in emotion-regulation strategy for women with metastatic breast cancer following supportive-expressive group therapy. *J Consult Clin Psychol* 2002;70:916–925.

201. Fawzy FI, Canada AL, Fawzy NW. Malignant melanoma: Effects of a brief, structured psychiatric intervention on survival and recurrence at 10-year follow-up. *Arch Gen Psychiatry* 2003;60: 100–103.

202. Goodwin PJ, Leszez M, Ennis M, et al. The effect of group psychosocial support on survival in metastatic breast cancer. *N Engl J Med* 345: 1719–26, 2001.

203. Evans DL, McCartney CF, Haggerty JJ Jr., et al. Treatment of depression in cancer patients is associated with better life adaptations: A pilot study. *Psychosom Med* 1988;50:73–76.

204. Costa D, Mogos I, Toma T. Efficacy and safety of mianserin in the treatment of depression of women with cancer. *Acta Psychiatr Scand Suppl* 1985;320.

205. Razavi D, Allilaire JF, Smith M, et al. The effect of fluoxetine on anxiety and depression symptoms in cancer patients. *Acta Psychiatr Scand* 1996;94:205–210.

206. van Heeringen K, Zivkov M. Pharmacological treatment of depression in cancer patients: A placebo-controlled study of miasnerin. *Br J Psychiatry* 1996;169:440–443.

207. Holland JC, Romano SJ, Heiligenstein JH, et al. A controlled trial of fluoxetine and desipramine in depressed women with advanced cancer. *Psychooncology* 1998;7:291–300.

208. Pezzella G, Moslinger-Gehmayr R, Contu A. Treatment of depression in patients with breast cancer: A comparison between paroxetine and amitriptyline. *Breast Cancer Res Treat* 2001;70:1–10.

209. Theobald DE, Kirsh KL, Holtsclaw E, et al. An open-label, crossover trial of mirtazapine (15 and 30 mg) in cancer patients with pain and other distressing symptoms. *J Pain Symp Manage* 2002;23:442–447.

210. Fisch MJ, Loehrer PJ, Kristeller J, et al. Fluoxetine versus placebo in advanced cancer outpatients: A double-blinded trial of the Hoosier Oncology Group. *J Clin Oncol* 2003;21:1937–1943.

211. Loprinzi CL, Sloan JA, Perez EA, et al. Phase III evaluation of fluoxetine for treatment of hot flashes. *J Clin Oncol* 2002;20:1578–1583.

212. Stearns V, Isaacs C, Rowland J, et al. A pilot trial assessing the efficacy of paroxetine hydrochloride (Paxil) in controlling hot flashes in breast cancer survivors. [see comments.]. *Ann Oncol* 2000;11:17–22.

213. Loprinzi CL, Kugler JW, Sloan JA, et al. Venlafaxine in management of hot flashes in survivors of breast cancer: A randomised controlled trial. [see comments.]. *Lancet* 2000;356:2059–2063.

214. Max MB, Lynch SA, Muir J, et al. Effects of desipramine, amitriptyline, and fluoxetine on pain in diabetic neuropathy. [see comments.]. *N Engl J Med* 1992;326:1250–1256.

215. Sumpton JE, Moulin DE. Treatment of neuropathic pain with venlafaxine. *Ann Pharmacother* 2001;35:557–559.

216. Semenchuk MR, Sherman S, Davis B. Double-blind, randomized trial of bupropion SR for the treatment of neuropathic pain. *Neurology* 2001; 57:1583–1588.

217. Evans DL, Mason K, Bauer R, et al. Neuropsychiatric manifestations of HIV-1 infection and AIDS. In: Charney D, Coyle J, Davis K, Nemeroff C (eds.), *Psychopharmacology: The Fifth Generation of Progress*. New York: Raven Press, 2002, pp. 1281–1300.

218. Goodnick PJ. Treatment of chronic fatigue syndrome with venlafaxine. *Am J Psychiatry* 1996; 153:294.

219. Goodnick PJ. Bupropion in chronic fatigue syndrome. *Am J Psychiatry* 1990;147:1091.

220. Goldstein DJ, Lu Y, Detke MJ, et al. Duloxetine in the treatment of depression: A double-blind placebo-controlled comparison with paroxetine. *J Clin Psychopharmacol* 2004;24:389–399.

221. Shen Y, Connor TJ, Nolan Y, et al. Differential effect of chronic antidepressant treatments on lipopolysaccharide-induced depressive-like behavioural symptoms in the rat. *Life Sci* 1999;65: 1773–1786.

222. Tran PV, Bymaster FP, McNamara RK, et al. Dual monoamine modulation for improved treatment of major depressive disorder. *J Clin Psychopharmacol* 2003;23:78–86.

223. Entsuah AR, Huang H, Thase ME. Response and remission rates in different subpopulations with major depressive disorder administered venlafaxine, selective serotonin reuptake inhibitors, or placebo. *J Clin Psychiatry* 2001; 62:869–877.

224. Grippo AJ, Francis J, Weiss RM, et al. Cytokine mediation of experimental heart failure-induced

anhedonia. *Am J Physiol Regul Integr Comp Physiol* 2003;284:R666–R673.

225. Lichtenstein GR, Bala M, Han C, et al. Infliximab improves quality of life in patients with Crohn's disease. *Inflamm Bowel Dis* 2002;8:237–243.

226. Opp MR, Krueger JM. Interleukin 1-receptor antagonist blocks interleukin 1-induced sleep and fever. *Am J Physiol* 1991;260:R453–R457.

227. Luheshi G, Miller AJ, Brouwer S, et al. Interleukin-1 receptor antagonist inhibits endotoxin fever and systemic interleukin-6 induction in the rat. *Am J Physiol* 1996;270:E91–E95.

228. Gomez-Reino JJ, Carmona L, Valverde VR, et al. Treatment of rheumatoid arthritis with tumor necrosis factor inhibitors may predispose to significant increase in tuberculosis risk: A multi-center active-surveillance report. *Arthritis Rheum* 2003;48:2122–2127.

229. Kroesen S, Widmer AF, Tyndall A, et al. Serious bacterial infections in patients with rheumatoid arthritis under anti-TNF-alpha therapy. *Rheumatology* 2003;42:617–621.

230. Kwon HJ, Cote TR, Cuffe MS, et al. Case reports of heart failure after therapy with a tumor necrosis factor antagonist. [summary for patients in *Ann Intern Med* 2003;138(10):I48;PMID:12755581]. *Ann Intern Med* 2003;138:807–811.

231. Miller AH, Vogt G, Pearce BD. The phosphodiesterase type 4 inhibitor, rolipram, enhances glucocorticoid receptor function. *Neuropsychopharmology* 2002;27:939–948.

232. Sephton SE, Dhabhar FS, Classen C, et al. The diurnal cortisol slope as a predictor of immune reactivity to interpersonal stress. *Brain Behav Immun* 2000;14:128.

233. Sephton S, Spiegel D. Circadian disruption in cancer: A neuroendocrine-immune pathway from stress to disease? *Brain Behav Immun* 2003;17:321–328.

CHAPTER 16

HIV/AIDS and Mood Disorders

JANE LESERMAN, DEAN G. CRUESS, AND JOHN M. PETITTO

▶ INTRODUCTION

Persons infected with human immunodeficiency virus (HIV) have reported high levels of current stress and past traumatic experiences.[1,2] The combination of past trauma and having a life-threatening illness, particularly one associated with central nervous system (CNS) involvement, may put HIV-infected individuals at heightened risk of developing mood disorders (e.g., major depression, subclinical depressive syndromes, and distress states). In an epidemiologic study of a nationally representative sample of 2864 HIV-infected patients, more than one-third screened positive for major depression and more than one quarter screened positive for dysthymia in the past year.[3] Although these rates were based on screening instruments that often significantly exceed more formal interview-based clinical assessments, HIV-infected individuals commonly report depressive symptoms and distress states throughout the course of the disease. Consequently, there is a need to formally assess for these types of mood disturbances and also to provide access to appropriate pharmacologic and psychologic treatments for depressed or distressed HIV-infected patients.

There are only a few controlled clinical trials of antidepressant medication among HIV-infected individuals, and to date, there are no large-scale, controlled studies of mood-stabilizing medications. The published controlled trials of antidepressant medication have documented their effectiveness among HIV-infected individuals, and the available evidence suggests that the selective serotonin reuptake inhibitors (SSRIs) reduce depressive symptoms and may be better tolerated by patients than older antidepressants.[4] However, careful monitoring must be undertaken to help limit the occurrence of drug interactions regardless of the medication prescribed for HIV-infected persons.

There is also some compelling evidence that not only mood disorders, such as major depression, but also subclinical depressive symptoms and distress states, have an adverse impact on the quality of life and the physical health status of HIV-infected individuals.[5] An accumulating number of published studies have examined the impact of depression and distress on neuroendocrine, sympathetic nervous system (SNS), and immune function as plausible pathways through which these psychologic factors may impact HIV disease progression and survival in this population.[5,6] Psychologic interventions including cognitive behavioral approaches may ameliorate the negative effects of stress, impact neuroendocrine activity, SNS, and immune function, and ultimately benefit the course of HIV disease.

This review summarizes the major studies examining the prevalence of mood disorders and the use of pharmacologic and psychologic interventions to treat depression and mania in the context of HIV disease. We show evidence that mood disorders are more prevalent in HIV-infected individuals than in the general population, and discuss some of the challenges in diagnosing mood disorders in HIV-infected persons. We will also reflect on important pharmacologic treatment considerations (e.g., efficacy, side effects, drug-drug interactions) in this population, and evaluate the evidence that pharmacologic and psychologic interventions can improve mood, reduce distress, and affect HIV disease indicators. In addition, we present the evidence that depression and stressful events may accelerate HIV disease progression, and consider some of the underlying physiologic mechanisms through which depression and distress might impact survival in HIV-infected individuals.

▶ DIAGNOSTIC CONSIDERATIONS

Psychiatric disorders, including mood disorders, are frequently unrecognized and untreated among HIV-infected individuals.[7,8] Diagnosing major depression is complicated by the fact that a number of depressive symptoms (e.g., fatigue, sleep disturbance, weight loss, difficulty concentrating) are also common symptoms of HIV disease.[9–11] Depressive symptoms may also reflect symptoms associated with a comorbid substance-related disorder.[12] Due to a number of overlapping symptom features, it is plausible that mood disorders may be under-diagnosed and inadequately treated in this population; thus, a thorough medical and psychiatric assessment is essential. Because of the potential for under-diagnosis, an inclusive approach in diagnosing depression is generally recommended in patients with a medical illness, such as HIV disease.

The assessment of mood disorders among HIV-infected persons poses other distinctive challenges, including that mood disorders may be considered primary or secondary to the medical illness. Treisman and colleagues[13] have stated that HIV-infected individuals with a primary mood disorder may or may not have a previous history of a mood disorder, but may have prevalence rates similar to traditional risk groups, such as homosexual men and intravenous drug users. On the other hand, individuals with a mood disorder secondary to HIV disease do not necessarily have a prior history or a familial history, and the mood disturbance most likely results from viral infection and CNS brain involvement. One must also consider the possibility of a spontaneous onset of first episode as well as a recurrence of depression in recently diagnosed HIV-infected individuals. Distinguishing between primary and secondary mood disorders among HIV-infected patients requires a thorough assessment of affective symptoms both current and past, and also a comprehensive evaluation of medical and neurologic contributions.

Researchers have addressed the issue of whether persons infected with HIV are at greater risk for developing a mood disorder compared to similar cohorts without HIV-infection. We know that persons at greatest risk for HIV (e.g., intravenous drug users, homosexuals, those in poverty) are also at greater risk for developing depression. The issue is whether HIV confers an added risk for depression over and above inclusion in these cohorts. Based on the most recent meta-analysis comparing HIV positive and HIV negative persons, those infected with HIV were shown to have twice the risk of having a current major depression.[14] Although the individual studies in the meta-analysis did not show that depression differed between serostatus groups, combined together, there was ample power to detect such differences. In the World Health Organization (WHO) study,[15] prevalence rates of major depression in two sites tended to be higher in the HIV-infected symptomatic individuals (17.4 and 18.4%) compared to seronegative controls (1.7 and 7.8%). Morrison and colleagues[16] examined women who were not current substance abusers including 93 HIV-infected and 62 noninfected controls. They found that the HIV-infected women had a significantly higher prevalence rate of major depressive disorder (19.4%) compared to the noninfected controls (4.8%). Like studies conducted mostly on men, this study suggests that HIV-infected women are at a significantly greater risk of major depressive disorder compared with demographically similar groups of noninfected women.

Similar to studies in younger populations, recent data from the 5-site Veterans Aging Cohort Study found that older HIV-infected veterans demonstrate greater prevalence of depressive symptoms than age-matched, noninfected veterans.[17] In addition, depressive symptoms appeared to decrease with age in the noninfected participants but not among the HIV-infected participants. Another recent study also found that unlike noninfected older adults (over 50 years of age) who exhibit a decline in depressive symptoms with age, older HIV-infected individuals do not show the same decline in depressive symptoms.[18] Thus, there is evidence that HIV confers a greater risk of depression for men and women, and young and old. Higher rates of depression in HIV-infected persons compared to the general population[3] may be due to both being in a high-risk group (e.g., intravenous drug user, homosexual) and to psychologic and physiologic factors associated with HIV infection.

Another issue is whether depression becomes more prevalent as HIV disease progresses. In other words, does advancing disease increase the risk of developing a major depression? The meta-analysis of cross-sectional studies found that persons with symptomatic disease had similar rates of depression compared to as asymptomatic HIV-infected persons.[14] This issue of whether depression becomes more prevalent as HIV progresses is better addressed with longitudinal studies. In addition, the question is more complex in that we must ask whether disease change leads to depression or vice versa.

Lyketsos and colleagues[19] reported an increase in depressive symptoms approximately 1.5 years before the onset of AIDS. In analyzing data out to 9 years, Leserman showed that AIDS clinical symptoms and $CD4^+$ cell count did not predict major depression[5]; however, depressive symptoms did predict increased risk of AIDS,[20] and

an AIDS clinical condition.[21] Rabkin et al.[22] found that depression did not increase despite worsening HIV infection across a 4-year period. To the contrary in another 3-year study, Rabkin et al.[23] found that those with fewer HIV symptoms had more psychologic improvement compared to those with more symptoms. An 8-year longitudinal study showed that depressive symptoms were associated with diminished performance on neuropsychologic measures of attention, executive functioning, and speed of information processing.[24] Neuropsychologic impairment is one indicator of HIV disease progression. A cross-sectional study examining HIV-infected depressed and nondepressed men found that the two groups did not differ on global neurocognitive impairment, although the depressed individuals exhibited greater memory impairment.[25] From this brief examination of studies, it seems that depression may be more likely to lead to clinical disease change than vice versa. We will discuss the evidence for this hypothesis in more detail later in this chapter.

▶ PREVALENCE OF MOOD DISORDERS IN HIV INFECTION

It is clear from the discussion above that in estimating prevalence of mood disorders we must consider whether the disorder is primary or secondary to HIV infection, the overlap between symptoms of HIV and depression, and the risk of depression in the cohort under investigation (e.g., gender, age, mode of infection). We will now present prevalence estimates for depressive disorders and mania.

Depression

HIV-infected individuals often report recurrent and sometimes severe depressive symptoms, but there has been a wide range of reported prevalence rates in this population. In a national representative sample of HIV-infected adults,

36% had a positive screen for current major depression and 26.5% screened positive for dysthymia during the previous year.[3] Based on the meta-analysis of 10 studies,[14] the overall prevalence of current (1–6 months) major depression in HIV-infected samples has been estimated at about 9%, with rates ranging from 5 to 20% across the majority of studies.[15,26–30] This variability in estimates is likely due to differences in measurement time frames, type of screening instrument used, and patient sample characteristics (e.g., gender, socioeconomic status, risk group, disease stage, treatment status, and comorbidity with other psychiatric conditions). For example, a recent study found significantly less depressive symptoms reported by patients taking highly active antiretroviral therapy (HAART) compared to those not prescribed the HAART regimen.[31] In comparing these prevalence studies, one should certainly consider the demographic and medical characteristics of the subjects studied. Despite variation in the estimates of depression, it is important to remember that even the lowest estimate of the rate of depression (5%) is more than twice that in the age- and sex-matched general population.[32]

One study estimated that 8% of HIV-infected homosexual men report a major depressive episode in the past month, and that approximately 6% develop a major depression in the following 6-month period.[28] Rabkin and colleagues[30] assessed 183 homosexual men infected with HIV and found that 17% had a current axis I depressive disorder. Although worse disease was not associated with more depression, dysthymia rates were elevated among men with CD4 cell counts <500. The majority of persons (mostly men) assessed in these studies seem to effectively adjust to HIV disease; however, a significant number may still experience mood disturbances.

It is well established that women report higher rates of depression than men in the general population,[33] however, the majority of the prevalence studies of depression in HIV disease have focused almost exclusively on men. In a study of HIV-infected IV drug users,[23,27] women were found to have more depressive symptoms at baseline and during 3-year follow-up compared to men, although the sexes did not differ on prevalence of major depression. High rates of depressive disorders in this study (33% for HIV-infected men and 26% for HIV-infected women) in part reflected the high rates for IV drug users (16% HIV negative men and 30% for HIV negative women).[27]

Although not including both sexes, a large-scale prevalence study of 765 HIV-infected women reported that 42% had chronic depressive symptoms and 35% had intermittent depressive symptoms.[34] Rates of depression among clinical HIV-infected samples have ranged from 1.9 to 35%,[35–38] and from 30 to 60% among community samples of HIV-infected women.[39,40] The wide variation in prevalence rates of depression among HIV-infected women is most likely the result of differing methodologies and study groups, and in some cases the use of relatively small sample sizes.

Our review has so far shown high rates of depression among persons infected with HIV, with rates that tend to be higher than their risk-matched controls. One study of IV-drug users (HIV-infected and noninfected) found that only 28% of the men and women diagnosed with an axis I depressive disorder reported receiving treatment for an emotional problem.[23] Thus, HIV-infected patients should be routinely assessed and, if necessary, appropriately treated for depression.

Mania

Mania can occur throughout the course of HIV disease, but often clusters into two categories: (1) a preexisting bipolar disorder that often develops early in the disease but that can occur later on and (2) the late-stage (or AIDS) mania, which is less likely to be associated with a preexisting condition or family history and most likely results from HIV dementia and related cognitive deficits.[13,41] Researchers note that AIDS mania (or secondary mania) seems to have a different clinical profile than traditional bipolar mania (or primary mania). This includes marked cognitive slowing or dementia that often complicates diagnosis, more pronounced irritable mood as opposed to euphoric states, and greater severity in presentation and course. The differences between the early-onset and late-onset types of mania may reflect different etiologies within the context of HIV disease and warrants further investigation.

The majority of studies report a relationship between the onset of manic symptoms and the development of cognitive impairment associated with CNS involvement. A chart review of HIV-infected patients found that manic syndromes affected roughly 8% of patients across a 17-month study period.[42] Patients with manic episodes, which tended to occur later in the disease course (e.g., CD4 cell counts <200), were less likely to have a family history of mood disorder and more likely to have concurrent dementia or other cognitive impairment than those with manic episodes occurring earlier on (e.g., CD4 cell counts >200). Kieburtz and colleagues[43] also described a manic syndrome among eight patients with AIDS, and suggested that the manic syndrome was secondary to HIV infection because the patients also developed simultaneous cognitive impairments. In a case-control study of 19 patients with HIV-associated mania and 57 HIV+ controls, incident AIDS dementia was significantly more common in patients with HIV associated mania.[44] Ellen et al[45] screened all patients referred to an HIV consultation-liaison psychiatry service over a 29-month period for manic symptoms and identified 23 patients with mania, of which 19 were considered to have secondary mania. The prevalence of secondary mania over the study period was 1.2% for HIV+ individuals, and 4.3% for those with AIDS. A recent study examining medical and psychiatric comorbidities among 881 HIV-infected veterans reported that 4% had mania.[46] Overall, these studies seem to indicate that the prevalence of mania is elevated among HIV-infected individuals, especially in the more advanced stages of HIV disease as CNS involvement becomes more pronounced.

Additional studies have also reported bipolar episodes in HIV-infected individuals. Perretta and colleagues[47] compared 46 HIV-infected patients with an index major depressive episode to an equivalent number of demographically matched noninfected index major depressive episode patients on rates of bipolar subtypes. The authors found that HIV-infected and noninfected clinic patients had a comparable history of familial mood disturbance, although the HIV-infected individuals had a higher family history of alcohol use. The authors also reported a significantly higher proportion of HIV-infected patients with lifetime bipolar II disorder (78%), and associated cyclothymic (52%) and hyperthymic (35%) temperaments. The authors posit that premorbid impulsive risk-taking traits associated with these temperaments may have played a role in needle-sharing drug use and/or unprotected sexual behavior. These associations warrant further investigation because the assessors were not blind to the affective diagnoses and family history of patients, and the comparison group was a convenience sample. A recent epidemiologic study of 4910 HIV-infected and 331,758 noninfected prison inmates reported a higher prevalence of bipolar disorder among both male and female HIV-infected inmates than their noninfected counterparts.[48] More large-scale, prospective studies are needed to determine the exact prevalence rates of mania and bipolar disorders among HIV-infected individuals.

Thus far, we have shown that HIV-infected persons are at higher risk for depression, mania, and bipolar illness. With the advancement of pharmacologic treatments for HIV disease, including HAART regimens, many infected individuals are living longer in the symptomatic stages of the disease. HIV is now often viewed as a chronic condition and effective long-term management is vital. Proper diagnosis and treatment of mood disorders is an essential part of the management of this disease. Next we will discuss issues concerning the pharmacologic treatment of mood disorders in HIV disease.

► PHARMACOLOGIC MANAGEMENT OF MOOD DISORDERS IN HIV INFECTION

Depression is associated with reduced adherence to HIV medication regimens[49]; adherence is extremely important to prevent HIV drug resistance. There is also evidence that depression and stress may impact the progression of HIV infection,[5] a topic that will be documented in greater detail later in this chapter. Thus, it is now apparent that antidepressant treatment in medically vulnerable patients may have important implications for reducing treatment nonadherence and medical morbidity, in addition to improving mood- and health-related quality of life.[7,50]

Although major depression is one of the most frequent psychiatric disorders reported among HIV-infected patients, other mood disorders such as dysthymia and mania also require appropriate assessment and intervention. Mood disorders unfortunately are often unrecognized and untreated in HIV-infected persons.[7]

Psychiatric assessment and treatment is complicated due to increased incidence and severity of side effects, and interactions of psychotropic medications with antiretroviral treatments and HIV medical conditions. Below is a brief summary of the essential data and issues relevant to the pharmacotherapeutic treatment of mood disorders in HIV-infected persons.

Ticyclic Antidepressants

Several studies have demonstrated that imipramine is an effective drug for treating depression in patients infected with HIV. In a double-blind, randomized placebo-controlled study of 97 HIV-infected patients, Rabkin et al.[51] found treatment with imipramine was efficacious in reducing depressive symptoms. At week 6 of treatment, they found that the response rates were 74% for the imipramine group and 26% for the placebo group. No changes in CD4[+] helper/inducer cell counts were found in imipramine treated sub-

jects. Adverse side effects, however, led to greater likelihood of discontinuation of imipramine within 6 months. Eliott et al.[52] blindly and randomly assigned 75 HIV-infected individuals to imipramine, paroxetine, or placebo. Of the 75 subjects enrolled, 75% completed 6 weeks, but only 45% completed the full 12-week trial. Although both antidepressants were equally efficacious at 6, 8, and 12 weeks, and were significantly more efficacious than placebo, side effects of ticyclic antidepressants (TCAs) markedly influenced attrition. The dropout rate in the imipramine group was 48% compared to 20% in the paroxetine group and 24% in the placebo group. Thus, although TCAs are efficacious, the apparent increased sensitivity of HIV patients to side effects, such as a significantly higher incidence of dry mouth complaints,[53] may interfere with compliance.

Selective Serotonin Reuptake Inhibitors

Consistent with psychopharmacologic studies of other medical conditions, SSRIs are as effective as TCAs but demonstrate a less problematic side effect profile in HIV-infected individuals. Rabkin and colleagues[54] enrolled HIV-infected depressed subjects who failed imipramine treatment (e.g., subjects who relapsed, did not tolerate side effects, no responders) in a 12-week open trial of fluoxetine. Although the baseline levels of depression severity were lower in the fluoextine study (HAM-D average score = 12.5) compared to the initial imipramine study (HAM-D average score = 15.8), 83% of subjects treated with fluoxetine (15–60 mg/day) responded and exhibited significant reductions in depressive symptoms. Fluoxetine treatment did not alter CD4[+] counts. The authors noted that fluoxetine was better tolerated than imipramine. In another study, Rabkin et al.[55] used a randomized placebo-controlled trial to compare treatment response to fluoxetine and placebo in HIV-infected patients with major depression. They found that 74% of the participants in this study responded to fluoxetine.

Interestingly, they also found a high response to placebo (47%). It is noteworthy that the intention-to-treat analysis showed that differences between treatment groups were less remarkable (57% of fluoxetine patients were responders compared to 41% of placebo group). Again, fluoxetine did not alter levels of $CD4^+$ cell counts. In an open trial of 28 depressed HIV-infected subjects, these same researchers also found a 70% response rate among subjects that completed the 8-week open trial with sertraline.[56] Side effects resulted in a loss of 18% of the total sample. Sertraline did not alter either $CD4^+$ cell counts or natural killer (NK) cell counts.

Ferrando et al.[57] performed a 6-week open trial comparing paroxetine, fluoxetine, and sertraline in 33 symptomatic HIV-infected individuals with depression. Overall, 73% completed the trial and 83% of those subjects were responders. Most of the subjects who dropped out of the study did so because of complaints of agitation, anxiety, and insomnia during the first half of the study. They found improvement in depression as well as somatic symptoms perceived to be related to HIV with SSRI treatment. Differences in the efficacy between the three SSRIs could not be ascertained reliably because of the design and small sample size (although the descriptive data suggested that fluoxetine was the most effective and well tolerated). A 6-week open trial investigation of the efficacy of paroxetine was conducted in 10 HIV-infected patients with major depression.[58] Significant improvement in HAM-D scores was noted between weeks 2 and 6 of the study. Finally, fluoxetine and group psychotherapy were more efficient than psychotherapy alone in HIV patients with major depression.[59]

Studies in women have been lacking, in part due to social factors with which they are faced (e.g., childcare for single-parent mothers, financial difficulties). More recently, a small open trial comparing fluoxetine ($n = 21$) and sertraline ($n = 9$) was performed exclusively in HIV-infected women.[60] Sixty percent of the women completed the trial, and 78% were responders (e.g., HAM-D decreased 50% or more).

Since HIV-infected individuals are commonly treated with protease inhibitors and nonnucleoside reverse transcriptase inhibitors, the interactions of these drugs with psychotropic medications is of paramount importance for treating physicians to consider. Protease inhibitors and nonnucleoside reverse transcriptase inhibitors can enhance or inhibit the activity of the CYP450 interacting with drugs metabolized by the same pathway in the liver including antidepressants, neuroleptics, and anticonvulsants.[61] DeSilva et al.[62] reported four cases of serotoninergic syndrome in patients receiving fluoxetine in combination with antiretroviral agents that included ritonavir, efavirenz, or saquinavir. A reduction of the initial dose of the SSRI, slow titration, and close monitoring for toxic reaction are recommended to avoid complications.

New Generation Antidepressants

Although newer generation antidepressants have promise for treating depression in the context of HIV disease, unfortunately, there are few studies testing their efficacy in HIV. In fact, much of what is available on the use of these agents in HIV-infected patients with depression pertains to their potential for untoward side effects.

Nefazodone was efficacious in an open trial of 15 HIV-infected outpatients; 73% of patients responded to treatment and relatively few adverse side effects were noted.[63] There is, however, significant potential for drug interactions between nefazadone and protease inhibitors, and nefazodone-induced hepatitis has also been reported.[63] Liver alterations may be partially due to the frequent comorbidity of HIV and viral hepatitis B and C.

Mirtazapine was shown to be an efficacious antidepressant with a profile that can benefit HIV+ patients by promoting weight gain and decreasing nausea,[64] although its sedating properties may complicate the frequent complaints of asthenia. Venlafaxine has demonstrated more limited effects at the level of the cytochrome

P450, decreasing the potential interaction with antiretroviral medication.[65] Several in vitro studies have shown that HIV medications including indinavir, saquinavir, and efavirenz, significantly interfere with the metabolism of bupropion by inhibiting CYP2B6.[66] Well-controlled studies are needed to examine further the effects of these types of new generation antidepressants among HIV-infected individuals.

Psychostimulants and Other Novel Therapies

In a randomized, double-blind treatment trial Fernandez et al.[67] compared desipramine to methylphenidate in depressed HIV-infected individuals. Both drugs showed approximately a 50% response rate; however, subjects treated with desipramine experienced more adverse side effects including dry mouth, anxiety, and insomnia. A placebo-controlled trial of dextroamphetamine for depression in HIV-infected individuals also showed a significant improvement in motivation (e.g., initiative) and mood in 73% of the patients assigned to the medication group compared to 25% of the participants in the placebo group.[68] In an open trial of dextroamphetamine among 24 AIDS patients diagnosed with depression and also exhibiting incapacitating low energy, Wagner and colleagues[69] found that 75% of the patients responded to treatment. In fact, improvement in mood and energy occurred in parallel with significant reductions in depression scores achieved as early as the second week of treatment. Although complete follow-up evaluations were unavailable, the authors found that treatment benefits (improved mood and energy) were maintained for up to 2 years in some patients. The use of stimulants in the treatment of depression in the context of HIV may be recommended in the later stages of the disease where a more rapid effect is desired; however, the use of these agents warrants further evaluation.

Testosterone has also been tested as a therapeutic agent because reductions in testosterone have been found to correlate with changes in mood, appetite, energy, and sexual dysfunction in HIV-infected men. In a double-blind placebo-controlled trial (6-week trial followed by 12-week open-label maintenance), Rabkin et al.[70] found that testosterone injections were effective in improving mood as well as libido, energy, and body muscle mass among 70 HIV-infected men with hypogonadal symptoms completing the study. The results of the double-blind placebo-controlled study of testosterone replacement therapy showed that 79% of subjects with depression reported a mood improvement, comparable to that of antidepressant therapy. These same investigators have also found that exercise may augment improvement in psychologic and nutritional status in HIV-infected individuals receiving testosterone replacement therapy.[71]

The adrenal steroid dehydroepiandrosterone (DHEA) has also been used to treat HIV-infected individuals. In an 8-week, open-label pilot study of 45 HIV-infected men, Rabkin and colleagues[72] reported that DHEA also demonstrated promise for improving mood as well as anabolic and androgenic parameters. Thus, androgen replacement and other novel therapies may hold promise in ameliorating depressive and other related symptoms among HIV-infected individuals.

Mood Stabilizers

The existing literature indicates that caution is warranted when prescribing mood stabilizers in the context of HIV infection. Parenti et al.[73] treated a group of 10 HIV-infected men with lithium using a serum concentration ranging from 0.5 to 1.5 meq/L. Although 7 of the 10 patients had to discontinue the treatment because of significant adverse side effects, no significant changes in CD4$^+$ cell counts or viral titers were reported. The authors found a significant decrease in the mixed lymphocyte reaction following treatment. An in vitro study, however, also showed that lithium had no effect on HIV replication and on virus-associated reverse transcriptase activity.[74] In another early investigation, el-Mallakh[75] described 14 cases of mania associated with AIDS, including data regarding chronologic appearance of signs and medical and psychiatric symptoms. The authors stated that when mania (or hypomania) occurred during HIV infection, it frequently happened once and did not recur. They also argued that AIDS-associated manic states were adequately responsive to available antimanic agents, however, AIDS patients with detectable changes in neurologic function (e.g., cognitive and neuroimaging changes) might be more prone to the deleterious side effects of these drugs. Furthermore, although mania or hypomania might be the presenting complaints that lead to the discovery of HIV-seropositive status, mania might be a signal of advanced signs of immunodeficiency.

Halman and colleagues[76] conducted a retrospective chart review identifying 11 patients with HIV presenting to an HIV/AIDS psychiatric service with an acute manic episode. Based on neurodiagnostic studies and treatment results, the authors posited that abnormal brain magnetic resonance imaging significantly predicted poor tolerance of lithium and neuroleptics. However, they found that the anticonvulsants were an effective alternative. A number of factors must be taken into consideration when prescribing these types of mood stabilizers among HIV-infected individuals. Although valproic acid has been shown to increase HIV replication in several in vitro studies,[77] there is clinical evidence indicating that valproic acid treatment does not affect viral load in vivo among HIV-infected patients receiving appropriate antiretroviral therapy.[78] Blood levels of valproate must be closely monitored, as well as conditions such as hypoalbuminemia and the simultaneous use of antibiotics (e.g., trimethoprim, sulfamethoxazole) since these can elevate the drug's blood concentration. It is particularly important for those taking valproate as well as other mood stabilizers that HIV disease status (e.g., viral load) be monitored systematically over the course of treatment in conjunction with the patient's infectious disease specialist or family doctor.

There is evidence of bidirectional interactions between carbamazepine and antiretroviral agents at the level of the cytochrome P450. On one hand, carbamazepine is a potent inducer of the CYP3A enzyme system increasing the metabolism of protease inhibitors such as indinavir[79] and non-nucleoside reverse transcriptase inhibitors such as delavirdine.[80] On the other hand, another protease inhibitor, ritonavir, is a potent inhibitor of the same enzymatic system that increases the risk of carbamazepine toxicity.[81]

Antipsychotic Agents and Mood Disorders

Mood disorders with psychotic features and primary psychotic disorders may occur in HIV-infected patients. Precautions must be taken when using antipsychotic medications in those infected with HIV as several reports have noted that HIV-infected patients may be more sensitive to the extrapyramidal side effects associated with the dopamine receptor antagonist.[82,83] It has been suggested that this may be related to subcortical motor slowing associated with advancing HIV disease. In a case series of 21 patients with psychotic symptoms (12 of whom had mania with psychotic features), risperidone was found to be efficacious and to possess fewer side effects than conventional antipsychotic drugs.[84] Some data suggest that AIDS patients may have increased sensitivity to the newer, atypical antipsychotic agents as well. An open-label study using clozapine reported improvement of psychotic symptoms among HIV-infected patients without extrapyramidal symptoms.[85] Compared to trials of antidepressants, there is a paucity of data from controlled studies on the effects of antipsychotic agents in HIV-infected persons.

Psychopharmacology in HIV: Clinical Considerations

Similar rules regarding the prescription of psychotropic drugs to medically healthy persons apply to treatment strategies among HIV-infected patients, although extra care is often required as HIV disease presents some unique challenges to prescribing physicians. Knowledge of pharmacology can often be used to therapeutic advantage as well to avoid adverse interactions. Factors including drug interactions related to psychotropic drug metabolism, protein binding, half-life, and effects on appetite require careful consideration particularly in more advanced HIV-infected patients. It is critical to carefully monitor significant interactions between psychotropic drugs and antiretroviral agents used in combination drug therapy. Mood stabilizers must be used cautiously in HIV-infected individuals, and the clinician should be mindful that psychotropic drugs, nonnucleoside reverse transcriptase inhibitors, and protease inhibitors all serve as substrates for various cytochrome P450 enzymes in the liver. Each of these classes of compounds possesses enzyme inducing and/or inhibiting properties, and drugs such as the protease inhibitor ritonavir can also simultaneously modify a number of these isoenzymes.[61] Antiretroviral agents frequently serve as substrates, inhibitors, and inducers of various liver cytochrome P450 enzymes involved in drug metabolism, particularly 2C19, 2D6, and 3A4. In addition, depression and substance abuse frequently cooccur in HIV-infected individuals, and the use of intravenous illicit drugs may further increase the risk of acquiring hepatitis C. Nontraditional, herbal agents used to treat psychiatric syndromes must also be monitored closely in HIV-infected patients. An open-label study revealed that the protease inhibitor, indinavir, was markedly reduced by the concomitant administration of St. John's Wort, and the magnitude of the reduction of indinavir levels was estimated to be significant enough to lead to drug resistance and result in treatment failure.[86]

Pain may be a frequently under-treated symptom among HIV-infected patients.[87] Although antidepressants are often effective in treating many chronic pain syndromes, it should be noted that AIDS patients may further suffer from neuropathic pain that is less responsive to antidepressant medication. Though placebo-controlled clinical trials have not demonstrated that stimu-

lants are effective in treating primary depression,[88] they may be useful adjunctive agents in the context of HIV disease. There may be potentially promising effects of glucocorticoid antagonists, such as RU486, as well as substance P antagonists in treating depression among medically healthy persons.[89,90]

Finally, since the majority of the antidepressant treatment trials had relatively small samples, trials with larger samples of patients and longer-term follow-up assessments of both mood and HIV disease progression are important. Further study is also warranted because of the potential drug interactions between medications used to treat mood disorders and those used for treating HIV infection.

In addition to the pharmacologic treatments for depression, there is also evidence that psychologic interventions (e.g., cognitive behavioral stress management, social support) may impact depression and quality of life in HIV disease. Before considering the role of these psychologic interventions, however, we will review the extensive literature on how depression and stress may affect HIV disease progression. Because the thrust of most of these psychologic intervention studies has been to examine their impact on HIV disease parameters, it makes sense to first establish the connection between depression and disease course.

▶ DEPRESSION AND HIV DISEASE PROGRESSION

There remains great variability in the course of HIV disease progression, despite recent advances in the treatment of this disease. Researchers have focused on the effects of depression and stress as possible mechanisms to explain variations in HIV disease course, in part due to the documented decrements in cellular immunity associated with psychosocial variables.[91–95]

Because HIV advances very slowly, the best evidence for a relationship between depression and HIV disease progression comes from longitudinal studies conducted over long time intervals. The San Francisco Men's Health Study, a 9-year longitudinal study of about 400 asymptomatic HIV-infected gay men, found that those who were depressed at study entry progressed to AIDS on average 1.4 years sooner than those who were not depressed.[96] These findings were unchanged when controlling for baseline demographic variables, CD4 T-lymphocyte count, HIV-related medical symptoms, and health habits. Earlier findings from this study after 5 years showed no relationship between baseline depression score and progression to AIDS, although depression was related to decline in $CD4^+$ T-lymphocytes.[97] Another analysis of this cohort after 7 years of follow-up showed that those who had elevated symptoms of depression at every visit had 1.7 times greater risk of mortality compared to those without elevated depression scores.[98] In a recent reanalysis of this data, Moskowitz[99] showed that men with positive affect had lower risk of mortality; positively worded items on the depression scale (e.g., hopeful, happy) were better predictors of survival than negative worded items (e.g., sad, lonely).

In another study of 414 HIV-infected gay men studied during 5 years, baseline depression score was associated with shorter time to death, but not significantly associated with change in $CD4^+$ count or AIDS.[100] Data from 1809 gay men in the Multicenter AIDS Cohort Study (MACS) found no relationship between depression at study entry and progression of HIV infection during 8 years of follow-up.[101] In a later analysis of these data after 13 years, depression scores at baseline, particularly somatic symptoms of depression, were associated with shorter time to dementia and survival.[102]

Interpretation of most longitudinal studies reported above is limited by the data analyses measuring depression at study entry rather than over time, and evaluating depression as a bivariate predictor versus a continuous variable. It would seem unlikely that a one-time measure of depression would predict disease progression many years later. A more robust test of the hypothesis that depressive symptoms may affect HIV disease progression might be examining depressive symptoms lagged during time intervals before disease change. Such an analysis (using Cox regression with time-dependent variables) lets the value of depressive symptoms (a continuous score) change at each time point, so that we can examine the cumulative effects of depression during time intervals before change in disease status.

Leserman and colleagues reported such an analysis from the Coping in Health and Illness Project (CHIP), a study of 96 initially asymptomatic HIV-infected gay men followed every 6 months for up to 9 years.[20,21] In an analysis after 5.5 years of follow-up,[20] increased risk of AIDS was associated with higher cumulative depressive symptoms, as measured by a modified Hamilton depression rating scale (HDRS).[103] Somatic symptoms of depression that could be related to HIV disease change were excluded. For every cumulative average increase of one severe depressive symptom (3-point increase on the HDRS), the risk of AIDS was doubled. An earlier analysis of the CHIP cohort after 2 years showed that depressive symptoms, especially in the presence of severe stress, were related to declines in several lymphocyte subsets (e.g., $CD16^+$ and $CD56^+$ NK cells, and $CD8^+$ cytotoxic-suppressor cells).[104] $CD8^+$ T-lymphocytes may inhibit HIV replication early in the infection,[105–107] and there is some evidence that NK cells may have clinical significance in suppressing HIV (e.g., low NK cell responsiveness to interferon-alpha has been linked to higher risk of death,[108] NK cells have been shown to lyse HIV-infected cells in vitro,[109] NK cells isolated from HIV-infected subjects have suppressed HIV entry and replication,[110] and NK cells have been negatively related to HIV viral load[111]).

CHIP data from 9 years showed that men with more cumulative depressive symptoms had increased risk of developing an AIDS clinical condition.[21] For each 3-point change in average depressive symptoms (equal to one severe symptom), the risk of developing a clinical AIDS condition was more than doubled. Figure 16-1 shows the Kaplan-Meir survival curves for continuing without an AIDS clinical condition for

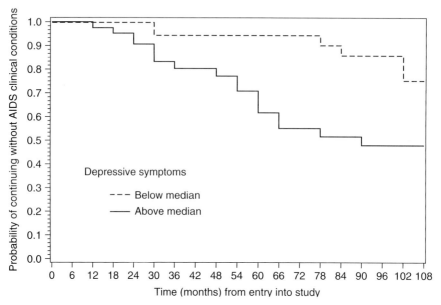

Figure 16-1. Kaplan-Meier estimate of the distribution of time (in months) until an AIDS clinical condition by depressive symptoms.

those above and below the median on depressive symptoms. These curves are only approximations, as they do not include control variables. The trajectory to an AIDS condition was about twice as fast among those above the median in depressive symptoms compared to those below the median. The 9-year CHIP analysis did not replicate earlier findings of a relationship between depressive symptoms and progression to AIDS (based on drop in CD4 <200 and/or and AIDS clinical condition).[20] At 7.5 years, there was a trend for depressive symptoms to predict progression to AIDS.[112] These findings from the CHIP study were unchanged when controlling for demographic variables, number of antiretroviral medications, and baseline values of both HIV RNA viral load and CD4+ lymphocyte count.

In the first study to examine the health effects of chronic depression in HIV-infected women ($N = 765$), Ickovics and colleagues found that women with chronic depressive symptoms were about two times more likely to die from HIV after 7 years, than those never experiencing

depression.[34] Mortality for those with intermittent depression was 1.6 times greater than those without depression. These analyses controlled for baseline CD4+ cell count, HIV RNA viral load, HIV-related symptoms, antiretroviral medication use, age, and employment status. The effects of depression on mortality were more pronounced among women who began the study with lower CD4+ counts, and thus were at greater risk of death. Ickovics and colleagues also found that chronic depression was associated with a greater decrease in CD4+ cell counts over time. In a cross-sectional analysis of HIV-infected women, Evans et al. found that depression and anxiety symptoms were correlated with lower NK cell activity, higher HIV RNA viral load, and higher activated CD8+ T-lymphocytes.[113] Activated CD8 cells (CD8+/CD38+/DR+) have been correlated with cytotoxic activity and HIV disease progression.[114–116] Similarly, another cross-sectional study of HIV-infected men and women showed that high psychologic stress was associated with lower number of helper T (memory) cells, but only for those with low levels of viral burden.[117] The authors focused on the memory subset of helper T-cells because these undergo more rapid decline with HIV disease progression.[118]

To summarize, a more robust relationship between depression and HIV disease progression is found in studies performed over long time intervals and those analyzing the chronic effects of depression. Despite this association, we need to question whether depression puts HIV-infected persons at greater risk for disease progression or whether changes in disease may be associated with increased risk of depression.

Direction of the Relationship between Depression and Disease Change

Studies have tried to address the chicken-egg issue of whether depression is a predictor or result of disease progression by measuring depression in the time intervals before AIDS or the development of medical symptoms. This approach helps to establish that the depressive symptoms occurred prior to changes in disease status. If disease changes are gradual, however, this strategy may not address the time ordering of events. In reexamining the 9-year longitudinal data from the CHIP study, Leserman showed that AIDS clinical symptoms and CD4[+] cell count did not predict major depression[5]; however, depressive symptoms did predict increased risk of having a drop in CD4[+] cell count consistent with AIDS,[20] and an AIDS clinical condition.[21] Thus, it appears that depression may more likely lead to clinical disease change than vice versa. More research is needed to address this issue.

▶ STRESS AND HIV DISEASE PROGRESSION

Another approach to determining if psychologic factors may impact on HIV disease progression, has been to examine the impact of stressful events, such as bereavement and other types of trauma, on changes in disease status. The stress of bereavement for instance, has been shown to correlate with subsequent development of depression.[119] The advantage of studying persons experiencing stress or trauma is that the direction of the relationship between stressful events and HIV disease change may be somewhat less ambiguous than the effects of depression on disease course, depending on the nature of the stressor studied.

Bereavement

Many studies have examined the stress of bereavement in HIV-infected persons, given that this population is at high risk for having a partner or close friend die. Kemeny and Dean showed that bereavement prior to study entry (having a close friend or lover who died of AIDS) was associated with more rapid decline in CD4[+] count over 3–4 years in 85 HIV-infected gay men.[120] These findings were not explained by differences in health habits, antiretroviral medication use, or age; however, bereavement, did not predict progression to AIDS or mortality. A later study among bereaved men reported that those who found meaning in bereavement showed less rapid decline in CD4[+] levels and lower rates of mortality due to AIDS during 2–3-year follow-up.[121] In analyzing a subsample from the MACS data, Kemeny et al.[122] found that recently bereaved men had increases in serum neopterin (an immune activation marker associated with increased risk of AIDS) and decreases in lymphocyte proliferative response to phytohemagglutinin (PHA) compared to a matched group of nonbereaved. In a 6-month study, Goodkin et al.[123] showed that bereaved HIV-infected men had decreased lymphocyte proliferative response to PHA, and decreased NK cell cytotoxicity compared to nonbereaved. Thus, bereavement appears to have a negative effect on the immune response of those infected with HIV, a response that may have clinical significance.

Other Trauma and Stressful Life Events

In addition to bereavement, researchers have focused on the negative health impact of other types of trauma and a wide variety of stressful life events. Ironson et al.[124] found that men with greater distress at the time of HIV serostatus notification had a greater chance of developing HIV-related clinical symptoms at 2-year follow-up. A study among 67 asymptomatic HIV-infected Black women, found that 62% of the sample had experienced a traumatic event during their lifetime (e.g., death of child, assault, rape).[1] Traumatic exposure, particularly among those with posttraumatic stress disorder, was associated with greater decrease in the $CD4^+/CD8^+$ ratio during 1-year follow-up. In a study of 618 HIV-infected children and adolescents (ages 1–20), having 2 or more stressful life events (e.g., family member's death, major illness, or loss) was associated with almost a threefold increased risk of immune suppression (decline in $CD4^+$ %) during 1-year follow-up.[125] Patterson et al. showed that HIV-infected gay men with less severe life adversity in combination with less depression were at lower risk for negative alternations in their immune status (e.g., $CD4^+$ %) during 6-month follow-up.[126] Other studies using short follow-up periods and/or questionnaire methods to assess life stress have generally not shown an association of stress with reduction in $CD4^+$ T-lymphocyte counts.[127–129]

Research on the adverse immunologic and health effects of stressful life events in HIV infection, has been consistently reported by the CHIP study during 9 years following the same cohort of gay men.[20,21,104,112,130–132] The CHIP stressful life events and difficulty measure is based on interviewer contextual ratings of stressful events that: (1) exclude stresses that could have resulted from disease progression (e.g., retirement due to HIV worsening) and (2) omit patient's ratings of distress to reduce the possibility that worsening disease could lead to poor coping and thus higher stress scores. At CHIP study baseline, men with more severe stressful life events in the previous 6 months were shown to have lower NK cell counts ($CD16^+$ and $CD56^+$) and fewer cytotoxic/suppressor cells ($CD8^+$ T-lymphocytes) compared to those with less stress.[130] In the same cohort, prior severe stress and depressive symptoms were independently associated with decreases in NK cell counts and $CD8^+$ T-lymphocytes after 2 years.[104] As noted above, decrements in these lymphocyte subsets may have clinical significance in HIV.[105–111]

The CHIP data also addressed the role of stressful life events on HIV clinical outcome. Severe stress was associated with greater risk for worsening HIV disease stage (e.g., drop in $CD4^+$ or development of HIV clinical symptoms) for men studied up to 3.5 years.[132] At 5.5,[20] 7.5,[112] and 9 years[21] of follow-up, Leserman and colleagues reported that higher average cumulative stressful events were predictive of faster progression to AIDS (decline in $CD4^+$ T-lymphocytes <200 and/or AIDS indicator condition). At these three time points, the study showed that for every increase in cumulative average stress equivalent to one severe stressor or two moderate stressors, the risk of AIDS was about doubled. The AIDS progression rate at the end of 8 years for those above the median in stress was 74% versus 40% for those below the median. Leserman et al.[21] also reported that for every increase in cumulative average stress equivalent to one severe stressor, the risk of developing an AIDS clinical condition (e.g., Kaposi sarcoma, pneumocystis pneumonia) was about tripled.

Limitations of the CHIP study include problems generalizing from a relatively small non-representative sample of gay men from North Carolina, most subjects progressing before wide spread use of HAART, and lack of control for length of time with HIV infection. Analyses did include controls for demographic variables, baseline $CD4^+$ T-cell count, baseline HIV RNA viral load, number of antiretroviral medications, and serum cortisol. Furthermore, measurement of cumulative average stress was lagged by 6 months before HIV disease progression, and stressors resulting from HIV disease changes were omitted. The association in the CHIP study of stressful life events with multiple measures of disease progression (e.g., AIDS, clinical AIDS condition, change in HIV disease stage, and T-lymphocyte subset decline) lends convergent validity to these stress/immune/disease progression findings.

Experimental Stress

Capitanio and colleagues[133] examined the effects of an experimentally manipulated social stress (e.g., unstable social group) on survival of male rhesus macaques infected with simian immunodeficiency virus (SIV). The unstable group animals (high stress) survived significantly shorter (169 days) compared to those in the stable group (low stress). Animals that received threats from other animals had higher SIV RNA levels (viral load), than those not receiving threats, regardless of social condition. Animals which engaged in grooming (less stressed) had lower SIV RNA levels.

Thus, studies in humans and one study in rhesus macaques indicate that stressful events and trauma may have a negative impact on HIV (SIV) disease progression. More consistent findings are associated with studying subjects over longer time periods, and examining actual stressors (e.g., bereavement) or using contextual-based interviews rather than questionnaire assessments of stress.

▶ PSYCHOLOGIC INTERVENTIONS

If stressful events, trauma, and depressive symptoms are related to HIV disease progression, what is the evidence that psychologic interventions (e.g., cognitive behavioral stress management, support groups) might improve immune markers and ultimately the health status of HIV-infected persons? In an early study of men waiting for serostatus notification, Antoni and colleagues[134] found that cognitive behavioral stress management appeared to buffer postnotification levels of depression and to increase CD4 lymphocytes, NK cell counts (CD56), and proliferative responses to PHA. Higher values on these immune markers were significantly and robustly associated with greater frequency of relaxation practice.

In another study of HIV-infected men, Antoni et al.[135] found that men randomized to a cognitive behavioral stress management intervention had reduced anxiety, anger, mood disturbance, and perceived stress, lower norepinephrine (NE) output (autonomic arousal), and higher T-cytotoxic/suppressor levels ($CD3^+CD8^+$) compared to those in a wait-list control condition. Higher T-cytotoxic/suppressor levels were associated with greater decreases in NE and more frequent home relaxation practice. Early on, the HIV virus is successful at escaping the immune response due to deficits in CD4 T-cell function, and increased levels of T-cytotoxic/suppressor cells found in peripheral blood are thought to comprise an important compensatory immune response to keep the virus in check.[136–138] Relative to a control group, cognitive behavioral stress management among HIV-infected gay men has also been associated with: (1) increases in transitional naive $CD4^+$ T-cells (a subset of CD4 T-helper cells that is vulnerable to decline) 6–12 months after the intervention,[139] (2) a decrease in salivary cortisol with a relative increase in dehydroepiandrosterone sulfate (DHEA-S) postintervention, two markers previously shown to be associated with HIV disease progression,[140,141] and (3) reductions in herpes simplex virus type 2 antibody titers (a virus extremely common among HIV-infected persons that may facilitate replication of HIV and faster disease progression).[142] These indicators of reduced risk for HIV disease progression (e.g., decrease in cortisol, increase in DHEA-S) were also associated with decreases in self-reported stress.[140,141,143] Ironson et al.[124] found that low adherence to a cognitive behavioral stress management intervention was associated with faster development of HIV symptoms and AIDS. Cognitive behavioral stress management has also been associated with increases in well-being, improved coping, and quality of life,[135,144,145] although these effects have not always been shown to be sustained over time.[146]

One study examining a stress management and relaxation intervention in HIV found no effect on immune change (CD4 cells, NK cell cytotoxicity, mitogen responsivity) compared to a wait-list control group.[147] Another small study failed to demonstrate that home practice of guided imagery or progressive muscle relaxation using a tape recording affected quality of life compared to a control group.[148]

Goodkin et al.[149,150] reported that a 10-week bereavement support group intervention was associated with higher CD4, larger decreases in HIV RNA viral load, greater number of total T-lymphocytes, decrease in plasma cortisol, and fewer health care visits compared to a standard care control condition. Increases in CD4 count were associated with higher group attendance and with decreases in cortisol among these HIV-infected gay men. In depressed men, one study showed that both a support group intervention and a cognitive behavioral treatment reduced depression, hostility, and somatization compared to a nonintervention control condition.[151] Another study found that HIV-infected persons randomized to interpersonal psychotherapy or supportive psychotherapy with imipramine had greater improvement on measures of depression than those receiving either supportive therapy or cognitive behavioral therapy.[152]

In the first study to examine emotional disclosure in HIV, those who wrote about their worst trauma had increased CD4+ lymphocyte count compared to those who wrote about mundane topics.[153] Another study found that long-term survivors of HIV tended to have greater emotional disclosure and depth processing when asked to write about trauma compared to a control HIV-seropositive comparison group.[154]

To conclude, most of the research indicates that psychologic interventions including cognitive behavioral stress management, supportive therapy, and emotional disclosure may ameliorate the negative effects of stress, and as such these types of interventions may have a benefi-cial impact on the course of HIV disease. More studies are needed comparing different types of psychologic interventions and the effects of such therapies combined with antidepressant medications.

▶ POTENTIAL-MEDIATING MECHANISMS

We have presented evidence that depression and stress may exacerbate HIV disease progression and that psychologic treatment may ameliorate some of these negative effects. The mechanisms mediating these psychoneuroimmune relationships are less clear. It is possible that poor health habits (e.g., smoking, substance abuse, risky sexual behavior, medication use) related to stress and depression might account for these findings; however, the relationships of stress and depression with HIV disease change persist even when controlling for these health variables.[34,96,120,122,123] In terms of biologic mediators, most HIV literature to date has focused on the hypothalamic-pituitary-adrenal (HPA) axis and SNS as possible mediators based on animal and human research linking immune status changes to dysregulation in these biologic systems.[155,156]

Neuroendocrine Pathway

Because disturbances of HPA axis function (e.g., increases in adrenocorticotrophin releasing hormone [ACTH] and cortisol) have been associated with stress and depression in humans, and such dysregulation may negatively impact the immune response, we will examine the evidence that glucocorticoids may be a mediating mechanism explaining the effects of depression and stress on HIV infection. Higher cortisol levels have been associated with worse stress and depression in some HIV studies. Gorman et al.[157] found that urinary cortisol was higher in HIV-infected persons who were depressed and anxious, and Goodkin et al.[123] found higher cortisol levels in the bereaved versus nonbereaved. Furthermore, among patients receiving cognitive behavioral therapy, decreases in perceived stress and anxiety were associated with declines in cortisol and the cortisol/DHEA ratio.[140–142] Serum cortisol, however, was not related to stress or depression in analyzing up to 9 years of natural history data from the CHIP study.[21] Furthermore, a 2-year study found that urinary cortisol was only associated with depressed and anxious mood at one assessment period.[158] Discrepant findings may be due to the time when cortisol was measured, the use of serum versus an integrated 24-hour urinary measure, the stage of HIV-infected persons studied, and the focus on chronic versus acute stress.

There are several pathways by which cortisol could affect changes in immune function and HIV disease progression. Cortisol may stimulate HIV viral replication,[159] modify programmed cell death, and alter the pattern of cytokines secreted (from Th1 to Th2),[159–162] changes that have been associated with HIV disease progression.[160,163] Clerici and colleagues[160] have suggested that increases in glucocorticoids and decreases in DHEA during HIV infection may alter the pattern of cytokines secreted by suppressing beneficial Th1 cytokines (e.g., interleukin [IL]-2, interferon-gamma) in favor of Th2 cytokines (e.g., IL-4, IL-6, IL-10). Reductions in the Th1 cytokines have been linked to HIV progression,[160,164] although the nature of these relationships in HIV remains controversial.[163,165]

An early study showed greatly increased HIV replication when hydrocortisone was added to the cell cultures of AIDS patients.[166] In another in vitro study, Nair et al.[167] found inhibition of NK cell activity when cortisol or ACTH was added to the cell cultures of AIDS patients. Glucocorticoids may affect HIV pathogenesis directly through increased viral replication or more indirectly by inhibiting the immune response to other pathogens.

Summarizing the results of five retrospective and prospective clinical studies, Christeff et al.[168] found that CD4[+] cell counts were negatively associated with serum cortisol and positively related to serum DHEA. Furthermore, cortisol was significantly higher in HIV positive than HIV negative men, especially during later stages of HIV infection. Goodkin et al.[149] showed that increased CD4[+] cell counts were associated with reductions in cortisol following a bereavement support group. Under conditions of stress, cortisol has been associated with decreases in mitogen response and lower lymphocyte functioning in HIV.[123,169] At baseline, the CHIP study found that the negative effects of stress on killer lymphocytes were amplified in those with high levels of cortisol.[131] Although longitudinally this study did not show that cortisol mediated the effects of stress on progression to AIDS; increases in cortisol were related to three markers of disease progression (e.g., AIDS, clinical AIDS condition, and mortality).[21,112] For every 3 μg/dL increase in cumulative average serum cortisol during 9 years of follow-up, there was a 40% increased risk of AIDS, and about a 2.5-fold increased risk of developing an AIDS clinical symptom or dying from HIV infection.[21] Increased plasma cortisol has also been linked to a social stressor in rhesus macaques and with accelerated SIV disease progression.[133] Other clinical studies, however, have not shown a relationship between CD4[+] T-lymphocytes and cortisol.[157,158] While there are some conflicting reports regarding the neuroimmunomodulatory effects of glucocorticoids, the majority of studies do show a relationship between cortisol and HIV disease markers. The causal direction of this relationship, however, remains controversial and more research is needed to clarify whether glucocorticoids have a mediating role in explaining the effects of stress and depression on HIV disease progression.

Sympathetic Nervous System Pathway

Chronic elevations of SNS activity (e.g., NE) among those infected with HIV may adversely affect immune system functioning (e.g., reduced lymphocyte proliferation, alteration in cytokine production). It has been suggested that NE may suppress Th1 type cytokines and increase Th2 type, changes associated with increased risk of HIV viral replication and increased vulnerability to opportunistic infections.[160,164,170,171] Cole et al.[172] have shown that HIV-infected gay men with higher baseline levels of autonomic nervous system (ANS) activity (e.g., systolic blood pressure, skin conductance, EKG interbeat interval) had poorer suppression of plasma RNA viral load and worse $CD4^+$ T-cell recovery after receiving HAART compared to men with lower levels of ANS activity. In vitro studies by the same investigator team have shown that NE can enhance HIV viral replication and viral gene expression.[171,172] Moreover, HIV-infected men who had greater declines in NE following a cognitive behavioral intervention had higher T-cytotoxic/suppressor lymphocytes compared to those with higher NE.[135]

Circulating catecholamines have also been shown to increase in response to psychologic stress and depression, and have long been associated with various alterations in the noradrenergic system.[173,174] Although difficult to assess in humans, such alterations may include changes in sympathetic pathways that innervate immune organs such as the spleen.[155,175] Although there is less HIV research on the immune effects of the SNS compared to the HPA axis, dysregulation in the SNS in response to stress and depression might be another significant mediating mechanism underlying the effects of stress and depression on HIV disease progression.

Substance P

Although the HPA axis and the SNS have been the most studied pathways mediating psychologic effects on HIV disease progression, neuropeptide substance P has also been implicated. A substance P antagonist has been efficacious for the treatment of depression,[176] and substance P may be involved in the modulation of HIV infection.[177] Plasma levels of substance P are higher in HIV-infected persons and are associated with decreased NK cell populations.[177] In addition, substance P has been shown to accelerate HIV replication in human peripheral blood monocyte-derived macrophages.[178] More research is needed on other possible pathways that may be responsible for conveying the effects of psychologic factors on HIV disease markers.

▶ SUMMARY

We have presented evidence that HIV-infected men and women are at increased risk for depression and other mood disturbance. This heightened risk seems to be due to both, HIV infection and membership in groups that are at high risk for depression (e.g., IV drug users, homosexuals). Despite the high levels of depression, mood disorders in HIV-infected patients often go untreated. Published controlled trials of antidepressant medication have documented their effectiveness among HIV-infected individuals, and the available evidence suggests that the selective SSRIs reduce depressive symptoms and may be better tolerated by patients than older antidepressants. In addition, cognitive behavioral stress management interventions and support groups have been shown to reduce distress and have a salutary effect on immune- and health-related measures in HIV-infected patients. It is important for clinicians treating HIV-infected patients to screen patients for depression and to provide adequate treatment when warranted, including both medication and psychologic treatment modalities.

Existing research provides some strong evidence that psychosocial factors such as chronic depression and stressful life events may affect HIV disease progression. It must be noted that the majority of the cited studies on psychologic moderators of HIV infection have been conducted on men, primarily before the advent of protease inhibitors. Therefore, this review may not be generalizable to women or to those currently taking HAART. The findings from recent studies among female samples, however, have been consistent with those conducted among men. Future studies should focus on these understudied populations, especially among those taking HAART.

Despite studies showing that depression and stress may impact HIV disease progression, we know little about the biologic mechanisms that may account for these relationships. There is some research to support the idea that alterations in the HPA axis and the SNS may play such a mediating role; however, more evidence is needed to elucidate these complex biologic relationships within the context of HIV infection. Furthermore, studies are needed on interventions aimed at modifying the deleterious effects of depression and stress among those infected with HIV.

Acknowledgment

Supported in part by NIH Grants MH-44618, AT002035, MH67687, HD37260, MH-55454, NS42216, and NS38179.

REFERENCES

1. Kimerling R, Calhoun KS, Forehand R, et al. Traumatic stress in HIV-infected women. *AIDS Educ Prevent* 1999;11:321.

2. Leserman J, Whetten K, Swartz M. How trauma and stressful events impact functional health status in HIV. *Am Psychosom Soc* 2004;A-60.

3. Bing EG, Burnam MA, Longshore D, et al. Psychiatric disorders and drug use among human immunodeficiency virus-infected adults in the United States. *Arch Gen Psychiatry* 2001;58:721–728.

4. Repetto MJ, Evans DL, Cruess DG, et al. Neuropsychopharmacologic treatment of depression and other neuropsychiatric disorders in HIV-infected individuals. *CNS Spectr* 2003;8:59–63.

5. Leserman J. HIV disease progression: Depression, stress, and possible mechanisms. *Biol Psychiatry* 2003;54:295.

6. Cruess DG, Petitto JM, Leserman J, et al. Depression and HIV infection: Impact on immune function and disease progression. *CNS Spectr* 2003;8:52–58.

7. Evans DL, Staab J, Ward H, et al. Depression in the medically ill: Management considerations. *Depress Anxiety* 1996–1997;4:199–208.

8. Treisman GJ, Angelino AF, Hutton HE. Psychiatric issues in the management of patients with HIV infection. *JAMA* 2001;286:2857–2864.

9. Norman SE, Chediak AD, Freeman C, et al. Sleep disturbances in men with asymptomatic human immunodeficiency (HIV) infection. *Sleep* 1992;15:150–155.

10. Perkins DO, Leserman J, Stern RA, et al. Somatic symptoms and HIV infection: Relationship to depressive symptoms and indicators of HIV disease. *Am J Psychiatry* 1995;152:1776–1781.

11. Vazquez-Justo E, Rodriguez Alvarez M, Ferraces Otero MJ. Influence of depressed mood on neuropsychologic performance in HIV-seropositive drug users. *Psychiatry Clin Neurosci* 2003;57:251–258.

12. Regier DA, Farmer ME. Comorbidity of mental disorders with alcohol and other drug abuse. *JAMA* 1990;264:2511–2518.

13. Treisman G, Fishman M, Schwartz J, et al. Mood disorders in HIV infection. *Depress Anxiety* 1998;7:178–187.

14. Ciesla JA, Roberts JE. Meta-analysis of the relationship between HIV infection and risk for depressive disorders. *Am J Psychiatry* 2001;158:725–730.

15. Maj M. Depressive syndromes and symptoms in subjects with human immunodeficiency virus (HIV) infection. *Br J Psychiatry* 1996;30:117–122.

16. Morrison MF, Petitto JM, Ten Have T, et al. Depressive and anxiety disorders in women with HIV infection. *Am J Psychiatry* 2002;159:789–796.

17. Justice AC, McGinnis KA, Atkinson JH, et al. Psychiatric and neurocognitive disorders among HIV-positive and negative veterans in care: Veterans Aging Cohort Five-Site Study. *AIDS* 2004;18(Suppl 1):S49–S59.

18. Rabkin JG, McElhiney MC, Ferrando SJ. Mood and substance use disorders in older adults with HIV/AIDS: Methodological issues and preliminary evidence. *AIDS* 2004;18(Suppl 1):S43–S48.

19. Lyketsos CG, Hoover DR, Guccione M, et al. Changes in depressive symptoms as AIDS develops. The Multicenter AIDS Cohort Study. *Am J Psychiatry* 1996;153:1430–1437.

20. Leserman J, Jackson ED, Petitto JM, et al. Progression to AIDS: The effects of stress, depressive symptoms, and social support. *Psychosom Med* 1999;61:397.

21. Leserman J, Petitto JM, Gu H, et al. Progression to AIDS, a clinical AIDS condition, and mortality: Psychosocial and physiological predictors. *Psychol Med* 2002;32:1059–73.

22. Rabkin JG, Goetz RR, Remien RH, et al. Stability of mood despite HIV illness progression in a group of homosexual men. *Am J Psychiatry* 1997;154:231–238.

23. Rabkin JG, Johnson J, Lin SH, et al. Psychopathology in male and female HIV-positive and negative injecting drug users: Longitudinal course over 3 years. *AIDS* 1997;11:507–515.

24. Baldewicz T, Leserman J, Silva SG, et al. Changes in neuropsychological functioning with progression of hiv-1 infection: Results of a 9-year longitudinal investigation. *AIDS Behav*, in press.

25. Goggin KJ, Zisook S, Heaton RK, et al. Neuropsychological performance of HIV-1 infected men with major depression. HNRC Group. HIV Neurobehavioral Research Center. *J Int Neuropsychol Soc* 1997;3:457–464.

26. Atkinson JJ, Grant I, Kennedy CJ, et al. Prevalence of psychiatric disorders among men infected with human immunodeficiency virus: A controlled study. *Arch Gen Psychiatry* 1988;45:859–964.

27. Lipsitz JD, Williams JB, Rabkin JG, et al. Psychopathology in male and female intravenous drug users with and without HIV infection. *Am J Psychiatry* 1994;151:1662–1668.

28. Perkins DO, Stern RA, Golden RN, et al. Mood disorders in HIV infection: Prevalence and risk factors in a non-epicenter of the AIDS epidemic. *Am J Psychiatry* 1994;151:233–236.

29. Williams JB, Rabkin JG, Remien RH, et al. Multidisciplinary baseline assessment of homosexual men with and without human immunodeficiency virus infection: Standardized clinical assessment of current and lifetime psychopathology. *Arch Gen Psychiatry* 1991;48:124–130.

30. Rabkin JG, Ferrando SJ, Jacobsberg LB, et al. Prevalence of axis I disorders in an AIDS cohort: A cross-sectional, controlled study. *Compr Psychiatry* 1997;38:146–154.

31. Starace F, Bartoli L, Aloisi MS, et al. Cognitive and affective disorders associated to HIV infection in the HAART era: Findings from the NeuroICONA study. Cognitive impairment and depression in HIV/AIDS. The NeuroICONA study. *Acta Psychiatr Scand* 2002;106:20–26.

32. Robins LN, Regier DA. *Psychiatric Disorders in America.* New York: Free Press, 1991.

33. Blazer DG, Kessler RC, McGonagle KA, et al. The prevalence and distribution of major depression in a national community sample: The National Comorbidity Survey. *Am J Psychiatry* 1994;151:979–986.

34. Ickovics JR, Hamburger ME, Vlahov D, et al. Mortality, CD4 cell count decline, and depressive symptoms among HIV-seropositive women. *JAMA* 2001;285:1466–1474.

35. Boland RJ, Moore J, Schuman P. The longitudinal course of depression in HIV-infected women. *Psychosomatics* 1999;40:160.

36. Goggin K, Engelson ES, Rabkin JG, et al. The relationship of mood, endocrine, and sexual disorders in human immunodeficiency virus positive (HIV+) women: An exploratory study. *Psychosom Med* 1998;60:11–16.

37. Taylor ER, Amodei N, Mangos R. The presence of psychiatric disorders in HIV-infected women. *J Counseling Develop* 1996;74:345–351.

38. McDaniel JS, Fowlie E, Summerville MB, et al. An assessment of rates of psychiatric morbidity and functioning in HIV disease. *Gen Hosp Psychiatry* 1995;17:346–352.

39. Moore J, Schuman P, Schoenbaum E, et al. Severe adverse life events and depressive symptoms among women with, or at risk for, HIV infection in four cities in the United States of America. *AIDS* 1999;13:2459–2468.

40. Smith DK, Moore JS, Warren D, et al. The design, participants, and selected early findings of the HIV Epidemiology Research Study. In: O'Leary A, Jemmott LS (eds.), *Women and AIDS: Coping and Care.* New York: Plenum Press, 1996, pp. 185–206.

41. Lyketsos CG, Schwartz J, Fishman M, et al. AIDS mania. *J Neuropsychiatry Clin Neurosci* 1997;9:277–279.

42. Lyketsos CG, Hanson AL, Fishman M. Manic episode early and late in the course of HIV. *Am J Psychiatry* 1993;150:326–327.

43. Kieburtz K, Zettelmaier AE, Ketonen L, et al. Manic syndrome in AIDS. *Am J Psychiatry* 1991;148:1068–1070.

44. Mijch AM, Judd FK, Lyketsos CG, et al. Secondary mania in patients with HIV infection: Are antiretrovirals protective? *J Neuropsychiatry Clin Neurosci* 1999;11:475–480.

45. Ellen SR, Judd FK, Mijch AM, et al. Secondary mania in patients with HIV infection. *Aust N Z J Psychiatry* 1999;33:353–360.

46. Kilbourne AM, Justice AC, Rabeneck L, et al. General medical and psychiatric comorbidity

among HIV-infected veterans in the post-HAART era. *J Clin Epidemiol* 2001;54(Suppl 1): S22–S28.

47. Perretta P, Akiskal HS, Nisita C, et al. The high prevalence of bipolar II and associated cyclothymic and hyperthymic temperaments in HIV-patients. *J Affect Disord* 1998;50:215–224.

48. Baillargeon J, Ducate S, Pulvino J, et al. The association of psychiatric disorders and HIV infection in the correctional setting. *Ann Epidemiol* 2003;13:606–612.

49. Starace F, Ammassari A, Trotta MP, et al. Depression is a risk factor for suboptimal adherence to highly active antiretroviral therapy. *J Acquir Immune Defic Syndr* 2002;31(Suppl 3):S136–S139.

50. Elliott AJ, Russo J, Roy-Byrne PP. The effect of changes in depression on health related quality of life (HRQoL) in HIV infection. *Gen Hosp Psychiatry* 2002;24:43–47.

51. Rabkin JG, Rabkin R, Harrison W, et al. Effect of imipramine on mood and enumerative measures of immune status in depressed patients with HIV illness. *Am J Psychiatry* 1994;151:516–523.

52. Elliot AJ, Karina KK, Bergam K, et al. Randomized, placebo-controlled trial of paroxetine versus imipramine in depressed HIV-positive outpatients. *Am J Psychiatry* 1998;155:367–372.

53. Younai FS, Marcus M, Freed JR, et al. Self-reported oral dryness and HIV disease in a national sample of patients receiving medical care. *Oral Surg Oral Med Oral Pathol Oral Radiol Endod* 2001;92:629–636.

54. Rabkin JG, Rabkin R, Wagner G. Effects of fluoxetine on mood and immune status in depressed patients with HIV illness. *J Clin Psychiatry* 1994;55:92–97.

55. Rabkin JG, Wagner G, Rabkin R. Fluoxetine treatment for depression in patients with HIV and AIDS: A randomized, placebo-controlled trial. *Am J Psychiatry* 1999;156:101–107.

56. Rabkin JG, Wagner G, Rabkin R. Effects of sertraline on mood and immune status in patients with major depression and HIV illness: An open trial. *J Clin Psychiatry* 1994;55:433–439.

57. Ferrando SJ, Goldman JD, Charness WE. Selective serotonin reuptake inhibitor treatment of depression in symptomatic HIV infection and AIDS: Improvement in affective and somatic symptoms. *Gen Hosp Psychiatry* 1997;19:89–97.

58. Grassi B, Gambini O, Graghentini G, et al. Efficacy of paroxetine for treatment of depression in the context of HIV infection. *Pharmacotherapy* 1997;30:70–71.

59. Zisook S, Peterkin J, Goggin KJ, et al. Treatment of major depression in HIV-seropositive men. HIV Neurobehavioral Research Center Group. *J Clin Psychiatry* 1998;59:217–224.

60. Ferrando SJ, Rabkin JG, de Moore GM, et al. Antidepressant treatment of depression in HIV-serpositive women. *J Clin Psychiatry* 1999;60: 741–746.

61. Tseng AL, Foisy MM. Significant interactions with new antiretrovirals and psychotropics. *Ann Pharmacother* 1999;33:461–473.

62. DeSilva KE, Le Flore DB, Marston BJ, et al. Serotonin syndrome in HIV-infected individuals receiving antiretroviral therapy and fluoxetine. *AIDS* 2001;15:1281–1285.

63. Elliot AJ, Karina KK, Bergam K, et al. Antidepressant efficacy in HIV-serpositive outpatients with major depressive disorder: An open trial of nefazadone. *J Clin Psychiatry* 1999;60:226–231.

64. Elliott AJ, Roy-Byrne PP. Mirtazapine for depression in patients with human immunodeficiency virus. *J Clin Psychopharmacol* 2000;20:265–267.

65. Ereshefsky L, Dugan D. Review of the pharmacokinetics, pharmacogenetics, and drug interaction potential of antidepressants: Focus on venlafaxine. *Depress Anxiety* 2000;12(Suppl): 30–44.

66. Hesse LM, von Moltke LL, Shader RI, et al. Ritonavir, efavirenz, and nelfinavir inhibit CYP2B6 activity in vitro: Potential drug interactions with bupropion. *Drug Metab Dispos* 2001;29:100–102.

67. Fernandez F, Levy JK, Samley HR, et al. Effects of methylphenidate in HIV-related depression: A comparative trial with desipramine. *Int J Psychiatry Med* 1995;25:53–67.

68. Wagner GJ, Rabkin R. Effects of dextroamphetamine on depression and fatigue in men with HIV: A double-blind, placebo-controlled trial. *J Clin Psychiatry* 2000;61:436–440.

69. Wagner GJ, Rabkin JG, Rabkin R. Dextroamphetamine as a treatment for depression and low energy in AIDS patients: A pilot study. *J Psychosom Res* 1997;42:407–411.

70. Rabkin JG, Wagner GJ, Rabkin R. A double-blind, placebo-controlled trial of testosterone therapy for HIV-positive men with hypogonadal symptoms. *Arch Gen Psychiatry* 2000;57:141–147.

71. Wagner G, Rabkin J, Rabkin R. Exercise as a mediator of psychological and nutritional effects

of testosterone therapy in HIV+ men. *Med Sci Sports Exercise* 1998;30:811–817.

72. Rabkin JG, Ferrando SJ, Wagner GJ, et al. DHEA treatment for HIV+ patients: Effects on mood, androgenic and anabolic parameters. *Psychoneuroendocrinology* 2000;25:53–68.

73. Parenti DM, Simon GL, Scheib RG, et al. Effect of lithium carbonate in HIV-infected patients with immune dysfunction. *J Acquir Immune Defic Syndr* 1988;1:119–224.

74. Evans DL, Smith MS, Golden RN. Antidepressants and HIV infection: Effect of lithium choride and desipramine on HIV replication. *Depression* 1993;1:205–209.

75. el-Mallakh RS. Mania in AIDS: Clinical significance and theoretical considerations. *Int J Psychiatry Med* 1991;21:383–391.

76. Halman MH, Worth JL, Sanders KM, et al. Anticonvulsant use in the treatment of manic syndromes in patients with HIV-1 infection. *J Neuropsychiatry Clin Neurosci* 1993;5:430–434.

77. Moog C, Kuntz-Simon G, Caussin-Schwemling C, et al. Sodium valproate, an anticonvulsant drug, stimulates human immunodeficiency virus type 1 replication independently of glutathione levels. *J Gen Virol* 1996;77:1993–1999.

78. Maggi JD, Halman MH. The effect of divalproex sodium on viral load: A retrospective review of HIV-positive patients with manic syndromes. *Can J Psychiatry* 2001;46:359–362.

79. Hugen PW, Burger DM, Brinkman K, et al. Carbamazepine-indinavir interaction causes antiretroviral therapy failure. *Ann Pharmacother* 2000;34:465–470.

80. Tran JQ, Gerber JG, Kerr BM. Delavirdine: Clinical pharmacokinetics and drug interactions. *Clin Pharmacokinet* 2001;40:207–226.

81. Berbel Garcia A, Latorre Ibarra A, Porta Etessam J, et al. Protease inhibitor-induced carbamazepine toxicity. *Clin Neuropharmacol* 2000;23:216–218.

82. Hriso E, Kuhn T, Masdeu JC, et al. Extrapyramidal symptoms due to dopamine blocking agents in patients with AIDS encephalopathy. *Am J Psychiatry* 1991;148:1558–1561.

83. Sewell DD, Jeste DV, Atkinson JH, et al. HIV-associated psychosis: A study of 20 cases. San Diego HIV Neurobehavioral Research Center Group. *Am J Psychiatry* 1994;151:237–242.

84. Singh AN, Golledge H, Catalan J. Treatment of HIV-related psychotic disorders with risperidone: A series of 21 cases. *J Psychosom Res* 1997;42:489–493.

85. Zirulnik L. Pilot study with clozapine in patients with HIV-associated psychosis and drug-induced parkinsonism. *Mov Disord* 1999;14:128–131.

86. Piscitelli SC, Burstein AH, Chaitt D, et al. Indinavir concentrations and St. John's wort. *Lancet* 2000;355:547–548.

87. Breitbart W, Rosenfeld BD, Passick SD, et al. The undertreatment of pain in ambulatory AIDS patients. *Pain* 1996;65:243–249.

88. Satel SL, Nelson JC. Stimulants in the treatment of depression: A critical overview. *J Clin Psychiatry* 1989;50:241–249.

89. Belanoff JK, Flores BH, Kalezhan M, et al. Rapid reversal of psychotic depression using mifepristone. *J Clin Psychopharmacol* 2001;21:516–521.

90. Stout SC, Owens MJ, Nemeroff CB. Neurokinin(1) receptor antagonists as potential antidepressants. *Annu Rev Pharmacol Toxicol* 2001;41:877–906.

91. Evans DL, Leserman J, Golden RN, et al. Immune correlates of stress and depression. *Psychopharmacol Bull* 1989;25:319.

92. Herbert TB, Cohen S. Stress and immunity in humans: A meta-analytic review. *Psychosom Med* 1993;55:364.

93. Herbert TB, Cohen S. Depression and immunity: A meta-analytic review. *Psychol Bull* 1993;113(3):472.

94. Stein M, Miller AH, et al. Depression, the immune system and health and illness. *Arch Gen Psychiatry* 1991;48:171.

95. Weisse CS. Depression and immunocompetence: A review of the literature. *Psychol Bull* 1992;111:475.

96. Page-Shafer K, Delorenze GN, Satariano, et al. Comorbidity and survival in HIV-infected men in the San Francisco Men's Health Survey. *Ann Epidemiol* 1996;6:420.

97. Burack JH, Barrett DC, Stall RD, et al. Depressive symptoms and CD4 lymphocyte decline among HIV-infected men. *JAMA* 1993;270:2568.

98. Mayne TJ, Vittinghoff E, Chesney MA, et al. Depressive affect and survival among gay and bisexual men infected with HIV. *Arch Intern Med* 1996;156:2233.

99. Moskowitz JT. Positive affect predicts lower risk of AIDS mortality. *Psychosom Med* 2003;65:620.

100. Patterson TL, Shaw WS, Semple SJ, et al. Relationship of psychosocial factors to HIV disease progression. *Ann Behav Med* 1996;18:30.

101. Lyketsos CG, Hoover DR, Guccione M, et al. Depressive symptoms as predictors of medical

outcomes in HIV infection. *JAMA* 1993;270(21): 2563.

102. Farinpour R, Miller EN, Satz P, et al. Psychological risk factors of HIV morbidity and mortality: Findings from the Multicenter AIDS Cohort Study (MACS). *J Clin Exp Neuropsychol* 2003;25:654.

103. Hamilton M. A rating scale for depression. *J Neurol Neurosurg Psychiatry* 1960;23:56.

104. Leserman J, Petitto JM, Perkins DO, et al. Severe stress, depressive symptoms, and changes in lymphocyte subsets in human immunodeficiency virus-infected men. *Arch Gen Psychiatry* 1997;54:279.

105. Price DA, O'callaghan CA, Whelan JA, et al. Cytotoxic T lymphocytes and viral evolution in primary HIV-1 infection. *Clin Sci* 1999;97:707.

106. Barker E. CD8+ cell-derived anti-human immunodeficiency virus inhibitory factor. *J Infect Dis* 1999;179(Suppl 3):S485.

107. Famularo G, Moretti S, Marcellini S, et al. CD8 lymphocytes in HIV infection: Helpful and harmful. *J Clin Lab Immunol* 1997;49:15.

108. Ullum H, Cozzi LA, Aladdin H, et al. Natural immunity and HIV disease progression. AIDS 1999;13:557.

109. Bandyopadhyay S, Ziegner U, Campbell DE, et al. Natural killer cell mediated lysis of T cell lines chronically infected with HIV-1. *Clin Exp Immunol* 1990;79:430.

110. Oliva A, Kinter AL, Vaccarezza M, et al. Natural killer cells from human immunodeficiency virus (HIV)-infected individuals are an important source of CC-chemokines and suppress HIV-1 entry and replication in vitro. *J Clin Invest* 1998;102:223.

111. Ironson G, Balbin E, Solomon G, et al. Relative preservation of natural killer cell cytotoxicity and number in healthy AIDS patients with low CD4 cell counts. AIDS 2001;15:2065.

112. Leserman J, Petitto JM, Golden RN, et al. The impact of stressful life events, depression, social support, coping and cortisol on progression to AIDS. *Am J Psychiatry* 2000;157: 1221.

113. Evans DL, Ten Have TR, Douglas SD, et al. Association of depression with viral load, CD8 T lymphocytes, and natural killer cells in women with HIV infection. *Am J Psychiatry* 2002;10:1.

114. Ho HN, Hultin LE, Mitsuyasu RT, et al. Circulating HIV-specific CD8+ cytotoxic T cells express CD38 and HLA-DR antigens. *J Immunol* 1993; 150(7):3070.

115. Liu Z, Cumberland WG, Hultin LE, et al. CD8+ T-lymphocyte activation in HIV-1 disease reflects an aspect of pathogenesis distinct from viral burden and immunodeficiency. *J Acquir Immun Defic Syndr* 1998;18:332.

116. Giorgi JV, Hultin LE, McKeating JA, et al. Shorter survival in advanced human immunodeficiency virus type 1 infection is more closely associated with T lymphocyte activation than with plasma virus burden or virus chemokine coreceptor usage. *J Infect Dis* 1999;179:859.

117. Motivala SJ, Hurwitz BE, Llabre MM, et al. Psychological distress is associated with decreased memory helper T-cell and B-cell counts in pre-AIDS HIV seropositive men and women but only in those with low viral load. *Psychosom Med* 2003;65:627.

118. Klimas NG, Caralis P, LaPerriere A, et al. Immunologic function in a cohort of human immunodeficiency virus type 1-seropositive and negative healthy homosexual men. *J Clin Microbiol* 1991;29:1413.

119. Bruce M. Psychological risk factors for depressive disorders in late life. *Biol Psychiatry* 2002;52:175.

120. Kemeny ME, Dean L. Effects of AIDS-related bereavement on HIV progression among New York City gay men. *AIDS Educ Prevent* 1995;7:36.

121. Bower JE, Kemeny ME, Taylor SE, et al. Cognitive processing, discovery of meaning, CD4 decline, and AIDS-related mortality among bereaved HIV-seropositive men. *J Consult Clin Psychol* 1998;66:979.

122. Kemeny ME, Weiner H, Duran R, et al. Immune system changes after the death of a partner in HIV-positive gay men. *Psychosom Med* 1995; 57:547.

123. Goodkin K, Feaster DJ, Tuttle R, et al. Bereavement is associated with time-dependent decrements in cellular immune function in asymptomatic human immunodeficiency virus type 1-seropositive homosexual men. *Clin Diagn Lab Immunol* 1996;3: 109.

124. Ironson G, Friedman A, Klimas N, et al. Distress, denial, and low adherence to behavioral interventions predict faster disease progression in gay men infected with human immunodeficiency virus. *Int J Behav Med* 1994;1:90.

125. Howland LC, Gortmaker SL, Mofenson LM, et al. Effects of negative life events on immune suppression in children and youth infected with human immunodeficiency virus type 1. *Pediatrics* 2000;106:540.

126. Patterson TL, Semple SJ, Temoshok LR, et al. Stress and depressive symptoms prospectively predict immune change among HIV-seropositive men. *Psychiatry* 1995;58:299.

127. Perry S, Fishman B, Jacobsberg L, et al. Relationships over one-year between lymphocyte subsets and psychosocial variables among adults with infection by human immunodeficiency virus. *Arch Gen Psychiatry* 1992;49:396.

128. Rabkin JG, Williams JBW, Remien RH, et al. Depression, distress, lymphocyte subsets, and human immunodeficiency virus symptoms on two occasions in HIV-positive homosexual men. *Arch Gen Psychiatry* 1991;48(2):111.

129. Kessler RC, Foster C, Joseph J, et al. Stressful life events and symptom onset in HIV infection. *Am J Psychiatry* 1991;148:733.

130. Evans DL, Leserman J, Perkins DO, et al. Stress-associated reductions of cytotoxic T lymphocytes and natural killer cells in asymptomatic HIV infection. *Am J Psychiatry* 1995;152:543.

131. Petitto JM, Leserman J, Perkins DO, et al. High versus low basal cortisol secretion in asymptomatic, medication-free HIV infected men: differential effects of severe life stress on parameters of immune status. *Behav Med* 2000;25:143.

132. Evans DL, Leserman J, Perkins DO, et al. Severe life stress as a predictor of early disease progression in HIV infection. *Am J Psychiatry* 1997; 154:630.

133. Capitanio JP, Mendoza SP, Lerche NW, et al. Social stress results in altered glucocorticoid regulation and shorter survival in simian acquired immune deficiency syndrome. *Proc Natl Acad Sci USA* 1998;95:4714.

134. Antoni MH, Baggett L, Ironson G, et al. Cognitive-behavioral stress management intervention buffers distress responses and immunologic changes following notification of HIV-1 seropositivity. *J Consult Clin Psychol* 1991;59:906.

135. Antoni MH, Cruess DG, Cruess S, et al. Cognitive-behavioral stress management intervention effects on anxiety, 24-hr urinary norepinephrine output, and T-cytotoxic/suppressor cells over time among symptomatic HIV-infected gay men. *J Consult Clin Psychol* 2000;68:31.

136. Walker BD, Plata F. Cytotoxic T lymphocytes against HIV. *AIDS* 1990;4:177.

137. Fauci AS. Mulfactorial nature of human immunodeficiency virus disease: Implications for therapy. *Science* 1993;262:1011.

138. Paul WE. Reexamining AIDS research priorities [see comments]. *Science* 1995;267:633.

139. Antoni MH, Cruess DG, Klimas N, et al. Stress management and immune system reconstitution in symptomatic HIV-infected gay men over time: Effects on transitional naive T cells (CD4(+) CD45RA(+)CD29(+)). *Am J Psychiatry* 2002;159: 143.

140. Cruess DG, Antoni MH, Kumar M, et al. Reductions in salivary cortisol are associated with mood improvement during relaxation training among HIV-seropositive men. *J Behav Med* 2000;23:107.

141. Cruess DG, Antoni MH, Kumar M, et al. Cognitive-behavioral stress management buffers decreases in dehydroepiandrosterone sulfate (DHEA-S) and increases in the cortisol/DHEA-S ratio and reduces mood disturbance and perceived stress among HIV-seropositive men. *Psychoneuroendocrinology* 1999;24:537.

142. Cruess S, Antoni M, Cruess D, et al. Reductions in herpes simplex virus type 2 antibody titers after cognitive behavioral stress management and relationships with neuroendocrine function, relaxation skills, and social support in HIV-positive men. *Psychosom Med* 2000;62:828.

143. Lutgendorf SK, Antoni MH, Ironson G, et al. Cognitive-behavioral stress management decreases dysphoric mood and herpes simplex virus-type 2 antibody titers in symptomatic HIV-seropositive gay men. *J Consult Clin Psychol* 1997;65: 31.

144. Lutgendorf S, Antoni MH, Schneiderman N, et al. Psychosocial counseling to improve quality of life in HIV infection. *Patient Educ Counsel* 1994;24:217.

145. Lutgendorf SK, Antoni MH, Ironson G, et al. Changes in cognitive coping skills and social support during cognitive behavioral stress management intervention and distress outcomes in symptomatic human immunodeficiency virus (HIV)-seropositive gay men. *Psychosom Med* 1998;60:204.

146. McCain NL, Munjas BA, Munro CL, et al. Effects of stress management on PNI-based outcomes in persons with HIV disease. *Res Nurs Health* 2003;26:102.

147. Coates TJ, McKusick L, Kuno R, et al. Stress reduction training changed number of sexual partners but not immune function in men with HIV. *Am J Public Health* 1989;79:885.

148. Eller LS. Effects of cognitive-behavioral interventions on quality of life in persons with HIV. *Int J Nurs Studies* 1999;36:223.

149. Goodkin K, Feaster DJ, Asthana D, et al. A bereavement support group intervention is longitudinally associated with salutary effects on the CD4 cell count and number of physician visits. *Clin Diagn Lab Immunol* 1998;5:382.

150. Goodkin K, Baldewicz TT, Asthana D, et al. A bereavement support group intervention affects plasma burden of human immunodeficiency virus type 1. Report of a randomized controlled trial. *J Hum Virol* 2001;4:44.

151. Kelly JA, Murphy DA, Bahr GR, et al. Outcome of cognitive-behavioral and support group brief therapies for depressed, HIV-infected persons. *Am J Psychiatry* 1993;150:1679.

152. Markowitz JC, Kocsis JH, Fishman B, et al. Treatment of depressive symptoms in human immunodeficiency virus-positive patients. *Arch Gen Psychiatry* 1998;55:452.

153. Petrie KJ, Fontanilla I, Thomas MG, et al. Effect of written emotional expression on immune function in patients with human immunodeficiency virus infection: A randomized trial. *Psychosom Med* 2004;66:272.

154. O'Cleirigh C, Ironson G, Antoni MH, et al. Emotional expression and depth processing of trauma and their relation to long-term survival in patients with HIV/AIDS. *J Psychosom Res* 2003;54:225.

155. Friedman EM, Irwin MR. Modulation of immune cell function by the autonomic nervous system. [Review] [125 refs]. *Pharmacol Therap* 1997;74:27.

156. Cupps TR, Fauci AS. Corticosteroid-mediated immunoregulation in man. *Immunol Rev* 2002; 65:133.

157. Gorman JM, Kertzner R, Cooper T, et al. Glucocorticoid level and neuropsychiatric symptoms in homosexual men with HIV infection. *Am J Psychiatry* 1991;148:41.

158. Kertzner RM, Goetz R, Todak G, et al. Cortisol levels, immune status, and mood in homosexual men with and without HIV infection. *Am J Psychiatry* 1993;150:1674.

159. Corley PA. Acquired immune deficiency syndrome: The glucocorticoid solution. *Med Hypotheses* 1996;47:49.

160. Clerici M, Trabattoni D, Piconi S, et al. A possible role for the cortisol/anticortisols imbalance in the progression of human immunodeficiency virus. [Review] [22 refs]. *Psychoneuroendocrinology* 1997;22(Suppl 1):S27.

161. Daynes RA, Meikle AW, Araneo BA. Locally active steroid hormones may facilitate compartmentalization of immunity by regulating the types of lymphokines produced by helper T cells. *Res Immunol* 1991;142:40.

162. Daynes RA, Araneo BA, Hennebold J, et al. Steroids as regulators of the mammalian immune response. *J Investig Dermatol* 1995;105:14S.

163. Maggi E, Mazzetti M, Ravina A, et al. Ability of HIV to promote a TH1 to TH0 shift and to replicate preferentially in TH2 and TH0 cells [see comments]. *Science* 1994;265:244.

164. Vago T, Clerici M, Norbiato G. Glucocorticoids and the immune system in AIDS. *Baillieres Clin Endocrinol Metab* 1994;8:789.

165. Graziosi C, Pantaleo G, Gantt KR, et al. Lack of evidence for the dichotomy of TH1 and TH2 predominance in HIV-infected individuals. *Science* 1994;265:248.

166. Markham PD, Salahuddin SZ, Veren K, et al. Hydrocortisone and some other hormones enhance the expression of HTLV-III. *Int J Cancer* 1986;37:67.

167. Nair MP, Saravolatz LD, Schwartz SA. Selective inhibitory effects of stress hormones on natural killer (NK) cell activity of lymphocytes from AIDS patients. *Immunol Investig* 1995;24:689.

168. Christeff N, Gherbi N, Mammes O, et al. Serum cortisol and DHEA concentrations during HIV infection. *Psychoneuroendocrinology* 1997;22 (Suppl 1):S11.

169. Antoni MH, Schneiderman N, Klimas N, et al. Disparities in psychological, neuroendocrine, and immunologic patterns in asymptomatic HIV-1 seropositive and seronegative gay men. *Biol Psychiatry* 1991;29:1023.

170. Cole SW, Kemeny ME. Psychobiology of HIV infection. *Crit Rev Neurobiol* 1997;11:289.

171. Cole SW, Korin YD, Fahey JL, et al. Norepinephrine accelerates HIV replication via protein kinase A-dependent effects on cytokine production. *J Immunol* 1998;161:610.

172. Cole SW, Naliboff BD, Kemeny ME, et al. Impaired response to HAART in HIV-infected individuals with high autonomic nervous system activity. *Proc Natl Acad Sci U S A* 2001;98:12695.

173. Dimsdale JE, Ziegler MG. What do plasma and urinary measures of catecholamines tell us about human response to stressors? *Circulation* 1991; 83:II36.

174. Ward MM, Mefford IN, Parker SD, et al. Epinephrine and norepinephrine responses in continuously collected human plasma to a series of stressors. *Psychosom Med* 1983;45:471.

175. Anand A, Charney DS. Norepinephrine dysfunction in depression. *J Clin Psychiatry* 2000; 61(Suppl 10):16.

176. Hokfelt T, Pernow B, Wahren J. Substance P: A pioneer amongst neuropeptides. *J Intern Med* 2001;249:27.

177. Douglas SD, Ho WZ, Gettes DR, et al. Elevated substance P levels in HIV-infected men. *AIDS* 2001;15:2043.

178. Ho WZ, Cnaan A, Li YH, et al. Substance P modulates human immunodeficiency virus replication in human peripheral blood monocyte-derived macrophages. *AIDS Res Hum Retroviruses* 1996; 12:195.

SECTION VI

Special Topics

CHAPTER 17

Chronic Pain Syndromes and Comorbid Mood Disorders

SAMANTHA MELTZER-BRODY AND ROBERT N. GOLDEN

► INTRODUCTION

Chronic pain is often treatment refractory and poses an enormous burden of suffering for the individual. The experience of constant pain may be viewed as a severe stress that is associated with the development of psychopathology, including depressive disorders, anxiety disorders, substance dependence, and personality disorders.[1–3] In 1981, Lindsay and Wyckoff labeled comorbid pain and depression as the "depression-pain syndrome."[4] More recently, studies have attempted to address the "chicken or the egg" issue of whether the emergence of psychopathology or chronic pain precedes the other. In either case, it is clear that many studies have demonstrated high rates of psychiatric disorders in patients with various types of chronic pain.[3]

Patients with major depression have a decreased ability to cope with chronic pain that can accompany medical illness.[5] Also, major depression is associated with a 50% increase in medical costs for chronic illness, even after controlling for severity of illness.[8] Patients with depression often present with a complicated range of symptoms, including both emotional and physical complaints, and frequently the physical complaints include unexplained pain.[6,7] Patients with depression are more likely to report their pain as severe, compared to those without depression, even when there is no apparent objective medical basis for the difference in pain intensity.[8]

In this chapter, we will discuss the growing literature of comorbid pain and depressive disorders and describe the psychologic and biologic models of how depression and pain interact. We will review specific chronic pain syndromes, beginning with chronic back pain, and then highlight four common functional somatic syndromes (FSS) that illustrate the relationship between chronic pain and comorbid depression and other psychiatric illness: chronic headaches, irritable bowel syndrome (IBS), fibromyalgia, and chronic pelvic pain (CPP). In addition, we will discuss the role of a history of abuse or trauma in the development of somatic symptoms and posttraumatic stress disorder (PTSD).

Comorbidity of Pain and Depression

A recent systematic evidence review of depression and pain comorbidity examined almost 60 articles in this area.[9] In this review, the mean prevalence of pain symptoms in patients with major depression was 65%, and conversely, the mean prevalence for concurrent major depression in patients identified as having a chronic pain syndrome was 52% for patients seen in pain clinics or programs, 38% in psychiatric consultation settings, and 27% in primary care settings.[11] At least half of the patients with major depression were not properly diagnosed and therefore not treated for depression in primary care settings, presumably because they presented with mostly somatic complaints (of which at least 60% were pain related) as opposed to psychologic complaints.[11] Additionally, greater pain severity at baseline has been associated with poor outcomes, including more severe depression, more pain-related functional limitations, and increased health care utilization.[10] Patients with pain and comorbid depression experience more pain and greater intensity and duration of pain.[11] Finally, in patients with depression and chronic pain who are treated with antidepressants, the baseline severity of the pain influences the response to antidepressant therapy.[11]

▶ PSYCHOLOGIC AND BIOLOGIC MODELS FOR THE IMPACT OF DEPRESSION ON CHRONIC PAIN

There are multiple theories that explore how depression and pain interact. Gatchel et al. have developed a three-stage conceptual model of the progression from acute pain to chronic disability with comorbid psychiatric distress.[12] This model describes a progression from acute (2–4 months) to chronic pain, and states that as the pain become more chronic, the patients undergo significant psychologic changes that produce a "layer of behavioral/psychologic problems over the original nociception or pain experience itself."[14] The literature also describes how comorbid depressive illness or other psychiatric disturbance may alter the perception of pain and increase pain intensity while decreasing the ability to tolerate the pain.[13] Fishbain et al. have summarized the five major hypotheses regarding chronic pain and depression interactions: (1) the " antecedent hypothesis," in which depression precedes the development of chronic pain, (2) the "consequence hypothesis," in which depression is a consequence of the chronic pain, (3) the "scar hypothesis," in which a previous history of depression before the onset of chronic pain predisposes the patient to a new depressive episode after the onset of chronic pain, (4) the "cognitive mediation" hypothesis, in which psychologic factors, such as poor coping strategies, are thought to mediate the interactions between chronic pain and depression, and (5) the "independent hypothesis," in which chronic pain and depression share some common etiologic mechanism but remain distinct diseases without causal interaction.[14]

Recently, the neuroanatomic and neurochemical processes associated with both depression and chronic pain have been a focus of study. The periaqueductal gray (PAG), appears to be a central anatomic site in the pain modulation system.[15,16] The PAG is an anatomic relay from limbic forebrain and midbrain structures to the brainstem.[11] These relay systems contain both serotonergic and noradrenergic neurons, important neurotransmitters in the regulation of mood and several of the neurovegetative and cognitive functions that are often altered in patients with depression. It appears that when there is a depletion of serotonin (5-HT) and/or norepinephrine (NE), the PAG system loses its modulatory effect so that minor signals from the body are amplified and more attention and emotion are focused on them. This may explain why patients with depression often have multiple somatic complaints.[11]

The hypothalamic-pituitary-adrenal axis (HPA) is felt to be involved in the experience of chronic pain.[17,18] It is believed that chronic stress caused by chronic pain leads to loss of negative glucocorticoid feedback on the HPA axis, resulting in downregulation of the glucocorticoid receptor within the brain and peripheral nervous system. This downregulation may lead to depressed mood.[16]

Antidepressant medications are often used to treat patients with chronic pain syndromes with varying degrees of success. These pharmacologic agents target either 5-HT and/or NE neurotransmitter levels, which as described earlier, both modulate descending, pain pathways. Historically, the tricyclic antidepressants, including amitriptyline, have been widely used.[19] The selective serotonin reuptake inhibitors (SSRIs) have also been shown to have modest efficacy in treating chronic pain, and more recently, the selective serotonergic and noradrenergic reuptake inhibitors (SNRIs) have shown strong potential as treatment for chronic pain disorders because of their dual action on both 5-HT and NE.[20–22] Throughout this chapter, we will discuss the use of antidepressant and other psychotropic medications in the treatment of chronic pain.

► CHRONIC BACK PAIN CBP

Epidemiology of Depressive Disorders in Chronic Back Pain (CBP)

Back pain is one of the most common complaints in patients presenting for care, and has an annual prevalence rate of 15–20% in adults.[23] Early studies of psychopathology in low back pain found rates of major depressive disorder ranging from 34 to 57% in patients with chronic low back pain.[24] Although these early studies were important in documenting the significant rates of psychiatric disorders in chronic pain patients, they contained some methodologic limitations, including the absence of a structured psychiatric interview for diagnostic purposes.[3] One study of patients with low back pain found a 64% lifetime prevalence of major depression, and reported that for those with a lifetime history of a psychiatric disorder and comorbid back pain, the former preceded the latter in 54% of those with major depression, 94% of those with substance abuse, and 95% of those with anxiety disorders.[25] Another study compared rates of psychopathology in patients with acute versus chronic low back pain, and found higher rates of psychopathology in the latter group.[26] The transition from acute to chronic back pain appears to be strongly influenced by

psychologic factors including distress, depressed mood, and somatization.[27]

Treatment of CBP and Comorbid Depression

Psychopharmacology

Antidepressant treatment of back pain is common, and it is estimated that 2–23% of patients with back pain are prescribed antidepressant medication.[28,29] Four systematic reviews of the efficacy of antidepressant therapy in the treatment of back pain have been conducted.[30–33] The two most recent reviews concluded that antidepressant therapy was effective in the treatment of back pain.[32,33] However, the latest systematic review concluded that the efficacy of antidepressant therapy was limited to those that inhibit NE reuptake (secondary amine tricyclics and tetracyclics), and this effect was independent of a comorbid diagnosis of depression.[33] In contrast, the SSRIs did not appear to be beneficial for patients with chronic back pain.[33]

Surgical Treatment

Surgical treatment of chronic back pain in patients with depression must be carefully considered. The decision to operate is based on the assumption that there is structural disease contributing to pain symptoms that is not purely explained by the psychopathology.[23] In order to optimize the benefits of surgery, it is recommended that prior to surgery, patients should be screened and aggressively treated for depression or other psychiatric disturbances.[34] In addition, as much as possible, an effort should be made to reduce environmental stressors including marital, occupational, fiscal, and legal issues prior to surgery.[23]

► FUNCTIONAL SOMATIC SYNDROMES

Functional somatic syndromes do not have any apparent underlying organic etiology, yet often cause considerable distress or impairment, and frequently require medical attention.[35] At least 33% of somatic symptoms are medically unexplained, are chronic or recurrent in 20–25% of patients, and are strongly associated with coexisting depressive and anxiety disorders.[36] Many somatic syndromes also have overlapping symptoms,[37] and often a history of abuse or trauma is associated with chronic somatic symptoms.

Abuse History, Somatic Symptoms, and PTSD

The long-term psychologic consequences among victims of sexual or physical abuse have been well documented, and include greatly increased rates of depression,[38–40] anxiety disorders, including PTSD,[41] and substance abuse.[42–44] Major depressive disorder and PTSD are often comorbid in victims of sexual abuse or trauma.[44–46] Recently, studies have also documented the long-term physical health effects of abuse.[47,48] Specifically, sexual and physical abuse have been shown to adversely impact the health of women with a variety of chronic health problems including gastrointestinal (GI) disorders,[49–53] neurologic conditions including headaches,[54] fibromyalgia,[55] and gynecologic complaints including CPP.[56]

A history of sexual and physical abuse has also been consistently shown to cause the highest rates of PTSD[57–59] which can lead to significant disability. Most abused women will not receive psychiatric evaluation or treatment, although the vast majority will receive health care during the period in which they have symptomatic PTSD. Women who are victims of rape or sexual assault are twice as likely to seek medical services than nonvictims[60,61] and seek medical services much more often than psychologic services in the year after being assaulted (72.6% compared with 19%).[62] Thus, obtaining an abuse and trauma history is a critical component of the comprehensive evaluation of a patient with a chronic somatic syndrome as well as an assessment for PTSD. A number of self-rated and observer-based rating scales have been developed and validated to facilitate screening for PTSD.[63–65] In particular, if the patient is

being seen in a nonpsychiatric setting, a self-rated screening scale can serve as a useful tool for triaging patients with a history of trauma and PTSD symptoms for further psychiatric evaluation.[66]

We will now discuss four common FSS: chronic headaches, IBS, fibromyalgia, and CPP. Each of these syndromes illustrates the relationship between chronic pain, comorbid psychiatric illness, and the potential role of a history of abuse or trauma in the development of chronic somatic complaints.

Headaches

Headache is the most common pain complaint and the most frequently seen medical concern in clinics.[67] The lifetime prevalence of headache in the general population is 93% for men and 99% for women.[68] Community-based epidemiologic studies have revealed that 14% of men and 29% of women experience some form of significant headache every few days.[69] Epidemiologic studies in the general population have confirmed high rates of comorbidity of psychiatric disorders in people suffering from headaches.

The *International Classification of Headache Disorders 2nd Edition* (ICHD) classifies three groups of headache disorders: primary headaches, secondary headaches, and all other cranial neuralgias including central and primary facial pain, and other nonspecific headaches. Types of primary headaches include migraine, tension-type headache, cluster headaches, trigeminal autonomic cephalalgias, and other less common primary headaches. Primary headaches account for approximately 90% of headache patients presenting for clinical care.[70] Although tension-type headache is the most common form of headache with a prevalence in the general population ranging from 30 to 80%, migraine headaches are the most costly type of headache and have been estimated to have a burden of disease of more than 13 billion dollars annually.[71] The largest epidemiologic studies of migraines, the American Migraine Studies I and II (AMS-I and AMS-II), demonstrated that 28 million U.S. residents have migraine and that one in four households have someone with migraine.[72] Additionally, migraine headache is the only type that has evidence of inherited susceptibility.[73] Rarely, abnormalities on chromosome 19 have also been identified in some patients with migraines.[74]

Secondary headaches, account for most of the other 10% of headaches seen in clinical practice and include: head or neck trauma, cranial or cervical vascular disorders, nonvascular intracranial disorders, substance abuse or withdrawal, infection, and structural disorders of the cranium, neck, eyes, ears, nose, sinuses, teeth, mouth, or other facial or cranial structures. Additionally, secondary headaches can often be the somatic presentation of a psychiatric disorder.

Tertiary headache disorders comprise a small number of total headaches seen in clinical practice and include other cranial neuralgias, central and primary facial pain, and all other headaches. Lastly, patients may suffer more than one type of headache disorder.[68]

Headaches as Chronic Pain

Headaches can become a chronic condition and some patients experience them daily. The IHS currently defines chronic daily headache (CDH) as a headache that occurs more than 15 days/month, is at least 4 hours in duration, and has persisted for at least 6 months. CDH can be divided into primary and secondary headaches and further characterized in headache lasting >4 hours versus those that last <4 hours. *Chronic migraine* patients have a history of episodic migraines and frequently have a family history of migraine exacerbation during the menstrual cycle, identifiable trigger factors, and unilateral headache. As many as 25% of migraine sufferers in the United States experience four or more severe migraine attacks per month, 35% experience one to four migraines per month, and 38% suffer from one or less severe attacks per month.[72]

Chronic tension-type headache (CTTH) is defined by a diffuse, bilateral pain, frequently involving the back of the head and neck, and may have some migraine-like features. The typical presentation is a middle-aged woman with a history of episodic-tension headaches that have turned into daily or almost-daily tension headaches. CTTH sufferers are often unresponsive to numerous treatment strategies.

Chronic Headaches and Comorbid Psychiatric Illness

Headache pain and psychiatric illness are often comorbid. The causative pathway is likely bidirectional: (1) headache pain may cause psychopathology and/or (2) headache pain may be a somatic manifestation of psychopathology. Headache is also the most frequent somatic complaint of people with major depression.[75] In children, somatic complaints of headaches that do not have an underlying organic etiology are often indicative of a depressive disorder.[76] Furthermore, headache that is comorbid with anxiety or depression worsens the prognosis of the headache condition, and worsens the perceived intensity of the headache activity and suffering.[77] Compared to nonheadache patients, headache patients are more frequently diagnosed with panic disorder, other somatoform disorders and adjustment disorders, sleep disorders, and axis II disorders, such as borderline personality disorder.[75]

Epidemiology and Risk Factors of Chronic Headache
CHRONIC DAILY HEADACHE
Chronic daily headache, especially chronic migraines, and CTTH, are characterized by the highest rates of comorbid depression and anxiety disorders. In a large population-based study in Western Europe ($n < 18,900$), 28.5% of women and 5.5% of men with CDH had both anxiety and depressive symptoms, and 21.3% of women and 5.5% of men with CDH had depressive symptoms.[78] Risk factors for CDH include: (1) analgesic overuse, (2) stressful life events, (3) headache or neck injury, (4) habitual snoring, and (5) excessive caffeine intake (more of a risk if <40 years old). Analgesic overuse can stem from stressful life events, such as depression, or head/neck injuries, which illustrates the close links even among the risk factors themselves.[79]

CDH is further characterized by the highest amount of psychiatric comorbidity compared with all other headache subtypes. One study found that 90% of those with CDH suffered from at least one psychiatric disorder. In this study, anxiety and depression were the most frequently diagnosed comorbid psychiatric illnesses.[80] Another study suggested that sleep disorders also occur concurrently in patients with CDH.[81]

CHRONIC MIGRAINE HEADACHE

Chronic migraines are often comorbid with psychiatric disorders. Breslau et al. found that migraine patients are four to five times more likely than those without migraines to have affective disorders, including dysthymia (4.4 times more likely), major depression (3.7 times more likely), manic episodes (5.4 times), and bipolar disorder (5.1).[82] The literature describes the bidirectional association of migraine and major depression. Major depression increases the risk for migraine, and migraine increases the risk for major depression. Migraine signals an increased risk for the first onset of major depression, and major depression signals an increased risk for the first time occurrence of migraine.[83] There is likely a common biology or mechanism underlying migraine and psychiatric disorder. Treatment of migraine headache includes a wide variety of agents including anticonvulsant medications which have "mood stabilizing" properties and appear to be effective in reducing migraine frequency.[84]

CHRONIC TENSION-TYPE HEADACHE

Chronic tension-type headache individuals frequently present with comorbid mood and anxiety disorders.[85] A recent epidemiologic study conducted in West Virginia and Ohio showed that CTTH sufferers were 3–15 times more likely than matched controls to receive a diagnosis of an anxiety or mood disorder and almost half of the CTTH patients exhibited clinically significant levels of anxiety and/or depression.[86] According to the 1998 American Headache Scientific Meeting, 50% of CTTH patients present with comorbid symptoms of anxiety or depression of "sufficient magnitude" that require treatment in order to manage the headache symptoms.[79]

Treatment of Chronic Headache and Comorbid Depression

Treatment with antidepressants may improve CTTH symptoms and reduce headache frequency. In several studies, including a large randomized placebo-control trial conducted from 1995 to 1998, tricyclic antidepressant medication and stress management therapy produced large reductions in the headache activity of CTTH sufferers, as well as reductions in analgesic medication use and headache-related disability as compared to placebo. In this study, the antidepressant medication alone yielded more rapid improvements in headache activity, but in combination with therapy, it was more likely to produce clinically significant reductions in headache scores than either one alone or a placebo.[87]

Fibromyalgia

Fibromyalgia is a common chronic musculoskeletal pain disorder characterized by widespread pain and generalized tender points as well as additional symptoms such as fatigue and sleep disturbances, irritable bowel and bladder syndromes, chronic headaches, paresthesias, hearing and vestibular dysfunctions, and chemical sensitivities. It is estimated that between 2 and 5% of the general population suffers from fibromyalgia,[88] 90% of whom are middle-aged women.[89] One large study estimated that 3.4% of women and 0.5% of men in the general population have symptoms of fibromyalgia.[90] This syndrome classically overlaps with other functional somatic disorders, particularly chronic fatigue syndrome, and with systemic lupus erthematosus. Current research suggests that stress plays a key role in the development of symptoms of fibromyalgia.[91] When considered as a discrete clinical disorder, fibromyalgia is characterized by the presence of two types of pain: diffuse, widespread pain, and trigger point tenderness.[92] Widely accepted diagnostic criteria calls for tender points at 11 of 18 musculoskeletal sites lasting at least 3 months.[92] However, there is some debate surrounding the inclusion of trigger point tenderness as being necessary for a diagnosis of fibromyalgia.[93]

Etiology of Fibromyalgia

Over the years there has been an ongoing debate as to whether fibromyalgia was simply a manifestation of somatized depression or a separate disorder. However, more recent research supports the belief that major depression does not fully explain FSS, such as fibromyalgia. While psychiatric comorbidity and life time stress play a great role in the clinical presentation of fibromyalgia, the other accompanying health conditions that often present with fibromyalgia—lowered pain threshold, IBS, tension headache, and temporomandibular disorders—suggest an underlying alteration in central nervous processing of nociceptive input for those with fibromyalgia.[94] There is evidence of abnormalities in the 5-HT and NE systems in patients with fibromyalgia.[95] The 5-HT and NE systems have been felt to mediate endogenous analgesic mechanisms via the descending inhibitory pain pathways in the brain and spinal cord.[96] Additionally, dysfunction of the 5-HT- and NE-mediated descending pain inhibitory pathways may play a role in the development of pain symptoms in fibromyalgia.[97] Other new studies have focused on what appears to be abnormal responsivity in the HPA axis.[98]

Fibromyalgia and Comorbid Mood Disorders

The literature clearly demonstrates that fibromyalgia is often comorbid with major depression and other psychiatric disorders, including PTSD.[98–100] A recent study of patients with fibromyalgia found prevalence rates of 42% for lifetime major depression, and 20% for lifetime PTSD.[101] Another recent study demonstrates that fibromyalgia coaggregates in families with both reduced pain thresholds and major mood disorders.[100] This suggests a possible genetic contribution to the etiology and has implications regarding the extent to which genetic and environmental factors may influence the development of fibromyalgia and mood disorders.[100]

Treatment of Fibromyalgia and Comorbid Mood Disorders

Antidepressant drug therapy has been shown to be efficacious in treating patients with fibromyalgia. There are data supporting the use of tricyclic antidepressants, SSRIs, and more recently the combined SNRIs. The tricyclic antidepressants have the most data available.[102,103]

Recently the SSRIs and SNRIs have drawn more attention as the first-line treatment modality for comorbid fibromyalgia and depression. A randomized, placebo-controlled, double-blind, flexible-dose study of fluoxetine in the treatment of fibromyalgia demonstrated that fluoxetine improved the overall functioning, including decreased pain, fatigue, and depression.[104] Some data suggest that the enhancement of both 5-HT and NE neurotransmission may be more effective in treating fibromyalgia than enhancement of either neurotransmitter alone.[105] The SNRIs, including venlafaxine and duloxetine show promise in treating patients with fibromyalgia.[106] One of the largest clinical trials for the treatment of fibromyalgia, which included an evaluation of the impact of comorbid major depression on response to treatment, found that duloxetine demonstrated significant efficacy, compared to placebo in patients with fibromyalgia, particularly for women.[97] Although approximately 38% of the patients in this study also had a current diagnosis of comorbid major depression, the effect of duloxetine on reduction of fibromyalgia symptoms was similar in patients with or without major depression.[97] In addition to antidepressant pharmacotherapy, cognitive-behavioral therapy (CBT) is also effective in treating fibromyalgia (as well as IBS, and other pain disorders).[36]

Irritable Bowel Syndrome

Epidemiology and Mechanism

Irritable bowel syndrome is a common and disabling functional GI disorder affecting 10-20% of the population. Women are affected more often than men.[107] IBS is usually referred to as a "functional GI disorder," a term used to define combinations of chronic or recurrent GI symptoms that do not have an identified underlying pathophysiology. Patients with IBS commonly experience chronic abdominal pain, bloating and altered bowel habits of either constipation or diarrhea. IBS is diagnosed by symptomatology according to the Rome criteria and the absence of organic disease.[108] The etiology of IBS is thought to result from dysregulation of the bidirectional communication systems between the GI tract and the brain. Neuroendocrine, immunologic and psychosocial factors have also been implicated.[107,108] For example, corticotrophin releasing hormone (CRH) appears to be an important mediator of the stress response in the "brain-gut" tract and may be linked to potential new treatments of IBS which include the CRH antagonists.[109]

Irritable Bowel Syndrome, Abuse History, and Comorbid Psychiatric Illness

Research has demonstrated a strong association between life stressors and IBS. Many studies have reported a high prevalence of self-reported physical and sexual abuse in patients with functional GI disorders.[49–52,110–113] One study of women patients seen within a gastroenterology practice demonstrated that those women with a sexual or physical abuse history report more pain, non-GI somatic symptoms, bed disability days, lifetime surgeries, psychologic distress, and functional disability compared to those without this history.[52] In addition to physical and sexual abuse, other lifetime losses or traumas, childhood family turmoil, and recent stresses all can contribute to poor health outcome in patients with IBS.[53] Severe life events or chronic social difficulties (e.g., bereavement, marital separation) are more frequently associated with functional bowel disorders than with organic GI disease.[114] In patients with IBS, those with sexual abuse were four times more likely to report pelvic pain than those without abuse.[52]

Although a history of physical or sexual abuse is not the sole etiology of the development of a functional GI disorder, it is associated with a tendency to communicate psychologic distress through somatic symptoms.[115] Patients who present with both a history of abuse and IBS usually have more severe symptoms and are treatment refractory to usual care.[116] These patients are also more likely to have a comorbid psychiatric disorder.[117]

Studies demonstrate that over 50% of patients with IBS who seek treatment have a psychiatric disorder, including major depression, panic disorder, generalized anxiety disorder, social phobia, and PTSD.[118] Furthermore, it appears that the psychiatric diagnosis usually precedes the diagnosis of IBS.[119] Studies suggest that IBS patients with greater depressive symptoms report greater pain severity because of the tendency to engage in catastrophic thinking and demonstrate less effective coping.[120,121]

Figure 17-1 illustrates the many factors that are relevant in a comprehensive formulation of a functional pain syndrome including biologic, psychologic, and social contributions. This model applies to both IBS as well as the other functional pain syndromes discussed. Our model begins by considering predisposing factors such as genetics and demographics, and then considers the role of a history of abuse or trauma and the individual's ability to cope with a severe stressor. Moderating variables include the type of coping strategy and the presence of psychiatric symptoms. All of these factors will ultimately impact on the emergence of somatic symptoms, treatment response, and functional health status.

Biopsychosocial Treatment Approach of Irritable Bowel Syndrome

The literature strongly supports a biopsychosocial treatment model of IBS for patients with persistent symptoms.[120–123] For the majority of patients with IBS (70%), the symptoms are episodic and usually managed by a primary care physician.[120] However, for patients with moderate to severe IBS in which the symptoms cause noticeable

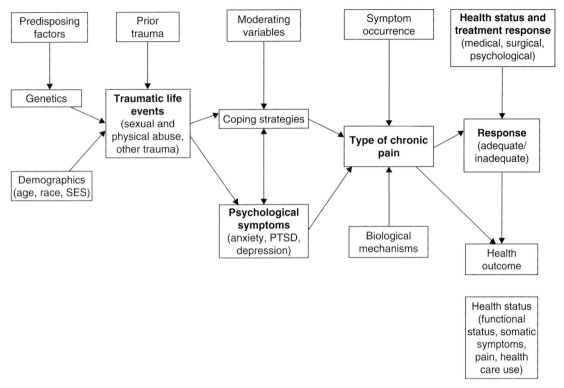

Figure 17-1. Schematic of the biopsychosocial model of chronic pain syndromes.

disruption in their lives and are associated with comorbid psychiatric symptoms, mental health intervention is indicated.[122] Most patients with moderate to severe IBS will have seen a gastroenterology specialist who can be instrumental in initiating a multidisciplinary treatment strategy. The field of gastroenterology now has specific recommendations that include: (1) establishing a therapeutic relationship so that the gastroenterologist practices active listening of the patient's concerns, responds in an empathic and nonjudgmental manner, (2) educating the patient about diagnosis, prognosis, and treatment alternatives, and (3) addressing psychosocial stressors and consulting a mental health professional who can address mood or anxiety disorder symptoms, screen for a history of abuse and trauma, and recommend appropriate pharmacotherapies and psychotherapies as needed.[123]

PSYCHOLOGIC TREATMENT STRATEGIES

A recent review of psychologic treatment interventions for IBS was conducted, including psychodynamic psychotherapy, hypnotherapy, and CBT interventions.[124] Some of these studies used GI symptoms as the outcome measure, while other studies used psychologic outcome measures such as mood and anxiety symptoms. Among the studies that address the efficacy of the psychotherapeutic intervention for treating both the GI and mood and anxiety symptoms associated with IBS, there is one positive study of psychodynamic psychotherapy,[125] and two positive studies of hypnotherapy.[126,127] The literature on CBT is significantly larger, although the results are mixed and there are a number of very small studies. However, in one of the largest CBT trials for the treatment of IBS (a three arm study comparing CBT vs. a psychoeducational group vs. routine medical care), the CBT group had significant reductions in symptoms of depression (as measured by the Beck depression inventory [BDI]),[128] and in the GI symptom of bloating, when compared to the control group receiving usual medical care, but did not differ when compared to the psychoeducational group on any measure.[129] Blanchard and colleagues have been studying CBT interventions for the treatment of IBS for many years, and have reported both positive and negative studies.[130,131] However, one study from this group compared cognitive therapy to a self-help support group and found significant improvement in IBS symptoms, depression, and anxiety in the cognitive therapy group that held up at a three-month follow-up assessment.[132]

PSYCHOPHARMACOLOGIC TREATMENT

There is a relatively small section of literature supporting the use of psychotropics in treating IBS. Although the SSRIs have been shown to be efficacious in the treatment of chronic pain,[133] there are only two case reports[134,135] and one recent controlled study of the efficacy of SSRIs in IBS.[136] In the controlled trial, patients received a high fiber diet with either paroxetine or placebo. Outcome measures included both GI symptoms, general well-being, and an assessment of mood (as measured by the BDI).[128] The results demonstrated that patients receiving the paroxetine had a significantly greater response compared to placebo on measures of well-being and depression, and this result remained significant for depressed versus nondepressed patients in the study (as assessed by baseline BDI score).[136] Interestingly, although paroxetine is currently classified as a selective 5-HT reuptake inhibitor, there is new evidence that it can act as both a 5-HT and NE reuptake inhibitor, which could partially explain its broad therapeutic efficacy.[137] Clearly, future studies are needed to confirm this preliminary finding and to evaluate other SSRIs in the treatment of IBS. In addition to the SSRIs, future studies should also focus on the SNRIs in the treatment of IBS, which as discussed earlier, have shown promising results in other functional pain disorders such as fibromyalgia.

Chronic Pelvic Pain

Epidemiology and Clinical Presentation

Chronic pelvic pain, defined as pelvic pain of at least 6 months duration, is a relatively common disorder with a prevalence of 15% among women of reproductive age.[138] It accounts for 10% of gynecologic consultations and 40% of diagnostic laparoscopies performed in general hospitals.[56,139] Women with CPP are often a distressed group and these patients have high rates of sexual and physical abuse, other trauma, and symptoms of depression.[140] The treatment of CPP is complex and challenging. Many women fail to respond to treatment, and relapse rates are high. CPP patients utilize a disproportionate amount of health care resources, comparable to patients with other similar chronic medical conditions such as IBS.[49]

As currently defined, CPP includes diverse symptoms of dysmenorrhea, dyspareunia, and other nonspecific complaints related to lower abdominal, pelvic floor, and vulvar pain.[138,140] It appears to be a heterogeneous disorder with multiple, and often unknown etiologies. Currently, there is no consensus concerning diagnostic categories of CPP within gynecology.[141] The challenge in the evaluation and management of patients with CPP is the often false assumption that the pain can be linked with some form of pathology or obvious tissue damage.[142] Because every structure in the abdomen and/or pelvis could have a role in the etiology of CPP, it is essential to think beyond the reproductive organs and consider other contributions, such as the peripheral and central nervous systems.

Current theories suggest that CPP is a biopsychosocial disorder in which psychologic events, such as sexual abuse and trauma interact with structural and physiologic factors to produce symptoms. These interactions determine how patients cope with their symptoms and how they respond to treatments, including psychologic as well as surgical and medical treatments. CPP is a challenging problem that is a major cause of disability and morbidity for women.[143] A recently published review of more than 100 articles on CPP concluded that there is no consensus on the definition of CPP, and that this deficiency reduces the ability to investigate causation and improve treatment.[141] Historically, three different operational definitions of CPP have been used in the literature: (1) durational: any type of pelvic pain that has lasted 6 months or longer, (2) anatomic: CPP that lacks apparent physical cause sufficient to explain the pain (usually meaning that laparoscopy disclosed minimal, if any, pathology), and (3) affective-behavioral: pain accompanied by significantly altered physical activity, including work, recreation, libido, as well as disturbance of mood.[144]

Chronic Pelvic Pain and History of Abuse

The association of CPP with childhood and/or adult sexual abuse has been well documented in the literature.[145–151] For example; studies by Lampe et al.[145] and Walker et al.[147] demonstrate a significant association between childhood sexual abuse (prior to age 15) and the later development of CPP. In a population-based survey of 1931 women in primary care practices, those with a history of childhood sexual abuse were more likely to report pelvic pain (23.5%) compared to those without abuse (11.2%).[39] Lechner et al.[149] showed that adult women in a family practice clinic with childhood sexual abuse were significantly more likely to have had surgical evaluation of pelvic pain (21.6%) compared to those without abuse (12.6%). Similarly, Springs et al.[150] reported a twofold increased odds ratio of having pelvic pain among those with a history of childhood abuse versus those without such a history. In addition, there is one study documenting significantly more depressed mood and illness behavior in women with CPP compared to those without pain just prior to undergoing an elective laparoscopy.[152]

Treatment of Chronic Pelvic Pain
PSYCHOLOGIC TREATMENT
Psychologic intervention studies for the treatment of CPP are extremely limited. The 2000 Cochrane Database Systematic Review identified only one study of sufficient quality that examined a psychologic intervention in the treatment of CPP. In this study, psychologic counseling paired with ultrasound scanning had a mild-moderate impact on the course of CPP.[153]

PSYCHOPHARMACOLOGY
Because many patients with CPP have comorbid depressive and anxiety symptoms, antidepressants have been tried as a treatment strategy. However, the efficacy of antidepressants in the treatment of CPP has been suboptimal, and a small double-blind study of the SSRI sertraline did not demonstrate clinical significance.[154] In clinical practice, the tricyclic antidepressants, other antidepressants including the SSRIs, and anticonvulsants are all used with modest success in the treatment of this frequently refractory group of patients.

The relationship between abuse, chronic pain, and psychiatric illness is complex and includes unanswered questions such as: What is the relationship between sexual abuse and pain? Is there a direct causal relationship? Is the pathway through an association with a psychiatric or other disorder? An integrative multidisciplinary approach has been thought to have the best chance for success with CPP; thus many suggest psychologic treatment in addition to traditional medical and surgical approaches.[143,155]

▶ CONCLUSIONS

Depressive disorders with comorbid chronic pain syndromes present a fascinating, although ultimately difficult treatment challenge to the clinician. Chronic pain is highly comorbid with depression and other psychiatric illness. Comorbid psychiatric illness appears to alter both the individual's perception of pain and ability to tolerate the pain. The FSS are a complex system of biologic, psychologic, and social factors. A psychiatric history is an important component of effectively treating this patient population, and the role of a history of abuse and potential comorbid PTSD must be kept at the forefront. The antidepressant medications have been shown to have efficacy in a variety of chronic pain syndromes and should be considered an important part of therapy, although further research is needed in order to confirm the efficacy of specific agents in specific patient populations. A collaborative team approach that includes mental health along with conventional medical or surgical therapies in the treatment of the chronic pain syndromes is critical because of the many psychologic factors that contribute to the individual's experience of pain.

REFERENCES

1. Katon W, Egan K, Miller D. Chronic pain: Lifetime psychiatric diagnoses and family history. *Am J Psychiatry* 1985;142:1156–1160.
2. Magni G, Caldieron C, Rigatti-Luchini S, et al. Chronic musculoskeletal pain and depressive symptoms in the general population: An analysis of the first national and nutrition examination survey data. *Pain* 1990;43:299–307.
3. Dersh J, Polatin PB, Gatchel RJ. Chronic pain and psychopathology: Research findings and theoretical considerations. *Psychosom Med* 2002;64:773–786.
4. Lindsay PG, Wyckoff M. The depression-pain syndrome and its response to antidepressants. *Psychosomatics* 1998;22:571–573.
5. Katon WJ. Clinical and health services relationships between major depression, depressive symptoms and general medical illness. *Biol Psychiatry* 2003;54:216–226.
6. Katon W, Sullivan M, Walker E. Medical symptoms without identified pathology: Relationship to psychiatric disorders, childhood and adult trauma, and personality traits. *Ann Intern Med* 2001;134:917–925.
7. Ohayon MM, Schatzberg AF. Using chronic pain to predict depressive morbidity in the general population. *Arch Geniatry* 2003;60(1):39–47.
8. Wilson KG, Mikail SF, D'Eon JL, et al. Alternative diagnostic criteria for major depressive disorder in patients with chronic pain. *Pain* 2001;91:2272–34.
9. Bair MJ, Robinson RL, Katon W, et al.. Depression and pain comorbidity: A literature review. *Arch Intern Med* 2003;163:2433–2445.
10. Von Korff M, Ormel J, Kaon W, et al. Disability and depression among high utilizers of health care: A longitudinal analysis. *Arch Gen Psychiatry* 1992;49:91–100.
11. Bair MJ, Robinson RL, Eckert GJ, et al. Impact of pain on depression treatment response in primary care. *Psychosom Med* 2004;66:17–22.
12. Gatchel RJ. Psychological disorders and chronic pain: Cause and effect relationships. In: Gatchel RJ, Turk DC (eds.), *Psychological Approaches To Pain Management: A Practitioner's Handbook.* New York: Guilford Press, 1996, pp.33–54.
13. Holzberg AD, Robinson ME, Geisser ME. The effects of depression and chronic pain on psychosocial and physical functioning. *Clin J Pain* 1996;12:118–125.
14. Fishbain DA, Cutler R, Rosomoff HL, et al. Chronic pain-associated depression: Antecedent or consequence of chronic pain. A review. *Clin J Pain* 1997;13:116–137.
15. Fields H. Pain modulation: Expectations, opioid analgesia and virtual pain. *Prog Brain Res* 2000;122:245–253.
16. Okada K, Murase K, Kawakita K. Effects of electrical stimulation of thalamic nucleus submedius and periaqueductal gray on the visceral nociceptive responses of spinal dorsal horn neurons in the rat. *Brain Res* 1999;834:112–121.
17. Blackburn-Munro G, Blackburn-Munro RE. Chronic pain, chronic stress and depression: Coincidence or consequence? *J Neuroendocrinol* 2001;13:1009–1023.
18. Clauw DJ, Chrousos GP. Chronic pain and fatigue syndromes: Overlapping clinical and neuroendocrine features and potential pathogenic mechanisms. *Neuroimmunomodulation* 1997;4:134–153.
19. Onghena P, van Houdenhove B. Antidepressant-induced analgesia in chronic non-malignant pain: A meta-analysis of 30 placebo-controlled studies. *Pain* 1992;49:205–219.
20. Briley M. Clinical experience with dual action antidepressants in different chronic pain syndromes. *Hum Psychopharmacol* 2004;19(Suppl 1): S21–S25.
21. Detke MJ, Lu Y, Goldstein DJ, et al. Duloxetine, 60 mg once daily, for major depressive disorder: A randomized double-blind placebo-controlled trial. *J Clin Psychiatry* 2002;63(4):308–315.
22. Rowbotham MC, Goli V, Kunz NR, et al. Venlafaxine extended release in the treatment of

painful diabetic neuropathy: A double-blind, placebo-controlled study *Pain* 2004;110(3): 697–706.

23. Loeser JD, Volinn E. Epidemiology of low back pain. *Neurosurg Clin North Am* 1991;2:713–718.

24. Kessler RC, Berglund P, Demler O, et al. The epidemiology of major depressive disorder: Results from the National Comorbidity Survey Replication (NCS-R). *JAMA* 2003;289(23):3095–3105.

25. Polatin PB, Kinney RK, Gatchel RJ, et al. Psychiatric illness and chronic low-back pain: The mind the spine—which does first? *Spine* 1993; 18:66–71.

26. Kinney RK, Gatchel RJ, Polatin PB, et al. Prevalence of psychopathology in acute and chronic low back pain patients. *J Occup Rehabil* 1993; 3:95–103.

27. Pincus T, Burton AK, Vogel S, et al. A systematic review of psychological factors as predictors of chronicity/diability in prospective cohorts of low back pain. *Spine* 2002;27(5):E109–E120.

28. Linton SJ. A review of psychological risk factors in neck and back pain. *Spine* 2000;25: 1148–1156.

29. DiIorno D, Henley E, Doughty A. A survey of primary care physicians practice patterns and adherence to acute low back pain problem guidelines. *Arch Fam Med* 2000;9:1015–1021.

30. Turner JA, Denny MC. Do antidepressant agents relieve chronic low back pain? *J Fam Pract* 1993;37:545–553.

31. Van Tulder MW, Koes BW, Bouter LM. Conservative treatment of acute and chronic nonspecific low back pain. *Spine* 1997;22:2128–2156.

32. Salerno SM, Browning R, Jackson JL. The effect of antidepressant treatment on chronic back pain. *Arch Intern Med* 2002;162:19–24.

33. Staiger TO, Gaster B, Sullivan MD, et al. Systematic review of antidepressants in the treatment of chronic low back pain. *Spine* 2003; 28:2540–2545.

34. Rush JA, Polatin P, Gatchel RJ. Depression and chronic low back pain: Establishing priorities in treatment. *Spine* 2000;25:2566–2571.

35. Malt EA, Berle JE, Olafsson S, et al. Fibromyalgia is associated with panic disorder and functional dyspepsia with mood disorders: A study of women with random sample population controls. *J Psychosom Res* 2000;49(5):285–289.

36. Kroenke K. Patients presenting with somatic complaints: Epidemiology, psychiatric comorbidity and management. *Int J Methods Psychiatr Res* 2003;12(1):34–43.

37. Nimnuan C, Rabe-Hesketh S, Wessely S, et al. How many functional somatic syndromes? *J Psychosom Res* 2001;51(4):549–557.

38. Molnar BE, Buka SL, Kessler RC. Child sexual abuse and subsequent psychopathology: Results from the National Comorbidity Survey. *Am J Public Health* 2001;91:753–760.

39. McCauley J, Kern DE, Kolodner K, et al. Clinical characteristics of women with a history of childhood abuse: Unhealed wounds. *JAMA* 1997;277 (17):1362–1368.

40. Felitti VJ. Long-term medical consequences of incest, rape, and molestation. *South Med J* 1991; 84:328–331.

41. Widom CS. Posttraumatic stress disorder in abused and neglected children grown up. *Am J Psychol* 1999;156:1223–1229.

42. Walker EA, Unutzer J, Rutter C, et al. Costs of health care use by women HMO members with a history of childhood abuse and neglect. *Arch Gen Psychiatry* 1999;56:609–613.

43. Wilsnack S, Vogeltanz N, Klassen A, et al. Childhood sexual abuse and women's substance abuse: National survey findings. *J Stud Alcohol* 1997;58:264–271.

44. Nixon RD, Resick PA, Nishith P. An exploration of comorbid depression among female victims of intimate partner violence with posttraumatic stress disorder. *J Affect Disord* 2004;82: 315–320.

45. Stein MB, Kennedy C. Major depressive and post-traumatic stress disorders comorbidity in female victims of intimate partner violence. *J Affect Disord* 2001;66:133–138.

46. Clum GA, Calhoun KS, Kimerling R. Associations among symptoms of depression and post-traumatic stress disorder and self-reported health in sexually assaulted women. *J Nerv Ment Dis* 2000;188:671–678.

47. Romans S, Belaise C, Martin J, et al. Childhood abuse and later medical disorders in women. *Psychother Psychosom* 2002;71:141–150.

48. Frothingham TE. Follow-up study eight years after diagnosis of sexual abuse. *Arch Dis Child* 2000;83:132–134

49. Drossman DA, Leserman J, Nachman G, et al. Sexual and physical abuse in women with functional or organic gastrointestinal disorders. *Ann Intern Med* 1990;113:828–833.

50. Leserman J, Drossman DA, Li Z, et al. Sexual and physical abuse history in gastroenterology practice: How types of abuse impact health status. *Psychosom Med* 1996;58:4–15.

51. Leserman J, Li Z, Drossman DA, et al. Impact of sexual and physical abuse dimensions on health status: Development of an abuse severity measure. *Psychosom Med* 1997;59:152–160.

52. Leserman J, Li Z, Drossman DA, et al. Selected symptoms associated with sexual and physical abuse history among female patients with gastrointestinal disorders: The impact on subsequent health care visits. *Psychol Med* 1998; 28:417–425.

53. Leserman J, Li Z, Hu YJB, et al. How multiple types of stressors impact on health. *Psychosom Med* 1998;60:175–181.

54. Golding JM. Sexual assault history and headache: Five general population studies. *J Nerv Ment Dis* 1999;187:624–629.

55. Walker EA, Keegan D, Gardner G, et al. Psychosocial factors in fibromyalgia compared with rheumatoid arthritis: II. Sexual, physical, and emotional abuse and neglect. *Psychosom Med* 1997;59:572–577.

56. Reiter RC. A profile of women with chronic pelvic pain. *Clin Obstet Gynecol* 1990;33:130–136.

57. Breslau N, Davis GC, Andreski P, et al. Traumatic events and posttraumatic stress disorder in an urban population of young adults. *Arch Gen Psychiatry* 1995;52:1048–1060.

58. Resnick H, Kilpatrick DG, Dansky BS, et al. Prevalence of civilian trauma and posttraumatic stress disorder in a representative sample of women. *J Consult Clin Psychol* 1993;61:984–991.

59. Breslau N, Davis GC, Andreski P, et al. Sex differences in posttraumatic stress disorder. *Arch Gen Psychiatry* 1997;54:1044–1048.

60. Golding JM. Sexual assault history and physical health in randomly selected Los Angeles women. *Health Psychol* 1994;13:130–138.

61. Waigandt A, Wallace DL, Phelps L, et al. The impact of sexual assault on physical health status. *J Trauma Stress* 1990;3:93–102.

62. Kimerling R, Calhoun KS. Somatic symptoms, social support, and treatment seeking among sexual assault victims. *J Consult Clin Psychol* 1994;62:333–340.

63. Meltzer-Brody S, Churchill E, Davidson JR. Derivation of the SPAN, a brief diagnostic screening test for post-traumatic stress disorder. *Psychiatry Res* 1999;88:63–70.

64. Breslau N, Peterson EL, Kessler RC, et al. Short screening scale for DSM-IV posttraumatic stress disorder. *Am J Psychiatry* 1999;156:908–911.

65. Brewin CR, Rose S, Andrews B, et al. Brief screening instrument for post-traumatic stress disorder. *Br J Psychiatry* 2002;181:158–162.

66. Meltzer-Brody S, Hartmann K, Miller WC, et al. A brief screening instrument to detect posttraumatic stress disorder in outpatient gynecology. *Obstet Gynecol* 2004;104:770–776.

67. Moriarty-Sheehan M. Headache evaluation and management. *Lippincotts Prim Care Pract* 2000;4(6):580–594.

68. Smith T. Epidemiology and impact of headache: An overview. *Prim Care* 2004;31:237–241.

69. Dupug HJ, Engel A, Devine BK, et al. Selected symtoms of psychological stress. U.S. Public Health Publication;1000:series 1137. National Centre for Statistics;1977.

70. Schappert S. National ambulatory medical care survey: Survey of 1989. National Center for Health Statistics. *Vital Health Stat* 1992;13:110.

71. Hu X, Markson L, Lipton R. Disability and economic costs of migraine in the United States: A population-based approach. *Arch Intern Med* 1999;159:813–818.

72. Lipton R, Stewart W. Migraine in the United States: A review of epidemiology and health care use. *Neurology* 1993;43(Suppl 3):S6–S10.

73. Russell MB, Andersson PG, Thomsen LL. Familial occurrence of cluster headache. *J Neurol Neurosurg Psychiatry* 1995;58(3):341–343.

74. Verin M, Rolland Y, Landgraf F, et al. New phenotype of the cerebral autosomal dominant arteriopathy mapped to chromosome 19: Migraine as the prominent clinical feature. *J Neurol Neurosurg Psychiatry* 1995;59(6):579–585.

75. Sheftell FD, Atlas S. Migraine and psychiatric comorbidity: From theory and hypotheses to clinical application. *Headache* 2002;42:934–944.

76. Lagges A, Dunn D. Depression in children and adolescents. *Neurol Clin* 2003;953–960.

77. Radat F. Psychopathology and headache. *Rev Neurol* (Paris) 2000;156(Suppl 4):S62–S67.

78. Bigel ME, Tepper SJ, Sheffell FD et al. Chronic daily headache: correlation between the 2004 and 1988 International Headache Society Diagnostic Criteria. *Headache* 2004;44(7):684–691.

79. Hutchinson S. Chronic daily headache. *Prim Care* 2004;31:353–367.

80. Verri AP, Proietti Cecchini A, Galli C, et al. Psychiatric comorbidity in chronic daily headache. *Cephalalgia* 1998;18(Suppl 21):45–49.

81. Guidetti V, Galli F, Cerutti R, et al. Chronic daily headache in developmental ages: Diagnostic issues. *J Head Pain* 2000;(Suppl 1):S89–S94.

82. Breslau N, Davis GC, Andreski P. Migraine, psychiatric disorders, and suicide attempts: An epidemiologic study of young adults. *Psychiatry Res* 1991;37:11–23.

83. Breslau N, Lipton RB, Stewart WF, et al. Comorbidity of migraine and depression: Investigating potential etiology and prognosis. *Neurology* 2003;60:1308–1312.

84. Chronicle E, Mullens W. *Cochr Database Syst Rev* 2004;(3):CD003226.

85. Breslau N, Schultz LR, Stewart WF, et al. Headache and major depression: Is the association specific to migraine? *Neurology* 2000;54:308–313.

86. Holroyd K, Stensland M, Lipchik G, et al. Psychosocial correlates and impact of chronic tension-type headaches. *Headache* 2000;40:3–16.

87. Holroyd KA, O'Donnel FJ, Stensland M, et al. Management of chronic tension-type headache with tricyclic antidepressant medication, stress management therapy, and the combination: A randomized controlled trial. *JAMA* 2001;285(17):2208–2215.

88. Neumann L, Buskila D. Epidemiology of fibromyalgia. *Curr Pain Headache Rep* 2003; 7(5):362–368.

89. Yunus, MB. Gender differences in fibromyalgia and other related syndromes. *J Gend Specif Med* 2002;5(2):42–47.

90. Wolfe FK, Ross J, Anderson Russell IJ, et al. The prevalence and characteristics of fibromyalgia in the general population. *Arthritis Rheum* 1995;8:19–28.

91. Van Houdenhove B, Egle UT. Fibromyalgia: A stress disorder? Piecing the biopsychosocial puzzle together. *Psychother Psychosom* 2004; 73(5):267–275.

92. Wolfe F, Smythe HA, Yunus U, et al. The American College of Rheumatology criteria for the classification of fibromyalgia: report of the multicenter criteria committee. *Arthritis Rheum* 1990;33:160–172.

93. Wolfe F. The relation between tender points and fibromyalgia symptom variables: Evidence that fibromyalgia is not a discrete disorder in the clinic. *Ann Rheum Dis* 1997;56(4):268–271.

94. Henningsen P, Derra C, Turp JC, et al. Functional somatic pain syndromes: Summary of hypotheses of their overlap and etiology. *Schmerz* 2004;18(2):136–140.

95. Russell IJ, Michalek JE, Vipraio GA, et al. Platelet 3H-imipramine uptake receptor density and serum serotonin levels in patients with fibromyalgia/fibrositis syndrome. *J Rheumatol* 1992;19: 104–109.

96. Millian MJ. Descending control of pain. *Prog Neurobiol* 2002;66:355–374.

97. Arnold LM, Lu YL, Crofford LJ, et al. for the Duloxetine Fibromyalgia Trial Group: A double-blind, multicenter trial comparing duloxetine with placebo in the treatment of fibromyalgia patients with or without major depressive disorder. *Arthritis Rheum* 2004;50(9):2974–2984.

98. McBeth J, Silman AJ. The role of psychiatric disorders in fibromyalgia. *Curr Rheumatol Rep* 2001;3(2):157–164.

99. Hudson JI, Pope HG Jr. The relationship between fibromyalgia and major depressive disorder. *Rheum Dis Clin North Am* 1996;22(2): 285–303.

100. Raphael KG, Janal MN, Nayak S, et al. Familial aggregation of depression in fibromyalgia: A community based test of alternate hypotheses. *Pain* 2004;110(1–2):449–460.

101. Roy-Byrne P, Smith WR, Goldberg J, et al. Posttraumatic stress disorder among patients with chronic pain and chronic fatigue. *Psychol Med* 2004;34(2):363–368.

102. Arnold LM, Keck PE Jr, Welge JA. Antidepressant treatment of fibromyalgia: A meta-analysis and review. *Psychosomatics* 2000;41(2):104–113.

103. Tofferi JK, Jackson JL, O'Malley PG. Treatment of fibromyalgia with cyclobenzaprine: A meta-analysis. *Arthritis Rheum* 2004;51(1):9–13.

104. Arnold LM, Hess EV, Hudson JI, et al. A randomized, placebo controlled, double-blind, flexible-dose study of fluoxetine in the treatment of women with fibromyalgia. *Am J Med* 2002;15; 112(3):191–197.

105. Fishbain D. Evidence-based data on pain relief with antidepressants. *Ann Med* 2000;32:305–316.

106. Ninan PT. Use of venlafaxine in other psychiatric disorders. *Depress Anxiety* 2000;12(Suppl):90–104.

107. Ringle Y, Sperber AD, Drossman DA. Irritable bowel syndrome. *Annu Rev Med* 2001;52:319–338.

108. Drossman DA. Irritable bowel syndrome. *Gastroenterologist* 1994;2(4):315–326.

109. Sagami Y, Shimada Y, Tayama J, et al. Effect of a corticotropin releasing hormone receptor

antagonist on colonic sensory and motor function in patients with irritable bowel syndrome. *Gut* 2004;53(7):958–964.

110. Delvaus M, Denis P, Allemand H, French Club of Digestive Motility. Sexual and physical abuses are more frequently reported by IBS patients than by patients with organic digestive diseases or controls: Results of a multicenter inquire. *Eur J Gastroenterol Hepatol* 1997;9:345–352.

111. Scarinci IC, McDonald-Haile JM, Bradley LA, et al. Altered pain perception and psychosocial features among women with gastrointestinal disorders and history of abuse: A preliminary model. *Am J Med* 1994;97:108–118.

112. Talley NJ, Helgeson S, Zinsmeister AR. Are sexual and physical abuse linked to functional gastrointestinal disorders? *Gastroenterology* 1992;102:A523.

113. Talley NJ, Fett SL, Zinsmeister AR. Self-reported abuse and gastrointestinal disease in outpatients: Association with irritable bowel-type symptoms. *Am J Gastroenterol* 1995;90:366–371.

114. Gaynes BN, Drossman DA. The role of psychosocial factors in irritable bowel syndrome. *Bailliere's Clin Gastroenterol* 1999;13(3):437–452.

115. Drossman, DA. Physical and sexual abuse and gastrointestinal illness: What is the link? *Am J Med* 1994;97:105–107.

116. Drossman DA, Corazziari E, Talley NJ, et al. *Rome II: The Functional Gastrointestinal Disorders*, 2nd ed. Lawrence, KS: Allen Press, 2000.

117. Walker EA, Katon W, Roy-Byrne PP, et al. Psychiatric illness and irritable bowel syndrome: A comparison with inflammatory bowel disease. *Am J Psychiatry* 1990;147:1656–1661.

118. Lydiard RB. Irritable bowel syndrome, anxiety and depression: What are the links? *J Clin Psychiatry* 2001;62(Suppl 8):38–45.

119. Toner BB, Garfinkel PE, Jeejeebhoy KN. Psychological factors in irritable bowel syndrome. *Can J Psychiatry* 1990;35:158–161.

120. Lackner JM, Quigley BM, Blanchard EB. Depression and abdominal pain in IBS patients: The mediating role of catastrophizing. *Psychosom Med* 2004;66(3):435–441.

121. Drossman DA, Li Z, Leserman J, et al. Association of coping pattern and health status among female GI patients after controlling for GI disease type and abuse history. *Psychosom Med* 1997;59:105.

122. Drossman DA, Thompson G. The irritable bowel syndrome: Review and a graduated multicomponent treatment approach. *Ann Intern Med* 1992;116:1009–1016.

123. Drossman DA. Psychosocial sound bites: Exercises in the patient-doctor relationship. *Am J Gastroenterol* 1997;92:1418–1423.

124. Blanchard EB, Scharff L. Psychosocial aspects of assessment and treatment of irritable bowel syndrome in adults and recurrent abdominal pain in children. *J Consult Clin Psychol* 2002;70(3):725–738.

125. Guthrie E, Creed F, Dawson D, et al. A controlled trial of psychological treatment for the irritable bowel syndrome. *Gastroenterology* 1991;100:450–457.

126. Whorwell PJ, Prior A, Colgan SM. Hypnotherapy in severe irritable bowel syndrome on quality of life. *Digest Dis Sci* 1984;41:2248–2253.

127. Houghton LA, Heyman DJ, Whorwell PJ. Symptomatology, quality of life and economic features of irritable bowel syndrome: The effect of hypnotherapy. *Aliment Pharmacol Therap* 1996;10:91–95.

128. Beck AT, Ward CH, Mendelson M, et al. An inventory for measuring depression. *Arch Gen Psychiatry* 1961;5:561–571.

129. Toner BB, Segal ZV, Emmott S, et al. Cognitive-behavioral group therapy for patients with irritable bowel syndrome. *Int J Group Psychother* 1998;48:215–243.

130. Greene B, Blanchard EB. Cognitive therapy for irritable bowel syndrome. *J Consult Clin Psychol* 1994;62(3):576–582.

131. Vollmer A, Blanchard EB. Controlled comparison of individual versus group cognitive therapy for irritable bowel syndrome. *Behav Therapy* 1998;29:19–33.

132. Payne A, Blanchard EB. A controlled comparison of cognitive therapy and self-help support groups in the treatment of irritable bowel syndrome. *J Consult Clin Psychol* 1995;63(5):779–786.

133. Jung AC, Staiger T, Sullivan M. The efficacy of selective serotonin reuptake inhibitors for the management of chronic pain. *J Gen Intern Med* 1997;12:384–389.

134. Kirsch MA, Louis AK. Paroxetine and irritable bowel syndrome. *Am J Psychiatry* 2000;157:1523–1524.

135. Emmanuel NP, Lydiard RB, Crawford M. Treatment of irritable bowel syndrome with fluvoxamine. *Am J Psychiatry* 1997;154:711–712.

136. Tabas G, Beaves M, Wang J, et al. Paroxetine to treat irritable bowel syndrome not responding to high-fiber diet: A double-blind placebo-controlled trial. *Am J Gastroenterol* 2004;914–920.

137. Gilmore ML, Owens MJ, Nemeroff CB. Inhibition of norepinephrine uptake in patients with major depression treated with paroxetine. *Am J Psychiatry* 2002;159(10):1702–1710.

138. Mathias SD, Kuppermann M, Liberman RF, et al. Chronic pelvic pain: Prevalence, health-related quality of life, and economic correlates. *Obstet Gynecol* 1996;87(3):321–327.

139. Howard FM. The role of laparoscopy in chronic pelvic pain: Promise and pitfalls. *Obstet Gynecol Surv* 1993;48(6):357–387.

140. Jamieson DJ, Steege JF. The association of sexual abuse with pelvic pain complaints in a primary care population. *Am J Obstet Gynecol* 1997;177:1408–1412.

141. Williams RE, Hartmann KE, Steege JF. Documenting the current definitions of chronic pelvic pain: Implications for research. *Obstet Gynecol* 2004;103(4):686–691.

142. Zondervan KT, Yudkin PL, Vessey MP, et al. The community prevalence of chronic pelvic pain in women & associated illness behavior. *Br J Gen Pract* 2001;51:541–547.

143. Gunter J. Chronic pelvic pain: An integrated approach to diagnosis and treatment. *Obstet Gynecol Surv* 2003;58:615–621.

144. Steege JF, Stout AL, Somkuti SG. Chronic pelvic pain in women: Toward an integrative model. Review. *Obstet Gynecol Surv* 1993;48(2):95–110.

145. Lampe A, Solder E, Ennemoser A, et al. Chronic pelvic pain and previous sexual abuse. *Obstet Gynecol* 2000;96(6):929–933.

146. Golding JM, Wilsnack SC, Learman LA. Prevalence of sexual assault history among women with common gynecologic symptoms. *Am J Obstet Gynecol* 1998;179:1013–1019.

147. Walker EA, Katon W, Harrop-Griffiths J, et al. Relationship of chronic pelvic pain to psychiatric diagnoses and childhood sexual abuse. *Am J Psychiatry* 1988;145:75–79.

148. Walker EA, Katon WJ, Neraas K, et al. Dissociation in women with chronic pelvic pain. *Am J Psychiatry* 1992;149:534–537.

149. Lechner ME, Vogel ME, Garcia-Shelton LM, et al. Self-reported medical problems of adult female survivors of childhood sexual abuse. *J Fam Pract* 1993;36:633–638.

150. Springs FE, Friedrich WN. Health risk behaviors and medical sequelae of childhood sexual abuse. *Mayo Clin Proc* 1992;67:527–532.

151. Beard RW, Belsey EM, Lieberman BA. Pelvic pain in women. *Am J Obstet Gynecol* 1977;128:566.

152. Hodgkiss AD, Watson JP. Psychiatric morbidity and illness behavior in women with chronic pelvic pain. *J Psychosom Res* 1993;38:3–9.

153. Stones RW, Mountfield J. Interventions for treating chronic pelvic pain in women. *Cochr Database Syst Rev* 2000;(4):CD000307.

154. Engel CC, Walker EA, Engel Al, et al. A randomized, double-blind crossover trial of sertraline in women with chronic pelvic pain. *J Psychosom Res* 1998;44(2):203–207.

155. Milburn A, Reiter RC, Rhomberg AT. Multidisciplinary approach to chronic pelvic pain. Review. *Obstet Gynecol Clin North Am* 1993;20(4):643–661.

CHAPTER 18

Complementary and Alternative Medical Approaches to Mood Disorder Treatment

Suzan Khoromi, Barbara E. Moquin, Jennifer M. Meegan,
and Marc R. Blackman

► INTRODUCTION

Numerous surveys reveal a marked increase in the usage of diverse complementary and alternative medicine (CAM) modalities during the last decade. Mood disorders, particularly major depressive disease, are among the most common conditions for which CAM treatments are employed. The three most commonly used CAM treatments for depression include relaxation, exercise, and herbal therapy. Other CAM treatments such as acupuncture, massage, yoga, art therapy, and transcranial magnetic stimulation (TMS) are used less often. CAM treatments are attractive to patients in part because they are perceived to be more empowering, less authoritatively derived, effective, and devoid of adverse effects. However, there is a dearth of rigorous research to substantiate the efficacy and safety of most CAM modalities currently used to treat patients with major depressive disorder (MDD) or other mood disorders. Major limitations in many of the reported studies have included small sample size, inconsistency in document-ing the diagnosis of MDD, failure to use placebo or other controls, lack of proper blinding, use of inadequate outcome measures, failure to control for confounders, inadequate duration of treatment, and intrusion of personal beliefs of the investigators themselves. The few well-controlled, large-scale clinical trials suggest that CAM modalities, when effective, are useful primarily in mild-moderate, rather than severe disease. The latter observations, along with the major public health importance of MDD, the substantial morbidity and mortality resulting from this chronic condition, and improvements in mainstream pharmacologic treatments suggest that validated CAM therapies of MDD will play an adjunctive, rather than primary, role in managing most patients. Given that there are few preclinical studies evaluating possible mechanisms by which various CAM modalities may exert their effects, there is a clear-cut need for more robust clinical and laboratory investigation to assure that the use of various CAM modalities in this patient population is grounded in contemporary evidence-based medicine.

Definition of Complementary and Alternative Medicine

Complementary and alternative medicine, as currently defined by the National Center for Complementary and Alternative Medicine (NCCAM), National Institutes of Health (NIH), refers to "practices that are unproven and not presently considered part of conventional medicine." This definition acknowledges the evolving nature of CAM, implying that as CAM practices are proven safe and effective, they may become part of mainstream health care.

The diversity of CAM modalities can be conceptually placed into four domains as follows:

- Mind-body medicine, such as hypnosis, meditation, spirituality, and the placebo effect
- Biologically based practices, such as herbs, botanicals, dietary supplements, and selected dietary practices
- Energy medicine, based on external electromagnetic fields or endogenous biofields that purport to extend healing from master practitioner to patient
- Manipulative and body-based practices, such as chiropractic, osteopathy, and therapeutic massage

Because whole medical systems of CAM, such as Indian Ayurvedic or Traditional Chinese Medicine (TCM), homeopathy, and naturopathy employ practices drawn from all the domains described above, it is more appropriate to treat these systems not as a domain, but as a category all their own, albeit one that shares features with each of the domains above.

▶ EPIDEMIOLOGY AND FREQUENCY OF CAM USE FOR DEPRESSION

Recent reports point to current use of one or more CAM modalities by 30–60% of the United States population, with continuing increases in usage with each successive major survey. Most CAM use is considered to be complementary, that is, in addition to mainstream interventions, whereas CAM modalities are less often used as an alternative to conventional treatment. Approximately 60% of CAM users in the United States do not discuss use of these modalities with their health care providers. This is of particular concern in patients with depression or other mental health disorders, in whom there is often an additional reluctance to discuss their behavioral disorders, and in whom there is an increased risk for adverse interactions between various CAM biologic agents and certain conventional drugs. For example, St. John's Wort (SJW), used commonly by persons with mild to moderate depression, stimulates the hepatic P450 enzyme system, and alters the metabolism of many allopathic medications.

In one survey, conducted in 1991, it was found that 34% of the U.S. population used at least one CAM treatment for 1 year.[1] In a subsequent report, 40% of 1035 respondents had used some form of alternative health care during 1996, and this utilization applied to both sexes and all racial, ethnic, income, and age groups. Depression was one of the most common reasons for using CAM therapies in both of these surveys.[2] A study of 312 primary care patients meeting criteria for major depression indicated that 6.4% used antidepressants and 3.5% used CAM treatments suggesting that self-medication to manage the morbidity of depression was common. Even more striking was the finding that the vast majority of depressed patients were untreated with either antidepressants or CAM treatments.[3] In a survey at the Medical University of South Carolina's outpatient clinic, 56% of 150 individuals evaluated had used herbal medicines within the previous month, of whom 32% reported using herbs to treat psychiatric symptoms.[4] In a national survey conducted between 1997 and 1998, 7.2% of the 2055 individuals reported suffering from "severe depression"; of these, 53.6% had used at least one CAM modality during the prior 12 months and 19.3% had visited a CAM therapist. Sixty-six percent of patients seen by conventional providers for severe depression had also used CAM to treat this condition.[5] In another study examining the relationship between psychiatric disorders and the use of CAM, 9585 households were evaluated in a telephone survey between 1997 and 1998, with 16.5% of respondents having used CAM during the prior 12 months. Twenty-one percent of these respondents met diagnostic criteria for one or more psychiatric disorders, as compared with 12.8% of respondents who did not report use of CAM. Individuals with major depression were significantly more likely to use CAM than those without this disorder.[6]

Characteristics of mental health visits to CAM providers were recently examined among a representative sample of acupuncturists, chiropractors, massage therapists, and naturopathic physicians in four states. Among 8933 reported visits to these providers, only 7–11% of the visits to acupuncturists, massage therapists, and naturopathic physicians were for a mental health complaint. Sixty-nine to eighty-seven percent of these patients were self-referred. In 6–20% of cases, treatment was discussed with conventional medical providers, but in only 1–5% of cases were actual referrals made to these providers. An additional 10–30% of patients acknowledged concomitant conventional medication usage to their CAM providers. Thus, for acupuncturists, massage therapists, and naturopaths, the proportion of visits for mental health concerns is similar to that in conventional primary care.[7]

In the most recent and largest survey reported to date, conducted as part of the Centers for Disease Control and Prevention's 2002 National Health Interview Survey, CAM use was evaluated in approximately 31,000 representative adults.[8] Nearly 62% of respondents claimed use of one or more CAM modalities during the preceding 12 months when CAM was defined as including use of prayer specifically for health purposes, whereas 36% reported using CAM when prayer was excluded. Depression and anxiety were among the most common reasons for the use of CAM modalities.

Depression and CAM Use in Elderly Populations

Depression is more common in older persons. To evaluate the predictors and patterns of CAM use among the elderly, Blue Shield Medicare conducted a 1-year mail-in survey of a population receiving Medicare coverage for acupuncture and chiropractic services. Of 728 respondents, 41% reported use of one or more CAM modalities, including herbs (24%), chiropractic (20%), therapeutic massage (15%), and acupuncture (14%). Results from this survey may not reflect the entire aged population, because trends in alternative medicine have shown that while many people will pay out-of-pocket for these expenditures, insurance coverage of CAM increases the probability of its use. Aged persons more likely to employ CAM modalities, like their younger counterparts, tend to be female, White, better educated, report depression, anxiety or arthritis, and are engaged in more disease prevention activities, such as exercise or frequent physician visits. To date, we are unaware of reports comparing the frequency and patterns of CAM use in older versus younger depressed patients.

Depression and CAM use in Ethnic Populations

Culture-specific symptoms sometimes lead to misinterpretation of psychologic distress.[9] Qualitative ethnographic research in clinical settings and the community currently explores the role of culture in psychopathology. Unlike in the United States where there is greater expression of interpersonal conflict and confrontation, many other cultures suppress internal distress, especially because these concerns are often seen as more sociomoral in nature. Thus, in worldwide primary care settings, the most common somatic symptoms, namely those of musculoskeletal pain and fatigue, are often indicative of underlying depression.[10] It is therefore important for the clinician to be knowledgeable concerning cultural meanings as it is likely that many somatic symptoms of ethnic patients may reflect psychosocial issues. The Diagnostic and Statistical Manual of Mental Disorders, DSM-IV-TR, includes a relevant appendix outlining 25 culturally related syndromes that may be associated with depression.

CAM use to assist with the management of depression varies among ethnic groups. In a 1999 survey, 60% of 184, mostly urban, Latino women responded regarding CAM use for depression, anxiety, and stress. More than half of the women were in their mid-30s and noted that herbs, minerals and vitamins, massage, and aromatherapy were most frequently chosen. Of note, 60% of the women reported that their health care providers did not ask about CAM use, and 40% stated that they did not discuss their CAM use.[11] In a pilot study of 39 Latino and Black women in New York City between the ages of 18 and 50, prayer and spiritual healing, meditation, and relaxation techniques were also found to be important.[12] Curanderismo is a diverse folk healing system of Latin America widely practiced by Mexican-Americans in the United States.[13] Given that Hispanics are the second largest and fastest growing minority group in the United States it is important to mention this centuries old practice that focuses on problems of psychologic, social, and spiritual nature usually not addressed by conventional health care providers.[13]

In a survey that over-sampled minorities,[14] 42.6% out of 1048 Blacks used at least one CAM remedy. Specificity of illness for CAM use was not reported. Blacks were more likely to report using herbs and home remedies than were other ethnic groups. In a study examining the management of depression and use of religion in elderly Blacks, no significant relationship was reported.[15] However, religion and spirituality are noted as the most common source of social and coping support for Blacks, and ritual, the power

of words in a narrative form, and dreams are often used in counseling and psychotherapy.[16]

In a paper exploring the experience of depression by elderly Korean immigrants in the United States,[17] the feeling of "having one's vital energy—ki-blocked" could further the development of Han or Hwabyung: folk illnesses similar to depression. Some Koreans consider depression to be a routine part of life as described by the Buddhist teaching, "life is a troubled sea.".[18] Thus, relating to their fate or a supernatural power is a common way of coping.

For the Japanese, there has been a greater social acceptability of anxiety versus depression. Thus, until recently there has been a low diagnostic rate of depression despite evidence of somatic symptoms. Japanese with symptoms of depression are still routinely treated with benzodiazepines, though with more widespread use of selective serotonin reuptake inhibitors (SSRIs), antidepressant use has increased.[9]

Though American Indians/Alaskan Natives (AI/ANs) constitute less than 1% of the total United States population, they number 280 cultural groups consisting of 478 tribes. Depression is often experienced in a combination of substance abuse, transgenerational trauma, and poverty in the AI/ANs families and communities.[19] In an interview of 300 Navajo Indian Health Service patients between the ages of 18 and 90, Kim and Kwok[20] found that 62% had used a native healer and that depression was one of the highest reasons for use. Garroutte et al.[21] studied 1456 AI Northern Plains members between the ages of 15 and 57 and found that commitment to native cultural spirituality, not Christianity, was significantly associated with a reduction in attempted suicide. The Medicine Wheel treatment approach has been utilized by AI/ANs to focus on a healthy balanced life incorporating spiritual, physical, social/cultural, and mental/emotional realms.[19]

Thus, viewing an individual from an ethnic population in a holistic context with family and community, offers a more accurate description and management of depression.

General Considerations

In the following chapter, we shall present an overview of selected CAM modalities that are commonly used in the management of patients with MDD. We recognize that, despite their widespread usage for hundreds or thousands of years, most CAM modalities have not been subjected to rigorously controlled scientific evaluations of their efficacy or safety. Moreover, in some trials of CAM treatment of depression, validation of the diagnosis of MDD using standardized (e.g., DSM) criteria is not always evident. Given that untreated MDD is associated with significant morbidity and mortality and that delaying proper treatment may be also associated with significant risks, it would appear prudent to await further studies to substantiate the usage of any of these modalities prior to recommending them as first line or complementary options in the treatment of patients with MDD.

THE PLACEBO EFFECT

Historically, a placebo has been considered to be an inactive or innocent management contrivance to encourage healing in the absence of specific therapeutics. As such, it has been relied upon to "control" for nonspecific effects that might confound calculation of the true benefits of a novel intervention. Of particular note is that the placebo effect may play an important role during the course of any mood-altering therapy. A recent meta-analysis suggested that the placebo effect occurs in as many as 30% of depressed patients undergoing clinical trials of major allopathic antidepressant medications, and that the incidence and prevalence of this phenomenon have increased during the past two to three decades.[22] In contrast, there has been little if any systematic inquiry into the frequency of the placebo effect in the context of CAM treatment of depression. This is a particularly important area for further study. Moreover, ethical considerations suggest that placebo-controlled clinical trials may not always serve to legitimately represent the benefit to the patient of certain CAM interventions wherein there is no apparent effect beyond that of a placebo.[23] Finally, there is broad consensus that more research into the biology of the placebo effect is warranted in depressed patients treated with both allopathic and CAM modalities.[24]

As to mood disorders other than MDD, surveys in patients with bipolar disorders regarding their usage of nonpharmacologic treatments indicate that prayer, exercise, avoidance of caffeine, meditation, relaxation, and guided imagery are some of most frequent techniques used for relief of symptoms. More than half of the 101 bipolar patients included in one survey[25] believed that these techniques were "a little to somewhat" helpful in reducing their symptoms, whereas 10–30% of patients believed that these modalities helped reduce their symptoms "a lot" or "completely." To our knowledge, there is one small, albeit well-conducted study suggesting that administration of a branched chain amino acid mixture to patients with bipolar disorder during manic episodes enhances the effect of standard treatments for mania.[26] This study requires confirmation before consideration of conducting a larger RCT to assess the effect of branched chain amino acids used in conjunction with other standard medical treatments in bipolar patients.

▶ TREATMENTS FOR PATIENTS WITH MAJOR DEPRESSIVE DISORDER

Mind-Body Medicine

Meditation

Meditation can be defined as an "intentional regulation of attention from moment to moment."[27] The attention is focused on a single repetitive phrase, word, sound, prayer, breath, or object.[28] When the mind becomes distracted, the meditator gently refocuses attention on the repetitive stimulus. Vipassana or mindfulness meditation, a Buddhist form of meditation with psychologic underpinnings, has been developed to train the mind to follow the mechanics of mental processing[27,28] and best illustrates the potential for meditation as a complement to psychotherapy. The major advantage seen by combining psychotherapy and meditation has been the intensification of the therapeutic process.[29]

Kutz et al.[29] studied 20 patients between 21 and 53 years of age who were involved in a 10-week mindfulness meditation program. Patients who had various psychiatric diagnoses, not specific for MDD and excluding psychosis, self-reported the largest decrease in depression and anxiety as measured by the SCL-90-R questionnaire. Six-month follow-up indicated that the improvements noted from the meditation program had continued.

Controlled studies of meditation in well-defined populations of patients with MDD are warranted. Brain imaging and neuroendocrine studies may be helpful in further evaluating the pathophysiologic mechanisms underlying the heightened sense of well-being experienced by meditators with or without a psychiatric diagnosis.

Guided Imagery

The only published information regarding the use of guided imagery as a treatment for depression derives from a study comparing the effects of muscle relaxation and guided imagery on anxiety, depression, and quality of life in 56 patients with advanced cancer.[30] No significant improvements in anxiety-related outcomes were detected after treatment, whereas depression scores and quality of life indices improved. To date, we are unaware of controlled studies using this modality in patients with MDD.

Relaxation Therapy

The "relaxation response" includes techniques that decrease heart rate, blood pressure and breathing rate, reduce serum lactic acid levels and oxygen consumption, often showing improvement in hypertension[31] and pain.[32] The relaxation response is not confined to any specific religious or secular practice, though may include hypnosis, autogenic training, meditation, prayer and yoga,[31] or simply involve focusing quietly on one's breathing pattern. The increased sym-

pathetic nervous system arousal associated with the stress response is more commonly seen in anxiety states.[33] However, because of the high comorbidity of anxiety and depression, relaxation therapy is often prescribed.

Though most of the studies investigating the effects of relaxation treatment for depression have utilized small sample sizes and short time periods, patients have reported beneficial physiologic and psychologic changes. To our knowledge, few RCTs have been reported assessing the efficacy of relaxation in patients with MDD. In one study of 30 outpatients with depression who were all taking antidepressant medication, the participants given relaxation therapy for 3 days showed significant improvement in symptom scores.[34] In another RCT of 37 patients with MDD receiving relaxation therapy, cognitive behavioral therapy, or tricyclic antidepressants (TCAs), the two CAM interventions resulted in significantly better Beck depression inventory (BDI) scores than did pharmacologic treatment, with no difference between cognitive and relaxation therapy.[35]

Thirty patients with unipolar depression diagnosed by a psychiatrist, received either medication (nortriptyline) alone (MA), relaxation therapy plus medication (RT&M), or cognitive therapy and medication (CT&M). The BDI and the Hamilton rating scale for depression (HRSD) were used to assess changes in depressive symptoms. CT&M and RT&M groups noted significantly fewer depressive symptoms than the MA group at discharge. In addition, the CT&M subjects were rated as less depressed at discharge than the RT&M and MA groups.[36]

Yoga

Multiple anecdotal reports attest to the beneficial effects of yoga on reducing anxiety and depression. In one randomized-controlled study,[37] 45 patients with melancholic depression based on DSM criteria were treated with one type of yoga practice, Sudarshan Kriya Yoga, electroconvulsive therapy (ECT), or imipramine for a period of 4 weeks. All three groups exhibited significant improvements on the BDI and the

HRSD scores. Remission rates based on total HRSD scores of seven or less were present at the end of the trial in 93, 73, and 67% of the ECT, imipramine, and yoga treatment groups, respectively. This well-conducted study is promising and further investigation of yoga in larger groups of patients with MDD is warranted.

Aromatherapy

Clinical aromatherapy refers to the use of aromatic and essential oils (EOs) from flowers and herbs for therapeutic purposes.[38] It is thought that EOs can alter a person's mood and behavior while facilitating physical, emotional, and mental well-being. People can respond immediately to scents with resultant calming, pain-reducing, sedating, and euphoric effects.[39] Aromatherapists often combine massage techniques with the use of EOs to produce pharmacologic effects with transdermal absorption.[40]

Though there is little objective evidence that aromatherapy can improve mood in depression, anecdotal reports suggest that patients experience it as helpful.[41] Bergamot, German chamomile, geranium, rosemary, and lavender are EOs most often suggested for relieving depressive symptoms.[38,42] Lavender has been studied the most by health care providers and shows some positive results for alleviating insomnia and reducing stress.[39]

Further research may add knowledge regarding mechanism of action of neurotransmitter release when individuals are exposed to various scents, as well as pairing EOs with specific physical and emotional illnesses.

Prayer

A belief in health having components of mental and spiritual factors has been an important predictor of CAM use.[43] One national survey found that 7% of persons surveyed regarding CAM use in the United States had used some type of spiritual healing: distant healing, prayer, Reiki, and/or therapeutic touch (TT). This was the fifth most commonly reported of all CAM therapies. Thirty-five percent of these same respondents noted that they had used prayer to address their health issues.[44] Another national survey reported that 82% of Americans in the United States believed in the healing power of prayer and 64% thought that physicians should pray with patients who requested it.[45]

Spiritual healing is a "broad classification of approaches involving the intentional influence of one or more persons upon another living system without utilizing known physical means of intervention."[46] Prayer includes: "intercessory—asking God, the universe or some higher power to intervene on behalf of an individual or patient; supplication—in which one asks for a particular outcome; and nondirected—in which one does not request any specific outcome."[47] Studies reported to date have not addressed the impact of prayer in patients with MDD.

Creative Arts Therapies

Music, dance, art, drama, and writing have always been vehicles for human expression. In recent decades, professionals in these fields have expanded knowledge, instituted training programs, and established accreditation systems for practitioners[48] and used these modalities to treat emotional and mental illnesses. Creative arts therapists "tap emotional rather than cognitive processes"[49] and this can more directly and immediately engage patients.[50] For some population groups with communication difficulties, either because of personal handicaps or unfamiliarity with the language of a psychotherapist, creative arts therapies can more easily reach emotional processes individually or in group settings. Underserved populations such as children, poor, minority, elderly, severely ill, and those with multiple handicaps often find traditional psychotherapy as "just talk"[48] and lacking relevance.

For the purposes of this chapter, music, dance, journaling, and color therapy used in depression will be highlighted. For some of these interventions (e.g., music, dance), clinical studies have been conducted in patients with well-defined MDD, whereas for others (e.g., journaling, color therapy), the reported literature derives from patients with less well-defined depressive symp-tomatology. Overall, there is a need to perform additional, carefully controlled studies of each of these creative therapies in patients with MDD and other mood disorders.

Music Therapy

Music therapy can transform the auditory aspect of an environment in ways that can assist the patient to make choices that are healthy and adaptive. It has been stated that "music improves the quality of life by providing meaningful and purposeful activities that are accessible, can be actively or passively employed by people who are well or people who have illness or disabili-ties."[51] These choices may be reality-based rather than flight into fantasy, interaction with others rather than withdrawal, increasing structure more than disorganization, increasing self-respect and competence, as well as stimulating the mind and body and relieving lethargy. Thoughtfully and sen-sitively used music can provide safe environments for remembering memories, expressing painful emotions, and providing a sense of release, clo-sure, and enhanced vitality.[52]

Although frontal and limbic system functions are hypothesized to be affected by music the mechanism of action is unknown.[53] A controlled trial comparing the results of cognitive therapy versus music therapy in nursing home residents with major depression found the cognitive ther-apy to be superior on the basis of BDI scores.[54] Another study incorporating a music psychoed-ucational tool examined 30 older adults diag-nosed with major or minor depression based on a structured interview using the schedule of affective disorders and schizophrenia. After being randomly assigned to one of three 8-week strategies: (1) a home-based program where the participants learned music stress reduction tech-niques with weekly visits by a music therapist; (2) a self-administered program where the par-ticipants applied the same techniques with a weekly telephone call from the therapist; and (3) a wait-list control group, participants in both music groups scored better than did the con-trols on standardized tests of depression, mood,

distress, and self-esteem. Of note, the results were clinically significant and were maintained during a 9-month follow-up period.[55]

Music therapists can contribute to research that highlights the power of music to enhance rest, restore peace and balance, activate and spir-itually uplift.

Dance Therapy

Individuals from various disciplines have devel-oped complementary and alternative movement therapies: eastern movement approaches (con-temporary yoga, Pilates-based methods, Feldenkrais), engineering (Hellerwork), physics (Feldenkrais), traditional rehabilitation (Con-ductive Education, body-mind centering), the performing arts (Alexander, dance therapy, body-mind centering), somatics (body-mind centering), and psychology (dance therapy). The proposed benefit of each therapy varies: it may be by improving functional status (Feldenkrais, Alexander), improving ease and awareness of movement (body-mind centering), achievement of a specific form (Pilates-based methods), or relief of emotional barriers (dance therapy).[56]

Dance/movement therapy (DMT) has been defined as "the psychotherapeutic use of move-ment as a process which furthers the emotional, cognitive, and physical integration of the indi-vidual" by the Association of Dance Therapy of America (1999). A theory explaining DMT is that dance can be an externalized form of inner feel-ings that cannot always be verbally or rationally expressed.[57] This is consistent with the concept that emotions are the link between body and psyche.[58] Chodorow[57] explains that, "an emo-tion by definition, is at once somatic and psychic. The somatic aspect is made up of bodily inner-vations and expressive physical action. The psy-chic aspect is made up of images and ideas. In psychopathology, the realms tend to split. By contrast, a naturally felt emotion involves a dialec-tical relationship—a union of body and psyche."

One study randomly assigned patients to receive dance therapy on some days and not on others. For each of the 12 patients with major depression, mood was compared regarding treatment versus no treatment. Some patients were found to have improved mood on treatment days, even though long-term effects on depression were not evaluated.[59] Further studies are needed to evaluate whether dance therapy can promote wellness by strengthening the immune and neuroendocrine systems through muscular action, physiologic processes, and the release of emotional distress.

Journaling

Writing about personal stressors or traumatic events has been associated with improvements in physical and emotional health.[60] Patients are able to become more proactive in their therapy and realize more personal responsibility for change.[61] Writing complements psycho-talk therapy as it assists therapists to obtain critical patient information more quickly and even more importantly, gives patients a feeling of staying connected with the therapist between sessions. Patients who have difficulty in one-to-one sessions can sometimes more easily communicate sensitive issues by journaling.[61] Self-mastery and self-reliance can be enhanced and journaling can provide a guide for navigating through future personal crises.[62] A journal may provide a path illuminating hidden opportunities involved in experiencing an illness.[62] Written dialogue with the self may provide an opportunity to make contact with a deeper, inner wisdom not always easily accessed through linear, logical means.[62]

The therapeutic use of journaling with verbal psychotherapy is seen as a means to affect a healing response.[62] Patients, who focus on both cognitive facts and emotions in the attempt to understand traumatic events, rather than just negative expression alone, have demonstrated the greatest improvements in health.[60] Further studies in well-defined populations of patients with MDD may add to our understanding of the reported improvements in immune system function[63] and decrease in depressive symptoms.[64]

Color Therapy

Color therapy refers to the use of color to heal physically, emotionally, mentally, and spiritu-

ally, and has been utilized for centuries in many parts of the world.[65] Color is "frequency within the visible spectrum of light, which composes a very small band of the total electromagnetic spectrum, from violet at 400 nm (higher energy photon) through red at 780 nm (lower energy photon). Each color of the spectrum is composed of a band of frequencies and therapeutic application of color to the body is accomplished by applying a single monochromatic wavelength within that band."

Colored light is thought to influence the autonomic nervous system at the level of the thalamus. A neurotransmitter chain reaction is established resulting in acetylcholine acting on the parasympathetic nervous system (decreasing muscle tension, heart rate, and blood pressure) and producing a physical relaxation response.[66] Colored light therapy, both through the eyes and applied to the body, is being studied and utilized in the fields of optometry, chiropractic, medicine, acupuncture, and psychology.[67]

Various studies have demonstrated that color exerts an impact on concentration, aggression, levels of stress, alertness, and depressive symptoms. Hospitals, prisons, and schools are using color therapy to enhance the quality of their environments.[65] Some of the most interesting studies to date, conducted in Germany, involve the combination of color and acupuncture. The investigators found that the "light was conducted within the body along the acupuncture meridians" and concluded that certain areas of the body were able to transfer light beneath the surface and that these areas corresponded to specific acupuncture points.[68] Many opportunities for continued multidisciplinary research exist in color therapy both as an individual modality and used in combination with other conventional and CAM treatments.

Biologically Based Practices

Vitamins

In countries such as China, Japan, and Australia, most people prefer treating major depression with CAM (i.e., traditional) versus allopathic (i.e., mainstream) therapies. In one national survey in Australia, 57% of people considered use of vitamins, minerals, and herbs as likely to help with depression, whereas only 29% of respondents believed antidepressants were likely to be helpful.[69] Despite their wide popularity and usage in many countries, including the United States, where nearly 30 billion dollars a year are spent on vitamins and over-the-counter herbal and mineral remedies, there is little evidence to support their beneficial usage in the treatment of MDD.

Deficiencies of B_{12} and folate are known to be associated with secondary depression, and there is some evidence that folic acid may serve as an adjunctive treatment for patients with primary depression. As many as 35% of depressed patients have folate deficiency[70] and this incidence may rise to 90% in elderly patients with depression.[71] In one recent U.S. survey of 2526 healthy individuals of various ethnic backgrounds, persons (n = 301) who met criteria of major depression based on DSM criteria, but not those (n = 121) diagnosed with dysthymia, had red blood cell folate levels that were lower than those of individuals without major depression.[72] In another study,[73] the relationship between folate and B_{12} and response to fluoxetine (20 mg/day for 8 weeks) was assessed during the treatment of patients with MDD based on DSM-IV criteria. Based on HAM-D scores, patients with low folate levels were more likely to have melancholic depression, and were significantly less likely to respond to fluoxetine. Alpert et al., reported significant improvement in mood in 22 patients with major depression and partial or nonresponse to an SSRI who were given supplemental folinic acid, regardless of their baseline folate levels, in addition to 15–30 mg of SSRI per day over a period of 8 weeks in an open-label trial.[74] This and other small studies suggest that folate supplementation may promote recovery from major depression independent of replenishment of low folate levels and may be useful in depressed patients who do not respond to antidepressant therapy. Folate also plays important roles in the chemical pathways leading to synthesis of *S*-adenosyl methionine (SAMe), the

principal methyl donor in a wide spectrum of neurochemical reactions. Likewise, it serves as a cofactor in the hydroxylation of phenylalanine and tryptophan, precursors to the synthesis of neurotransmitters such as norepinephrine and serotonin that are believed to play a key role in the pathogenesis of depression.

Dietary Restrictions

Nutritional status can exert a significant impact on emotional well-being. Diets too low in complex carbohydrates can deplete serotonin levels and contribute to depression, whereas increased protein and essential fatty acid intake may increase alertness and uplift spirits.

In one small randomized, controlled study in depressed patients, restriction of sugar and caffeine intake, but not of red meat and artificial sweeteners,[75] was associated with significant improvement in depressive symptoms. Four out of ten patients assigned to the study group were sensitive to sugar. In contrast, in another small study, carbohydrate intake was associated with a short-term improvement in depression.[76]

Alcohol cessation has been associated with rapid relief of depression in alcoholic patients admitted to alcohol rehabilitation programs.[77,78] In comparison, moderate alcohol intake may be associated with lower levels of depression in some people who do not have alcohol abuse problems.[79] Further investigation is warranted to elucidate the role of alcohol intake or abstention in patients with MDD.

Herbal Treatments

Despite the widespread use of herbs and plants such as SJW, ginseng, wild oats, lemon balm, basil, and for the treatment of depression, only a few of these treatments have been rigorously studied.

St. John's Wort

St. John's wort belongs to the genus hypericium of which there are more than 370 species. Not only do SJW flowers, leaves, and stems have varying chemical compositions but factors such as time of harvest, plant processing, and extraction methods also add to this variability.

To date, no single active chemical substance has been unequivocally identified as being most directly associated with the mood elevating properties of SJW. Approximately seven groups of pharmacologically active compounds have been identified from preparations of SJW including phenylpropanes, flavonol glycosides, biflavones, tannins and proanthrocyanidins, xanthones, phloroglucinols, EOs, amino acids, and naphthodianthrones. SJW's suggested modes of action include monoamine oxidase (MAO) inhibitor inhibition, and modulation of GABAergic activity,[80] monoamine reuptake,[81] and upregulation of 5HT1A and 5HT2A receptors.[82] Attempts to find the one ingredient that would mediate the mood effects of SJW to date have not been definitive and the active ingredient is presently considered the whole hypericium extract even though some evidence indicates that hyperforin may play a key role. Therefore, it is customary to standardize SJW's effect on hyperforin as a measure of its potency. Because the pharmacologically active ingredient has not yet been clarified, it is difficult to make dose recommendations. Most studies have used doses ranging from 350 to 1800 mg.

Neuroendocrine Effects

Acute administration of oral hypericum to healthy human subjects in a dose of 2700 mg has been associated with an increase in growth hormone and decrease in prolactin levels, suggesting increased dopaminergic transmission.[83] Quantitative electroencephalography studies of healthy human volunteers treated with acute doses of hypericum have revealed increases in alpha, theta, and delta bands[84] suggesting enhancement in serotonergic, noradrenergic, and cholinergic activity, respectively. In one placebo-controlled, single blind study assessing the acute effects of oral administration of Hypericum perforatum extract (WS 5570) to 12 healthy men in doses of 600–1200 mg was associated with increases in ACTH secretion, a trend toward increased GH secretion[85] and no changes in cortisol and prolactin secretion.

Clinical Effects of St. John's Wort in Patients with Depression

In a placebo-controlled study comparing the effects of SJW, amitriptyline, and placebo on EEG, cognitive function, and potential cardiac side effects in 12 healthy men for 14 days, SJW did not affect heart rate variability whereas amitriptyline showed a significant decrease. Neither SJW nor amitriptyline exerted significant effects on cognitive functions such as choice reaction, psychomotor coordination, short-term memory, and responsiveness to distractive stimuli. Both drugs caused significant EEG changes: SJW increased theta power density and amitriptyline increased theta as well as fast alpha power density.[86]

Multiple randomized-controlled trials have been conducted to assess the relative efficacy of SJW as compared with a placebo, TCAs, and SSRIs in thousands of depressed patients. Several meta-analyses and review articles evaluating the quality of these trials[87] have found no systematic biases in these studies.

Many of the randomized-controlled trials comparing SJW with placebo report that SJW is superior to placebo in terms of valid endpoints of clinical depression such as the Hamilton depression scale.[88] These studies were mostly directed toward patients with mild to moderate symptoms of major depression at the time of enrollment in the study. In patients with major depression of moderately severe degree, one multicenter study[89] in 200 patients revealed that SJW, at a dose of 900 mg/day orally for a period of 8 weeks was not superior to a placebo. In another study, neither a daily oral dose of SJW of 800 mg nor a daily dose of fluoxetine 20 mg/day were found to be more effective than a placebo during a 6-week treatment course in 149 elderly patients with mild to moderate depression. More recently an NIH multicenter study failed to demonstrate significant improvement in psychologic outcome measures in patients with major depression of mild to moderate severity who were randomly assigned to take SJW, a placebo, or a standardized antidepressant.[90]

Some studies were not placebo-controlled, but directly compared SJW with a standard antidepressant. Thus, SJW was compared with imipramine at doses of 100 mg/day[91,88] and 150 mg/day,[92] as well as with amitriptyline 30 mg/day[93] and maprotiline 75 mg/day.[94] Doses of hypericium used in these studies averaged from 900 to 1800 mg given in three divided doses. Most of these studies suggested that SJW's effect was equivalent to that of TCAs with a significantly better side effect profile.

A few trials also have compared the efficacy of SJW with that of SSRIs. When compared with sertraline 75 mg/day, SJW (doses averaging 900 mg/day) was found to be equally efficacious and well tolerated[95] in 30 patients with mild to moderate depression over a 7-week study period. Noninferiority trials that did not include a placebo arm should be interpreted with caution, however, as this effect is quite large in studies assessing the mood elevating effects of any treatment for depression.

SJW's tolerability and side effect profile appear to be quite acceptable in most studies. Reported side effects include headache, dizziness, photosensitivity, abdominal pain and discomfort, dry mouth, and fatigue. There are a few reports of mania or submania in some patients and therefore it has been suggested that SJW should not be prescribed along with SSRIs, TCAs, and MAOIs.[96] Unfortunately, numerous drug interactions have been reported, including those with cyclosporine,[97] protease inhibitors, and nonnucleoside reverse transcriptase inhibitors, such as efavirenz and nevirapine, used for HIV infection.[98] Most importantly, SJW interacts with the hepatic P450 enzyme system that contributes to metabolism of many drugs, contributing to clinically significant, adverse botanical-drug interactions with oral contraceptives, anticoagulant, immunosuppressant, and chemotherapeutic drugs.

Thus, based on data from multiple clinical trials, controversy remains as to whether SJW is effective in alleviating signs and symptoms of major depression of mild to moderate degree, and with fewer side effects than encountered with conventional antidepressant medications. Additional studies are being conducted to examine its potential utility in patients with symptoms of minor depression of mild-moderate degree, social phobia, and seasonal affective disorder (SAD). In this context, NCCAM and the National Institute of Mental Health are cosponsoring a study of the efficacy and safety of SJW versus citalopram in the treatment of patients with minor depressive disorder.

S-Adenosyl-L-Methionine (SAMe)

This naturally occurring substance and most important methyl donor in the central nervous system, has showed significant antidepressant activity in several clinical trials. First developed in 1973, it has been extensively marketed for improving mood and emotional well-being.[99,100] The rationale for using SAMe in response to depression stems from its role in the metabolism of serotonin, dopamine, and melatonin. Oral and intravenous SAMe supplementation has been shown to significantly increase SAMe levels in cerebrospinal fluid, indicating SAMe's crossover through the blood-brain barrier.[101] Like other antidepressant drugs, SAMe has been found to be able to increase the cAMP-dependent phosphorylation of microtubule-associated protein-2 in the somatodendritic compartment.[102]

In one multicenter 4-week long, double-blind study, Pancheri et al.,[103] compared intramuscular SAMe (400–1200 mg/day) with the conventional antidepressant, imipramine (25–150 mg) orally and inactive control in 287 patients with MDD of varying severity. Before study enrollment, all patients were accessed and diagnosed with major depression according to DSM-IV criteria (mean baseline HAMD 24.3; moderately severe symptom level), with a unipolar course, without psychotic symptoms. No significant difference in efficacy was found between SAMe and imipramine based on HAM-D scores, whereas SAMe was associated with fewer adverse effects and better tolerability as compared with imipramine. This is the largest study evaluating the effects of SAMe and imipramine for antidepressive effects, which also indicates a greater outcome in terms of clinical benefit, equivalence, and better tolerability profile.

In another, similarly designed multicenter study,[104] the efficacy and tolerability of oral versus intramuscular administration of SAMe were compared with that elicited by 150 mg of imipramine given orally. In this study, 143 patients were randomized to receive oral SAMe 1600 mg/day whereas 138 patients were provided imipramine for 6 weeks, and 147 patients who received SAMe intramuscularly were compared with 148 patients who took imipramine for 4 weeks. Prior to enrollment, these patients were also categorized with MDD by DSM-IV criteria. Overall, there were no significant differences in efficacy measures between SAMe and imipramine. As in the prior study, there were fewer adverse events and better tolerance with SAMe versus imipramine. It was concluded that the antidepressive efficacy of oral SAMe and 400 mg of intramuscular SAMe were comparable to that of 150 mg of oral imipramine. These data suggested that SAMe might be useful in clinical settings where it is crucial to ensure antidepressant activity without adverse effects.

In a meta-analysis, Mischoulon and Fava[100] reviewed the evidence of a small number of clinical trials evaluating SAMe doses versus placebo and standard antidepressants. This review focused on the relationship between dosage and the type and severity of depression. In addition, the analysis suggested that with SAMe, of the onset olfaction may occur a few days to 2 weeks sooner than with TCAs. After excluding studies with insufficient statistical power, poor design, lack of inclusion of a placebo, unclear clinical objective diagnostic criteria, the authors concluded that in 6 of at least 8 placebo-controlled studies with sample sizes ranging from 40 to 100, SAMe was superior to placebo and was equivalent to placebo in the other two studies. It was also found that in 6 out of the 8 comparison studies with TCAs, SAMe was equivalent in efficacy and more effective than was imipramine in the study by Pancheri et al.[103]

In the studies evaluated, SAMe was administered in doses ranging from ≥200 mg/day by parenteral route to ≥1600 mg/day by oral route. SAMe exerted a comparable antidepressant effect with that of TCAs, and was more effective than placebo.

SAMe is well-tolerated and relatively free of adverse effects. Possible side effects include mild insomnia, loss of appetite, constipation, nausea, dry mouth, sweating, dizziness, and nervousness. Recommended doses have ranged from 400 to 1600 mg/day, although some patients have used doses greater than 3000 mg/day to alleviate depression.[100] Overall, the data regarding SAMe's antidepressant effect would appear to warrant further research to assess the long-term benefits and adverse effects. It might also be beneficial to compare it with newer antidepressants. In that regard, NCCAM is currently sponsoring a clinical trial of the potential utility of SAMe in management of patients with MDD.

Ginkgo Biloba

Ginkgo biloba is a botanical agent that is purported to alleviate some of the symptoms of depression. It has been speculated that use of extracts of ginkgo biloba leaves (EGb 761) might be particularly effective in older individuals with mild depression resulting from cognitive decline or poor quality of sleep. In addition to increasing blood flow to the brain, animal studies have shown an increase in the number of serotonin receptor sites after supplementation with ginkgo. The latter effect, if validated in humans, could prove to be of special benefit in the elderly. In one controlled trial, ginkgo was shown to elicit improvement in resistant major depression when used as a complementary agent to conventional antidepressant activity.[105]

Lingjaerde et al. conducted a 2-year, placebo-controlled study to access whether winter depression can be prevented by ginkgo biloba. After meeting the criteria for major depression, patients were randomized to receive either oral Bio-Biloba, twice daily or placebo for 10 weeks, or until they developed symptoms of winter depression. No significant differences were observed in the development of winter depression symptoms between the two treatment groups.[106] This was the first controlled study on a possible effect of ginkgo extract in patients with SAD.

Use of ginkgo biloba has been associated with relatively few adverse effects, such as headache, nauseas, vomiting, and/or other gastrointestinal symptoms. Clearly, more research is required to evaluate the efficacy and safety of gingko biloba as a treatment for patients with MDD or SAD.

Tryptophan and 5-Hydroxytryptophan

5-Hydroxytrytophan or 5-HTP contributes to the physiologic processes of feeding, sleep, sexual behavior, mood, vigilance, and learning, all of which are modified to varying factors in human depression.[107] 5-HTP is considered a natural treatment, not only because of its presence in the body, but also because of its extraction from an African plant (*Griffonia simplicifolia*).[108] Typically, it is sold either as a crude extract of the plant or in pills with a content of 25, 50, or 100 mg.

A meta-analysis of the literature related to 5-HTP and tryptophan, two precursors to serotonin,[109] evaluating 180 studies between 1966 and 2000, concluded that most studies were not rigorous because they combined these amino acids with other supplements; were not randomized, blinded, or placebo-controlled; or included heterogeneous groups of patients with depression. Only one study of 5-HT[110] was considered to be rigorously controlled and satisfied inclusion criteria for analysis. In the latter study, patients were diagnosed with MDD by formal psychiatric evaluation, and 5-HT was found to be superior to placebo in relieving mood symptoms in depression based on changes in scores on standardized psychometric evaluations.

There may be safety issues related to the use of these compounds and their contaminants. L-Tryptophan may interact adversely with MAO inhibitors and with high doses of fluoxetine (50–100 mg/day).[111] Side effects include hypomania and delirium. The combination of lithium, phenelzine, and L-tryptophan has resulted in fatalities.[112] In contrast, 5-HTP appears to be much better tolerated and has been used successfully in combination with MAO inhibitors[113] and SSRIs.[114]

In 1990, more than 1500 patients with eosinophilia-myalgia syndrome and approximately 40 deaths were reported in this country among people ingesting tryptophan for various reasons, including sleep disorders and depressive symptoms.[115]

Based on these results further well-controlled clinical trials of 5-HTP in patients with clearly defined MDD appear warranted.

Kava Kava & Lavendula

To date anecdotal reports from a small number of European studies suggest that Kava Kava may reduce symptoms of anxiety, but be associated with an increased risk of serious hepatotoxicity. Thus, at the present time, further evaluation of the use of Kava Kava in treating patients with MDD does not appear warranted. Lavendula has been reported to be beneficial as a mood elevator both anecdotally in patients with depression[116] and in a small but well-conducted RCT. In the latter, addition of 60 drops/day of lavendula tincture to imipramine 100 mg/day over a 4-week period reportedly enhanced significantly the effect of imipramine based on HRSD scores. The latter findings require confirmation before consideration of instituting larger-scale studies of lavendula tincture as a possible adjunctive treatment to a standard antidepressants.

Dietary Supplements

OMEGA-3 FATTY ACIDS

Several epidemiologic studies have established a robust inverse correlation between intake of seafood and the prevalence of major psychiatric illnesses. In this context, in a survey of multiple countries, a nearly 60-fold cross-national difference in prevalence of major depression has been attributed in part to the strong negative correlation with the amounts of sea food consumed.[117] To date, however, there are no rigorously controlled clinical intervention trials[118] to support these important epidemiologic data. Given the encouraging preclinical and epidemiologic findings, and the generally nontoxic and nutritionally based nature of omega-3 fatty acid (OFA) treatment, more clinical research appears warranted to ascertain whether administration of OFAs will benefit patients with MDD.

DHEA

Studies in adults and adolescents with MDD have revealed a blunted dehydroepiandrosterone (DHEA) circadian variation, with low DHEA and high cortisol/DHEA ratio at 8:00 a.m. Anecdotal reports suggest that administration of DHEA can improve mood, energy, confidence, activity levels, and interest. Antidepressant effects and responses appear to be directly correlated with treatment-induced increases in plasma DHEA and DHEA-S levels.[119] Two small RCTs suggest that DHEA monotherapy in doses of 30–90 mg/day may help in significantly alleviating symptoms of major depression[120] and dysthymia[121] based on psychometric scores. One caveat in the study of MDD patients was that some patients were medication free, whereas others were taking stable doses of antidepressants. In all studies, DHEA was well tolerated by subjects and none dropped out because of side effects. Thus, it would appear that DHEA should be further evaluated as a possible adjunctive therapy in the management of patients with MDD and dysthymia.

Other Active Metabolites

Both phenylethylamine (PEA), an endogenous neuroamine, and inositol, an essential nutrient required for cellular growth and survival, have been studied in an open-label fashion in small groups of patients with major depression.[122,123] To date, however, there is insufficient evidence to warrant the use of either metabolite in patients with MDD.

Energy-Based Therapies

Transcranial Magnetic Stimulation

Transcranial magnetic stimulation delivers a magnetic pulse through a hand-held coil applied to the head and induces neuronal depolarization by creating an electrical current in desired regions of the cortex.[124] This safe and noninvasive technique has been widely explored in patients with depression: 15 placebo-controlled clinical studies in nearly 200 subjects with MDD based on DSM criteria or bipolar disorder in the depressed phase and two meta-analyses of TMS in depression have been conducted to date.[125,126] Changes in activity in brain regions remote from the site of stimulation have been shown from single sessions of TMS delivered to the left prefrontal cortex in depressed patients[127] and normal volunteers.[128] Variables influencing study results include: localization, frequency, and duration of repetitive TMS (rTMS) treatment, and the number of interventions per day. The majority of sham-controlled studies using rTMS have used high frequency left frontal cortex stimulation over 2 weeks, using Hamilton depression scores as a primary indicator of efficacy.

Studies using single-pulse TMS via a large coil placed on the vertex allowing stimulation of broad regions of the bilateral frontal and parietal cortices have also reported significant antidepressant effects in patients with MDD based on DSM criteria.[129] Single pulse TMS and 1 Hz stimulation carry a much better safety profile in terms of decreasing seizure threshold than does high frequency TMS.[130]

Attempts have been made to localize the optimal site of cortical stimulation to enhance recovery from depression.[131] Only the active stimulation of the left prefrontal cortex resulted in improvement of mood in "medically resistant" psychotic depressed patients after 1 week of daily treatments with a return to pretreatment state within 2 weeks in one study and after 2 weeks of stimulation at low frequency TMS in depressed patients in another study.[132] Other studies have shown mixed results. Loo et al.[133] failed to find a difference between 2 weeks of sham and active TMS at low frequency in 18 medication resistant depressed patients.

In a meta-analysis of 23 controlled studies, Burt et al. reported an average percent improvement with active TMS of 29% as compared with nearly 7% in sham-treated individuals.[126] However, few patients met standard criteria for clinical response or remission in any of these studies. The same meta-analysis failed to find a significant difference between effect sizes in low and high frequency studies. Some studies suggest an inverse relationship between frequency of stimulation and mood improvement, e.g., 1 Hz TMS as compared to 20 Hz,[134] or with 5 Hz compared to 20 Hz.[135]

In comparison, right prefrontal stimulation with rTMS at low frequency has been associated with significant improvement as compared to left prefrontal stimulation in treating mania in a small group of patients.[136]

Safety of TMS

Seizures are the most serious side effect associated with TMS. However, existing treatment guidelines can help in selecting parameter combinations that minimize this risk. Other less serious adverse effects include headache and neck pain.

Based on the aforementioned results, a larger-scale trial RCT of TMS use in patients with well-defined MDD appears warranted.

Acupuncture

Both acupuncture and electroacupuncture have been shown to accelerate the synthesis and release of serotonin and norepinephrine in the CNS of experimental animals.[137] In addition, insertion of needles in acupuncture points (or meridians) has been associated with increased endorphin levels which may also play a role in depressed individuals.[138] There are few studies assessing the effects of acupuncture in patients with MDD, and they suffer from inadequate grouping of patients with depressive symptomatology,[137] poor design,[139] and lack of significant differences between the sham acupuncture and true acupuncture arms.[140–142] Based on the studies reported to date, acupuncture and electroacupuncture cannot be recommended for the treatment of MDD at this time.

Reiki

Reiki is described as a biofield modality that "intends to affect energy fields that purportedly surround and interpenetrate the human body." These therapies, which include Reiki, Qigong, and TT, involve touch or placement of the hands in or through the biofields, the existence of which have not been conventionally scientifically proven. Reiki may reduce stress by relaxation and reequilibrating the autonomic nervous system. Some practitioners of Reiki believe that this may lead to improved immune system function and enhanced endorphin production.[143] Generally, recipients feel a sense of well-being, peace, relaxation, and pain relief.

Biofield therapies, such as Reiki, are generally experienced as noninvasive and low-risk despite the mechanism(s) of action currently being unknown. Health care providers are increasingly integrating Reiki into patient care. Numerous hospital-based programs routinely offer Reiki to patients, family members, and staff. Some of the medical settings include but are not limited to psychiatric settings, emergency rooms, hospice, rehabilitation centers, care for HIV/AIDS, hospice, and nursing homes.

Though Astin and colleagues[47] identified more than 100 clinical trials investigating distant healing involving Reiki, only 23 met the criteria for placebo-control, published in peer-reviewed journals, and were clinical rather than experimental. Though there were no studies specifically focusing on Reiki treatment and depression,[144] study of the effects of 30 min of Reiki on biologic markers related to the stress response, salivary IgA, cortisol, and blood pressure in 23 healthy subjects revealed biochemical changes in relaxation and immune responsivity, a drop in systolic blood pressure, and an increase in salivary IgA levels. There was a nonsignificant reduction in salivary cortisol. Further research is required to determine whether Reiki use exerts beneficial effects in patients with MDD.

Therapeutic Touch

Therapeutic touch is an "intentionally directed process of energy exchange during which the practitioner uses the hands as a focus to facilitate the healing process."[145] TT was developed in the 1970s by Dr. Dolores Krieger after nearly 10 years of research on healing, clinical practice, and teaching at New York University.[146] Though TT originated from the nursing profession, it is a modality that can be easily learned and practiced by health care providers from other disciplines. Healing touch (HT) is another biofield therapy that combines a group of noninvasive techniques including TT. Specific differences among the biofield therapies, particularly Reiki and TT, are usually described as pertaining to philosophy and training, rather than to outcome measurements. Practitioners can also describe personal qualitative experiential differences when providing these modalities.[147]

Multiple experiments with electrophotography have revealed differences in the emission of electromagnetic radiation from the hands of various individuals, biotherapists, as well as non-skilled controls.[148] Further multidisciplinary research utilizing physicists, biomechanical engineers, and biotherapists may provide some explanation for the mechanism of action evidenced in outcome measures of clinical practice.

More than 30 years of nursing research suggests clinical efficacy when TT is used to decrease anxiety and pain. However, many studies continue to be qualitative with limited sample size and no studies specifically address effects in patients with MDD. TT use with psychiatric patients has only recently been explored, possibly due to continued controversy regarding use of touch in psychiatric settings.[149]

The effects of TT on hormonal, neurotransmitter, mood, and anxiety indicators were investigated in 41 healthy female volunteers from 30 to 64 years of age. There was a significant reduction in mood disturbance across three sessions in patients using TT versus the control group. There were no significant effects on catecholamines or cortisol, whereas there was a reduction in nitric oxide in the third session, suggesting that results of TT could be cumulative. The latter study suggests changes in mood disturbance that warrant further investigation.

Manipulative and Body-Based Practices

Massage Therapy

The few reported controlled trials assessing the efficacy of massage therapy in depressed patients are small, poorly designed, and indicate a modest effect on anxiety, but not depression.[150,151] Therefore, at this time, therapeutic massage cannot be recommended as an effective adjunctive modality in the treatment of patients with major depression.

Whole Medical Systems

Although TCM, Ayurvedic Medicine, naturopathy, and other Whole Medical Systems have been widely used to manage symptoms and signs of depression, there is a paucity of scientific literature validating the utility of these multifaceted approaches for the treatment of patients with MDD. Thus, in the present chapter, focus has been placed upon discussing those components of these Systems, such as meditation, acupuncture, yoga, where systematic studies have been conducted. These medical systems are based on a qualitatively distinctive concept of biosystems such as the "Yin" and "Yang" in TCM. Many of the treatments proposed in these systems are based on the purported balancing of "body energies" and "detoxification."

Other Therapies

Light Therapy for Seasonal Affective Disorder

Seasonal affective disorder is a seasonal mood disorder, typified by the appearance of symptoms of depression in the autumn and winter, with spontaneous remission in the spring and summer. Mania can rarely occur as well, as can a summer form of SAD. Not surprisingly, most of the literature comes from Scandinavian countries such as Finland, where SAD is a significant public health problem, particularly in women.

Numerous articles have addressed the usefulness of light therapy in patients with SAD. The etiology of SAD was first believed to be due to abnormalities in the secretion or metabolism of melatonin; however, more recent research indicates that abnormal serotonin function may be a more important factor contributing to SAD.[152] The intensity of light originally recommended for usage in SAD was in the range of 2000–2500 lx for periods of about 2 hours a day, as this intensity was believed to be effective in suppressing nocturnal melatonin secretion.[153] However, a brighter light of 7,000–10,000 lx leads to more rapid symptom remission suggesting a dose-response relationship of phototherapy in patients with SAD. Several randomized trials and a meta-analysis of 39 well-conducted studies of phototherapy for SAD[154] conclude that different light intensities may be associated with different effects in reducing the typical symptoms of SAD, with stronger light being more effective in controlling the typical symptoms of a depression but not the atypical symptoms characterizing SAD.

Studies using light visor for SAD have shown no evidence that brighter visors (6000 lx) are more effective than dim visors (400 lx).[155] This suggests that light source from a light box, which is placed a distance from the subject may have a lesser likelihood of the photons hitting the retina whereas a dim light emitted from a light visor providing a dose as low as 60 lx may be sufficient to saturate the equilibrium of the unknown photochemical reaction underlying the antidepressant effect of light therapy.[154] Dim light from a visor may provide sufficient photons to be absorbed by the user's retina. The timing of phototherapy (early morning vs. midday) does not seem to significantly affect symptom responses in patients with SAD. Symptom remission usually starts within 4 days of using phototherapy, often with a complete resolution of vegetative symptoms after 1 week of light therapy. In one study, 67% of patients with mild depression exhibited remission after 1 week of treatment as compared with 40% of patients with severe depressive symptoms.[152] Symptoms can recur if light therapy is discontinued. Reported side effects are minor and include eyestrain and headache. One major problem with many clinical studies of phototherapy in patients with SAD relates to the difficulty in designing appropriate placebo controls.

Aerobic Exercise Training

Exercise is one of the best studied treatment modalities in patients with depression, with more than a thousand trials and several reviews.[156,157] Most studies indicate significant improvement in depressive scores regardless of the type of exercise program used.[158,159]

A meta-analysis of 80 well-conducted studies[160] suggests that exercise is associated with decreases in depression scores of more than 50%, versus a much lesser response in patients in the no exercise groups. In one recent study,[161] the effectiveness of a 16-week aerobic exercise program was compared with standard medication in older patients with MDD. One hundred and fifty-six men and women aging from 50 to 77 years with MDD diagnosed by DSM-IV criteria were randomly assigned to an aerobic exercise program, a conventional antidepressant medication, or a combination of exercise and antidepressant medication. All three treatments resulted in significant declines in the mean HAM-D and BDI scores. Patients with moderate and severe depression (based on BDI and HAM-D scores) who were randomly assigned to the antidepressant medication alone subgroup, exhibited a more significant decline in depressive symptoms when compared with those assigned to the other two subgroups. The subgroup of mildly depressed patients, assigned to exercise plus antidepressant medication exhibited better scores and a better response than the patients assigned to other two subgroups. Based on these reviews and meta-analysis, exercise appears to be an effective adjunctive treatment in patients with mild MDD.

Future Research and Considerations

Despite numerous advances in the understanding of the pathophysiology of MDD and other mood disorders, and the introduction of new antidepressants with improved efficacy and safety profiles, as many as 30–40% of patients with MDD are either refractory to treatment with antidepressants or cannot tolerate them. Not surprisingly, many patients utilize one or more CAM modalities to treat their depression and other mood disorders, despite the dearth of scientific evidence to support the efficacy and/or safety of many of these treatments. Most depressed patients do not discuss their CAM use with their health care providers, and there is a need for improved patient communication and education regarding this topic. Clearly, there is a compelling rationale to devise novel, rigorous, contemporary paradigms to systematically identify and evaluate the most promising CAM modalities for the treatment of various populations of depressed patients. Nonetheless, in view of the high morbidity and mortality associated with MDD, CAM treatments, even when proved effective and safe, are most likely to be useful when used in patients with MDD of minor to moderate severity, or as adjunctive treatments to allopathic interventions in patients with more serious disease. Whether CAM modalities will exert therapeutic benefit(s) in patients with minor depressive disease, chronic dysthymia, and other mood disorders, remains to be clarified.

REFERENCES

1. Eisenberg DM, Kessler RC, Foster C, Norlock et al. Unconventional medicine in the United States. Prevalence, costs, and patterns of use. *N Engl J Med* 1993;328(4):246–252.

2. Astin JA. Why patients use alternative medicine: Results of a national study. *JAMA* 1998;279(19):1548–1553.

3. Druss BG, Rohrbaugh R, Kosten T, et al. Use of alternative medicine in major depression. *Psychiatr Serv* 1998;49(11):1397.

4. Emmanuel NP, Cosby C, Crowford M, et al. *Prevalence of Herbal Products Use by Subjects Evaluated for Pharmacological Clinical Trials.* Boca Raton, FL: 38th Annual Meeting of the New Clinical Drug Evaluation Unit Program, 1998.

5. Kessler RC, Soukup J, Davis RB, et al. The use of complementary and alternative therapies to treat anxiety and depression in the United States. *Am J Psychiatry* 2001;158(2):289–294.

6. Unutzer J, Klap R, Sturm R, et al. Mental disorders and the use of alternative medicine: Results from a national survey. *Am J Psychiatry* 2000; 157(11):1851–1857.

7. Simon GE, Cherkin DC, Sherman KJ, Eisenberg et al. Mental health visits to complementary and alternative medicine providers. *Gen Hosp Psychiatry* 2004;26(3):171–177.

8. Barnes PM, Powell-Griner E, McFann K, et al. Complementary and alternative medicine use among adults: United States, 2002. *Adv Data* 2004(343):1–19.

9. Kirmayer LJ. Cultural variations in the clinical presentation of depression and anxiety: Implications for diagnosis and treatment. *J Clin Psychiatry* 2001;62(Suppl 13):22–28; discussion 29–30.

10. Simon GE VM, Piccinelli M, et al. An international study of the relation between somatic symptoms and depressiion. *N Engl J Med* 1999; 341:1329–1336.

11. Staff J. *JAMWA* and *Latina* Magazine Collaborate in Complementary and Alternative Medicine Survey. *JAMWA* 2000;55(2):104–105.

12. Cushman LF WC, Factor-Litvak P, Kronenberg F. Use of complementary and alternative medicine among African-American and Hispanic women in New York City: A pilot study. *J Am Womens Assoc* 1999;54(4):193–195.

13. Trotter R. Curanderismo. A picture of Mexican-American folk healing. *J Altern Complement Med* 2001;7(2):129–131.

14. Mackenzie ER, Taylor L, Bloom BS, et al. Ethnic minority use of complementary and alternative medicine (CAM): A national probability survey of CAM utilizers. *Altern Ther Health Med* 2003;9(4):50–56.

15. Nelson PB. Ethnic differences in intrinsic/extrinsic religious orientation and depression in the elderly. *Arch Psychiatr Nurs* 1989;3(4):199–204.

16. Parks F. The role of African American folk beliefs in the modern therapeutic process. *Clin Psychol Sci Pract* 2003;10(4):456–467.

17. Pang KY. Symptoms of depression in elderly Korean immigrants: Narration and the healing process. *Cult Med Psychiatry* 1998;22(1):93–122.

18. Obeyesekere G. Depression, Buddhism, and the Work of Culture in Sri Lanka. In: Kleinman AaG B (ed.), *Culture and Depression: Studies in the Anthropology and Cross-Cultural Psychiatry of*

Affect and Disorder. Berkeley, CA: University of California Press, 1985, pp. 134–152.

19. Gray NN. American Indian and Alaska native substance abuse: Co-morbidity and cultural issues. *Am Indian Alsk Native Ment Health Res* 2001;10(2):67–84.

20. Kim CaK. Navajo use of native healers. *Arch Intern Med* 1998:2245–2249.

21. Garroutte E, Goldberg J, Beals J, et al. Spirituality and attempted suicide among American Indians. *Soc Sci Med* 2003;56:1571–1579.

22. Walsh BT, Seidman SN, Sysko R, et al. Placebo response in studies of major depression: Variable, substantial, and growing. *JAMA* 2002; 287(14):1840–1847.

23. Miller FG, Emanuel EJ, Rosenstein DL, et al. Ethical issues concerning research in complementary and alternative medicine. *JAMA* 2004; 291(5): 599–604.

24. Guess H, Kleinman A, Kusek JW, et al. The science of the placebo; Toward an interdisciplinary research agenda *Br Med J* 2002.

25. Dennehy EB, Gonzalez R, Suppes T. Self-reported participation in nonpharmacologic treatments for bipolar disorder. *J Clin Psychiatry* 2004;65(2):278.

26. Scarna A, Gijsman HJ, McTavish SF, et al. Effects of a branched-chain amino acid drink in mania. *Br J Psychiatry* 2003;182:210–213.

27. Kabat-Zinn J. An outpatient program in behavioral medicine for chronic pain patients based on the practice of mindfulness meditation: Theoretical considerations and preliminary results. *Gen Hosp Psychiatry* 1982;4(1):33–47.

28. Goleman D. *The Varieties of Meditative Experience*. New York: Dutton, 1977.

29. Kutz I, Borysenko JZ, Benson H. Meditation and psychotherapy: A rationale for the integration of dynamic psychotherapy, the relaxation response, and mindfulness meditation. *Am J Psychiatry* 1985;142(1):1–8.

30. Sloman R. Relaxation and imagery for anxiety and depression control in community patients with advanced cancer. *Cancer Nurs* 2002;25(6): 432–435.

31. Benson H, Beary JF, Carol MP. The relaxation response. *Psychiatry* 1974;37(37).

32. Caudill M, Schnable R, Zuttermeister P, et al. Decreased clinic use by chronic pain patients: Response to behavioral medicine intervention. *Clin J Pain* 1991;7:305–310.

33. Benson H, Frankel FH, Apfel R, et al. Treatment of anxiety: A comparison of the usefulness of self-hypnosis and a meditational relaxation technique. *Psychother Psychosom* 1978;30:229–242.

34. Broota A aDR. Efficacy of two relaxation techniques in depression. *J Pers Clin Stud* 1990;6: 83–90.

35. Murphy GE, Carney RM, Knesevich MA, et al. Cognitive behaviour therapy, relaxation training, and tricyclic antidepressant medication in the treatment of depression. *Psychol Rep* 1995;77:403–420.

36. Bowers WA. Treatment of depressed in-patients. Cognitive therapy plus medication, relaxation plus medication, and medication alone. *Br J Psychiatry* 1990;156:73–78.

37. Janakiramaiah N, Gangadhar BN, Naga Venkatesha Murthy PJ, et al. Antidepressant efficacy of Sudarshan Kriya Yoga (SKY) in melancholia: A randomized comparison with electroconvulsive therapy (ECT) and imipramine. *J Affect Disord* 2000;57(1–3):255–259.

38. Wood K. The promise of aromatherapy. *Provider* 2003;29(3):47–48.

39. Jones JE, Kassity N. Varieties of alternative medicine experience: Complementary care in the neonatal intensive care unit. *Clin Obstet Gynecol* 2001;44(4):750–768.

40. Ernst ER, Stevinson J, Complementary therapies for depression: An overview. *Arch Gen Psychiatry* 1998;55:1026–1032.

41. Alexander B. *The Place of Complementary Therapies in Mental Health: A User's Experiences and Views*. Nottingham, England: Nottingham Patients' Council Support Group, 1993.

42. Zand J. The natural pharmacy: Herbal medicine for depression. In: Strohecker J, Strohecker SN (ed.), *Natural Healing for Depression*. New York: Perigee, 1999.

43. Astin J. Why patients use alternative medicine: Results of a national study. *JAMA* 1998;279: 1548–1553.

44. Eisenberg DM, Ettner RB, Appel SL, et al. Trends in alternative medicine use in the United States, 1990-1997: Results of a follow-up national survey. *JAMA* 1998;280:1569–1575.

45. Wallis C. Faith and healing: Can prayer, faith and spirituality really improve your physical health? A growing and surprising body of scientific evidence say that they can. *Time* 1996;147.

46. Benor D. Survey of spiritual healing research. *Complement Med Res* 1990;4:9–33.

47. Astin J, Harkness E, Ernst E. The efficacy of "distant healing": A systematic review of randomized trials. *Ann Intern Med* 2000;132:903–910.

48. Gibson R. The creative arts therapies. *Curr Psychiatr Therap* 1982:185–188.

49. Schubert D. Creativity and the ability to cope. *Creat Psychiatry* 1975;5.

50. Zwerling I. The creative arts therapies as "real therapies." *Hosp Commun Psychiatry* 1979;30(12).

51. Clair A. *Therapeutic uses of Music with Older Adults*. London: Health Professions Press, 1996.

52. Lane D. Music therpay: An effective instrument in palliative care. *Palliat Matters* 1997;8:2–3.

53. Field T, Martinez A, Nawrocki T. Music shifts frontal EEG in depressed adolescents. *Adolescence*. 1998;33:109–116.

54. Zerhusen J, Boyle K, Wilson W. Out of the darkness: Group congnitive therapy for depressed elderly. *J Psychosoc Nurs Ment Health Serv*. 1991;29:16–21.

55. Hanser SB, Thompson LW. Effects of a music therapy strategy on depressed older adults. *J Gerontol*. 1994;49(6):P265–P269.

56. Cotter A. Western movement therapies. *Phys Med Rehabil Clin Northern Am*. 1999;10(3):603–616.

57. Chodorow J. *Dance Therapy and Depth Psychology*. New York: Routledge & Kegan Paul, 1991.

58. Pert C. *Molecules of Emotion*. New York: Scribner, 1997.

59. Stewart N, Mc Mullin LM, Rubin LD. Movement therpay with depressed inpatients: A randomized multiple single case design. *Arch Psychiatr Nurs* 1994;8:22–29.

60. Ullrich PM, Lutgendorf SK. Journaling about stressful events: Effects of cognitive processing and emotional expression. *Ann Behav Med* 2002; 24(3):244–250.

61. McGihon N. Writing as a therapeutic modality. *J Psychosoc Nurs Mental Health Serv* 1996;34(6): 31–35.

62. Day A. The journal as a guide for the healing journey. *Nurs Clin North Am* 2001;36:131–142.

63. Petrie K, Booth RJ, Pennebkaer JW, et al. Disclosure of trauma and immune response to a hepatitis B vaccination program. *J Consult Clin Psychol* 1995;63:787–792.

64. Lepore S. Expressive writing moderates the relation between intrusive thoughts and depressive symptoms. *J Pers Soc Psychol* 1997;73:1030–1037.

65. Demarco A, Clarke N. An interview with Alison Demarco and Nichol Clarke: Light and colour therapy explained. *Complement Ther Nurs Midwifery* 2001;7:95–103.

66. Barber C. The use of music and colour theory as a behaviour modifier. *Br J Nurs* 1999;8(7): 443–448.

67. Breiling B (ed.), *Light Years Ahead: The Illustrated Guide to Full Spectrum and Colored Light in Mindbody Healing*. Berkeley, CA: Celestial Arts, 1996.

68. Pankratov S. Meridians conduct light. *Raum und Zeit (in German)* 1991;35(88):16–18.

69. Jorm AF, Korten AE, Jacomb PA, et al. Mental health literacy: A survey of the public's ability to recognise mental disorders and their beliefs about the effectiveness of treatment. *Med J Aust* 1997;166(4):182–186.

70. Godfrey PS, Toone BK, Carney MW, et al. Enhancement of recovery from psychiatric illness by methylfolate. *Lancet* 1990;336(8712): 392–395.

71. Abalan F, Subra G, Picard M, et al. Incidence of vitamin B 12 and folic acid deficiencies on old aged psychiatric patients. *Encephale* 1984;10(1):9–12.

72. Morris MS, Fava M, Jacques PF, et al. Depression and folate status in the US Population. *Psychother Psychosom* 2003;72(2):80–87.

73. Fava M, Borus JS, Alpert JE, et al. Folate, vitamin B12, and homocysteine in major depressive disorder. *Am J Psychiatry* 1997;154(3): 426–428.

74. Alpert JE, Mischoulon D, Rubenstein GE, et al. Folinic acid (Leucovorin) as an adjunctive treatment for SSRI-refractory depression. *Ann Clin Psychiatry* 2002;14(1):33–38.

75. Christensen L, Burrows R. Dietary treatment of depression. *Behav Ther* 1990;21:183–193.

76. Benton D, Donohoe RT. The effects of nutrients on mood. *Public Health Nutr* 1999;2(3A):403–409.

77. Brown SA, Schuckit MA. Changes in depression among abstinent alcoholics. *J Stud Alcohol* 1988; 49(5):412–417.

78. Brown SA, Inaba RK, Gillin JC, et al. Alcoholism and affective disorder: Clinical course of depressive symptoms. *Am J Psychiatry* 1995;152(1): 45–52.

79. Power C, Rodgers B, Hope S. U-shaped relation for alcohol consumption and health in early adulthood and implications for mortality. *Lancet* 1998;352(9131):877.

80. Cott JM. In vitro receptor binding and enzyme inhibition by Hypericum perforatum extract. *Pharmacopsychiatry* 1997;30(Suppl 2): 108–112.

81. Neary JT, Bu Y. Hypericum LI 160 inhibits uptake of serotonin and norepinephrine in astrocytes. *Brain Res* 1999;816(2):358–363.

82. Teufel-Mayer R, Gleitz J. Effects of long-term administration of hypericum extracts on the affinity and density of the central serotonergic 5-HT1 A and 5-HT2 A receptors. *Pharmacopsychiatry* 1997;30(Suppl 2):113–116.

83. Franklin M, Chi J, McGavin C, et al. Neuroendocrine evidence for dopaminergic actions of hypericum extract (LI 160) in healthy volunteers. *Biol Psychiatry* 1999;46(4):581–584.

84. Schellenberg R, Sauer S, Dimpfel W. Pharmacodynamic effects of two different hypericum extracts in healthy volunteers measured by quantitative EEG. *Pharmacopsychiatry* 1998;31(Suppl 1):44–53.

85. Schule C, Baghai T, Sauer N, et al. Endocrinological effects of high-dose Hyperricum perforatum extract WS 5570 in healthy subjects. *Neuropsychobiology* 2004;49(2):58–63.

86. Siepmann M, Krause S, Joraschky P, et al. The effects of St John's wort extract on heart rate variability, cognitive function and quantitative EEG: A comparison with amitriptyline and placebo in healthy men. *Br J Clin Pharmacol* 2002;54(3):277–282.

87. Whiskey E, Werneke U, Taylor D. A systematic review and meta-analysis of Hypericum perforatum in depression: A comprehensive clinical review. *Int Clin Psychopharmacol* 2001;16(5):239–252.

88. Philipp M, Kohnen R, Hiller KO. Hypericum extract versus imipramine or placebo in patients with moderate depression: Randomised multicentre study of treatment for eight weeks. *Br Med J* 1999;319(7224):1534–1538.

89. Shelton RC, Keller MB, Gelenberg A, et al. Effectiveness of St John's wort in major depression: A randomized controlled trial. *JAMA* 2001;285(15):1978–1986.

90. Effect of Hypericum perforatum (St John's wort) in major depressive disorder: A randomized controlled trial. *JAMA* 2002;287(14):1807–1814.

91. Akhondzadeh S, Kashani L, Fotouhi A, et al. Comparison of Lavandula angustifolia Mill. tincture and imipramine in the treatment of mild to moderate depression: A double-blind, randomized trial. *Prog Neuropsychopharmacol Biol Psychiatry* 2003;27(1):123–127.

92. Woelk H. Comparison of St John's wort and imipramine for treating depression: Randomised controlled trial. *Br Med J* 2000;321(7260):536–539.

93. Bergmann RL, Forster J, Schulz J, et al. Atopic family history. Validation of instruments in a multicenter cohort study. *Pediatr Allergy Immunol* 1993;4(3):130–135.

94. Harrer G, Hubner WD, Podzuweit H. Effectiveness and tolerance of the hypericum extract LI 160 compared to maprotiline: A multicenter double-blind study. *J Geriatr Psychiatry Neurol* 1994;7(Suppl 1):S24–S28.

95. Brenner R, Azbel V, Madhusoodanan S, et al. Comparison of an extract of hypericum (LI 160) and sertraline in the treatment of depression: A double-blind, randomized pilot study. *Clin Ther* 2000;22(4):411–419.

96. Rodriguez-Landa JF, Contreras CM. A review of clinical and experimental observations about antidepressant actions and side effects produced by Hypericum perforatum extracts. *Phytomedicine* 2003;10(8):688–699.

97. Ruschitzka F, Meier PJ, Turina M, et al. Acute heart transplant rejection due to Saint John's wort. *Lancet* 2000;355(9203):548–549.

98. Henney JE. From the Food and Drug Administration. *JAMA* 2000;283(13):1679.

99. Saletu B, Anderer P, Linzmayer L, et al. Pharmacodynamic studies on the central mode of action of S-adenosyl-L-methionine (SAMe) infusions in elderly subjects, utilizing EEG mapping and psychometry. *J Neural Transm* 2002;109(12):1505–1526.

100. Mischoulon D, Fava M. Role of S-adenosyl-L-methionine in the treatment of depression: A review of the evidence. *Am J Clin Nutr* 2002;76(5):1158S–1161S.

101. Morelli V, Zoorob RJ. Alternative therapies: Part I. Depression, diabetes, obesity. *Am Fam Physician* 2000;62(5):1051–1060.

102. Zanotti S, Mori S, Radaelli R, et al. Modifications in brain cAMP- and calcium/calmodulin-dependent protein kinases induced by treatment with S-adenosylmethionine. *Neuropharmacology* 1998;37(8):1081–1089.

103. Pancheri P, Scapicchio P, Chiaie RD. A double-blind, randomized parallel-group, efficacy and safety study of intramuscular S-adenosyl-L-methionine 1,4-butanedisulphonate (SAMe)

versus imipramine in patients with major depressive disorder. *Int J Neuropsychopharmacol* 2002; 5(4):287–294.

104. Delle Chiaie R, Pancheri P, Scapicchio P. Efficacy and tolerability of oral and intramuscular S-adenosyl-L-methionine 1,4-butanedisulfonate (SAMe) in the treatment of major depression: Comparison with imipramine in 2 multicenter studies. *Am J Clin Nutr* 2002;76(5):1172S–1176S.

105. Wong AH, Smith M, Boon HS. Herbal remedies in psychiatric practice. *Arch Gen Psychiatry* 1998;55(11):1033–1044.

106. Lingjaerde O FA, Magnusson A. Can winter depression be prevented by ginkgo biloba extract? A placebo-controlled trial. *Acta Psychiatr Scand* 1999;100:62–66.

107. Moret C, Briley M. The possible role of 5-HT(1B/D) receptors in psychiatric disorders and their potential as a target for therapy. *Eur J Pharmacol* 2000;404(1–2):1–12.

108. Young SN. Are SAMe and 5-HTP safe and effective treatments for depression? *J Psychiatry Neurosci* 2003;28(6):471.

109. Shaw K, Turner J, Del Mar C. Tryptophan and 5-hydroxytryptophan for depression. *Cochr Database Syst Rev* 2002(1):CD003198.

110. Van Praag J, Korf J, Dols L, et al. A pilot study of the predictive value of the probenicid test in applicaton of 5-hydroxytryptophan as antidepressant. *Psychopharmacology* 1972;25: 14–21.

111. Steiner W, Fontaine R. Toxic reaction following the combined administration of fluoxetine and L-tryptophan: Five case reports. *Biol Psychiatry* 1986;21(11):1067–1071.

112. Staufenberg EF, Tantam D. Malignant hyperpyrexia syndrome in combined treatment. *Br J Psychiatry* 1989;154:577–578.

113. Alino JJ, Gutierrez JL, Iglesias ML. 5-Hydroxytryptophan (5-HTP) and a MAOI (nialamide) in the treatment of depressions. A double-blind controlled study. *Int Pharmacopsychiatry* 1976; 11(1):8–15.

114. Nardini M, De Stefano R, Iannuccelli M, et al. Treatment of depression with L-5-hydroxytryptophan combined with chlorimipramine, a double-blind study. *Int J Clin Pharmacol Res* 1983;3(4):239–250.

115. Hertzman PA, Blevins WL, Mayer J, et al. Association of the eosinophilia-myalgia syndrome with the ingestion of tryptophan. *N Engl J Med* 1990;322(13):869–873.

116. Buchbauer G, Sunara A, Weiss-Greiler P, et al. Synthesis and olfactoric activity of side-chain modified beta-santalol analogues. *Eur J Med Chem* 2001;36(7–8):673–683.

117. Hibbeln JR. Fish consumption and major depression. *Lancet* 1998;351(9110):1213.

118. Stoll AL, Severus WE, Freeman MP, et al. Omega 3 fatty acids in bipolar disorder: A preliminary double-blind, placebo-controlled trial. *Arch Gen Psychiatry* 1999;56(5):407–412.

119. Fabian TJ, Dew MA, Pollock BG, et al. Endogenous concentrations of DHEA and DHEA-S decrease with remission of depression in older adults. *Biol Psychiatry* 2001;50(10):767–774.

120. Wolkowitz OM, Reus VI, Keebler A, et al. Double-blind treatment of major depression with dehydroepiandrosterone. *Am J Psychiatry* 1999; 156(4):646–649.

121. Bloch M, Schmidt PJ, Danaceau MA, et al. Dehydroepiandrosterone treatment of midlife dysthymia. *Biol Psychiatry* 1999;45(12):1533–1541.

122. Sabelli H, Fink P, Fawcett J, et al. Sustained antidepressant effect of PEA replacement. *J Neuropsychiatry Clin Neurosci* 1996;8(2):168–171.

123. Levine J, Barak Y, Gonzalves M, et al. Double-blind, controlled trial of inositol treatment of depression. *Am J Psychiatry* 1995;152(5):792–794.

124. Hallett M, Epstein CM, Berardelli A, et al. Topics in transcranial magnetic stimulation. *Suppl Clin Neurophysiol* 2000;53:301–311.

125. Martin JL, Barbanoj MJ, Schlaepfer TE, et al. Repetitive transcranial magnetic stimulation for the treatment of depression. Systematic review and meta-analysis. *Br J Psychiatry* 2003;182: 480–491.

126. Burt T, Lisanby SH, Sackeim HA. Neuropsychiatric applications of transcranial magnetic stimulation: A meta analysis. *Int J Neuropsychopharmacol* 2002;5(1):73–103.

127. Szuba MP, O'Reardon JP, Rai AS, et al. Acute mood and thyroid stimulating hormone effects of transcranial magnetic stimulation in major depression. *Biol Psychiatry* 2001;50(1):22–27.

128. George MS, Wassermann EM, Williams WA, et al. Changes in mood and hormone levels after rapid-rate transcranial magnetic stimulation (rTMS) of the prefrontal cortex. *J Neuropsychiatry Clin Neurosci* 1996;8(2):172–180.

129. Kolbinger HH G, Hufnagel A, Moller H-J, et al. Transcranial magnetic stimulation (TMS) in the treatment of major depression: A pilot study. *Hum Psychopharmacol* 1995;10:305–310.

130. Wassermann EM, Grafman J, Berry C, et al. Use and safety of a new repetitive transcranial magnetic stimulator. *Electroencephalogr Clin Neurophysiol* 1996;101(5):412–417.

131. O'Connor M, Brenninkmeyer C, Morgan A, et al. Relative effects of repetitive transcranial magnetic stimulation and electroconvulsive therapy on mood and memory: A neurocognitive risk-benefit analysis. *Cogn Behav Neurol* 2003;16(2):118–127.

132. George MS, Wassermann EM, Kimbrell TA, et al. Mood improvement following daily left prefrontal repetitive transcranial magnetic stimulation in patients with depression: A placebo-controlled crossover trial. *Am J Psychiatry* 1997;154(12): 1752–1756.

133. Loo CK, Mitchell PB, Croker VM, et al. Double-blind controlled investigation of bilateral prefrontal transcranial magnetic stimulation for the treatment of resistant major depression. *Psychol Med* 2003;33(1):33–40.

134. Kimbrell TA, Little JT, Dunn RT, et al. Frequency dependence of antidepressant response to left prefrontal repetitive transcranial magnetic stimulation (rTMS) as a function of baseline cerebral glucose metabolism. *Biol Psychiatry* 1999; 46(12):1603–1613.

135. George MS, Nahas Z, Molloy M, et al. A controlled trial of daily left prefrontal cortex TMS for treating depression. *Biol Psychiatry* 2000;48(10):962–970.

136. Grisaru N, Chudakov B, Yaroslavsky Y, et al. Transcranial magnetic stimulation in mania: A controlled study. *Am J Psychiatry* 1998;155(11): 1608–1610.

137. Hans J. Electroacupuncture: An alternative to antidepressants for treating affective diseases? *Int J Neurosci* 1986;29(1–2):79–92.

138. Han JS, Terenius L. Neurochemical basis of acupuncture analgesia. *Annu Rev Pharmacol Toxicol* 1982;22:193–220.

139. Luo H. Progress in the treatment of depression with new electroacupuncture. *Zhongguo Zhong Xi Yi Jie He Za Zhi* 2000;20(11):806–807.

140. Roschke J, Wolf C, Muller MJ, et al. The benefit from whole body acupuncture in major depression. *J Affect Disord* 2000;57(1–3):73–81.

141. Yang X, Liu X, Luo H, et al. Clinical observation on needling extrachannel points in treating mental depression. *J Tradit Chin Med* 1994; 14(1):14–18.

142. Luo H, Meng F, Jia Y, et al. Clinical research on the therapeutic effect of the electroacupuncture treatment in patients with depression. *Psychiatry Clin Neurosci* 1998;52(Suppl): S338–S340.

143. Miles PaT, G. REIKI-review of a biofield therapy history, theory, practice and research. *Altern Ther* 2003;9(2):62–72.

144. Wardell DaE, J. Biological correlates of Reiki touch healing. *J Adv Nurs* 2001;33(4):439–445.

145. NH-PA. Theraputic touch. Accessed at: www. therapeutic-touch.org.

146. Krieger D. *The Therapeutic Touch: How to Use Your Hands to Help or to Heal.* New York: Prentice-Hall, 1986.

147. Potter P. What are the distinctions between reiki and therapeutic touch? *Clin J Oncol Nurs* 2003; 7(1):89–91.

148. Berden M, Jerman I, Skarja M. A possible physical basis for the healing touch (biotherapy) evaluated by high voltage electrophotography. *Acupunct Electrother Res.* 1997;22:127– 146.

149. Hughes P, Grochowski RM, Harris CND. Therapeutic touch with adolescent psychiatric patients. *J Holistic Nurs* 1996;14(1):6–23.

150. Platania-Solazzo A, Field TM, Blank J, et al. Relaxation therapy reduces anxiety in child and adolescent psychiatric patients. *Acta Paedopsychiatr* 1992;55(2):115–120.

151. Field T, Grizzle N, Scafidi F, et al. Massage and relaxation therapies' effects on depressed adolescent mothers. *Adolescence* 1996;31(124): 903–911.

152. Partonen T, Lonnqvist J. Seasonal affective disorder. *Lancet* 1998;352(9137):1369–1374.

153. Eastman CI, Lahmeyer HW, Watell LG, et al. A placebo-controlled trial of light treatment for winter depression. *J Affect Disord* 1992;26(4): 211–221.

154. Lee TM, Chan CC. Dose-response relationship of phototherapy for seasonal affective disorder: A meta-analysis. *Acta Psychiatr Scand* 1999;99(5): 315–323.

155. Rosenthal NE. *Winter Blues: Seasonal Affective Disorder. What it is and how to Overcome it.* New York: Guilford Press, 1993.

156. Glenister D. Exercise and mental health: A review. *J R Soc Health* 1996;116(1):7–13.

157. Byrne A, Byrne DG. The effect of exercise on depression, anxiety and other mood states: A review. *J Psychosom Res* 1993;37(6):565–574.

158. Martinsen EW. Benefits of exercise for the treatment of depression. *Sports Med* 1990;9(6):380–389.

159. Martinsen EW. Physical fitness, anxiety and depression. *Br J Hosp Med* 1990;43(3):194, 196, 199.

160. North TC, McCullagh P, Tran ZV. Effect of exercise on depression. *Exerc Sport Sci Rev* 1990;18:379–415.

161. Blumenthal JA, Babyak MA, Moore KA, et al. Effects of exercise training on older patients with major depression. *Arch Intern Med* 1999;159(19):2349–2356.

CHAPTER 19

Comorbidity of Mood Disorders and Substance Abuse

CHARLES P. O'BRIEN

▶ INTRODUCTION: DEFINING COMORBIDITY

Dual diagnosis is a term usually defined as the combination of a mental disorder with substance abuse. Because substance abuse and addiction are also mental disorders, it is preferable to speak of "substance abuse in combination with other mental disorders." It should also be noted that other medical illnesses cooccur with mental illness and this can be thought of as another form of comorbidity. The most efficient way of managing a health care system often involves having common mental illnesses such as depression and anxiety disorders treated in general medical clinics along with diabetes, hypertension, and asthma. Psychiatric consultation can be obtained when necessary. Another approach when the psychiatric disorder is severe consists of allowing psychiatric physicians to manage coexisting uncomplicated medical problems in their patients. Patients often suffer from multiple chronic diseases and in some settings such as the VA health-care system, a "one stop shopping" approach is ideal. Long-term medical care for patients dually diagnosed with common medical, psychiatric, and substance use disorders should be treated in the most efficient way possible and with the least inconvenience to the patient.

The remainder of this chapter will be focused on the management of mood disorders complicated by substance abuse. There are etiologic factors to consider. Some cases of substance abuse or addiction begin with an attempt to self-medicate the symptoms of anxiety or depression. The patient takes whatever drug happens to be available whether it is marijuana, stimulants, alcohol, opiates, or nicotine. This self-medication with nonprescribed drugs may produce some alleviation of symptoms at first. Subsequently, however, the drug use may become out of control and the patient then has a new problem in addition to the original psychiatric disorder. In this sequence, the psychiatric problem occurs first and it is subsequently complicated by self-medication leading to substance abuse or addiction. In other cases, the substance abuse occurs first and the psychiatric disorder is a complication of the social stress caused by the drug use and/or the biologic effects of chronic drug use on the brain.

▶ EPIDEMIOLOGY

The prevalence of cooccurring substance use disorders and other mental disorders for the United States has been derived from two surveys over the past two decades, the epidemiologic catchment area (ECA) survey administered during 1980 through 1984[1] and the National Comorbidity Survey (NCS) administered between 1990 and 1992.[2] In the ECA Survey 47% of individuals with schizophrenia also had a substance use disorder and 61% of individuals with bipolar disorder also had a substance use disorder. Of those with antisocial personality disorder, 84% had a coexisting substance use disorder. Viewed from the other direction, surveys within substance abuse clinics show even higher prevalence of serious mental illness (SMI) in patients being treated for substance use disorders. The 2001 National Household Survey on Drug Abuse (NHSDA) found a strong relationship between substance use disorders and other types of mental illness.[3]

Based on a variety of epidemiologic studies it would appear that between 7 and 10 million persons have cooccurring substance use and other mental disorders and up to 66% of drug addicts have one or more psychiatric diagnoses during their lifetimes.[4] One out of four persons with major depression is a substance abuser.[5] Persons with mood disorders are up to eight times more likely to have a substance abuse problem and when compared to the general population, women with bipolar disorder are seven times more likely to be alcoholics.[6] The relationship between depression and nicotine use is complex and not fully understood.[7, 8] Smokers with a history of depression experienced more withdrawal symptoms[9] and have lower rates of smoking cessation.[10] DSM-III-R-defined nicotine dependence signaled a threefold increased risk for major depression.[11]

► COMMON DIAGNOSTIC COMBINATIONS

Depression and Nicotine Dependence

Symptoms of depression and anxiety are associated with nicotine dependence. Available data suggest that tobacco use and nicotine dependence are more common among adolescents who experience depression symptoms[12] particularly those with more serious psychiatric conditions.[13] Adolescents with attention-deficit hyperactivity disorder are at greater risk for tobacco use.[14] And weight concerns appear to promote smoking initiation and current smoking in female adolescents.[15]

Nicotine has some useful properties in that it produces a sense of calming with increased alertness and muscle relaxation. In dependent smokers, one of the motivational forces driving smoking is the suppression of nicotine withdrawal symptoms (Table 19-1). This suppression of withdrawal effect is especially noticeable with the first cigarette in the morning. The average one pack per day smoker takes 10 puffs per cigarette or 200 puffs per pack. Each puff amounts to a discrete reinforcement by a small dose of nicotine. Nicotine absorbed rapidly via the lungs reaches the left side of the heart through the pulmonary circulation and then is ejected through the aortic arch through the carotids into the brain very rapidly. The pulmonary route is the most efficient pathway to the brain, even more rapid than intravenous injection. Thus, a typical smoker has had millions of reinforcements by the time they attempt quitting. This produces an intense learning paradigm with nicotine craving associated with people, places, and situations in which the smoker has activated the brain by nicotine many times over the years. Quitting produces nicotine withdrawal symptoms and the learned cues provoke conditioned cigarette craving even years after the last dose of

► **TABLE 19-1** NICOTINE WITHDRAWAL SYNDROME

Irritability, impatience, hostility
Anxiety
Dysphoric or depressed mood
Difficulty concentrating
Restlessness
Decreased heart rate
Increased appetite or weight gain

nicotine. During nicotine withdrawal, depressive symptoms may appear or, in an already depressed person, become more acute. Many patients cite depressive symptoms as the reason that they resumed smoking after a quit attempt.

Treatment of Nicotine Dependence Complicated by Depression

Nicotine dependence has been the subject of numerous clinical trials in recent years and effective medications are available with several more in the process of being evaluated for FDA approval. The general procedure involves beginning the patient on a long-term relapse prevention medication, setting a quit date after the medication has reached therapeutic levels, and then using nicotine replacement therapy to treat nicotine withdrawal symptoms. Nicotine replacement therapy comes in the form of a patch, chewing gum, or nasal spray. Nicotine blocks the withdrawal symptoms and it can be tapered over 5–10 days. Some heavy smokers find that they need to continue the nicotine replacement for several months because of prolonged withdrawal symptoms. Prior to stopping smoking, bupropion (Zyban) should be started at a dose of 150 mg twice daily to reduce nicotine craving. Bupropion should be continued for at least 3 months. Bupropion is also used to treat depression and thus it can reduce the depressive symptoms in smokers who are dually diagnosed with depression and nicotine dependence. Bupropion, however, is different from other antidepressants in that it also reduces the craving for nicotine and thus it should be used even with nondepressed smokers. Often depression becomes much worse after smoking is stopped and the patient may need intensive psychotherapy in addition to medication. Cognitive behavioral psychotherapy has been found to be effective for depression and it can be administered in combination with the medications as described above.

Nicotine addiction is so common that all physicians should become familiar with treating it according to the guidelines mentioned above. It is also, however, one of the most difficult addictions to treat and so a patient who does not respond to the treatment prescribed above or who has frequent relapses should be referred to a speciality program. Even with the best combinations of medications and cognitive behavioral therapy, the success rate (stable abstinence at 1 year), is in the neighborhood of 30%. In randomized clinical trials, the control group (placebo) shows less than 10% success at 1 year.

Nicotine dependence is a worldwide problem and in recent years, the pharmaceutical industry has actively engaged in the development of novel medications to aid in smoking cessation. One such novel medication is rimonabant, a cannabinoid (CB-1) receptor antagonist. In clinical trials, this medication has been found to reduce relapse in smokers as well as reduce weight in obese patients. This medication is currently in the FDA approval process and will likely join nicotine replacement therapy and bupropion as an additional option to aid in the treatment of nicotine addiction.

Depression with Opiate Addiction

Depression is found among opiate addicts following several different scenarios. Patients suffering from chronic pain often become depressed and occasionally they may seek the mood elevating or antidepressant effects of their prescribed opiates instead of limiting them for pain relief. While addiction developing in the course of opiate therapy for chronic pain is relatively uncommon, the association with depression is one of the danger signals that the treating physician should look for. Appropriate antidepressant medication is indicated.

A totally different scenario occurs in street heroin addicts. Often when they present for treatment they are in partial opiate withdrawal and they complain of symptoms of depression. They may even meet criteria for major depressive disorder. The most common treatment for heroin treatment is methadone maintenance. Recently another maintenance option, buprenorphine, became available. This has increased the availability of treatment because buprenorphine can be prescribed by authorized physicians from their private office instead of requiring a specialized treatment program, as is the case with methadone. After 2–3 weeks on a stable dose of methadone or buprenorphine, the depressive symptoms frequently disappear; for those patients who do not respond to methadone or buprenorphine maintenance, antidepressants may be combined with their maintenance medication.[16]

Treatment of Opiate Addiction

The medications used to treat opiate addiction do not in any way interfere with the mechanism of action of antidepressants and mood stabilizers. Opiates themselves have antidepressant effects and thus patients newly started on an opiate agonist or partial agonist treatment such as methadone or buprenorphine should not be given antidepressants until after they are stabilized on the opiate maintenance medication. If depressive symptoms persist, then standard antidepressant therapy is indicated. Patients with bipolar disorder can be treated with mood stabilizers such as lithium, valproic acid, carbamazepine, or lamotrigine. In general, the results of treatment have been positive in that depressive symptoms are relieved and mood is stabilized; however, the treatment of the mood disorder does not necessarily benefit the addictive disorder. Addiction is a chronic disease that requires long-term treatment and attention to mood disorders is important, but not curative for the addiction.

Another form of treatment for opiate addiction involves the opiate antagonist, naltrexone. This medication blocks opiate receptors and makes relapse to opiate addiction impossible as long as naltrexone is present. This treatment requires a detoxification first and often the newly abstinent heroin addict has numerous depressive symptoms. Naltrexone can be initiated to prevent relapse and it can also be given in combination with an antidepressant. There is no adverse interaction between naltrexone and SSRIs or tricyclic antidepressants and the antidepressant helps in the treatment of the overall heroin addiction syndrome. There have been reports of increased levels of antidepressants when given to patients on naltrexone, but the increase is usually not of a magnitude that requires dose adjustment. In every case the best treatment for opiate addiction is a combination of medication and psychotherapy either agonist or antagonist approaches. A variety of psychotherapy techniques have been found effective and all seem to combine well with medications. Therapy techniques include cognitive behavioral and supportive expressive psychotherapy.

Depression and Stimulant Addiction

Stimulants such as cocaine and methamphetamine produce excitation, elation, and in general, feelings that are the opposite of depression. However, on abrupt cessation, these drugs produce a serious withdrawal syndrome that is marked by depression, sometimes very severe with suicidal thoughts. Thus, the treatment of cocaine addiction often involves the simultaneous treatment of depression. As with other addictions it is also important to work on relapse prevention. The patient realizes that returning to cocaine or amphetamine will at least temporarily relieve the painful, depressive symptoms. This will only perpetuate the cycle of intoxication followed by depression.

The chronic use of stimulants, both cocaine and amphetamine, is associated with the development of depressive symptoms over time. Many of the original effects that were considered desirable show tolerance with time. The effects on sexual arousal that initially produced enhancement of sexual function gradually evolves into reduced sexual arousal. Erectile dysfunction in chronic male users is not unusual.

Treatment of Stimulant Addiction

Antidepressant medications help with depressive symptoms in the treatment of cocaine addiction. There have been studies demonstrating the benefits of tricyclics such as desipramine and SSRIs such as fluoxetine, but the results are far from consistent. In order to reduce the likelihood of relapse, a program of relapse prevention psychotherapy is important. Counseling by an experienced addiction counselor has been found to be effective.[17] Cognitive behavioral psychotherapy has been found to be effective when combined with medication. Thus far, no medication has been approved by the FDA for the treatment of cocaine addiction or amphetamine addiction. However, there are several medications that are approved for other indications. Recently, in randomized clinical trials, these medications have been found to reduce relapse. Such medications may ultimately be approved by the FDA for the treatment of cocaine addiction but further research is needed. Medications that have been reported to be effective in preventing relapse when combined with appropriate counseling are: modafinil,[18] topiramate,[19] baclofen,[20] and propranolol.[21] Fewer studies of amphetamine addiction have been published. Thus far, no medication has shown promising results.

Depression among cocaine addicts may have arisen spontaneously and then cocaine and other stimulants are used in an attempt to self-medicate or depression may be a complication of long-term stimulant usage. Bipolar disorder is also frequently associated with cocaine abuse or addiction. Mood stabilizers should be utilized in combination with one of the medications described above for relapse prevention.

Depression and Alcoholism

While depressive symptoms are very common among individuals with alcoholism, there is no evidence that depression increases the risk of developing alcoholism. By the time patients with alcoholism present for treatment, it is often difficult to determine when the depressive symptoms began. Did they antedate the alcoholism (primary depression) or did they arise later in the course of chronic alcohol use? As discussed in the introduction to this chapter it is often not clear whether alcohol use predates the mood disorder or whether the alcoholism develops as a result of an attempt at self-medication of a mood disorder. Many of the symptoms of alcoholism overlap with symptoms of depression thus causing diagnostic confusion. Continued drinking during alcohol-induced depression is a result of alcohol addiction, not necessarily a primary major depression.

Schuckit and his colleagues have demonstrated that while many alcoholics appear depressed at the beginning of treatment, these symptoms will remit in a large proportion after detoxification and a period of abstinence from alcohol. Therefore, these authors[22] recommend detoxifying the patient from alcohol and waiting several weeks to see if the depressive symptoms go into remission. Unfortunately, in the current managed care environment with short or no hospital stay permitted, there is usually no opportunity to wait to determine whether the symptoms remit. When antidepressant treatment is instituted early, it will be impossible to know whether the symptoms would have remitted with the passage of time in an alcohol-free state.

Suicide Risk

It is well known that suicide risk is elevated in all patients suffering from a mood disorder. When the mood disorder is complicated by substance abuse, the risk goes up still further.[23] The suicide attempt is often an impulsive act with no premeditation and may occur during a period of intoxication. The treating physician must be alert to this risk and discuss the potential for self-harm with the patient and, when appropriate, with family members. Also, prescriptions should not be written for a quantity of medication that could be lethal as these patients may impulsively consume the entire bottle.

Treatment of Alcoholism

The treatment of cooccurring mood disorders and alcoholism requires addressing both disorders from the start. Patients who are alternately intoxicated or in withdrawal cannot participate effectively in psychotherapy sessions. Thus, cessation of drinking is essential. Detoxification of an alcohol-dependent person can be accomplished with the aid of medications such as benzodiazepines (Table 19-2). If detoxification is to occur on an outpatient basis, a benzodiazepine with a relatively low abuse potential such as oxazepam is recommended. A dose of 15–30 mg every 4–6 hours can be used to suppress alcohol withdrawal symptoms. After the patient has been detoxified, relapse prevention measures can be undertaken as well as the initiation of treatment for the mood disorder. Three medications are currently available to prevent relapse to alcohol drinking. All of them can be combined with antidepressant medication.

Disulfiram (Antabuse) blocks alcohol metabolism producing a noxious byproduct, acetaldehyde, if the patient ingests any alcohol. While this treatment can be very effective, it is poorly accepted by patients. Controlled clinical trials have not found a significant advantage for this medication. It can be useful in specific cases where ingestion of the medication can be

▶ **TABLE 19-2** ALCOHOL WITHDRAWAL SYNDROME

Alcohol craving
Tremor, irritability
Nausea
Sleep disturbance
Tachycardia
Hypertension
Sweating
Perceptual distortion
Seizures (12–48 h after last drink)
Delirium tremens (rare in uncomplicated withdrawal)
Severe agitation
Confusion
Visual hallucinations
Fever, profuse sweating
Tachycardia
Nausea, diarrhea
Dilated pupils

observed by a spouse or other monitor on a daily basis.

Another treatment option is naltrexone, a medication that blocks opiate receptors thus, depriving the patient of some of the reward from drinking alcohol. Patients with a family history of alcoholism tend to have a very sensitive endogenous opioid system that is activated by alcohol. This produces a rush and a high from alcohol mediated by endogenous opioids. This high is blocked by naltrexone thus decreasing alcohol craving and risk of relapse. Most but not all randomized clinical trials have found naltrexone to effectively prevent relapse in combination with counseling or psychotherapy.

The FDA has recently approved a new medication called acamprosate. It works on the NMDA/glutamate system to reduce alcohol craving. The choice among these three medications should be made with the collaboration of the patient who should also be put into a program for treatment of the depressive disorder. Other medications are in clinical trials but not yet approved for the treatment of alcoholism. Topiramate, a GABA enhancer, has FDA approval for the treatment of seizure disorders. It was found in a controlled clinical trial to reduce relapse among alcohol-dependent individuals.[24]

Bipolar Disorder and Alcoholism

The lifetime prevalence of alcoholism in patients with bipolar disorder is higher than it is for any other axis I diagnosis. More than 50% of bipolar patients suffer from alcoholism.[25] When alcoholism occurs with bipolar disorder, the risk of suicide is greatly enhanced.[6] Moreover, patients with this combination are especially difficult to manage.

Treatment of the bipolar disorder should follow the same guidelines as outlined in Chapter 3 on pharmacotherapy of mood disorders. The major difference is that in the face of alcoholism, the alcoholism use must be addressed at the same time that the patient is started on a mood stabilizer. Relapse prevention treatment for alcoholism should be instituted as described above with medication and psychotherapy.

Other Diagnoses Frequently Cooccurring with Substance Abuse

Anxiety Disorders and Alcohol

Anxiety disorders are common psychiatric syndromes and they frequently cooccur with alcoholism. Although there is controversy as to whether there is a true association,[26] the average clinician will see many patients with this form of comorbidity. The possible etiologic mechanisms are described above. Patients may attempt to relieve their anxiety symptoms using alcohol as a medication. There also may be increased risk for developing anxiety disorders after years of chronic alcohol use. While generalized anxiety disorder, social phobia and agoraphobia are found regularly in association with alcoholism, in recent years there has been increased interest in posttraumatic stress disorder (PTSD). This anxiety disorder has been reported to have an important association with alcoholism. Approximately 60% of men and 50% of women in the United States have experienced at least one severe trauma in their lives.[27] PTSD, a common response to trauma, occurs in 10–13% of U.S. women and 5–6% of men.[28, 29] Estimates of childhood or adult trauma among substance abusers range from 30 to 90% with rates of PTSD estimated at between 30 and 50%.[30] Both the prevalence and severity of alcoholism are related to severity of PTSD.[31] Despite this established association between PTSD and alcoholism, PTSD is under-diagnosed in treatment seeking substance abusers.[30]

There is a functional relationship between alcohol use and anxiety symptoms among PTSD patients who report using alcohol to reduce their anxiety symptoms. Alcohol is also used to facilitate falling asleep and to suppress trauma-related nightmares. During treatment, alcohol withdrawal may aggravate PTSD symptoms due to the autonomic arousal that is associated with the alcohol withdrawal syndrome (Table 19-2).

Borderline Personality Disorder with Substance Abuse

Patients with borderline personality disorder are notoriously difficult to treat. They experience alterations in mood and tend to be impulsive, suicidal, and unpredictable. Substance abuse is very common in this group of patients. Dulit et al.[33] found 67% of a population of borderline personality disorder patients had the cooccurring diagnosis of substance use disorder.

No clinical trials of the treatment of substance abuse among patients with personality disorder have been conducted. Management of the substance abuse problem, however, is often the focal point of treatment of borderline patients. Psychotherapy, of course, is virtually impossible when patients are actively abusing drugs. Common drugs involved with borderlines are alcohol and cocaine. Treatment of this combination should be approached as described in the section on treatment of cocaine addiction and treatment of alcoholism. The drug abuse must be brought under control in order for the treatment of the borderline personality disorder to be successful. Substance abuse is considered a poor prognostic indicator in borderline patients and it is recommended that the therapy focus first on the substance abuse problems and then on the psychotherapy of the borderline condition.[34]

Marijuana and the "Amotivational Syndrome"

Amotivational syndrome is not an official diagnosis but it has been repeatedly associated with marijuana use, particularly in adolescents. These patients have many of the symptoms of a mood disorder and they may carry the diagnosis of major depression. Marijuana has long been a commonly used illegal drug in the United States and its usage was even more wide spread in the 1970s than it is today. There are, however, a significant number of people who wish to stop their marijuana use and they may consult a physician for help. They may be seen by pediatricians, family practitioners, or by psychiatrists. These patients usually meet criteria for dependence on marijuana and they may have a syndrome that is characterized by lack of motivation, low productivity, and lack of interest in anything except "getting stoned." Recently, there have been clinical trials of specific psychotherapies for the treatment of marijuana dependence.[35] The etiologic relationship between marijuana dependence and lack of motivation is controversial and certainly not proven. It is an association without a known causal linkage. No medication has been found to be effective in the treatment of marijuana withdrawal symptoms or prevention of relapse to marijuana use. Other psychiatric syndromes have also been reported in association with marijuana dependence especially depression.[36]

▶ SUMMARY

Substance abuse and addiction in combination with other mental disorders are very common clinical problems. In general, they are best approached by an integrated treatment program that combines treatment of the addiction with treatment of the additional mental disorder. Attention to both problems is essential. Management of the addictive disorder is not successful if the accompanying mental disorder is not also treated with special medications and with effective psychotherapy. Similarly, treatment of the mental disorder without also simultaneously addressing the substance abuse will be uniformly unsuccessful. For both addictive disorders and other mental disorders there are effective psychotherapies and medications. In the case of mood disorders, treatment with antidepressants or mood stabilizers can be instituted as indicated. There are no contraindications to combining these treatments. Of course, the presence of comorbidity adds complexity to the clinical problems and is a negative prognostic indicator. In particular, the presence of substance abuse increases the likelihood of suicide attempts. For the clinician, these patients represent a difficult clinical problem, but such patients are very common and thus all clinicians

must be prepared to treat both sides of the coin: the substance abuse and the mood disorder.

REFERENCES

1. Regier DA, Farmer ME, Rae DS, et al. Comorbidity of mental disorders with alcohol and other drug abuse. *JAMA* 264(19):2511–2518,1990.
2. Kessler RC, McGonagle KA, Zhao S, et al. Lifetime and 12-month prevalence of DSM-III-R psychiatric disorders in the United States. Results from the National Comorbidity Survey. *Arch Gen Psychiatry* 1994;51(1)8–19.
3. Substance Abuse and Mental Health Services Administration (SAMSHA). Report to Congress on the Prevention and Treatment of Co-Occurring Substance Abuse Disorders and Mental Disorders, 2002.
4. Kessler RC, Nelson CB, McGonagle KA, et al. The epidemiology of co-occurring addictive and mental disorders: Implications for prevention and service utilization. *Am J Orthopsychiatry* 1996;66:17–31.
5. Kessler RC. The epidemiology of dual diagnosis. *Biol Psychiatry* 2004;56(10):730–737.
6. Frye MA, Altshuler LL, McElroy SL et al. Gender differences in prevalence, risk, and clinical correlates of alcoholism comorbidity in bipolar disorder. *Am J Psychiatry* 2003;160(5):883–889.
7. Farrell M, Howes S. Bebbington P, et al. Nicotine, alcohol and drug dependence and psychiatric comorbidity; Results of a national household survey. *Br J Psychiatry* 2001;179:432–437.
8. Fergusson DM, Goodwin RD, Horwood LF. Major depression and cigarette smoking: Results of a 21-year longitudinal study. *Psychol Med* 2003; 33(8):1357–1367.
9. Convey LS, Glassman AH, Stetner F. Depression and depressive symptoms in smoking cessation. *Comprehen Psychiatry* 1990;31(4):350–354.
10. Glassman AH, Helzer JE, Covey LS, et al. Smoking, smoking cessation, and major depression. *JAMA* 1990;264(12):1546–1549.
11. Breslau N, Johnson EO. Predicting smoking cessation and major depression in nicotine-dependent smokers. *Am J Public Health* 2000;90(7): 1122–1127.
12. Escobedo LG, Kirch DG, Anda RF. Depression and smoking initiation among us latinos. *Addiction* 1996;91(1):113–119.
13. Breslau N. Psychiatric comorbidity of smoking and nicotine dependence. *Behav Genet* 1995; 25(2):95–101.

14. Milberger S, Biederman J, Faraone S, et al. ADHD is associated with early initiation of cigarette smoking in children and adolescents. *J Am Acad Child Adolesc Psychiatry* 1997;36(10):37–44.

15. French SA, Perry CL, Leon GR, et al. Weight concerns, dieting behavior and smoking initiation among adolescents: A prospective study. *Am J Public Health* 1994;84(1):1818–1820.

16. Woody G, O'Brien CP, Rickels K. Depression and anxiety in heroin addicts. *Am J Psychiatry* 1975; 132:447–450.

17. Crits-Christoph P, Siqueland L, Blaine J, et al. Psychosocial treatments for cocaine dependence: National Institute on Drug Abuse collaborative cocaine treatment study. *Arch Gen Psychiatry* 1999;56(6):493–502.

18. Dackis CA, Kampman KM, Lynch KG, et al. A double-bind, placebo-controlled trial of modafinil for cocaine dependence. *Neuropsychopharmacology* 2005;30:205–211.

19. Kampman KM, Pettinati HM, Volpicelli JR, et al. Cocaine dependence severity predicts outcome in outpatient detoxification from cocaine and alcohol. *Am J Addict* 2004;13(1):74–82.

20. Shoptaw S, Yang X, Rotheram-Fuller EJ, et al. Randomized placebo-controlled trial of balofen for cocaine dependence: preliminary effects for individuals with chronic patterns of cocaine use. *J Clin Psychiatry* 2003;64(12):1440–1448.

21. Kampman KM, Volpicelli JR, Mulvaney FD, et al. Cocaine withdrawal severity and urine toxicology results from treatment entry predict outcome in medication trials for cocaine dependence. *Addic Behav* 2002;15(1):251–260.

22. Raimo EB, Schuckit MA. Alcohol dependence and mood disorders. *Addict Behav* 1998;23(6):933–946.

23. Goldberg JF, Singer TM, Garno JL. Suicidality and substance abuse in affective disorders. *J Clin Psychiatry* 2001;62(Suppl 25):35–43.

24. Johnson BA, O'Malley SS, Ciraulo DA, et al. Dose-ranging kinetics and behavioral pharmacology of naltrexone and acamprosate, both alone and combined, in alcohol-dependent subjects. *J Clin Psychopharmacol* 2003;23(3):281–293.

25. Salloum IM, Thase ME. Impact of substance abuse on the course and treatment of bipolar disorder. *Bipolar Disord* 2000;2:269–280.

26. Schuckit MA. Low level of response to alcohol. *Am J Psychiatry* 1994;151(2):184–189.

27. Kessler RC, Sonnega A, Bromet E. Posttraumatic stress disorder in the National Comorbidity Survey. *Arch Gen Psychiatry* 1995;52(12):1048–1060.

28. Breslau N, Peterson EL, Schultz LR, et al. Major depression and stages of smoking. A longitudinal investigation. *Arch Gen Psychiatry* 1998;55(2): 161–166.

29. Kessler RC, Nelson CB, McGonagle KA. The epidemiology of co-occurring addictive and mental disorders: Implications for prevention and service utilization. *Am J Orthopsychiatry* 1996;66(1): 17–31.

30. Dansky BS, Brady KT, Saladin ME. Victimization and PTSD in individuals with substance use disorders: Gender and racial differences. *Am J Drug Alcohol Abuse* 1996;22(1):75–93.

31. Breslau N, Davis GC. Posttraumatic stress disorder in an urban population of young adults: Risk factors of chronicity. *Am J Psychiatry* 1992;149(5): 671–675.

32. Osher FC, Drake RE, Noordsy DL, et al. Correlates and outcomes of alcohol use disorder among rural outpatients with schizophrenia. *J Clin Psychiatry* 1994;55(3):109–113.

33. Dulit RA, Fyer MR, Haas GL, et al. Substance use in borderline personality disorder. *Am J Psychiatry* 1990;147(8):1002–1007.

34. Links PS, Heslegrave RJ, Mitton JE, et al. Borderline personality disorder and substance abuse: Consequences of comorbidity. *Can J Psychiatry* 1995;40(1):9–14.

35. Stephens RS, Babor TF, Kadden R, et al. (2002). The marijuana treatment project: Rationale, design and participant characteristics. *Addiction* 2002; 97(Suppl 1):109–124.

36. Arendt M, Munk-Jorgensen P. Heavy cannabis users seeking treatment- prevalence of psychiatric disorders. *Soc Psychiatry Psychiatr Epidemiol* 2004;39(2):97–105.

CHAPTER 20

Orienting Treatment to Recovery Principles

SUSAN R. BERGESON

"I must be crazy to be in a loony-bin like this." (McMurphy in *One Flew Over The Cuckoo's Nest*, 1975)[1]

"The concept of recovery is rooted in the simple yet profound realization that people who have been diagnosed with mental illness are human beings" (Pat Deegan, Ph.D., Psychiatrist, consumer and author 1996).[2]

"The challenge . . . is to bring about a fundamental shift in the way in which chronic diseases and long-term conditions are managed—a shift which will empower and liberate patients to play a central role in decisions about their illness." (*The Expert Patient—A New Approach to Chronic Disease Management.* Department of Health and Human Services, September 2001)[3]

"Recovery is about individuals taking control of their own lives and not having others determine their care or treatment. The concept has evolved to mean the process by which an individual comes to terms with their disability and learns how to cope. Recovery does not imply a cure but a life long journey and process." (A. Kathryn Power, M. Ed., Director, Center for Mental Health Services, Substance Abuse and Mental Health Services Administration, Department of Health and Human Services, 2004)[4]

The way mental health is viewed and the way people living with mental illnesses are treated is undergoing a seismic shift. From the *Cuckoo's Nest* to the President's New Freedom Commission on Mental Health; from passive maintenance to active patient-directed treatment plans; the expectations of physicians are changing dramatically.

It is now recommended that physicians orient their practices toward recovery. The groundbreaking Surgeon General's Report on Mental Health in 1999 indicates that treatment must be oriented to recovery.[5] The President's New Freedom Commission on Mental Heath Care's final report in 2003 states that recovery is the goal of treatment.[6] The Evidence-Based Practices for Mental Health recently adopted by the Center for Mental Health Services (CMHS), a division of the Substance Abuse and Mental Health Services Administration (SAMSHA), identify recovery as the first evidence-based practice upon which the remaining five are built.[7] The Institute of Medicine, in its follow up to its landmark report "*Crossing the Quality Chasm,*" has identified patient-centered, recovery-oriented treatment as important to improving the quality of mental health care in the United States.[8]

But what is recovery and how can physicians do much beyond medication and symptom reduction within a busy practice?

Since the mid-1980s, a great deal has been written about mental health recovery from the perspective of the patient (consumer), family member, and health care professional. Early research by Courtney Harding (1987 citation)[9] and others challenged the belief that stability is the best outcome one could hope for persons with mental illnesses. They discovered there are several outcomes possible for persons with severe mental illnesses and that many people did progress beyond mere stability. Mental health professionals drew on this research to formulate theoretical and practical models of recovery that could be adapted for use in psychosocial rehabilitation.

Mueser et al. summarized 121 research studies that focused on recovery and recovery skills ranging from greater knowledge of psychiatric illness and its treatment, to coping skills, and relapse prevention strategies.[10]

Recovery refers both to a process and an outcome. However, physicians may be more used to thinking in terms of outcomes, i.e., the goal of treatment is the reduction or elimination of symptoms. Recovery goes beyond this medical outcome, it encompasses a process and an orientation "that regardless of their state of illness of health, people can have hope, feel capable of expanding their personal abilities, and make their own choices."[11]

A. Kathryn Power, M.Ed., Director of the Center for Mental Health Services, Substance Abuse and Mental Health Services Administration, defines recovery as

"The processes by which people are able to live work, learn, and participate fully in their communities."

- The ability to live a fulfilling and productive life despite a disability.
- A reduction or complete remission of symptoms.
- The ability to make important decisions affecting one own life."[12]

Orienting treatment to recovery means that individuals living with mental illnesses are not just partners in care with professionals but ultimately in control of their own lives. It positions health care professionals not as providers of care but as guides pointing out options and sharing insights from their perspectives that may or may not become a part of recovery process selected by the person in recovery. Ultimately, recovery is seen as a life-long process.

Recovery is not a return to the state prior to the onset of illness. The nature of mental illnesses as life-long, chronic, recurring conditions may mean there is no healthy "before" for a patient's return journey. The lessons learned through the recovery process may move the patient forward to an awareness and state far better than any experienced before the onset of illness. The goal of recovery therefore is not return. Caras writes: "I am not recovered. There is no repeating, regaining, restoring, recapturing, recuperating, retrieving. There was not convalescence. I am not complete. What I am is changing and growing and integrating and learning to be myself. What there is, is motion, less pain, and a higher portion of time well-lived."[13]

Jacobson and Greensley, in their work creating a recovery model for use within the Wisconsin Mental Health System, define recovery as a combination of "internal conditions—the attitudes, experiences, and processes of change of individuals who are recovering—and external, conditions—the circumstances, even policies, and practices that may facilitate recovery."[14]

The internal and external conditions outlined here are a useful framework within which physicians can orient their practices to recovery.

▶ INTERNAL CONDITION 1: HOPE

Having hope is critical to getting better. However, years of living with a mental illness and/or the cognitive dysfunction that is part of the illness, leaves patients devoid of hope. Central to hope is the belief that recovery is possible. This belief is based on recognizing and accepting the illness, committing to change, identifying and building on individual strengths instead of weaknesses to implement change, focusing on the future instead of the past, seeking and celebrating change in small steps, focusing and refocusing on value-based priorities, and avoiding negative self-talk while practicing optimism.

By focusing on strengths and possibilities, and working on wellness goals, people living with mental illnesses, no matter how ill, can move forward toward wellness. Physicians are important purveyors of hope. Patients and family members are sensitive to the physician's beliefs, stated or unstated about their ability to recover. As one family member put it:

> "We were all huddled around her bed in the hospital. Her doctor pulled my father and aside and told him that most frequently people with bipolar II disorder end up killing themselves. I watched my family as one by one my father took each person aside and solemnly told them this news. I watched as the hope they were holding onto so tightly was extinguished from their faces. I watched my sister too, and though nobody said a word about what the doctor had told them, I could literally see the fight go out of her in that short half hour of time. Being the good and obedient daughter she had always been, she killed herself a few weeks later." (E-mail to DBSA, 2004)

PHYSICIAN ACTIONS

1. Convey hope that recovery is possible regardless of the patient's condition.
2. Help the patient and family build on patient's strengths such as a desire to work, the love for a child, an interest in gardening, and so on to motivate and guide change rather than focusing on the negatives of the current situation.
3. Celebrate small steps on the recovery journey with the patient.

▶ INTERNAL CONDITION 2: HEALING

Professionals may be uncomfortable with the idea of recovery because it may be viewed as unrealistic or naive. However, recovery is not synonymous with cure. Recovery may be better considered in terms of healing. Healing, as used

here, has two main components: defining a self apart from illness, and regaining control.

Estroff notes that people who have psychiatric disabilities often find that they lose their "selves" inside mental illness.[15] Healing occurs when the person sees the illness not as their entire self-definition but as only part of their reality. As patients learn who they are apart from their illnesses, and build on their strengths, they gain confidence and can continue to expand their goals and dreams.

The second process within this definition of healing is control. Jacobson and Greensley define control as reducing symptoms of the illness, medication being a successful strategy, but also through self-care practices, such as adopting a wellness lifestyle or using symptom monitoring and response techniques.[14]

The other issue central to control is who directs the course of recovery. The physician's role is to provide medical knowledge, guidance, and advice. However, it is the patient who ultimately must adopt, adjust, or reject this information. As a patient advocacy organization, the Depression and Bipolar Support Alliance (DBSA) often listens with skepticism as physicians talk about patient's lack of "compliance" with medication regimens. The word compliance itself reflects a hierarchy of power where the physician decrees and the patient fulfills the decree. The reality is that if the physician has not outlined options and listened carefully to patient preferences, and has not worked with patients to jointly select a treatment option which may or may not include medication, then it is naïve to assume the patient will adhere, let alone "comply." Psychiatric medications, like the illnesses they treat, carry widespread stigma. For many patients, it takes time, education, and living with non-medication-based treatments before they will determine that a medication option is one they chose to select and one to which they will adhere.

PHYSICIAN ACTIONS

4. See the patient as more than the illness, communicate this with every action and treatment recommendation.

5. Reflect in every action that the patient, not the physician, has ultimate control over the treatment strategy selected.

▶ INTERNAL CONDITION 3: EMPOWERMENT

Jacobson and Greensley note three components of empowerment. The first is the ability to *act autonomously*, which occurs as consumers build their knowledge base and self-confidence, and are therefore able to choose among meaningful options. The next is *courage* defined by a willingness to take risks and speak authentically about their illness and experiences. The third is *responsibility*, defined by patient/consumers as developing goals, working with professionals, family, and friends to make plans to reach these goals, take on decision-making tasks, and engage in self-care.

Physicians promote empowerment by providing meaningful choices and respecting the right of patients to make those choices. Or as Bill Anthony from Boston University states, "professionals do not hold the key to recovery—consumers do. The task of professionals is to facilitate recovery; the task of consumers is to recover."[16]

PHYSICIAN ACTIONS

6. Encourage autonomy.
7. Support courageous acts.
8. Reinforce the need for and support the patient's actions to create goals and plans for self-care.

▶ INTERNAL CONDITION 4: CONNECTION

Connection captures the aspect of recovery having to do with rejoining the social world through activities, relationships, and/or work. Larry Fricks, noted consumer advocate, states that year after year when surveying consumers within Georgia, there are three things mental health consumers consistently want—a home, a job, and a date. (The Nineteenth Annual Rosalynn Carter Symposium On Mental Health Policy,

lecture "Recovery-Based Innovation" Nov. 6, 2003.)[16] It is interesting to note that all three of these relate to connection. Consumers want a place in the community, a meaningful role within the community, and the potential for an intimate relationship. Physicians orienting their practice toward recovery must think beyond medication management and encourage patients to set and work on goals to help them reestablish connections. Physicians should ask about those goals in all subsequent appointments. Its is not up to physicians to determine these goals, but it is a part of a recovery orientation to discuss their importance and the progress toward their achievement.

PHYSICIAN ACTIONS

9. Encourage patients to connect through a job, the creation of friendships, and the development of social activities.
10. Monitor progress made toward these goals in the same way side effects are monitored and medication adherence is checked.

Jacobson and Greensley also note three external conditions that can be used to orient a physician's practice to recovery.

▶ EXTERNAL CONDITION 1: A HUMAN RIGHTS ORIENTATION

As Deegan notes, mental health consumers are first and foremost human beings.[2] As such, they have rights and should be treated with dignity. This calls into question the use of involuntary commitment, involuntary treatment, the use of restraints, or any other forced treatment. Physicians should discuss advance directives with patients and their families so patients can plan in advance what will and will not occur in case of an adverse event.

PHYSICIAN ACTIONS

11. Encourage patients and their families to create advance directives.

12. Ensure the basic human rights of patients are honored in every situation, advocating on behalf of patients whose rights are abrogated.

▶ EXTERNAL CONDITION 2: A POSITIVE CULTURE OF HEALING

In a positive culture of healing, professionals believe that everyone can achieve hope, healing, empowerment, and connection, regardless of their current status. This belief leads the physician to focus on the person, not the illness, and on their strengths and goals. In a positive culture of healing, health care professionals collaborate with patients on decisions about the services used to support the patients' recovery. Collaboration implies that the consumer is an active participant, that he or she is presented with a range of options and given the opportunity to choose from among them, and that providers allow the patient to take some risks with the choices he or she makes. Patients have the opportunity to make choices other than those the provider might have made for them.

Physician Actions

13. Engage the patient as an active participant in his/her treatment decisions.
14. Respect the fact that it is the patient who is living with the mood disorder and as such, the patient has the right to make treatment decisions that the physician may not fully agree with.

▶ EXTERNAL CONDITION 3: RECOVERY-ORIENTED SERVICES

The Boston University Center for Psychiatric Rehabilitation defines recovery-oriented services as those directed at symptom relief, crisis intervention, case management, rehabilitation, enrichment, rights protection, basic support, and self-help.[17] The recovery orientation in these services is reflected in the actions and attitudes of all the staff who come in contact with patients.

Physician Actions

15. Lead the rest of the staff by exhibiting recovery-oriented attitudes and actions.
16. Ensure the entire staff exhibits recovery-oriented attitudes and actions.

The 16 actions outlined above can help physicians orient their practices toward a recovery model. Most are attitudinal and few take any significant additional time within the usual busy, time constrained practice. If a physician has the ability to start with just one or two changes, the following information direct from patients can help prioritize physician actions.

A consumer group in Ohio developed a set of criteria to rate the impact of mental health professionals on their recovery. Clients in the mental health system rated these from most to least impact as follows.

1. Encourage my independent thinking
2. Treat me in a way that helps my recovery process
3. Treat me as an equal in planning my services
4. Give me freedom to make my own mistakes
5. Treat me like a person who can shape my own future
6. Listen to me and believe what I say
7. Look at and recognize my abilities
8. Work with me to find the resources or services I need
9. Be available to talk to me when I need to talk to someone
10. Teach me about the medications I am taking.[18]

Encouraging patients to think independently is the single most important action physicians can implement to orient their practices to recovery. But patients want and deserve the maximum, not the minimum physicians have to offer. Patients want "the right atmosphere or organizational climate in your mental health organization— one that is sensitive to consumers, and values the independence of the individual. It allows consumers to risk, to fail. It holds that every consumer has a right to the same pleasures, passions, and pursuits of happiness that we have. It looks at potential, not deficits."[19]

The clock will never be turned back. Patients are not going to return to the cuckoo's nest. Recovery means avoiding over protection, under valuation, and the inadvertent fostering of learned helplessness. Recovery means life—with all the pain and all the benefits any one else experiences.

Physicians want the very best for their patients and providing care for a patient with a mood disorder can be challenging. Orienting your practice to recovery builds on the findings of the Surgeon General, the President's New Freedom Commission, and the Center For Mental Health Services' Evidence Based Practices. A recovery orientation can be as simple as encouraging patients to think independently or as comprehensive as the 16 actions listed within this chapter. Ultimately, patients are asking physicians, to work "with us"; not "for us," not "in our best interest" and not "on our behalf"; but truly "with us," so patients can live full and rich lives.

REFERENCES

1. Kesey K. *One Flew over the Cuckoos Nest*. Viking Press, New York, NY: 1977.
2. Deegan PE. Recovery as a journey of the heart. *Psychosoc Rehabil J* 1996;19(3):91–97.
3. Department of Health, *The Expert Patient: A New Approach to Chronic Disease Management*, 2001.
4. Power AK. Achieving the promise transforming the public mental health system through technical assistance. U.S. Department of Health and Human Services, Substance Abuse and Mental Health Services Administration, Center for Mental Health Services, 2004.
5. U.S. Department of Health and Human Services. *Mental Health: A Report of the Surgeon General—Executive Summary*. Rockville, MD: U.S. Department of Health and Human Services, Substance Abuse and Mental Health Services Administration, Center for Mental Health Services, National Institutes of Health, National Institute of Mental Health, 1999.
6. President's New Freedom Commission on Mental Health Achieving the Promise: Transforming Mental Health Care in America. Accessed August 20, 2004. Online at: http://www.mentalhealthcommission.gov/reports/FinalReport/toc.html
7. Evidence based practices shaping mental health services toward recovery. U.S. Department of Health and Human Services, Substance Abuse and Mental Health Services Administration, Center for Mental Health Services. Accessed August 20, 2004. Online at: http://www.mentalhealthpractices.org/index.html
8. Institute of Medicine. Crossing the Quality Chasm A New Health System for the 21st Century Committee on Quality of Health Care in America National Academy Press, Washington, DC, 2003.
9. Harding CM, Brooks GW, Asolaga T SJ, et al.. Courtney Harding. The Vermont longitudinal study of persons with severe mental illness. *Am J Psychiatry* 1987;144:718–726.
10. Mueser, Kim T, et al. A review of the research. *Psychiatr Serv* 2002;53(10):1272–1284.
11. Resnick S, Rosenheck R, Lehman A. An exploratory analysis of practices of recovery. *Psychiatr Serv* 2004;55(5):540–546.
12. Power AK. Achieving the promise transforming the public mental health system through technical assistance. U.S. Department of Health and Human Services, Substance Abuse and Mental Health Services Administration, Center for Mental Health Services, 2004.
13. Ralph RO. Review of Recovery Literature: A Synthesis of a Sample of Recovery Literature. Alexandria, VA: National Technical Assistance Center. Retrieved August 20, 2004 from http://www.nasmhpd.org/general_files/publications/ntac_pubs/reports
14. Jacobson, Greensley MSW, Diane F. What is recovery? A conceptual model and explication. *Psychiatr Serv* 2001;52(4):482–485.
15. Estroff SE. Self, identity, and subjective experiences of schizophrenia: In search of the subject. *Schizophr Bull* 1989;15:189–196.
16. Anthony W. *Psychiatr Rehabil J* 2000;24(2):159–168.
17. Anthony WA. Recovery from mental illness: The guiding vision of the mental health service system in the 1990's. *Psychosoc Rehabil J* 1993;16(4): 11–23.

18. Ralph RO, Lambric TM, Steele RB. Recovery issues in a consumer developed evaluation of the mental health system. In: *Proceedings of the Fifth Annual National Conference on Mental Health Services Research and Evaluation*. Alexandria, VA: National Association of State Mental Health Program Directors (NASMHPD) Research Institute. Retrieved August 20, 2004 from http://www.nasmhpd.org/general_files/publications/ntac_pubs/reports/ralphrecovweb.pdf

19. Allott P, Loganathan A. Discovering hope for recovery from a British perspective. Retrieved August 20, 2004 from http://www.herefordshire-mentalhealth.info/recovery/recovery_lit.pdf

Index

Page numbers followed by *f* or *t* indicate figures or tables, respectively.